PRAISE FOR *BECOMING VEGAN: COMPREHENSIVE EDITION*

"Over 600 pages of in-depth science on vegan nutrition. This is more than a book about **Becoming Vegan,** it is a primary and comprehensive text book on nutritional science that should be studied by all health professionals in America.

Joel Fuhrman, MD, New York Times best-selling author of *Eat to Live*

"Brenda Davis and Vesanto Melina are authoritative and influential leaders in nutrition, and this is one of the most valuable resources health professionals and nutrition enthusiasts will ever own. *Becoming Vegan: Comprehensive Edition* clearly and meticulously demonstrates how a well-designed plant-based diet provides tremendous power for health at every stage of the life cycle. "

Neal Barnard, MD, adjunct associate professor of medicine,
George Washington University, president of PCRM

"*Becoming Vegan: Comprehensive Edition* is THE go-to book on vegan nutrition. It is meticulously researched, clear and insightful. If you have nutrition questions, this is the book you can trust for the answers.

Michael Greger, MD, public health director, The Humane Society of the United States

"Plant-based registered dietitians and authors extraordinaire, Brenda Davis and Vesanto Melina have done it again! This book is without peer for anyone seeking a sound, rational foundation for a plant-based dietary lifestyle.

Michael Klaper, MD, consultant, educator, and physician with True North Health Center

"*Becoming Vegan* is stunningly comprehensive, totally up-to-date, and a terrific gift to our world. If you're interested in how to be optimally healthy on a vegan diet, this is THE resource you want."

John Robbins, author of *Diet For A New America and The Food Revolution*

"This book is the bible of nutrition, filled to the brim with knowledge, facts, and pure wisdom.

Julieanna Hever, MS, RD, CPT, author of *The Vegiterranean Diet*
and host of *What Would Julieanna Do?*

"All of your questions about plant-based nutrition answered—guaranteed! Clearly written and packed with information—truly everything you need to know about vegan diets— *Becoming Vegan: Comprehensive Edition* is a remarkable one-of-a-kind guide. Whether you're a long-term vegan or new to this way of eating, this is a book you'll turn to again and again for helpful information.

Virginia Messina, MPH, RD, author of *Vegan for Life* and *The Dietitian's Guide to Vegetarian Diets*

"If ever there was a book that told you EVERYTHING you ever needed to know about being (or becoming) vegan, this one is it! I highly recommend it as an evergreen addition to your bookshelf!

Kathy Freston, New York Times best-selling author of *The Lean, Veganist,* and *Quantum Wellness*

BECOMING VEGAN

COMPREHENSIVE EDITION

the complete reference to plant-based nutrition

Brenda Davis, RD

Vesanto Melina, MS, RD

BOOK PUBLISHING COMPANY

Summertown, Tennessee

Library of Congress Cataloging-in-Publication Data

Davis, Brenda, 1959-
    Becoming vegan : the complete reference on plant-based nutrition / Brenda
Davis, RD, and Vesanto Melina, MS, RD. — Comprehensive edition.
        pages cm
    Includes bibliographical references and index.
    ISBN 978-1-57067-297-2 (pbk.) — ISBN 978-1-57067-900-1 (e-book)
    1. Veganism—Health aspects. 2. Veganism. 3. Nutrition. I. Melina,
Vesanto, 1942- II. Title.
    RM236.D38 2014
    613.2'622—dc23

                                                    2014018034

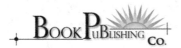

We chose to print this title on sustainably harvested paper stock certified by the Forest
Stewardship Council,® an independent auditor of responsible forestry practices. For more
information, visit us.fsc.org.

Cover art: Julia Ruffles, http://www.juliaruffles.co.uk/
Cover and interior design: John Wincek

Printed in the United States

Book Publishing Company
P.O. Box 99
Summertown, TN 38483
888-260-8458
bookpubco.com

ISBN 13: 978-1-57067-297-2

23 22 21 20   9 10 11 12

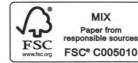

To the visionaries before us and beside us, who have dedicated their lives to making this world a kinder, gentler place:

- Donald Watson, Dr. Frey Ellis, and the founders of the vegan movement;

- Jay and Freya Dinshah, and others who started vegan organizations throughout the world;

- Bob and Cynthia Holzapfel, and the hundreds of courageous plant-based pioneers at The Farm;

- Jane Goodall, John Robbins, Albert Schweitzer, and all those who have guided our paths to compassion;

- Michael Klaper, Neal Barnard, Michael Greger, Joel Fuhrman, William Harris, and the many other physicians who have dedicated their lives to assisting others toward healthful vegan lifestyles;

- Virginia Messina, Reed Mangels, Sue Havala, Winston Craig, Jack Norris, George Eisman, and the countless dietitians who laid the foundations of vegan dietary wisdom.

CONTENTS

ACKNOWLEDGMENTS

We're most grateful for our brilliant and dedicated colleagues at Book Publishing Company, including publisher Bob Holzapfel, editors Cynthia Holzapfel and Carol Kroskey, and marketing and support team Anna Pope, Thomas Hupp, John Schweri, and Rhiannon Wolfe.

Our deepest thanks go to the insightful colleagues and friends who provided invaluable feedback, thoughtful commentary, support, and inspiration: Reed Mangels, Jack Norris, Ginny Messina, Paul Shapiro, Mark Rifkin, Margie Colclough, Margie Roswell, Andres and Lily Vallejo, Heather Waxman, John Pierre, Ruth Heidrich, James Chicalo, Carolyn Johnston, Andrea Frisque, Stephane Lahaye, and Daneen Agecoutey.

Many thanks for the time and expertise of our gracious advisors: Paul Appleby, Luciana Baroni, Winston Craig, Michael Greger, Michael Klaper, Kristen Yarker, Joe Millward, Melvin H. Williams, Ricardo Uauy, Ailsa Welch, Jagoda Ambroszkiewicz, Francesca Crowe, Undurti N. Das, John Davis, Jill Wallace, and Freya Dinshah.

We appreciate the supportive energy of our research assistants: Renee Webb-Pelchat, Deanna Ibbitson, Carole Douglas, Katherine Jassman, and Hana Tahae.

Boundless love and gratitude to our partners, Paul Davis and Cam Doré, for their continued dedication and support. Special thanks to Cam for his brilliant and ongoing assistance with technical challenges.

Richest blessings to our cherished and supportive family members: Brenda's mother, Doreen Charbonneau; her mother-in-law, Linda Davis; her children, Leena Markatchev and Cory Davis; and her son-in-law, Nayden Markatchev, and to Vesanto's children, Xoph Crawford and Kavyo Crawford; her son-in-law, Stefan Shielke; her dear grandson, Chance Shielke, and to Claire and Audra Doré.

Photographic credits and appreciation go to Kevin Trowbridge (Kevin Trowbridge.com) and his assistant Katherine Jassman.

We're also grateful to the companies that generously shared their excellent products for recipe testing—Sunrise Soya Foods, Garden Protein International (Gardein), Manitoba Harvest Hemp Foods, Omega Nutrition, Nature's Path Foods, and LeSaffre Yeast Corporation—and to ESHA Research for its outstanding nutritional analysis program, *The Food Processor*.

BECOMING VEGAN

COMPREHENSIVE EDITION

the complete reference to plant-based nutrition

CHAPTER 1

Widening the Circle of Compassion

Our lives begin to end the day we become silent about things that matter.

MARTIN LUTHER KING, US CIVIL RIGHTS LEADER

I t takes immense inner strength to oppose the status quo. It takes courage to resist the pressure to accept what the influential people in your life consider morally and culturally reasonable, and perhaps even necessary. Yet, if people didn't rise up against social injustice, slavery still would be legal, the poor would remain uneducated, and women wouldn't be able to vote.

What does a vegan lifestyle have to do with social justice? Nothing—if animals are regarded as resources; everything—if animals are recognized as sentient beings. It's possible that the greatest social injustice of our time doesn't involve humans at all, but rather our fellow beings—nonhuman animals. Becoming vegan is about taking a stand against this injustice.

The seeds of vegan ethics were sown by philosophers and spiritual leaders in the East, where prevalent religions, such as Buddhism, Jainism, and Hinduism, emphasized compassion toward animals and included vegetarianism as a part of their core doctrines. These seeds were nurtured and spread in the West by Pythagoras, a sixth-century BC Greek philosopher and mathematician. Pythagoras shunned the consumption of animal flesh and directed his followers to do the same.[1]

While many other notable thinkers followed suit, including Plato, Plutarch, Seneca, Ovid, and Socrates, it wasn't until the mid-1800s that the moral roots of vegetarianism were firmly established in Western culture. The epicenter was England, and the driving forces were moral leaders of select Christian churches. Although the movement became well-grounded in the West, when contrasted with the practices and teachings of the East, its early influence was limited.

Vegan Awakenings

T he ethics of consuming dairy products were hotly debated within the burgeoning British vegetarian movement, but it wasn't until 1944 that a small, like-minded group of individuals decided to develop a new branch of vegetarianism, one whose practitioners consumed no animal products.

The father of the contemporary vegan movement, Donald Watson (1910–2005), and his compatriots recognized that the flesh-food industry and the egg and dairy-product industries were inextricably linked, because animals raised to produce eggs and milk were eventually slaughtered and eaten when they were no longer productive. These British vegans contended that the case against these industries rivaled the indictment of the meat industry, so the use of dairy products and eggs was no longer justifiable for ethical vegetarians. Their intent was to eliminate the exploitation of animals and to move closer to a truly humane society.

To do so, they founded the first Vegan Society in 1944; initially, it had only twenty-five members.[2] In the 1950s, London physician Frey Ellis joined their ranks and significantly strengthened the scientific understanding of vegan health.

In 1948, Dr. Catherine Nimmo and Rubin Abramowitz established America's first vegan society in Oceano, California. The group continued gathering members until 1960, when a national organization, the American Vegan Society (AVS), was founded by H. Jay Dinshah. As a strong vote of support, Nimmo became the first paying member and encouraged her former group to join AVS.[3, 4] Although Jay passed on in 2000, AVS remains vibrant under the guidance of his wife, Freya Dinshah, who has been with the organization since its inception.

AVS has consistently encouraged the active practice of *ahimsa* (a Sanskrit word meaning dynamic harmlessness) as a part of a vegan lifestyle. Members embrace ahimsa as an urgent worldwide necessity and advocate six pillars—one for each letter of ahimsa:[5]

Abstinence from animal products

Harmlessness with reverence for life

Integrity of thought, word, and deed

Mastery over oneself

Service to humanity, nature, and creation

Advancement of understanding and truth

However, it wasn't until 1987 that the vegan movement entered mainstream America. John Robbins provided the catapult with the release of his groundbreaking book, *Diet for a New America*. This work included the first hard-hitting exposé of the consequences of factory farming for food animals, the environment, and human health. Today, vegan groups and societies are present in more than fifty nations worldwide. The Vegan World Network support members by providing contact information online along with news about events, forums, and health issues.[6]

Vegan: The Founder and the Word

Donald Watson coined the word *vegan* to describe a particular variant of vegetarianism that excluded the use and consumption of all animal products. A vegetarian for 81 years and vegan for 63, he successfully avoided any need for medication—conventional or herbal—and had hardly a day's illness during his lifetime. His longevity had not been inherited; his father had passed on at the age of 63, and few other relatives survived beyond 70.[7] As he aged, not only did he remain physically healthy but also mentally alert. Many of Watson's most celebrated interviews were conducted after he turned 90, and he continued to grant interviews until shortly before his death at the age of 95.

How Is Vegan Pronounced?

The correct pronunciation is "vee-gan" or "vee-gen" with the stress on the first syllable. It's not pronounced "vai-gan," "vey-gn," or "vee-jan."

Vegan Defined

 A *vegan* is an individual who embraces the philosophy of veganism and seeks to follow a vegan lifestyle.

Veganism is a philosophy that promotes reverence for life and compassion for all living beings and rejects the notion that animals are resources to be exploited.

A *vegan lifestyle* excludes, as far as is possible and practical, all forms of animal exploitation. Vegans avoid consumer products derived from animals, including foods of animal origin; clothing produced from fur, leather, wool, or silk; and animal-derived ingredients in personal-care and cleaning products. Instead, animal-free alternatives arc promoted. Vegans also avoid activities that involve the mistreatment of animals, including animal research and animal-based entertainment.

A *vegan diet* excludes meat, poultry, fish, dairy products, eggs, gelatin, and other foods of animal origin (except human breast milk). Vegan diets include all foods of plant origin, including vegetables, fruits, legumes, grains, nuts, and seeds.

A *pure vegetarian* is someone who follows only a vegan diet, not a vegan lifestyle. Sometimes pure vegetarians are referred to as "dietary vegans." These individuals use nondietary animal products, such as leather. They also may support the use of animals in research and have no objection to the use of animals for entertainment. In such cases, their choice to consume a vegan diet is generally motivated by personal health concerns rather than by any ethical objections to eating animals. However, pure vegetarians may become vegan as they learn more about vegan philosophy.

HOW VEGAN DO I NEED TO BE TO CALL MYSELF A VEGAN?

Being vegan isn't about personal purity or about moral superiority. It's about making a conscious choice to widen your circle of compassion by avoiding

Vegetarian Roots

The word "vegetarian" was coined by the founders of the British Vegetarian Society in 1842. The word comes from the Latin word *vegetus,* which means "lively, fresh, and vigorous."[8]

There's good evidence that the first people to call themselves vegetarians actually followed what is now referred to as a vegan diet. Historical records show that between April 1842 and September 1847, vegetarians consumed only plant foods.[9]

animal exploitation, as far as is possible and practical. It's about becoming more other-centered and less self-centered. If you strive to avoid animal products and activities that exploit animals, you already are vegan, even if you slip on occasion. There are no vegan police scrutinizing card-carrying vegans. If there were, our numbers would rapidly diminish.

In today's world, it's virtually impossible to be 100 percent "cruelty-free." For example, one might discover insect-derived natural red dye #4 in a piece of candy, or drink a glass of wine that had been clarified using isinglass from the membranes of fish bladders. Unfortunately, traces of animal products lurk in phones, match heads, sandpaper, color gels in theatrical lighting, photographic film, cars, bicycles, planes, computers, and more.

Efforts to live compassion-centered lives count far more than proficiency at avoiding the trace amounts of animal products that permeate marketplaces. Indeed, there are occasions during which the use of a decidedly nonvegan product results in a greater reduction in animal suffering than would avoiding its use. Think back to the predigital camera era. Had the use of film been avoided, thousands of individuals who were moved by graphic images of exploited animals would have unknowingly continued to contribute to their exploitation. A vegan lifestyle is a means to an end (which is to reduce animal suffering), not the end itself.

IS HONEY VEGAN?

Technically, honey isn't vegan, because it's a product made by bees for bees. This is also true for other bee products, such as beeswax, bee pollen, honeycomb, propolis, and royal jelly. When we take bee products from bees, we're taking what these beings have labored to produce and what they rely on for their survival. Vegans strive to avoid the exploitation of *all* living beings—including bees. Considering the numerous alternative sweeteners available, there seems little justification to use honey.

While it sounds like an open-and-shut case, the issue of whether to use honey is a contentious one within the vegan community. The debate isn't so much about whether or not honey is an animal product—it is. The debate is more about whether having to avoid honey might deter potential vegans from a committed vegan lifestyle. To the average person, avoiding honey seems extreme, perhaps even a little crazy. After all, we're talking about insects here, and plenty of insects are harmed in daily life, even in the harvesting of plants. So, the thought is that if vegans relaxed about the honey issue, people might be a little more open to the possibility of becoming vegan themselves.

Both sides have valid arguments. It's virtually impossible to avoid killing insects in daily life, but it seems reasonable to avoid their purposeful exploitation. Then again, if a rigid stance on honey keeps people from taking meat and milk off their menus, it seems counterproductive. Instead, it makes sense to first focus public-education efforts on the issues surrounding the production of meat, eggs, and milk. It also makes sense to inform people who wish to minimize animal exploitation about the concerns surrounding other animal-derived commodities, such as honey, silk, and wool. In the end, we each need to do what we can in the quest for a more compassionate world.

Why Vegan?

Albert Einstein recognized that the separate existence we feel as individuals is in fact an illusion—that along with all beings, we're a part of the universe at large. He explained, "A human being is part of a whole, called by us the universe, a part limited in time and space. He experiences himself, his thoughts and feelings, as something separated from the rest—a kind of optical delusion of his consciousness. This delusion is a kind of prison for us, restricting us to our personal desires and to affection for a few persons nearest us. Our task must be to free ourselves from this prison by widening our circles of compassion to embrace all living creatures and the whole of nature and its beauty."

This vision captures the very essence of "why vegan." Becoming vegan is about making an ethical decision to become more aware of our connections to fellow creatures and to widen our circles of compassion to respect their right to exist and lead pain-free lives. It requires taking a stand against deeply rooted customs and traditions—customs and traditions that are often practiced by people we love, respect, and admire.

For most of us, considering this choice triggers a long, hard battle with our conscience. Fortunately, for most of us, our conscience prevails.

Coauthor Brenda Davis waged this battle as a young child, as do many people. She recalls:

> "I'll never forget the shock and devastation that engulfed me on a vacation with my family in Spain. My parents had decided to attend a bullfight featuring Spain's most celebrated bullfighter. Ten thousand cheering fans erupted in thunderous applause when he entered the stadium. I suspected that this beautifully dressed man was going to fight a bull, and I found the thought quite distressing. But I could never have imagined that he was going to kill the bull. During this exhibition, I was stunned by the spectacle of this innocent animal being tortured and couldn't believe that not a single soul came to his rescue. I found it confusing and horrifying at the same time.
>
> "However, despite this natural compassion for animals, I somehow became desensitized to their plight as years passed. As I ate the flesh of animals, donned

their skins, and enjoyed their circus performances, their suffering didn't weigh as heavily on my mind as it did during that bullfight. In adulthood, however, I began to question the party line, and vegetarianism intrigued me. After graduating from university with a major in human nutrition, I became increasingly convinced that a plant-rich diet was optimal.

"Still, my battle with my conscience wasn't fully reignited until a rather remarkable incident. A friend had asked if he could drop by for coffee on his way to hunt deer. After dispensing with the usual trivialities, I asked him how he could justify pulling the trigger on such a beautiful animal. I pointed out that it wasn't fair—deer had no defense against his bullets. And I asked him if it made him feel like more of a man to shoot and kill another creature.

"His response stunned me—and changed the course of my life. He said, 'You have no right to criticize me. Just because you don't have the guts to pull the trigger doesn't mean you're not responsible for a trigger being pulled every time you buy a piece of meat camouflaged in cellophane in the grocery store. You're simply paying someone to do the dirty work for you. At least the deer I eat have had a life. I doubt very much you can say the same for the animals sitting on your plate.'

"I was silenced, because he was absolutely right. In that instant, I vowed to take responsibility for the food I bought and to find out about the lives of the animals I ate. What I learned filled me with shame, guilt, and outrage, but more importantly, it reawakened my compassion for animals.

"When I think back, I realize I understood at an early age that animals have their own feelings and their own purposes. Still, it didn't fully prepare me for the interaction I was to have with my son at the same tender age. One day, he asked me if we could buy a McDonald's hamburger. I suspected that he pictured a lovely grove of hamburger trees behind every McDonald's restaurant. I explained that while our burgers at home were made of plants, such as beans, the McDonald's hamburgers were made of cows. He looked at me as though I had completely lost my mind and replied quite emphatically, 'Mommy, people do not eat cows.' He seemed shocked I'd say such a strange thing. When I explained that people do eat cows, he began to cry. Finally, in an exasperated voice, he asked, 'Mommy, them have eyes. Don't they know that cows are people too?'

"I understood. He could see that cows think, feel, smell, hear, eat, sleep, and love—just like people. He couldn't see why that wasn't enough for us to treat them like people."

Many people believe that being vegan is only about eschewing hamburgers and ice cream. It's not. Being vegan is about widening our circles of compassion to include those who are commonly excluded, whether they're humans or non-human animals. It's about understanding that our choices have consequences for ourselves, and beyond ourselves. It's about recognizing that eating animals and animal products is both unnecessary and potentially harmful.

As we'll see, the modern animal agriculture industry causes unspeakable suffering to animals, as well as potentially massive ecological devastation. Intensive animal agriculture reduces land for food production, contributes to global warming, and depletes natural resources. If everyone on the planet ate lower on the food chain, hunger could essentially be eradicated, many diet-related diseases could be avoided, environmental destruction could be reversed, and animal suffering would ease. Being vegan is about making choices that are a true reflection of our ethical and moral principles, and acknowledging that custom and tradition justify nothing.

The vision of a truly ethical universe is captured brilliantly by the words of Dr. Albert Schweitzer, Nobel Peace Prize recipient and esteemed humanitarian: " . . . the time is coming when people will be amazed that the human race existed so long before it recognized that thoughtless injury to life is incompatible with real ethics. Ethics is in its unqualified form extended responsibility with regard to everything that has life."

To begin to live ethically, the first critical step is to take the blinders off. Many exceptional books and documentaries explore the topic of animal rights and include exhaustive examinations of industries that exploit animals for retail products, entertainment, experimentation, and medical research. However, the industry most responsible for animal suffering is the food industry. More than 95 percent of all animals purposefully killed by people are killed to be eaten.

NONHUMAN ANIMALS—THEIR PLIGHT, OUR POWER

Some people view everything on this planet as a resource here for the taking. To them, animals exist for the express purpose of serving humans in some way. This logic is used to defend the exploitation of animals for fashion, entertainment, experimentation, research, and food. Some controversy exists about how animals should be treated, but the actual use of animals isn't a point of contention for the vast majority of people in our society.

However, the standard rules of use vary, depending on the creature and the culture. For example, in America, kittens and puppies are beloved pets. In China, they might be dinner; in some restaurants, patrons can select an individual kitten or puppy. Without a second thought, the chef efficiently skins and boils the animal alive. While Americans may be disgusted by the treatment of cats and dogs in China, treating lobsters in a similar manner seems perfectly acceptable.

Some people would argue that dogs and cats are more intelligent than lobsters, so they deserve to be treated more kindly. That might seem like a logical argument, except that our treatment of pigs, which have been shown to be more intelligent than dogs, is arguably worse than our treatment of lobsters. Yet, these intelligent animals are seldom treated as pets. Instead, they're treated like raw materials for the food industry's meat machine.

The Making of Meat Machines

People in the food industry didn't deliberately set out on the path to cruel animal husbandry practices. But in the name of efficiency, that's the direction in which the industry developed. Consider that in 1900, 41 percent of Americans lived on farms; one hundred years later, that number had dropped to

1.9 percent.[10] Meanwhile, the population grew from 76,094,000 in 1900 to more than 281,422,000 in 2000, increasing demand for food. As a result, the consumption of animal products rose.

How is it possible to supply sufficient meat and milk to satisfy so many people with so few farmers? In a word, agribusiness. Unfortunately, the model developed by agribusiness transforms animals into production units, with the goal of generating the greatest amount of meat for the least amount of money. The most efficient way to accomplish this task is not to raise the animals in fields but in specialized facilities that allow the industry to minimize the time it takes to prepare them for slaughter. Called concentrated animal feeding operations (CAFOs) by the industry, agribusiness facilities that treat animals as production units are more commonly known as factory farms.

Every year in North America, approximately eleven billion land animals are slaughtered for food.[11, 12] Of these, 99.9 percent of chickens, 97 percent of laying hens, 99 percent of turkeys, 95 percent of pigs, and 78 percent of cattle are raised on CAFOs.[13] Average consumers understand so little about these establishments that they easily forget that the meat at the grocery store is the flesh of an animal. Fattened on cheap feed, bred for rapid growth, treated with antibiotics to control disease and with hormones to stimulate appetite and maximize weight gain, and immobilized in small spaces that allow little movement during their short lives, these animals, so effectively hidden from view, endure unspeakable suffering.

A MODERN PIG'S LIFE

In some ways, an animal's intelligence and awareness makes its treatment at CAFOs even more horrifying. Pigs have been shown to be more intelligent than dogs or three-year-old children.[14] For example, Professor Stanley Curtis of Penn State University discovered that pigs have remarkably long memories and are highly skilled at video games, which they play with a joystick designed for them. He added that pigs learn to play simple games every bit as quickly as primates.[15]

In addition, the traditional view that pigs are just filthy animals may be quite far from the truth. When in their natural environment, pigs are surprisingly clean. They're very particular and have discrete sites for eating, sleeping, grooming, and elimination. Although pigs do roll in mud, this behavior is necessary to regulate their body temperature, because they lack sweat glands and are prone to heat stress. The mud also protects them from insects and sunburn.

But most of today's pigs can't roll in mud or explore their talent at video games. Instead, in the United States, an estimated 110 million pigs were slaughtered for food in 2010.[16] In China, hog production is estimated at five times that of the United States.[17] According to the United Nations Food and Agriculture Organization (FAO), each year, 1.3 billion of these intelligent animals end up on people's plates.[18] Although the natural life span of a pig is ten to fifteen years, pigs raised for food in America live approximately six months—and in an environment that can in no way be called "natural."

Breeder sows, which continually produce litters, live until their productivity wanes, generally about three to four years. Most of this time is spent in gestation or farrowing crates, which provide insufficient room for the sows to turn around while they're pregnant or after they've given birth. In their natural setting, piglets wean at about 15 weeks. But on a CAFO, after only two to four weeks of nursing, the piglets are removed to be fattened more quickly, and the sow is reimpregnated.

Weanlings spend the next six weeks in "nurseries," or wire cages stacked one on top of the other. Piglets that don't grow fast enough (the runts of the litter) are generally euthanized by 3 weeks of age. Although workers employ a variety of methods to kill the runts, among the more common are blunt trauma to the head and "thumping"; piglets are picked up by their hind legs and slammed onto a concrete floor until they die.

Healthy piglets don't fare much better. Most undergo a variety of mutilations, including ear-notching, tail-docking, teeth-clipping, and, for males, castration. Done primarily to reduce stress-related behaviors, these procedures are performed without the use of anesthetics, causing needless and agonizing pain. During their time in the cages, piglets also receive medication to prevent the diarrhea that results from eating solid foods they're too young to properly digest.

The piglets destined for meat production are then transferred to cramped pens and fed until they reach a slaughter weight of 240 to 300 pounds. The pigs are crammed in together, in single stalls or groups, with no room for rooting, exploring, nesting, or other standard social behaviors. The floors commonly are metal grid systems, which allow urine, feces, and vomit to fall into a huge pit below. As a result, the air inside these facilities is permeated with ammonia fumes and other noxious gases from which the pigs have no escape. The cramped conditions also prevent regular cleaning, so dust and dander also riddle the air.

Not surprisingly, respiratory diseases are endemic under such conditions. Pig factories are fertile breeding grounds for communicable diseases, such as swine influenza, enzootic pneumonia, infectious atrophic rhinitis, and porcine reproductive and respiratory syndrome. To ensure that the pigs survive until it's time for slaughter, antibiotics, hormones, and other pharmaceuticals are routinely added to their feed.

The pigs that do survive must endure more suffering. In America alone, an estimated one million pigs die en route to slaughter each year, from crushing, freezing, dehydration, or disease. When they reach the slaughterhouse, if they're frightened and resist loading, unloading, or moving forward in the facility's chutes, they're prodded with electric rods set to a painfully high voltage. In some cases, the pigs are beaten with metal pipes or kicked by frustrated handlers.

The slaughtering process is hardly more humane. The first step is to render the pigs unconscious by stunning them using electricity or suffocating them with carbon dioxide (CO_2). The pigs are then dragged upside down using chains or ropes wound around their back feet. Unfortunately, electrical stunning isn't always effective, and reports of conscious pigs squealing and kicking wildly while hanging are not uncommon. Next comes the "sticker," or the person who slits the pig's throat to bleed her out. If the sticker is unsuccessful, the still-living—and possibly conscious—pig continues along the disassembly line to the scalding tank, where she is boiled alive for hair removal.[13, 19-24]

Every time consumers buy a pound of bacon or a few slices of ham from a grocery store, they provide a financial incentive to the pig industry to continue these kinds of activities and, however unknowingly, give these actions an implied seal of approval.

CHICKEN LITTLE WAS RIGHT

Of course, pigs aren't the only animals processed in such a fashion. The treatment of chickens and other poultry, while not exactly the same, also needs to be examined more closely by consumers who may be unaware of industry practices.

The poultry industry includes chickens, turkeys, ducks, geese, pheasants, quail, and other fowl. More than nine billion of these animals are slaughtered in North America every year for food; chickens comprise the vast majority.[11] They're raised either for meat (broilers) or eggs (layers)—and more than 95 percent are raised in total confinement from birth to death. (For "free-range" conditions, see page 19.) But this treatment is contrary to the way chickens live in a more natural setting.

Chickens are social animals that live communally in flocks. Each flock has a well-established pecking order in which dominant individuals are given priority when it comes to food and nesting areas. Each individual knows his or her place in the flock and remembers the faces and ranks of up to ninety other birds.[25] Chickens have unique personalities; some are timid and fearful, while others are bold and gregarious. Hens prefer to lay eggs in the same location and often share their nesting site with one or more other hens.

Chickens are far more intelligent than most of us realize. Research suggests that they're better at math, logical reasoning, and self-control than toddlers.[26] Chickens learn by observation, can anticipate events, and can predict outcomes. They have a sense of object permanence (the ability to understand that if an object is moved out of sight, it still exists), and can use sounds and gestures to communicate with one another.[27] When we begin to understand chickens' complex nature, the cruelty of their short and brutal existence in a CAFO becomes even more evident.

Broilers

Broiler chickens are generally raised on open floors in huge metal sheds that often house 20,000 or more birds per shed and 150,000 to 300,000 birds per operation. The average space allotted per animal is less than 1 square foot. The overcrowding causes the chickens extreme stress, escalating their risk of injury and disease. Some starve to death because they can't access food or water; some die of heart attacks or organ failure.

Because of the popularity of white breast meat, these birds are selectively bred for bigger breasts. As a result, they're almost twice as heavy at slaughter as their relatives from the 1950s. However, selective breeding of this type causes muscle growth to surpass bone growth, resulting in deformities, fractures, tears, and ruptures. Many birds are literally crippled by their own weight.

At only 6 or 7 weeks of age, the birds have reached market weight and are gathered to be transported for slaughter. At the slaughterhouse, chickens are dumped onto conveyor belts and hung upside down on a movable rack. There's no requirement for them to be stunned before slaughter, because chickens are exempt from the Humane Methods of Slaughter Act that applies to cattle, sheep, and pigs. Instead, they're subjected to an electric water bath that paralyzes them but doesn't always render them unconscious. Before they're plunged into scalding water to loosen their feathers, their throats are slit so they can bleed out and die. In some cases, the process is unsuccessful, and these unfortunate birds drown in the near-boiling water.[28–30]

Layers

Although they live longer, hens raised to lay eggs may be worse off than broilers. They live their lives in wire battery cages that restrict their movement while still allowing them to lay eggs. The entire system, from feeding and watering to egg collection, is typically fully automated. The cage floors slope forward so that eggs roll onto a conveyor belt, which transports the eggs directly from the layers to the cleaning stations.

These egg-laying hens are packed into the wire cages so tightly that they're given less than half the space of broilers, or approximately 67 square inches per bird (slightly more than half the size of a standard sheet of paper). This degree of overcrowding makes it impossible for the birds to carry out any natural behaviors. For perspective, a hen needs about 72 square inches of space to be able to stand up straight, 178 square inches to preen, and 291 square inches to flap her wings.

The inability to perform any of these activities causes the chickens to behave abnormally. To prevent the birds from pecking one another to death, workers use a heated blade to sear off about one-third to one-half of a chicken's beak. This amputation is conducted without an anesthetic and causes severe nerve injury, as well as acute and even chronic pain.

Most egg factories also subject their birds to the practice of forced molting in an effort to induce another egg-laying cycle. During this time, food is either completely withheld (starvation regimen) or restricted (low-nutrient diet) for ten to fourteen days, causing weight losses of up to 35 percent of body weight.

These birds are productive for twelve to twenty-four months. After that, egg production drops below the level that would provide an economic return. Because laying hens typically are genetically selected for efficient egg production and have low meat yields, they have little value to meat processors. Traditionally, such spent hens were used for soup and school lunch programs, but with the large supply of broilers available, there's little demand for these smaller birds. Today, it's not uncommon for producers to dispose of the birds on-site by gassing them. Then, they're either incinerated, or ground up and incorporated into animal feed given to other animals—including future generations of chickens.

To keep the industry going, these layers must be constantly replaced. So, at 1 day old, chicks are sexed to determine their fate. Female chicks go on to become egg layers. But because they can't lay eggs and are poor meat producers, the 260 million male chicks born each year in the United States have no economic value to the industry and are immediately disposed of. The most common disposal methods are maceration (chicks are ground up alive), gassing (CO_2, argon, or both), suffocation (chicks are thrown into garbage cans, bags, or dumpsters), and electrocution (chicks are sucked through pipes onto a kill-plate).[27, 31, 32]

CATTLE, COWS, AND CALVES

Humans domesticated cattle about eight thousand years ago. Today, domestic cattle provide humans with about half of their red meat, about 80 percent of their leather, and 95 percent of their animal milk.

Cattle

Although beef cattle are branded and dehorned (and males are castrated)—all without anesthetic or pain relief—their lives seem rather enviable when contrasted with those of pigs or chickens. Beef cattle are among the few food animals that spend their lives outdoors. Conventionally raised cattle are pastured during their first seven to nine months of life, and when they reach about 650 pounds, they're taken to a feedlot for "finishing." Although most of these facilities house more than 1,000 head of cattle, larger facilities can accommodate 30,000 to 150,000 animals at any one time. At the feedlot, they receive a high-energy, grain-based diet designed to pack about 400 pounds on to their frames in three to four months.

Of course, adding about 100 pounds per month on an unnatural diet has consequences for an animal's health. Cattle evolved on a forage-based diet, which is extremely high in fiber and low in starch. When cattle eat a grain-based diet, microflora in their rumen (first stomach) produce organic acids, driving down the rumen pH. This causes a variety of health problems and, in severe cases, can lead to bloat, acidosis, and liver abscesses. As a result, the feed is routinely laced with antibiotics not only to reduce the risk of diseases induced by these intensive feeding systems but also to help promote rapid growth.[11, 33, 34]

In fact, about 70 percent of all antibiotics used in the United States are given to livestock. This overuse of antibiotics contributes to the increasing problem of antibiotic-resistant bacteria.[35] In 2011, a study published in the journal *Clinical Infectious Diseases* analyzed 136 samples of meat and poultry taken from twenty-six grocery stores in five US cities. Of those, 77 percent of the turkey samples, 42 percent of the chicken samples, and 37 percent of the beef samples (almost half the total samples taken) tested positive for the disease-causing bacteria *Staphylococcus aureus*. Ninety-six percent of these staph bacteria were resistant to at least one antimicrobial agent. Even worse, 52 percent were multidrug-resistant, demonstrating resistance to three or more classes of antimicrobial agents.[36]

People who eat beef consume more than just these antibiotics. In the United States, growth hormones have been given to beef cattle since the 1950s. According to a Congressional Research Service report, approximately two-thirds of all US cattle—and about 90 percent of feedlot cattle—receive growth hormones. In large commercial feedlots, they are given to close to 100 percent of the animals. The report adds: "Cattle producers use hormones because they allow animals to grow larger and more quickly on less feed and fewer other inputs, thus reducing production costs, but also because they produce a leaner carcass more in line with consumer preferences for diets with reduced fat and cholesterol."[37]

Hormone pellets are implanted under the ear skin when cattle arrive at feedlots and again about halfway through the fattening period. In people who eat feedlot-fattened beef, hormone residues that remain in the beef may act as endocrine disruptors, interfering with the actions of natural hormones in the body. Some experts suggest that these compounds may affect fertility, the age of the onset of puberty, and the risk of certain cancers in humans eating the meat. Hormones also wind up in feedlot waste, eventually making it into waterways. To avoid these problems, the European Union banned hormone-treated beef in 1989, which initiated a long-standing trade dispute with the United States.[37, 38]

The final journey for cattle is to the slaughterhouse, where they file one by one up a ramp to be stunned, hoisted into the air, have their throats slit, and be sent down the disassembly line.

Slaughterhouses pose hazards for humans, as well. Many large slaughterhouse operations process more than three hundred head of cattle per hour.[39] Over the years, line speeds have escalated and accidents have multiplied. Because meatpacking plants receive fines for high injury rates, plant managers and owners have an incentive to falsify safety records. Some have been caught keeping records that misrepresent the actual occurrence of injury and illness by as much as 1,000 percent.[40] In addition, most plants are nonunionized, the pay is low, and workers are largely immigrants. Not surprisingly, slaughterhouses are among the most dangerous workplaces in North America.

Cows and Their Calves

Many people become vegetarians to express their compassion for animals. Yet, some believe that drinking milk and eating eggs are reasonable choices because the animals don't have to die for us to take their milk or eggs. While this is true, in practice they're virtually always slaughtered once they become unproductive. Current intensive methods of milk and egg production occasion no less suffering and death than meat production (and in the case of egg production, probably more).

In the 1950s, most farm families had at least two dairy cows to ensure year-round dairy products for the family. Typical dairy farms had about a dozen cows, and the very largest farms boasted 50 to 100 cows. Today, standard dairy farms exceed 100 cows, with many large facilities housing 700 to 1,000 animals and the largest facilities accommodating 40,000 animals.[41]

Along with the increase in farm size came an increase in milk production. In the early 1900s, the average cow produced about 3,000 pounds of milk in a year. By 1950, milk production had almost doubled to more than 5,000 pounds annually, and today, each animal produces more than 17,000 pounds of milk per year. This is a biological miracle of sorts—a sixfold increase in milk production in about 100 years. Unfortunately, this "miracle" has been achieved at a high cost for cows and their offspring.

Dairy cows begin their cycle of milk production by being impregnated (generally by artificial insemination) at about 13 to 16 months of age. They give birth to a calf after a nine-month gestation period and continue to be impregnated once a year to ensure steady production of milk. In most cases, calves are separated from their mothers within a day of birth. While the separation is extremely traumatic for both mother and calf, it seems that allowing more time together serves only to strengthen their bond and heighten the stress of the eventual separation.

Female offspring are raised to replace the spent cows. Male calves are of no value to the dairy industry, except for a few that are used for breeding. These fortunate breeder calves are funneled into the beef industry; the rest are used to produce veal. In the United States, this generally means "special-fed veal" (also called white veal or milk-fed veal). The calves' flesh color is very light because they're exclusively fed an iron-deficient milk replacement; their flesh is very tender because most veal calves are tethered at the neck in small stalls so they can't turn around and develop their muscles. These animals are slaughtered at the age of 16 to 18 weeks. About 15 percent of US veal is called "bob veal" and comes from newborn calves ranging from 2 to 3 days to 2 to 3 weeks of age.[42, 43]

Every aspect of dairy farming—whether breeding, feeding, impregnating, medicating, or milking—is designed to maximize production and profit. More than 80 percent of US dairy cows are confined in indoor systems, although some have access to outdoor strawyards. Less than 10 percent of US dairy cows are raised on pasture. Some cows are reared in stalls where they're tethered at the neck, while others are in freestalls and are able to roam within the barn.

These methods of rearing trigger two conditions: lameness and mastitis. Lameness, the leading cause of cow deaths, occurs in an estimated 14 to 25 percent of cows and is caused primarily by hoof lesions associated with concrete flooring and insufficient physical activity. Mastitis, or painful swelling of the mammary glands, is triggered by the demands of extremely high milk production and bacterial infections due to poor sanitation. It's the most common medical condition reported in US dairy cows and the second leading cause of death.

One factor strongly associated with both lameness and mastitis is the use of recombinant bovine somatotropin (rBST or bovine growth hormone). Bovine growth hormone, a genetically engineered hormone designed to increase milk yields, is injected into cows at many of the larger US dairies. Although the tremendous increase in milk production over the years is mostly due to successful breeding for this trait, the use of rBST further increases milk yields by 10 to 15 percent, giving milk producers an incentive for its use despite the consequences for the cows.

Most Holstein cows in the United States average about 729 days of milk production (enduring two to three pregnancies to achieve this) before their production wanes and they're no longer of use to the industry. Nearly all dairy cows go to slaughter at 4 years of age. In contrast, their natural lifespan would be more than 20 years.[42, 43]

SOMETHING FISHY

As a food, fish is widely viewed as the best of protein sources and the only significant source of important long-chain omega-3 fatty acids. As a result, fish and fishing have been put on a pedestal of sorts. For example, national and international health authorities recommend that people consume at least two servings of fish per week to reduce their risk of heart disease. In addition, people in developing countries are being advised to multiply their fish intake by two to three times.

Globally, an estimated one trillion fish are caught each year, excluding illegal catches and bycatch.[44] Where do all these fish come from? The commercial fishing industry is divided into two sectors—capture fisheries (commercial fishing fleets that target wild fish and seafood) and aquaculture ("farms" that raise fish and aquatic animals in confined areas). Today, the total weight of fish and other aquatic animals consumed by humans is provided relatively equally by these two sectors.[45]

But concerns about exploitation of these creatures are growing by the year. Despite the expansion of aquaculture, more than 90 percent of the global predatory fish population has been wiped out.[46] Of all the remaining monitored fish stocks in the wild, more than half are now fully exploited, meaning that the stock cannot sustain further expansion of fishing. Another quarter is overexploited, depleted, or slowly recovering.[45]

Overfishing is rapidly devastating marine ecosystems. Each decade since the 1950s, the number of collapsed fish stocks has increased exponentially. Experts predict that if current trends in fishing continue, by 2048 there will be a total global collapse of all stocks currently fished.[47] Yet, despite this looming ecological crisis, consumers are urged to eat more fish, encouraging the industry to continue its destructive practices.

Capture Fisheries

Capture fisheries employ a wide range of catching techniques. Potassium cyanide and other poisons are routinely applied to coral reefs to paralyze or stun reef fish for aquariums or to capture exotic species for live-fish restaurants, killing the reefs in the process. Other methods include the highly malicious, such as dynamiting coral reefs, and the excessively—and cruelly—efficient, such as bottom-trawling, long-lining, gill-netting, and purse-seining.

Bottom-trawling is one of the most ecologically devastating activities in which humans engage. The ocean depths are among the most pristine ecosystems that remain on planet earth and are the home of many yet-unnamed species that may well become extinct before they've even been discovered. Because it involves dragging huge nets—equipped with metal plates at each end and metal wheels along the bottom edges—along the ocean floor, bottom-trawling has been deemed the underwater equivalent of clear-cutting forests. The comparison may be overly generous to bottom-trawlers, because they're more like giant underwater bull-dozers that demolish bottom-dwelling communities. In 2006, the United Nations (UN) Secretary General reported that 95 percent of damage to seamount ecosystems is the result of deep-sea bottom-trawling.[48]

Bottom-trawling is also wasteful. Among the worst offenders are shrimp trawlers, which unintentionally kill up to 20 pounds of nontarget marine life for every pound of shrimp plucked from the trawling net.[49] The creatures trapped inside these nets are dragged upward, along with rocks, coral, and other fragments of ocean habitat. On ascent, they experience rapid decompression, causing vital organs to rupture. This bycatch, which includes sea turtles, dolphins, sharks, and numerous other aquatic species, is commonly tossed overboard.

Although less destructive to the ocean floor than bottom-trawling, the long-line industry is notorious for the collateral mortality of millions of marine animals, including birds, dolphins, sharks, and turtles. Fish and other animals captured by long lines can be dragged behind a boat for hours or even days. Long-lining uses one or more main lines from which dangle short branch lines with hooks at the ends. Lines can be as long as 75 miles and hold hundreds or thousands of baited hooks. They're set at varying depths in the water, depending on the target species, but this tactic doesn't prevent other animals from being hooked.

In contrast, gill-netting uses huge floating nets to snare target fish. The nets, measuring from hundreds of feet to more than a mile wide, have weighted foot ropes at the bottom and buoyant floats at the top. By adjusting the balance of weights to floats, fishers can set the nets to any desired depth. The nets' mesh is sized precisely to snare the target species. Targeted fish attempt to swim through the openings, but their gills become trapped and they can't escape. Nontarget species are small enough to swim through or large enough that their gills aren't caught. Still, gill nets are often left unmonitored for long periods, so trapped fish can slowly suffocate.

Purse-seining also employs a large net. It's called a "purse" seine because the rope that passes through a series of rings that run along the bottom of the net can be pulled to completely close the net, like a giant drawstring bag. The catch is then hauled to the surface. Purse-seining is the preferred method for capturing fish that congregate in schools near the water's surface. However, a primary concern is that dolphins are commonly trapped in purse seines and can drown. In addition, fish are often still alive when they're pulled on deck and are conscious when their gills are slit and they're gutted.

Less environmentally destructive systems, such as hand lines and traps, are also commonly used in the capture industry but often are no less cruel. Sharks, for example, are individually caught using hooks, but they're not humanely killed.

Do Fish Suffer?

Until recently, the sentience of fish wasn't given much consideration by animal scientists. Few believed that fish had much capacity to think, and even fewer believed that they had the capacity to feel. Since the 1990s, however, a steady stream of studies has forced us to rethink these beliefs.

Using multiple approaches to investigate behavior and stress responses, scientists confirm that fish demonstrate myriad complex behaviors and skills. Fish form relationships, recognize other individuals, pass on knowledge and skills, have long-term memories, solve problems, collaborate in hunting, use tools, strategize, feel fear and distress, and avoid situations that past experience suggests are risky. Fish also have the neurotransmitters and pain receptors necessary to feel pain, and they demonstrate physiological and behavioral responses to painful stimuli. While the issue is still one that is hotly debated among scientists, most experts contend that fish do feel pain, but because it's expressed differently, comparing the extent of their suffering to that of mammals is difficult.[50–53]

Because shark fins—a delicacy in Asian cuisine—fetch a premium price, only their fins are cut off. The still-living animals are then returned to the ocean where they slowly suffocate, unable to use their fins to swim or gills to breathe (for sharks to breathe, water must be moving over their gills).

Aquaculture as an Alternative

The killing of wild fish and other sea life has become so efficient that it now exceeds these populations' ability to replenish themselves at replacement rates. The imminent global collapse of wild fish stocks has been driving a massive shift from capture fisheries to culture fisheries, otherwise known as aquaculture or aquafarming. Aquaculture is the fastest-growing animal-based food sector in the world. In 1980, aquaculture provided an estimated 9 percent of global fish stocks (by weight); by 2008, the figure was about 46 percent.[54, 55]

Culture fisheries raise fish and other aquatic animals in controlled facilities known as fish farms. Some are land based and raise fish in ponds, pools, tanks, or raceways; others are near ocean shorelines, where fish are held in nets, pens, or cages. All are intensive operations, similar to CAFOs for land animals.

The goal of fish farming is no different than that of intensive chicken, pig, or cattle farming—to generate the greatest amount of meat for the least amount of money. As a result, fish farms maintain a density of animals never seen in the wild. Growth accelerators are used to speed weight gain, and antibiotics are used to contain the spread of disease. The consequences of these intensive operations are widespread and severe:

- **Fish welfare.** Poor conditions in aquaculture operations (e.g., crowding, inappropriate physical environment, polluted water, disease outbreaks) can cause stress, fear, discomfort, and pain in these animals.

- **Environmental damage.** Ecologically sensitive areas, such as mangroves, coastal estuaries, and salmon migration routes, can be seriously threatened by fish-farm outputs, including nitrogenous waste (mainly from fish feces), food pellets, and drug residues. Released into the ocean, this untreated waste affects water quality and other sea life and also fuels harmful algal blooms, a proliferation of toxin-producing algae that can cause massive die-offs of fish, shellfish, marine mammals, seabirds, and animals further up the food chain who consume them.

- **Pressure on wild fish stocks.** The strongest argument used to justify fish farming is the protection of wild fish. Paradoxically, by raising these carnivorous animals, fish farming endangers wild fish. It actually takes 2.5 to 5 pounds of wild fish used as feed to yield 1 pound of farmed carnivorous fish.[56, 57] In addition, cultured fish that escape fish farms can transfer serious diseases, sea lice, and other parasites to wild fish stocks. When nonnative or exotic species escape into nearby waters, they can devastate native fish populations. For example, when cultured Atlantic salmon reproduce in Pacific waters, they spread disease to native stocks and compete for limited resources, such as food and habitat.

- **Genetic engineering.** While not yet approved for sale, genetically altered salmon, prawns, and abalone are currently being cultured. For example, growth-hormone genes from Chinook salmon have been added to Atlantic salmon, allowing for year-round growth. These transgenic salmon reach market size in half the time it takes conventional salmon. There's concern that these genetically modified animals could escape into the wild (as many fish farmed in open systems do), posing a significant threat to native species.[58, 59]

The "Humane" Myth

Vegans are often challenged by people who consume products derived from "humanely treated" animals and who wonder what could possibly be wrong with eating them.

However, there's an important distinction in ethical perspectives between vegans and conscientious meat consumers about what's "humane." Vegans are ethically opposed to *any* exploitation of animals. Vegans don't view animals as humanity's to use and reject the notion that if they're treated "humanely" before being slaughtered, people are justified in killing and eating them.

Slavery provides a good analogy. Most people would agree that it's preferable to treat slaves kindly than to subject them to all manner of cruelty. However, for those who oppose slavery as ethically and morally wrong, simply treating slaves well can't justify the practice of slavery itself.

In addition, although the majority of people agree that animals raised for food should be treated humanely, only a small percentage seems to be willing to pay more for meat, milk, and eggs produced under such conditions. Consumers who profess to prefer humane products also can be easily swayed back to regular products if the humane products are unavailable or too costly, or when eating out.

Still, even consumers who commit to humane products, regardless of price or convenience, can be misled. While some obtain humanely raised products directly from small local farmers, most shop at grocery stores. In stores, consumers must rely on food labels to determine whether or not products come from animals treated in an acceptable manner. Catchphrases that suggest these animals were treated well include "free-range," "free-roaming," "cage-free," "pasture-raised," "grass-fed," "organic," "humanely raised," "certified humane," and "animal-compassionate."

However, most farms that purport to meet these standards aren't independently inspected to verify that their practices meet consumer expectations. On many "humane" farms, animals are still generally bred by the thousands, kept in crowded conditions, and removed from their mothers shortly after birth. Chickens are still debeaked and male offspring still disposed of. Even in facilities that offer access to the outdoors, the access may only be a small opening to an outdoor enclosure that's inaccessible to many of the animals crowded into the facility.

Of course, in the end, all animals raised for meat, milk, or eggs—regardless of how they're treated—meet the same fate. While a few are slaughtered on small farms, most "humanely raised" animals are transported to and slaughtered in the same facilities that process animals raised on factory farms.

Perhaps the greatest advantage of "humane" meat is its cost. Higher price tags on meat could eventually tame the taste buds of meat eaters, ultimately reducing the number of animals slaughtered for food. Again, it's certainly preferable that farm animals suffer less than more. But the fact that they may have suffered less than most other farm animals still doesn't justify their exploitation in the first place.

We've just scratched the surface of the animal-rights argument; search the Internet for excellent websites and books on this topic. Also see Resources on pages 450 to 452.

Animal Agriculture—Paying the Price with Our Planet

There's no question that intensive animal agriculture is among the most notorious polluters of air, water, and soil and the greatest contributor to deforestation, desertification, and species extinction. While a shift toward a vegan diet may well be the most powerful step an individual can take toward the preservation of this planet, it also may be an ecological imperative.

The human species is consuming the earth's resources more rapidly than its reserves can be replenished, and food choices may be the greatest contributor to this depletion. By 2050, there will be an estimated 9.3 billion people on the planet, and if we continue on our current trajectory, we'll have insufficient food to sustain this population. Leading authorities have examined the diets of different nations, and the results show that if every person ate the same foods as the average American, we'd need 3.74 Earths to sustain the world's population in 2050.[60] Even if every individual consumed a plant-rich diet similar to the diet of today's average Malaysian, we'd still need 2.48 planets.[61]

The ecological crisis we face is a reflection of sheer numbers. The global population is growing by a staggering 250,000 people per day,[62] or 166 per second. Our fragile planet is ill-equipped to handle an exponentially escalating population of human beings. Humanity's annual demand on the earth's natural resources has been exceeding the planet's renewal capability since the 1970s. In 2008, experts estimated that it would take 1.5 years for the earth to regenerate the renewable resources that people used—and to absorb the CO_2 waste they produced—in that year. This 50 percent deficit means that our current manner of living isn't sustainable for future generations.[61]

People are slowly coming to realize that the laws of nature aren't up for grabs. All life on this planet, regardless of its position in the web of existence, depends on these laws for survival. Within this web lies a complex food matrix. The lowest level of the food matrix sustains plants, which in turn sustain animals, all of which constantly recycle nutrients back into the soil. Humans have altered the food matrix to such an extent that other levels must adapt or perish.[63] The problem is that eventually the toll of these alterations will become so great, the entire system will collapse. While some believe that we're already beyond the point of no return, we must do what we can within the laws of Mother Nature.

In 2010, to determine the relative ecological impact of human activities, the International Panel for Sustainable Resource Management of the United Nations Environmental Program (UNEP) examined all available scientific data on the topic. The panel concluded that two activities have a disproportionately large effect on the planet's life-support systems: animal agriculture, especially the raising of livestock for meat and dairy products, and the use of fossil fuels.[64] They suggested a global shift toward a vegan diet to protect the world from hunger, poverty, and the worst impacts of climate change.[65]

HOW TO REDUCE GLOBAL WARMING

Global warming is accelerating at a rate that has exceeded most predictions. The consequences are most obvious in the Far North, where the ice is melting and polar bears are losing essential habitat. Although its effects are less obvious in other parts of the world, global warming has been linked to an increase in extreme weather conditions, such as tropical storms, floods, droughts, and heat waves.[67-69]

The culpability of intensive animal agriculture in contributing to global warming is no longer a matter of debate among environmentalists. In a groundbreaking United Nations FAO report, "Livestock's Long Shadow," livestock were found to be responsible for 18 percent of greenhouse-gas emissions—more than all forms of transportation combined.[70] In 2008, people raised close to 68 billion land animals for consumption, according to the FAO.[71] Experts estimate that this figure will double by 2050. Inherently tied to greenhouse-gas emissions—the fundamental cause of global warming—this number is important.[72]

According to the Kyoto Protocol, the main greenhouse gases are CO_2, methane, nitrous oxide, and three groups of fluorinated gases.[73] Efforts to curb global warming, both nationally and internationally, have concentrated largely on reducing or capping CO_2 emissions. Advocates have advised consumers to

Resolving Human Hunger

Ethical arguments for a vegan diet often focus on issues related to animal rights. However, persuasive arguments can also be made regarding human rights. All people have the right to food, which means being free from hunger, food insecurity, and malnutrition. Sadly, when land is used to grow crops to feed "livestock," the very poorest people often go hungry.

The 1983–1985 Ethiopian famine provides a rather poignant example. During this period, while hundreds of thousands of people starved to death, Ethiopia continued to export grains to feed livestock in developed nations—to service the interest on its debt. Tragically, the vast majority of the world's starving children live in nations that routinely export grains for animal feed.

In addition, many of these nations are actively trying to expand their own meat and dairy supplies in an effort to provide animal protein for their people. But, by reducing food available to starving people, this practice only widens the gap between rich and poor.

A global shift toward a vegan diet could provide a viable solution to human hunger. According to UNEP's International Panel for Sustainable Resource Management, "Impacts from agriculture are expected to increase substantially due to population growth and increasing consumption of animal products. Unlike fossil fuels, it is difficult to look for alternatives: people have to eat. A substantial reduction of impacts would only be possible with a substantial worldwide diet change, away from animal products." [64]

Currently, 60 percent of the food supply is grown for human consumption. Switching to all-plant diets would increase the global calorie supply by an estimated 50 percent, which could effectively wipe out human hunger. [66] Even if only one in ten people stopped eating animals, sufficient food would be available to sustain the one billion people who currently suffer from hunger.

use alternative energy sources, select fuel-efficient appliances, and drive low-emission vehicles.

But when compared to CO_2, the global-warming effects of methane are 23 times greater and those of nitrous oxide are 296 times greater. [70] Emissions related to methane and nitrous oxide are most strongly linked to the red meat and dairy industries. Surprisingly, few experts have thought to suggest eating veggie burgers instead of hamburgers to combat these emissions.

Those who do recognize intensive animal agriculture as a factor in global warming often blame cow flatulence for increasing methane levels, but livestock leave their mark in many other ways. People increase CO_2 emissions when they run farm machinery, bring in feed, transport animals, or clear forests to make room for food animals. Fertilizers generate nitrous oxide, and manure releases more methane. The UN estimates that one-fifth of human-generated greenhouse-gas emissions—9 percent of the CO_2, 37 percent of the methane, and 65 percent of the nitrous oxide—comes from livestock production. [70]

It may come as a surprise to learn that the majority of these household greenhouse-gas emissions are due to food *production* rather than food *miles*, as is commonly believed. When people think about going green with their diet, most often they focus on sourcing food locally. The idea is that the fewer miles food travels in transport trucks, the less fossil fuel is used, thus reducing the food's carbon footprint. However, local animals are typically fattened on transported fodder, trucked to slaughter, processed, and shipped to retail outlets.

Still, researchers at Carnegie Mellon University discovered that food delivery accounts for only 4 percent of food-related greenhouse-gas emissions, and transportation, as a whole (including food delivery), for just 11 percent. Food wholesaling and retailing were found to account for another 5 percent. Ultimately, the researchers found that average consumers could reduce their carbon footprint more effectively by eating 100 percent vegan *one* day a week than by eating 100 percent local *seven* days a week.[74]

Meanwhile, at 83 percent, food production accounted for the vast majority of emissions within the food industry. Within this category, 44 percent was due to CO_2 emissions, 23 percent to methane, 32 percent to nitrous oxide, and 1 percent to hydroflourocarbons and other industrial gases. Thus, the impact of food production on climate change is due mainly to the more-destructive, non-CO_2 greenhouse gases.

The word is spreading. In September 2008, Rajendra Pachauri, chair of the UN Intergovernmental Panel on Climate Change, suggested that people should aim for one meat-free day a week, then continue to decrease the amount of meat they eat.[75] Dr. Pachauri estimated that if everyone in the United Kingdom (about 50 million people) followed this advice, the reduction in CO_2 emissions would be greater than it would be if five million cars were taken off the road. In the United States—assuming the entire 2013 population of 315 million ate a meat-free diet one day a week—the equivalent reduction in CO_2 emissions would exceed that delivered by eliminating 31.5 million cars.[76]

In addition, if land use were reappraised and plant foods were raised for direct consumption, the global face of malnutrition could be transformed. Currently, approximately 80 percent of the world's soybeans and more than 50 percent of the corn is fed to livestock.[72] However, it takes about 15 pounds of feed to yield 1 pound of beef, 6 pounds for 1 pound of pork, and 5 pounds for 1 pound of chicken.[77] The bottom line is that raising livestock consumes far more food than it yields.

KEEPING THE WATER CLEAN

The food supply—indeed, the entire ecosystem—depends on fresh water. The increase in freshwater demand parallels human population growth, but water availability is shrinking. For example, approximately 45 percent of fresh water in the United States has been deemed unfit for drinking or recreational use because of contamination by dangerous microorganisms, pesticides, and fertilizers.[78] Water shortages now impact more than one billion people worldwide, and water pollution affects many more by boosting rates of infectious disease.

Besides threatening drinking water and human food supplies, water shortages and water pollution severely reduce biodiversity.[79] In the *Living Planet Report 2010,* the state of the earth's biodiversity was assessed and assigned a

Living Planet Index (LPI). This index provides a solid measurement of the effect of humanity's demands on the earth's resources over time. The assessment of water systems tracked changes in 2,750 animal populations, including 714 species of fish, birds, reptiles, amphibians, and mammals found in temperate and tropical freshwater ecosystems. The report indicates that the global freshwater LPI declined by 35 percent between 1970 and 2007, and the tropical freshwater LPI declined by almost 70 percent.[61]

What caused this drastic decline? Mostly, it's animal agriculture, which is recognized as one of the leading threats to water systems. It's estimated that agricultural production consumes 70 percent of global fresh water.[79] According to David Pimental, professor of ecology and agriculture at Cornell University, it takes about 43 times more water to produce 1 pound of beef than to produce 1 pound of cereal grain when the water used to produce the animal feed is factored in—about 43,000 liters of water per kilogram of beef versus 1,000 liters of water per kilogram of cereal grains.[79]

In addition, the US Environmental Protection Agency (EPA) warns that the agricultural industry is "the leading contributor to identified water quality impairments in the nation's rivers and streams, lakes, ponds, and reservoirs."[80] Although human waste released into water systems must first be treated, no such requirements exist for animal waste. This can have devastating consequences.

In the United States, confined food animals produce approximately 500 million tons of raw waste every year, or about triple that of the human population.[80] In fact, a farm with 2,500 dairy cows produces about the same amount of waste as a city of 411,000 people.[81] On factory farms, manure is stored in open-air pits or huge holding tanks, presenting a potential hazard. Manure from animals raised on CAFOs contains pathogenic organisms; pharmaceuticals, such as hormones and antibiotics; chemical contaminants, such as heavy metals and nitrates; and excessive nutrients, such as phosphorus and nitrogen—all of which can threaten water quality. Concrete manure pits can crack, and if laid in sand or gravel, manure can leak out and work its way into groundwater; holding tanks can overflow and pollute nearby surface water.

If leaks are avoided, after a holding period of about six months, the manure is spread on farm fields as fertilizer.[82] If it's applied in an amount greater than the soil and crops can absorb and utilize, the excess can contaminate waterways and release toxic gases into the environment.[83] It's also estimated that crops absorb only one-third to one-half of the nitrogen in the manure applied.

Runoffs, polluted by the nitrogen and phosphorus in manure, can cause "dead zones" in water systems by nourishing algal blooms that deplete oxygen and choke out aquatic life.[84] According to the US Department of Agriculture, poultry operations bear the brunt of the responsibility for the pollution in these runoffs, contributing 64 percent of excess nitrogen and 52 percent of excess phosphorus.[85]

In addition, pathogenic bacteria can end up in nearby rivers and streams that may, in turn, be used to irrigate vegetable crops. In fact, most outbreaks of vegetable-related food-borne illness can be traced back to animal farming operations, which can contaminate plant foods grown nearby.

According to the EPA, as much as 80 percent of the antibiotics routinely administered orally to livestock ends up in their manure—unchanged.[82] This is a significant concern for human health. Routine subtherapeutic use of antibiotics in animals can lead to antibiotic resistance in pathogenic bacteria—and the reduced effectiveness of antibiotics for people who become infected with these organisms.[83, 86]

There are also serious concerns about the health consequences of administering hormones to livestock. In 2010, a panel of experts led by Samuel Epstein, MD, chairman of the Cancer Prevention Coalition, filed a US Food and Drug Administration petition seeking an immediate ban on the use of hormones in meat production. According to Dr. Epstein, their use is directly linked to increased rates of hormonal cancers, specifically breast, prostate, and testicular cancers.[87] Unfortunately, both antibiotics and hormones (natural and synthetic) end up in surface water and groundwater when released in manure.[81]

USING LAND MORE WISELY

Water isn't the only resource affected negatively by animal agriculture. According to the FAO, "Livestock production accounts for 70 percent of all agricultural land and 30 percent of the land surface of the planet."[70] Livestock production has a massive impact on both the quality and quantity of available soil, by damaging and depleting reserves.

Although soil is commonly thought of as little more than dirt, it's actually a complex system dependent on living and organic materials, such as decaying plants, worms, bacteria, algae, and other microorganisms. Unfortunately, intensive farming and monocrop agriculture cause nutrient depletion and soil erosion, while overapplication of fertilizers and pesticides causes serious contamination. Soil forms only at a rate of about 1 centimeter every 150 to 500 years (or 1 inch every 381 to 1,270 years), so if it's rapidly depleted, soil regeneration will not occur for many generations. Experts believe that the planet can sustain losses of 1 ton of soil per hectare per year. However, every year, approximately 90 percent of US cropland loses soil at a rate thirteen times higher; ranges and pastures lose soil at a rate six times higher.

Livestock production is a primary culprit in desertification, or the deterioration of useable semiarid land into nonproductive deserts. Overgrazing strips the land of plants that anchor topsoil, leading to irreversible soil loss, reduction in biodiversity, and the invasion of alien species.[88] Overgrazing is also a factor in climate change; it drives up CO_2 emissions by reducing the carbon sink provided by desert plants and increases methane generated by livestock. An estimated 60 percent of American pastureland is overgrazed.[89]

These are grim statistics. In a 2006 report to the US Senate, the Nutrition Security Institute estimated that if soil loss continues at present rates, the planet has only enough topsoil to last for 48 more years.[90] In other words, if some dramatic changes to the current food production system aren't made, by 2054, the earth's farmable topsoil will be gone, as will the primary method of providing food to the 9 billion people expected to occupy this planet by then. If we don't change the current trajectory, we'll end up where we're heading.

Soil depletion isn't the only worry. Raising livestock is among the leading causes of deforestation globally, particularly in rain forests, such as those in the Amazon.[61, 70] The Amazon has been described as a valuable carbon sink because of the amount of carbon that its plants assimilate from atmospheric CO_2 during the process of photosynthesis.[91] However, when people burn forests to clear land for livestock, carbon stored in the trees and plants is immediately released as CO_2. It's estimated that deforestation contributes about 15 percent of annual global CO_2 emissions.[92, 93]

After centuries of habitation by humans with minimal impact, the Amazon rain forest has been mercilessly exploited; in just a few decades, approximately 17 percent has been cleared.[94] Since 1970, an area about the size of Texas—almost 725,000 square kilometers—has been lost.[95] An estimated 91 percent of these deforested areas is used for livestock production, with the resulting increase in methane, as well.[70, 96] Brazil's thriving soybean industry, dedicated largely to animal feed, is also encroaching on rain forests.[97] If people continue to destroy rain forests, the planet could eventually reach a tipping point where the entire ecosystem collapses.

Global deforestation also threatens the existence of millions of plant and animal species, causing the global loss of an estimated 50,000 species each year, or 137 plant species a day.[93, 98] The Amazon rain forest alone is a region of unparalleled biodiversity, housing more than 10 percent of all the species on earth, including numerous endemic and endangered species. Many of these species are likely not yet identified; in a single decade (1999 to 2009), more than 1,200 new plants and vertebrates were discovered in the Amazon alone—that's one new species every three days.[94] Many undiscovered species may be beneficial to humans, but if they're extinguished before they're discovered, we'll never know what we lost. While the human race can recover within a few generations from economic hardships, natural disasters, and even wars, species extinction is permanent. As the rate of extinction accelerates, the safety net for our own species disintegrates.

AIR-QUALITY ISSUES

Although we must be concerned about the future, livestock production creates health hazards for humans today. Factory farms stink—both figuratively and literally. While their horrific stench has long been viewed as an inconvenience in the eyes of the industry and the courts, evidence suggests that the impact is far more insidious. Researchers have established that odors from factory farms are associated with nausea, vomiting, headache, shallow breathing, coughing, sleep disorders, upset stomach, appetite depression, irritated eyes, nose and throat irritation, and mood disturbances (including agitation, annoyance, and depression) in both farm workers and residents of nearby communities.

Whether animal waste is stored or spread on fields, it undergoes decomposition, releasing noxious fumes. More-severe respiratory symptoms, including bronchitis, occupational asthma, mucous membrane irritation, organic dust toxic syndrome, and long-term lung damage, are frequently reported in farm workers.[99] Nearly 70 percent of workers employed at swine CAFOs report at least one respiratory symptom, while 58 percent experience chronic bronchitis.[82] Manure pits are especially problematic, posing confined-space hazards due to CO_2 levels that lead to oxygen deficiency, and toxic gases, including methane, ammonia, and hydrogen sulfide. For their own safety, farm workers are advised to never enter a manure pit without wearing a self-contained breathing apparatus.[100]

ADDING UP THE COSTS

Each passing day brings us a little closer to the realization of a Native North American saying: "When all the trees have been cut down, when all the animals have been hunted, when all the waters are polluted, when all the air is unsafe to breathe, only then will you discover you cannot eat money."

A typical fast-food burger costs about $2. Because of the deleterious effects of current livestock production, experts suggest that the real cost is closer to $200.[101] If we want to stand a fighting chance, we must stop subsidizing the livestock industry and deflating the price of animal products. If we subsidize anything, it should be vegetables.

Vegan Goes Mainstream

Until the early to mid-1980s, the word *vegan* conjured up images of hippies wasting away on diets of roots and shoots. The only place "vegan" ever appeared on a product label was in a health food store. If you happened to mention your vegan diet to a doctor or dietitian, they would try to "educate" you about the risks of eliminating two of what were considered to be essential food groups: meat and dairy. University textbooks warned soon-to-be doctors and dietitians that vegan diets were downright dangerous.

Fortunately, the tables have turned. In 2010, *Businessweek* featured an article called "Power Vegan." The first paragraph obliterated the old vegan stereotype:[102]

> "It used to be easy for moguls to flaunt their power. All they had to do was renovate the chalet in St. Moritz, buy the latest Gulfstream jet, lay off 5,000 employees, or marry a much younger Asian woman. By now, though, they've used up all the easy ways to distinguish themselves from the rest of us—which may be why a growing number of America's most powerful bosses have become vegan. Steve Wynn, Mort Zuckerman, Russell Simmons, and Bill Clinton are now using tempeh to assert their superiority. As are Ford Executive Chairman of the Board Bill Ford, Twitter cofounder Biz Stone, venture capitalist Joi Ito, Whole Foods Market Chief Executive Officer John Mackey, and Mike Tyson. Yes, Mike Tyson, a man who once chewed on a human ear, is now vegan."

There's no denying it—the vegan lifestyle is now on mainstream America's radar. By winning international titles, vegan bodybuilders have blown away the image of "skinny weakling" vegans. Elite endurance athletes are gaining a competitive edge by fueling their bodies with plants. (For more on vegan athletes, see chapter 13.) Executive chefs are dazzling judges with extraordinarily colorful and creative vegan masterpieces. Models, musicians, and movie stars are strutting their vegan stuff. Peer-reviewed articles that examine the therapeutic value of vegan diets are making headlines. Even doctors and dietitians are now endorsing plant-based diets as ideal for the prevention and treatment of lifestyle-induced chronic diseases.

As a result, increasing numbers of average Americans are exploring meat-free diets. For example, 56 percent of the more than 1,800 chefs polled in a National Restaurant Association survey cited vegan entrées as a hot trend.[103] *USA Today* listed becoming flexitarian (a person who occasionally includes meat or fish in a predominantly vegetarian diet) as one of the top ten consumer food trends. In fact, close to half the American population is trying to reduce overall meat consumption.[104]

Poll numbers back this up. In 2012, the Vegetarian Resource Group commissioned Harris Interactive to survey Americans who followed vegetarian or vegan diets, or who regularly ate vegetarian meals. The poll showed an estimated 4 percent of Americans follow a vegetarian diet (never consume meat, poultry, or fish), and 1 percent (two million Americans) follow a vegan diet (never consume meat, poultry, fish, dairy, or eggs). In addition, about 15 percent of Americans avoid meat, poultry, and fish at many of their meals (but less than half the time), and 14 percent avoid these foods at more than half their meals. This would suggest that about a third of Americans choose vegetarian meals on a regular basis.[105]

Although three decades ago many consumers associated the word *vegan* with risky fad diets, today it's linked with conscious personal, ethical, and ecological choices. A burgeoning movement is demanding food produced responsibly and sustainably. Consumers are drawn to eating styles that provide a solution to the crushing escalation in obesity, diet-induced diseases, and health care costs.

Not surprisingly, the market is responding. Vegan restaurants are popping up everywhere, and products featured in mainstream grocery stores are using the word *vegan* on labels as a marketing tool. Vegan lifestyles are topics of conversation on wildly popular talk shows. Vegan books, shoes, cosmetics, and specialty products are exploding into the marketplace. The shift in the perception of the masses is palpable—and the future hopeful.

Yes, challenges remain. They boil down to a rather cynical version of the Golden Rule: "Them that got the gold make the rules." Businesses that earn hefty profits from animal exploitation wield a great deal of power. These industries have tremendous influence on government policy and are key recipients of agricultural subsidies. Consumers also are constantly bombarded with commercial advertising that makes leather, suede, silk, steak, and lobster seem attractive, sexy, sophisticated, and highly desirable.

Fortunately, we have a choice. We can allow ourselves to fall into a hypnotic consumer trance, or we can honor our inner moral compasses and withhold the gold. Better still, we might consider embracing the original Golden Rule: "Do unto others as you would have others do unto you." In this older, wiser form, the Golden Rule serves as a core principle for every major world religion and as a foundation for humanity.

Humankind is beginning to entertain the idea of expanding its definition of "others" to include our nonhuman brethren. The first steps have been taken. Scientists are now submitting declarations to protect the rights of animals that exhibit the traits of a "person," such as self-awareness, creativity, communication, and intentionality. Perhaps the day will come when simply being a sentient being—able to think, feel, and suffer—is enough.

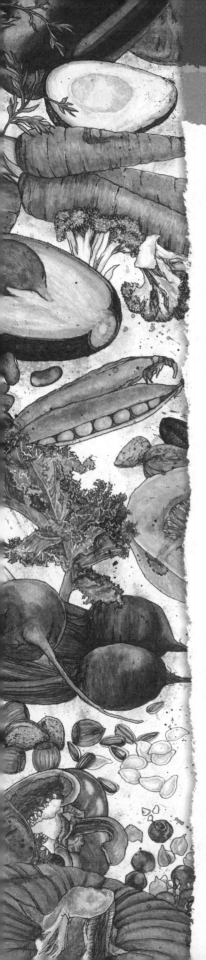

CHAPTER 2

The Great Vegan Advantage

He that takes medicine and neglects diet wastes the skills of the physician.

CHINESE PROVERB

A few short decades ago, scientific communities viewed vegan diets as downright dangerous, and health practitioners warned against their use. Gradually, research studies provided compelling evidence for their safety, and attitudes began to shift. Today, the views of the medical establishment are clearly reflected in the official position of the Academy of Nutrition and Dietetics (formerly the American Dietetic Association): "It is the position of the American Dietetic Association that appropriately planned vegetarian diets, including total vegetarian or vegan diets, are healthful, nutritionally adequate, and may provide health benefits in the prevention and treatment of certain diseases."[1]

Vegan diets have not only been vindicated, but they're also being hailed as health heroes, and for good reason. They provide a simple solution for the global epidemic of chronic disease. Well-designed vegan diets afford powerful protection against an imposing list of noncommunicable diseases and serve as safe, economical, and highly effective treatment tools.

Vegan Nutrition: The Big Picture

The primary criticism leveled against vegan diets is that they're nutritionally inadequate and that, relative to non-vegan diets, they increase the risk of malnutrition. People assume meat is necessary for protein, iron, and zinc, and dairy products are required to meet calcium needs.

However, people who eat well-designed plant-based diets have little difficulty meeting recommended intakes for these and most other nutrients. The single exception is vitamin B_{12}—plants aren't reliable sources. However, many vegan foods are fortified with vitamin B_{12}, and supplements are inexpensive and widely available. In addition, everyone older than 50 (including nonvegetarians) is advised to use fortified foods and supplements for B_{12}—just as vegans do. (For more on vitamin B_{12}, see pages 214 to 222.) Both vegan and omnivorous diets have the potential to adequately nourish a population, if appropriately planned, and to be risky, if poorly planned.

While "malnutrition" is generally associated with *undernutrition* (insufficient access to food, or hunger), actually, more people in the world experience another form of malnutrition: *overnutrition* (overconsumption of calories). By 2010, the number of people suffering from overnutrition exceeded the number of people suffering from undernutrition.[2]

Vegan diets rarely lead to under- or overnutrition. Research has consistently confirmed a greater prevalence of overnutrition, overweight, and obesity within general populations than within vegan populations.[3-7] In the United States, an estimated 68 percent of the general population suffers from overnutrition, leading to overweight or obesity.[8] This, in turn, increases the risk of type 2 diabetes, coronary artery disease, stroke, hypertension, nonalcoholic fatty liver disease, gallbladder disease, gout, osteoarthritis, sleep apnea, some cancers, and complications of pregnancy.[9]

A third type of malnutrition, *micronutrient deficiency,* overlaps with both under- and overnutrition. Micronutrient deficiencies are common across all dietary groups. They can result from insufficient access to food, poor variety in the diet, and/or excess consumption of fat and sugar, which crowds out more-nutritious foods. In vegan populations, micronutrient deficiencies—especially vitamin B_{12} deficiency—are more prevalent in people who consume overly restrictive diets.

VEGAN NUTRITION INTAKES AND STATUS

Research to date that assesses the overall dietary intakes and nutritional status of vegans provides reassurance that well-planned vegan diets supply adequate nutrition. Generally, vegan diets contain greater amounts of iron, folate, thiamin, magnesium, potassium, manganese, fiber, beta-carotene, and vitamins B_6, C, and E than omnivorous diets. However, they may contain lower amounts of zinc, iodine, calcium, selenium, riboflavin, and vitamins B_{12} and D, so it's important for vegans to include reliable sources of these nutrients. The bottom line is that animal products aren't necessary for healthful and nutritionally adequate diets.

Table 2.1 provides a summary of research that addresses the overall nutritional adequacy of vegan diets for adults and adolescents. (Research on single nutrients is discussed in upcoming chapters, as is research pertaining to infants and children.) The studies included in table 2.1 focus specifically on vegans rather than on the broader vegetarian community.

TABLE 2.1. Summary of vegan research (adults): body mass index (BMI), overall nutrient intakes, and status

LEAD AUTHOR(S), LOCATION (OR STUDY), AND YEAR	PARTICIPANTS/ METHODS	RESULTS	CONCLUSIONS/ COMMENTS
Rizzo, AHS-2, 2013[3]	71,751 participants (5,694 vegans*). Compared diet, BMI, and lifestyles of nonvegetarians, semivegetarians, pescovegetarians, vegetarians, and vegans.	BMI was highest in nonvegetarians and lowest in vegans. Calorie and protein intakes were similar among the groups. Fat, saturated fat, and trans fat intakes were highest among nonvegetarians and lowest among vegans. Fiber, beta-carotene, magnesium, and potassium intakes were highest among vegans. Intakes of vitamin B_{12}, vitamin D, vitamin E, calcium, and zinc were lowest among vegans, but the intakes of all but vitamin D and calcium were well within the recommended range. Vegan calcium intakes averaged 933 mg per day.	BMI was lowest among vegans, and vegans had the lowest rates of overweight and obesity. Although nutrient intakes were within the recommended range for most vegans, the lower tails of some nutrient distributions suggested inadequate intakes by a portion of the subjects.
Spencer, UK EPIC-Oxford, 2003[5]	37, 875 participants (1,553 vegans). Compared diet, BMI, and lifestyles of meat eaters, fish eaters, vegetarians, and vegans.	BMI was highest among meat eaters and lowest among vegans, with fish eaters and vegetarians having similar BMIs. 50% of the BMI difference was attributed to macronutrient intakes (energy, protein, fat, carbohydrate, fiber, sugar, alcohol). 5% of the difference was attributed to lifestyle factors (e.g., smoking, physical activity, education).	Vegans had the lowest BMI, least overweight, and least obesity. Dietary factors most strongly linked to increased BMI were high protein and low fiber.
Davey, UK EPIC-Oxford, 2002[10]	65,429 participants (2,596 vegans). Questionnaire, interviews, seven-day food diary. Compared lifestyle and nutrient intakes of meat eaters, fish eaters, vegetarians, and vegans.	Vegans had the highest intakes of thiamin, vitamin C, vitamin E, folate, magnesium, iron, and fiber. Vegans had the lowest intakes of retinol (preformed vitamin A), vitamins B_{12} and D, calcium, and zinc. Vegan intakes exceeded recommended intakes, except for vitamin B_{12} and calcium (excluding supplements). Iron intakes were low in premenopausal women in all dietary groups.	All four diet groups were close to recommended intakes for nutrients. Significant differences were noted in macronutrient and fiber intakes.

LEAD AUTHOR(S), LOCATION (OR STUDY), AND YEAR	PARTICIPANTS/ METHODS	RESULTS	CONCLUSIONS/ COMMENTS
Larsson, Sweden, 2002[11]	60 adolescent participants (30 vegans, 30 nonvegetarians). Examined nutritional intake and status of adolescents. Diet history was validated by measuring nitrogen, sodium, and potassium excretion in urine. Measured serum B_{12}, iron, and folate.	Average vegan food intakes of riboflavin (males only), vitamin D (females only), vitamin B_{12}, calcium, and selenium did not meet recommended intakes; when supplements were factored in, only calcium and selenium were low. Average nonvegetarian food intakes of selenium (females only) did not meet recommended intakes. There was no significant difference in proportion with low iron status between vegans (20%) and omnivores (23%). Vegans consumed more vegetables, legumes, and fiber, and less fat, saturated fat, cholesterol, and sodium.	Swedish vegan adolescents may consume insufficient calcium and selenium, even with supplements. Vegans need to replace milk products with calcium-rich vegan foods. Vegan adolescents may have lower risk of heart disease. Poor iron status appears to be more a female problem than a vegan problem.
Haddad, United States, 1999[12]	45 participants (25 vegans, 20 nonvegetarians). Compared dietary intake (4-day food intake) and selected biochemical and hematologic measures in vegans and similar nonvegetarians.	Vegans had higher intakes of fiber, vitamin C, folate, iron, copper, magnesium, and manganese; lower intakes of zinc; and lower BMI. When supplements were factored in, the dietary groups had similar vitamin B_{12} intakes. Lab results: Iron status: Similar in both dietary groups; vegans had lower storage iron (ferritin). B_{12} status: Mean serum B_{12} and homocysteine did not differ between dietary groups; 10/25 vegans had at least one indicator of suboptimal B_{12} status. Immune status: There was no difference in functional measures of immune response; however, vegans had lower leukocyte, lymphocyte, and platelet counts. Protein status: Vegans had higher serum albumin, but 10/25 vegan women did not meet recommended protein intake of 0.8 g/kg body weight.	Vegan diets were lower in total fat and cholesterol and higher in fiber and most nutrients, except for vitamin B_{12} (although intakes were about the same with supplements factored in). Protein intakes were low for some vegan women. Although immune function was similar, there was a question about whether lower leukocyte, lymphocyte, and platelet counts could be a result of the low body weights of vegans.

LEAD AUTHOR(S), LOCATION (OR STUDY), AND YEAR	PARTICIPANTS/ METHODS	RESULTS	CONCLUSIONS/ COMMENTS
Draper et al., United Kingdom, 1993[13]	124 participants (38 vegans, 52 vegetarians, and 34 meat avoiders (semivegetarians). Compared dietary intakes using 3-day weighed intakes and food-frequency questionnaires.	Vegan intakes of iodine, riboflavin, and vitamin B_{12} were below recommended values (but were met by other dietary groups); vegan intakes of magnesium, iron, copper, vitamin B_6, and vitamin E were significantly higher than for other groups; vegan intakes of riboflavin, iodine, calcium, vitamin B_{12}, and vitamin D were significantly lower.	Vegans need to increase their intake of vitamin B_{12}, also probably of riboflavin and possibly iodine and vitamin D (perhaps through supplementation).
Lockie, UK, 1985[14]	37 participants (10 vegans, 9 vegetarians, 8 whole-food "healthy eating") nonvegetarians, and 10 regular nonvegetarians). Compared food intakes and lab assessments of vegans, lacto-ovo vegetarians, whole-food omnivores, and regular omnivores.	Vegans met at least 95% of the recommended intakes for all nutrients except riboflavin, vitamin B_{12} (although no clinical evidence of deficiency was found), and vitamin D (none of the groups met the RDA for vitamin D). Vegan intakes of fiber, thiamin, folate, vitamin C, and iron were significantly higher than nonvegetarian intakes.	The vegan diet met the recommended intakes for almost all nutrients without the aid of dietary supplements, and came closer to meeting approved dietary goals than other dietary groups.
Ellis, Path, and Montegriffo, UK, 1970[15]	50 participants (26 vegans and 24 nonvegetarians). Compared detailed physical assessments and blood work.	Average vegan weights were 4.5 kg (10 lb) lower in males and 3.6 kg (8 lb) lower in females than in nonvegetarian controls. Average total cholesterol was lower in male vegans than in controls (181 mg/100 ml vs. 240 mg/100 ml); there were no differences between females. Serum B_{12}: 9 vegans had low B_{12} (< 140 pg/mL); 3 were B_{12} deficient (< 80 pg/mL). Serum folate: vegans had higher folate levels (mean 14.4 ng/mL vs. 5.2 ng/mL for nonvegetarians). 5 nonvegetarians were folate deficient (< 3 ng/mL).	No significant differences in the average clinical status of vegans and nonvegetarians were found.
Guggenheim, Weiss, and Fostick, Jerusalem, 1962[16]	119 vegan participants. Assessed dietary intakes.	The only nutrient significantly below recommended intakes in vegan diets was riboflavin. While calcium intakes were below recommended intakes, they were comparable to nonvegetarian intakes at 825 mg per person per day.	The general level of nutrient consumption was satisfactory except for riboflavin, which fell significantly below the RDA.

LEAD AUTHOR(S), LOCATION (OR STUDY), AND YEAR	PARTICIPANTS/ METHODS	RESULTS	CONCLUSIONS/ COMMENTS
Hardinge and Stare, United States, 1954[17]	85 participants (25 vegans, 30 vegetarians, and 30 omnivores). Compared nutritional adequacy of three types of diets.	Only a few vegan subjects had protein, calcium, and riboflavin intakes below recommended levels. Vegan diets were significantly higher in iron, thiamin, and vitamins A and C than the other dietary patterns.	The vegan diets were generally well balanced.

Sources:[3, 5, 10–17]

*Vegans were listed as "strict vegetarians" in this study and defined as individuals who reported consuming each of the following not at all or less than one time per month: meat (red meat, poultry), fish, eggs, milk, and dairy products.

When interpreting these results, it's important to recognize potential limitations. First, the strength of the evidence is reduced when few subjects are followed. Second, while the most revealing evidence would come from lifelong vegans, currently, few individuals fit this bill. Third, vegans, like vegetarians or omnivores, aren't a homogeneous group. Researchers don't always tease out which vegans eat heathfully and which do not; nor do they distinguish vegans who adopted their diets in an effort to overcome an existing medical condition.

Finally, some methods used to obtain dietary information are far from foolproof. Often, diet recalls or food-frequency questionnaires are used; responses may provide only very rough estimates of food intake. In addition, participants may be followed for too short a time to obtain sufficient information about changes in their nutritional status.

Chronic Disease and the Vegan Advantage

Evidence regarding disease rates in vegan populations continues to flow into scientific journals at ever-increasing rates. Much of this data is sourced from studies of two large populations, both of which compare vegans to similar health-conscious vegetarians, semivegetarians, fish eaters, and meat eaters. The first population comprises members of the Seventh-day Adventist (SDA) church. The Adventist Health Study-1 (AHS-1) followed 34,198 California Adventists between 1974 and 1988, resulting in dozens of research papers. The Adventist Health Study-2 (AHS-2), which began in 2002, includes Adventists from across the United States and Canada, and is ongoing. Of the 96,000 participants in AHS-2, 28 percent are vegetarian and 8 percent are vegan. While some preliminary results from AHS-2 have been released, findings are expected to be published for several years.

The second large population participates in the European Prospective Investigation into Cancer and Nutrition (EPIC). With approximately 520,000 participants from ten European countries, EPIC is the largest cohort study of diet and health to date. The United Kingdom's EPIC-Oxford is one of twenty-three EPIC centers; it's unique among the centers because it purposefully recruited as many vegetarians and vegans as possible. Of the 65,500 people enrolled in EPIC-Oxford, approximately 29 percent were vegetarian and 4 percent were vegan when they enrolled. Research on this cohort is ongoing, although several reports have already been published. Other smaller but significant cohorts from the United Kingdom (Health Food Shoppers and Oxford Vegetarian Study) and Germany (Heidelberg Study) have also been followed.

Chronic diseases, such as cardiovascular diseases (CVD), diabetes, cancers, and lung diseases, are responsible for more deaths worldwide than all other causes combined. In 2008, 63 percent of global deaths were due to these conditions.[18] According to the World Health Organization (WHO), by 2020, chronic diseases will be responsible for almost three-quarters of deaths globally.[19]

According to the 2010 WHO *Global Status Report on Noncommunicable Diseases*, the four primary causes of the epidemic are an unhealthy diet, physical inactivity, tobacco use, and alcohol consumption.[18] Simply put, the majority of premature deaths globally are self-inflicted. This is no revelation—the alarm was sounded decades ago.

In 1990, a WHO technical report, *Diet, Nutrition, and the Prevention of Chronic Diseases*, singled out two food categories as being largely responsible for the epidemic of diet-induced chronic disease: energy-dense foods of animal origin and foods processed or prepared with added fat, sugar, and salt.[20] The foods most strongly linked to disease-risk reduction were whole plant foods, namely vegetables, fruits, cereals, and legumes. Since then, evidence supporting the benefits of plant-based diets has continued to mount.

In response, health organizations have revised diet and nutrition recommendations to reflect the current state of knowledge. For example, the 2010 *Report of the Dietary Guidelines Advisory Committee on the Dietary Guidelines for Americans* suggests four major action points for Americans.[21] These include eating less; exercising more; reducing intakes of refined grains and foods with added sugars, solid fats, and sodium; and shifting to a more plant-based diet that emphasizes vegetables, beans, peas, fruits, whole grains, nuts, and seeds.

Recent studies suggest that vegans come closer to meeting international and national nutrition recommendations for total fat, saturated fat, cholesterol, trans-fatty acids, and fiber than other dietary groups.[1, 22] In addition to being low in saturated fat, high in fiber, and cholesterol-free, vegan diets provide abundant antioxidants and protective phytochemicals. Not surprisingly, AHS-2 reported a 15 percent reduced mortality rate in vegans and a 9 percent reduced mortality rate in lacto-ovo vegetarians compared to similar health-conscious nonvegetarians.[23] It's little wonder that vegan diets are rising stars in the quest to combat chronic disease.

CARDIOVASCULAR DISEASE

In 2005, CVD accounted for 30 percent of all deaths and still is a leading cause of death worldwide.[24] However, years of scientific research have established that plant-based diets have a beneficial effect on CVD risk.[25] The data also confirm significant risk reduction in vegetarian populations.[26–29]

In 2013, both EPIC-Oxford and AHS-2 released data on vegetarian and vegan rates of CVD. EPIC-Oxford found that vegetarians (including both lacto-ovo vegetarians and vegans) had a 32 percent lower risk of ischemic heart disease compared to meat and fish eaters when adjusted for confounding variables, except body mass index (BMI), and a 28 percent lower risk when BMI was factored in.[30] AHS-2 reported a 19 percent risk reduction for ischemic heart disease in vegetarians (including lacto-ovo vegetarians and vegans), and a 13 percent risk reduction for CVD compared to nonvegetarians. The most significant findings were for vegan men, who experienced a 55 percent risk reduction in ischemic heart disease and a 42 percent risk reduction in CVD compared to nonvegetarians. (Vegan women experienced no risk reduction compared to non-vegetarian women.) Because men are at higher risk and often consume larger portions of meat, it's possible they enjoy a greater benefit from consuming a plant-based diet.[23]

In a 1999 meta-analysis of five prospective studies of health-conscious populations (vegetarians, vegans, fish eaters, and meat eaters), death rates for vegans were reported for four of the five studies (one study didn't separate vegans from vegetarian participants). Ischemic heart disease mortality in vegans was 26 percent lower than for participants who regularly ate meat (compared to 34 percent lower mortality for both vegetarians and fish eaters). However, vegans had a 30 percent lower risk of cerebrovascular disease (compared to 13 percent lower for vegetarians and 4 percent higher for fish eaters), although due to the small number of events, this finding was not statistically significant.[25]

While the 1999 meta-analysis suggested that vegan diets provide a stronger protective effect against stroke compared to all other dietary patterns, both vegetarians and fish eaters enjoyed greater protection against ischemic heart disease. It's interesting to note that the 2013 EPIC-Oxford study found no lower risk of ischemic heart disease in fish eaters compared to meat eaters. Although the reason for this finding isn't clear, it's possible that fried fish, a favorite in the United Kingdom, could have predominated in the diets of the fish eaters.

Although there's no question that meat eaters have a more ominous cluster of cardiovascular risk factors than vegans, one might have expected vegans to fare even better than they did.[31] The results might have been more impressive if the vegans in these studies had been lifelong vegans, or at least longtime vegans (ten years or more). Of course, vegan diets may favorably affect some CVD risk factors, while negatively affecting others. As a result, it's important for vegans to be aware of any potential dietary pitfalls that may increase CVD risk and take steps to avoid them.

There are many known risk factors for CVD, some of which are modifiable by diet and lifestyle changes and others that aren't (e.g., age, gender, and family history). Among the risk factors that can be controlled, some are considered "major" modifiable risk factors, while others are classified as "emerging" risk factors. Although all the major modifiable risk factors are favorably impacted by vegan diets, the effects on emerging risk factors are more variable.

Major Modifiable Risk Factors

Elevated Blood Cholesterol Levels The dietary factors linked to elevated blood cholesterol levels are saturated fat, trans-fatty acids, and to a lesser extent, dietary cholesterol.[32] It's estimated that for every 1 percent decrease in cholesterol levels, there's a 2 to 4 percent decrease in heart disease risk.[22] The most effective cholesterol-lowering food components are soluble fiber, plant protein, plant sterols and stanols, polyunsaturated fats, and phytochemicals—all of which are found exclusively or predominantly in plant foods. Vegans consume no cholesterol, have the lowest saturated-fat intake of all dietary groups, and have lower trans-fatty acid intakes.[22, 33, 34] While there's good evidence that replacing saturated fat with polyunsaturated fat significantly reduces CVD risk, replacing saturated fat with refined carbohydrates (e.g., white-flour products, white rice, and sugar-sweetened beverages and treats) elevates CVD risk.[35] Although intakes of refined carbohydrates vary in vegan diets, vegans generally consume a higher proportion of carbohydrates from unrefined foods than do nonvegetarians.

Not surprisingly, in twenty-four studies of vegan, lacto-ovo vegetarian, and nonvegetarian populations conducted from 1978 to 2007, the total blood cholesterol levels of vegans were shown to be lower than those of any other dietary group, averaging approximately 150 mg/dl (3.9 mmol/L).[22] This compares to 187 mg/dl (4.84 mmol/L) for the lacto-ovo vegetarians and 193 mg/dl (5 mmol/L) for the nonvegetarians in these studies (see table 2.2 on page 38).

The vegan average of 150 mg/dl (3.9 mmol/L) is a bit of a magic number in the medical world. According to Dr. William Castelli, former director of the Framingham Heart Study (the longest-running epidemiological study ever conducted) and current medical director of the Framingham Cardiovascular Center, "In the first fifty years of Framingham, only five subjects with a cholesterol level less than 150 mg/dL developed coronary artery disease."[36]

Although there was a significant difference in the low-density lipoprotein cholesterol (LDL) levels of vegans compared to those of other dietary groups, the differences in high-density lipoprotein cholesterol (HDL) were small. The LDL levels of vegans averaged approximately 85 mg/dl (2.2 mmol/L), compared to 105 mg/dl (2.7 mmol/L) for lacto-ovo vegetarians and 119 mg/dl (3.1 mmol/L) for nonvegetarians (see table 2.2). The HDL levels of vegans averaged approximately 49 mg/dl (1.27 mmol/L), compared to 52 mg/dl (1.35 mmol/L) for lacto-ovo vegetarians and 54 mg/dl (1.4 mmol/L) for nonvegetarians.[22] It's important to note that most study participants (regardless of their dietary group) were from health-conscious populations, making these differences less pronounced than they would have been had vegans been compared to the population at large.

In addition to having lower cholesterol levels, vegans also appear to be at an advantage when it comes to cholesterol metabolism. A 2011 study from Brazil found that vegans experienced increased removal of artery-clogging remnants (specifically cholesterol) and reduced cholesterol ester transfer, both of which favor atherosclerosis prevention.[37]

Dietary cholesterol has been shown to increase the susceptibility of LDL to oxidation by nearly 40 percent.[38, 39] When cholesterol becomes oxidized, it has negative effects on arteries, promoting plaque formation and causing hardening of the arteries (reducing their elasticity). The susceptibility of LDL to oxidation can be reduced by the presence of antioxidants, such as vitamin E, carotenoids, vitamin C, flavonoids, and polyphenolic compounds.

Antioxidants come primarily from whole plant foods and are generally more concentrated in typical vegan diets, compared to typical omnivorous diets.[22, 28, 40] Limited evidence suggests that adopting a vegan diet or other plant-based diet improves antioxidant status and decreases the oxidation of lipids (fats).[41–44] In addition, some evidence suggests that high intakes of heme iron (iron from meat, as opposed to nonheme iron from plants) may act as a prooxidant, increasing LDL oxidation and atherosclerosis.[45, 46] Vegans don't consume heme iron, possibly providing further protection against CVD.

Table 2.2 shows CVD-related lab values and dietary intakes, which compare the averages from studies of vegan, lacto-ovo vegetarian, and nonvegetarian populations conducted between 1979 and 2008. The figures were not weighted according to the number of participants in each study.

Elevated Triglyceride Levels One common criticism of plant-based diets has been that they can increase blood triglyceride levels. However, this tends to occur only when refined carbohydrates (sugars and flour products) are overconsumed, because the body converts them into triglycerides for storage purposes. Other dietary factors linked to elevated triglycerides are more strongly associated with omnivorous diets; these include overconsumption of calories and excessive intakes of total fat, saturated fat, trans-fatty acids, cholesterol, and alcohol.

TABLE 2.2. Average CVD-related lab measures and dietary intakes

MEASURE	VEGAN	LACTO-OVO VEGETARIAN	NONVEGETARIAN (MEAT EATERS)
LAB MEASURES			
Total cholesterol	150 mg/dl (3.9 mmol/L)	187 mg/dl (4.84 mmol/L)	193 mg/dl (5 mmol/L)
LDL	85 mg/dl (2.2 mmol/L)	105 mg/dl (2.7 mmol/L)	119 mg/dl (3.1 mmol/L)
HDL	49 mg/dl (1.27 mmol/L)	52 mg/dl (1.35 mmol/L)	54 mg/dl (1.4 mmol/L)
Triglycerides	83.5 mg/dl (0.94 mmol/L)	107.8 mg/dl (1.2 mmol/L)	95.5 mg/dl (1.1 mmol/L)
DIETARY INTAKES			
Saturated fat (% of calories)	6.9	10.6	12
Cholesterol (mg/day)	0	153	266
Fiber (g/day)	43	30	22

Source: [22]

Many lifestyle factors can help to keep triglycerides in check, including physical activity; abstaining from alcohol; minimizing intake of sugar and products made with white flour; and eating a low-fat, high-fiber, omega-3-rich plant-based diet. Research suggests that vegans have the lowest triglyceride levels of all dietary groups. In sixteen studies conducted between 1979 and 2007, vegan triglyceride levels averaged 83.5 mg/dl (0.94 mmol/L), compared to 107.8 mg/dl (1.2 mmol/L) for lacto-ovo vegetarians and 95.5 mg/dl (1.1 mmol/L) for meat eaters.[22]

Hypertension (High Blood Pressure) Blood pressure in vegans is generally within a healthy range, and few vegans have high blood pressure.[47–53] Studies have consistently reported differences in blood pressure in vegetarians compared to nonvegetarians, ranging from 5 to 10 mmHg systolic and 2 to 8 mmHg diastolic.[54–56]

A 2009 AHS-2 report found that, compared to nonvegetarians, the incidence of hypertension was 75 percent lower for vegans. Although hypertension was self-reported in this study, it had been diagnosed by a physician and treated within the previous twelve months.[52] In 2012, further findings of AHS-2 were released.[53] While the risk reduction wasn't quite as strong as in the 2009 report, the later study reported that vegans had a 63 percent reduction in the risk of developing hypertension compared to nonvegetarians.

In EPIC-Oxford, self-reported, age-adjusted, physician-diagnosed hypertension in study participants ranged from 5.8 percent in male vegans to 15 percent in male meat eaters and 7.7 percent in female vegans to 12.1 percent in female meat eaters.[51] While an individual's BMI is strongly associated with his or her blood pressure levels, it was estimated that only about half the variation in hypertension could be attributed to the study subjects' BMI. The remainder was attributed to dietary factors, such as intakes of fat, saturated fat, sodium, alcohol, and fiber, and nondietary factors, such as physical activity.

Increasing the intake of long-chain omega-3 fatty acids (mainly through fish consumption) has been shown to be effective in reducing hypertension.[58] However, EPIC-Oxford didn't report an advantage for fish eaters compared to vegans, suggesting that other factors have a greater impact.[51]

In addition, although omega-3 fatty acids from fish may be protective, fish is also the most concentrated food source of mercury. It's possible that if contaminated fish are consumed, the protection against hypertension afforded by long-chain omega-3 fatty acids could be offset by mercury. The potential consequences of mercury toxicity include a number of cardiovascular diseases, as well as renal dysfunction, insufficiency, and proteinuria.[59]

Overweight and Obesity Vegans have a decided advantage in maintaining healthy body weight and composition when compared to similar health-conscious nonvegetarians. Since 1990, more than twenty studies have consistently reported that vegans are leaner than people in other dietary groups and have both a lower BMI and a lower percentage of body fat.[22]

The two largest studies are AHS-2 and EPIC-Oxford. In the British EPIC-Oxford studies, although average BMIs for all dietary groups were within the healthy BMI range, meat eaters had the highest BMIs, while vegans had the lowest.[5] In four American AHS-2 reports, only the average BMI of vegans falls within this optimal BMI range. The mean BMI for vegans was between 23.6 and 24.1 in these studies, compared to 28.2 to 28.8 for meat eaters—a 4.6 to 4.7 point difference.[3, 4, 30, 60] EPIC-Oxford found a 1.92-point difference between male vegans and meat eaters and a 1.54-point difference between female vegans and meat eaters.[5] However, age-adjusted obesity rates (BMI > 30) were 2.6 times higher in male meat eaters compared to male vegans and 3.2 times higher in female meat eaters compared to female vegans.

In the EPIC-Oxford study, nondietary lifestyle factors, such as smoking and exercise, explained only about 5 percent of the difference in BMI between the dietary groups; their effects may have been diluted because of the health-conscious nature of the cohort. In contrast, energy and macronutrient intakes (i.e., calories, fat, protein, and carbohydrate) explained about half the difference.

The dietary factors judged to be most strongly linked to a higher BMI were low fiber and high protein intake (as a percentage of calories). Although high protein intake itself isn't commonly associated with weight gain, study authors suggested that hormonal changes induced by diets rich in protein may alter metabolic systems to favor weight gain.[5] Meanwhile, increasing fiber intake appears to improve satiety, reduce fat absorption, and promote better insulin control, thereby resulting in lower BMIs.

Relative fiber and protein intakes were significantly associated with BMIs in all dietary groups except vegans. The absence of an association within the vegan group was thought to be related to small variations in intakes within this group. The authors suggested that in the case of protein, it's possible that only high intake of animal protein is associated with increased BMI, so for vegans, varying the percentage of plant protein in their diets wouldn't affect BMI.[5]

Emerging Risk Factors That Are Favorably Affected by Vegan Diets

Inflammation Chronic inflammation can make arterial plaque vulnerable to rupture and thrombosis, heightening the risk of a coronary event. Generally, lifestyle factors, such as smoking, inactivity, being overweight, and poor food choices, can contribute to such inflammation and elevate blood levels of high-sensitivity C-reactive protein (hs-CRP), a predictor of cardiac risk. An hs-CRP of less than 1 mg/L is considered low risk for CVD, 1 to 2.9 mg/L suggests intermediate risk, and above 3 mg/L is associated with high risk.[61] Although levels of hs-CRP in vegans aren't well-known, four of five studies assessing hs-CRP levels in vegetarians showed significantly lower inflammation frequency in vegetarians compared to omnivores.[62–66]

The only study assessing vegan hs-CRP levels found markedly lower levels in vegans (0.57 mg/L) compared to endurance athletes (0.75 mg/L) and those who followed standard Western diets (2.61 mg/L).[67] Although this study was small (63 participants), the differences were striking. In addition, the vegan diet in this study was largely raw.

Poor Antioxidant Status Although the relationship between antioxidant status and CVD risk remains uncertain, vegans and vegetarians, who generally consume larger amounts of antioxidants than nonvegetarians, may be at an advantage.

Several studies have reported better antioxidant status in vegetarians, vegans, and raw vegans than in nonvegetarians, although in some studies, benefits were limited to some, but not all, measures of antioxidant status.[43, 68–75] It's important to note that although antioxidants from food appear to be protective, research on antioxidant supplements has been less encouraging.

Increased Carotid Intima-Media Thickness (Carotid IMT) There's evidence to suggest that dietary changes can affect carotid IMT (a measure of the thickness of artery walls and of arterial stiffness and damage to the blood vessels). Diets high in meat and low in fiber can increase arterial stiffness, and vegan or near-vegan diets can decrease it.[67, 76, 77] In addition, a recent study from Hong Kong reported improved arterial function (including carotid IMT) in vegetarians who have been provided vitamin B_{12} supplementation to treat low B_{12} levels.[78]

High Trimethylamine N-Oxide (TMAO) TMAO is produced when intestinal bacteria ingest carnitine and produce trimethylamine (TMA), which is taken to the liver and converted to TMAO. Although research on TMAO is very preliminary, this is an emerging risk factor worth noting. Researchers suggest that high TMAO levels may accelerate atherosclerosis and hardening of the arteries, increasing the risk of major cardiac events.

Diets determine the amount of TMAO a body makes. The carnitine used for its formation is found in animal products—mainly red meat. Omnivores who regularly consume red meat are ideal hosts for TMA-producing bacteria; regular meat consumption encourages their growth and increases TMAO production. Vegans have none of these bacteria. Even when vegans are fed carnitine supplements, they don't produce TMA because they lack the bacteria to do so. Avoiding meat gradually reduces the gut bacteria that turn carnitine into TMA, and ultimately TMAO, providing a further incentive to adopt a vegetarian or vegan diet.[79]

Emerging Risk Factors That May Be Negatively Affected by Vegan Diets

Elevated Homocysteine Levels Although the amino acid homocysteine occurs naturally in humans, elevated homocysteine damages blood vessel walls—triggering blood clots, oxidative stress, and inflammation—and has been shown to be highly predictive of CVD and coronary events.[80, 81] Three B vitamins—folic acid, vitamin B_6, and vitamin B_{12}—serve as the standard treatment for elevated homocysteine, but research results have been inconsistent, and the value of B-vitamin therapy for reducing CVD risk has come into question.[82–96]

While the utility of B-vitamin therapy for reducing homocysteine and CVD risk continues to incite lively debate, we do know that poor folate, B_6, and B_{12} status is associated with elevated homocysteine. While vegans generally have excellent folate and vitamin B_6 status, their vitamin B_{12} status tends to be low, especially if they don't use supplements. Although it isn't known precisely how low serum B_{12} must be to compromise homocysteine metabolism, one study suggested that when serum B_{12} falls below 300 pg/ml (222 pmol/L), homocysteine levels rise.[97] Experts recommend that patients with serum B_{12} below 400 pg/ml should be further tested for vitamin B_{12} deficiency, including tests for homocysteine and serum methylmalonic acid (MMA).[98] Levels above 400 pg/ml (300 pmol/L) are considered safe; thus, this seems a prudent target for vegans.

Finally, researchers have reported a significant positive correlation between poor omega-3 fatty-acid status and elevated homocysteine, particularly in subjects who had high blood levels of adrenic acid, a long-chain omega-6 fatty acid, and low blood levels of docosahexaenoic acid (DHA), a long-chain omega-3 fatty acid.[31, 99] Treatment with DHA has successfully lowered homocysteine levels in DHA-depleted subjects.[31]

Abnormal Blood Coagulation Several scientific studies have examined markers for the tendency to form blood clots in vegetarians, including vegans and near-vegans. Few of these studies have included enough vegans to make those results statistically significant, but three of four studies reported lower levels of the coagulation protein, factor VII, in vegetarians compared with nonvegetarians,[100–102] two of four studies reported lower levels of fibrinogen in vegetarians compared to nonvegetarians,[101, 103] and two studies found no significant difference.[104, 105] Better fibrinolysis in vegetarians and vegans compared to nonvegetarians was reported in one study,[103] while another found better blood fluidity in vegetarians.[104]

Surprisingly, two relatively recent studies using sensitive test methods reported higher platelet aggregation in vegetarians than in nonvegetarians.[101, 102] The negative findings for platelet aggregation are contrary to expectations because many dietary factors associated with increased platelet aggregation, such as saturated fat and cholesterol, are reduced in vegetarian and vegan diets. In addition, intake of some dietary factors known to diminish platelet aggregation (such as phytochemicals in vegetables, fruits, and herbs) tend to be increased in vegetarian and vegan diets.

Experts suggest that most plausible explanation for this discrepancy is that some vegetarians have poor omega-3 status and high intakes of omega-6 fatty acids. (For more on fatty acids, see pages 117 to 134.) A recent review study suggests that vegetarians—especially vegans—would benefit from eating more omega-3 fatty acids and improving the balance between omega-3 and omega-6 fatty acid intakes.[31]

Poor Vitamin D Status Several large epidemiological studies have confirmed that suboptimal vitamin D status causes significant increases in CVD risk.[106–108] Although this is a concern for all dietary groups, it's well-known that vegan populations tend to have reduced levels of vitamin D, which could have adverse consequences for their cardiovascular health.

Using Vegan and Near-Vegan Diets to Treat High Cholesterol Levels and CVD

Vegan and near-vegan diets have been used in a variety of trials to improve specific CVD markers, such as high blood lipid levels and high blood pressure, and to treat severe coronary artery disease (CAD).

The Vegan Verdict

A well-planned vegan diet offers, quite arguably, the most powerful protection against cardiovascular disease (CVD) that can be provided by any diet. However, the degree of protection can vary considerably, depending on the overall quality of the vegan diet. A poorly planned vegan diet may not provide any advantage over a nonvegetarian diet and could end up increasing CVD risk. To provide maximum protection against lipid abnormalities and cardiovascular disease, vegan diets should include unprocessed, whole plant foods as dietary staples and reliable sources of vitamin B_{12}, vitamin D, and omega-3 fatty acids.

A review study reporting on data collected between 1975 and 2007 found that lacto-ovo vegetarian dietary interventions resulted in total and LDL cholesterol reductions of 10 to 15 percent. Vegan dietary interventions were associated with decreases of 15 to 25 percent, while vegan diets rich in specific protective components (e.g., plant sterols, viscous fiber, soy protein, and nuts) resulted in reductions of 20 to 35 percent.[109] Generally, vegan or near-vegan diets also slightly reduce HDL cholesterol, but observational studies suggest lower HDL levels don't increase cardiovascular risk when associated with a low-fat plant-based diet. While some trials reported increases in triglyceride levels, the reverse was true for trials that featured diets rich in whole high-fiber plant foods.[109]

Two researchers have demonstrated that very low-fat vegan or near-vegan diets can effectively reverse established CAD. In 1983, Dr. Dean Ornish used a combination of diet (10 percent fat, near-vegan), exercise, and stress management to treat 23 patients, comparing them with 23 controls who were asked to make no lifestyle changes. This pioneering work provided initial evidence that comprehensive diet and lifestyle changes could actually reverse CAD.[110]

In 1990, Ornish published his landmark study, The Lifestyle Heart Trial.[111] In this study, 28 participants were randomized to a lifestyle intervention group and 20 to a control group. The participants making lifestyle changes similar to those in his 1983 study experienced dramatic improvements in cardiac health. Eighty-two percent of the experimental group experienced regression of their coronary blockages, while 53 percent of the control group experienced progression. Angina frequency fell 91 percent in the experimental group and jumped 165 percent in the control group. LDL cholesterol dropped approximately 37 percent in the experimental group, compared to 6 percent in the control group. In a five-year follow-up, more improvements were reported, including further regression in arterial blockages. By then, experimental participants had 2.5 times fewer cardiac events than control-group participants.[112, 113]

The second researcher, Dr. Caldwell Esselstyn, used a very low-fat, near-vegan diet plus cholesterol-lowering medications (if necessary) to treat 24 patients with severe CAD. At the five-year follow-up, none of the 18 patients who adhered to the program had experienced a cardiac event. Of 11 patients who had undergone angiography, none had progression of their blockages—and eight had significant regression. No one on the program experienced disease progression, a cardiac event, or cardiac interventions; one person temporarily left the program, but returned when symptoms reappeared.[113]

In 2014, Dr. Esselstyn released a study that followed 198 patients with established CVD, 177 who were compliant with a very low-fat vegan diet and 21 who were not. Of the compliant patients, one individual had a cardiac event (a stroke)—a recurrence event rate of 0.6 percent. Thirteen of the 21 noncompliant patients experienced a cardiac event—a recurrence rate of 62 percent.[114]

No current studies exist on whether higher-fat vegan or near-vegan diets cause positive changes in artery lesions and blockages. However, case reports dating back to the mid-1970s suggest significant improvements in coronary health with the use of higher-fat vegan diets. British researchers Dr. Frey Ellis and Thomas Sanders published reports of patients suffering from severe angina who completely eliminated symptoms after a few months on a strict vegan (but not low-fat) diet.[115, 116] Canadian researcher David Jenkins successfully and dramatically lowered lipids in patients using his trademark "portfolio diet," a vegan program that maximizes plant sterols and viscous fiber and includes soy foods and nuts.[117–121] Investigators have also reported remarkable improvements in cardiovascular markers in participants who consume higher-fat raw diets.[67, 122–125]

There's no doubt that very low-fat vegan diets are particularly effective in treating severe CAD. However, a question that remains is how the addition of nuts, seeds, or avocados would affect the results. It's possible that bioactive compounds and nutrients in these foods and their beneficial effect on nutrient absorption could reduce inflammation, drive down triglyceride levels, increase HDL levels, and further improve outcomes. Of course, it's also possible that dietary fat intake from any source needs to be minimized to reverse coronary blockages. Ongoing research will eventually answer these questions. For now, whole-foods vegan diets are powerful allies in the battle against the world's leading killer.

CANCER

Cancer, the most dreaded of all chronic diseases, is currently the second largest cause of death globally, and the rates are rising.[126, 127] Although perhaps its onset is less predictable than heart disease or type 2 diabetes, cancer is no indiscriminate killer. Surprisingly, a mere 5 to 10 percent of cancers are determined by individuals' genes; the remaining 90 to 95 percent of cancers are products of their environment.

Although it's tempting to assume that populations with low cancer rates will always be protected, migration often wipes out any advantage within a generation or two. One study that followed Japanese women who migrated to Hawaii reported a nearly threefold increase in breast cancer rates in the first generation to reside in Hawaii and a fivefold increase in the second generation. Rates of colon cancer in these migrants also jumped almost fourfold within the first generation (it didn't increase further in the second).[128]

TABLE 2.3. Estimated contribution of diet to cancer deaths

TYPE OF CANCER	PERCENT OF DEATHS LINKED TO DIET
Prostate	75
Colorectal	70
Breast, endometrial, gallbladder, and pancreatic	50
Gastric (stomach)	35
Lung, larynx, pharynx, esophagus, mouth, and bladder	20
Other	10

Source:[129]

Evidence suggests that diet is the linchpin, accounting for an estimated 30 to 35 percent of all cancers. Beyond food choices, an estimated 25 to 30 percent of cancers (87 percent of lung cancers) are primarily due to smoking, 15 to 20 percent are linked to infections, 10 to 20 percent are triggered by obesity, and 4 to 6 percent are tied to alcohol ingestion. The balance is thought to be caused by a variety of factors, such as radiation, stress, inadequate physical activity, and environmental contaminants.[129]

The degree to which diet serves as a causative factor varies according to the type of cancer. As shown in table 2.3, the impact of diet varies with the cancer type or site and is particularly high in the hormone-related and intestinal (colorectal) cancers prevalent in those following Western diets.

In a laudable effort to reduce the global burden of cancer, the World Cancer Research Fund and the American Institute of Cancer Research (WCRF/AICR) convened two expert panels to determine the strength of the existing evidence linking diet and lifestyle factors to cancer. Foods, food components, supplements, dietary patterns, physical activity, body composition, and body fatness were all factored in and scrutinized. The reports present judgments regarding these factors and their relative impact on cancer risk for seventeen potential cancer sites. Released in 1997 and 2007, these reports are considered the most authoritative and influential in this field to date.[130, 131] WCRF/AICR's Continuous Update Project (CUP) also monitors scientific findings on an ongoing basis and maintains a central database of evidence. This allows the panel to review and revise recommendations as new evidence presents itself.

Table 2.4 (page 46) provides an abbreviated version of the 2007 findings as they relate to six of the cancers most directly impacted by food choices. Evidence listed as "convincing" or "probable" was deemed strong enough to include in public health goals (meant for health professionals) and personal recommendations (meant for communities, families, and individuals). Evidence listed as "limited" or "suggestive" was considered insufficient as a basis for public health goals and personal recommendations, although it was strong enough to show a generally consistent trend toward either reducing or increasing cancer risk.

TABLE 2.4. Dietary and other factors that affect cancer risk

CANCER SITE	EFFECT ON RISK	EVIDENCE: CONVINCING	EVIDENCE: PROBABLE	EVIDENCE: SUGGESTIVE OR LIMITED
Breast	Decreases risk	Lactation	Physical activity (postmenopause)	Physical activity (premenopause)
	Increases risk	Alcoholic drinks		Total fat (postmenopause)
Colorectal	Decreases risk	Foods with fiber,* physical activity	Garlic, milk, calcium in supplements	Nonstarchy vegetables, fruits, foods with folate, fish, foods with selenium, selenium in supplements
	Increases risk	Red meat, processed meat, alcoholic drinks (men), body fatness, abdominal fatness	Alcoholic drinks (women)	Cheese, foods with animal fat, foods with sugar
Esophageal	Decreases risk		Nonstarchy vegetables, fruits, foods with vitamin C	Foods with fiber, foods with folate or vitamin E, physical activity
	Increases risk	Alcoholic drinks, body fatness		Red meat, processed meat at high temperatures, drinks
Lung	Decreases risk		Fruits, foods with carotenoids	Nonstarchy vegetables, foods with selenium, foods with quercetin, selenium in supplements
	Increases risk	Beta-carotene in supplements, body fatness (postmenopause)	Abdominal fatness (postmenopause)	Red meat, processed meat, butter, total fat
Prostate	Decreases risk		Foods with lycopene, foods with selenium, selenium in supplements	Legumes, foods with vitamin E, foods with quercetin, vitamin E supplements
	Increases risk		High-calcium diets	Processed meat, milk or dairy products
Stomach	Decreases risk		Nonstarchy vegetables, fruits	Legumes, foods with selenium
	Increases risk	Salt, salted and salty foods		Processed meat, smoked foods, grilled or barbecued animal foods

Source:[131, 134]

*In the 2007 report, the evidence was probable; however, in 2011, the panel strengthened the judgment to convincing.

Recommendations for Cancer Risk Reduction

The WCRF/AICR Panel established a set of public health goals and personal recommendations based on probable and convincing findings that would be most likely to provide the greatest protection against cancer. These recommendations are provided below, along with brief comments regarding rationale, mechanisms, and/or current state of knowledge.[131]

Body Fatness Be as lean as possible within the normal range of body weight. Ideally, body weight throughout childhood and adolescence should be at the lower end of the normal BMI range. Maintain body weight within the normal range from age 21. Avoid weight gain and increases in waist circumference throughout adulthood.

Although carrying some body fat appears to protect against premenopausal breast cancer, excessive increases in body fatness are associated with cancers of the esophagus, colorectum, pancreas, breast (postmenopause), kidney, gallbladder, and liver. Increased body fatness causes changes in hormones and hormone-like chemicals, such as insulin-like growth factor 1 (IGF-1), insulin, leptin, and sex steroids, and leads to increases in insulin resistance—all of which can trigger inflammatory sequences associated with cancer risk.

Physical Activity Be physically active as a part of everyday life. Be moderately physically active, aiming for an activity level equivalent to brisk walking for at least 30 minutes every day. As fitness improves, aim for 60 minutes or more of moderate activity or for 30 minutes or more of vigorous physical activity every day. Limit sedentary habits, such as watching television.

Some evidence links inactivity to cancers of the lung and pancreas. Consistent data suggest that physical activity protects against cancers of the colon, breast (postmenopause), and endometrium, and it likely protects against cancers associated with excess body fatness. The mechanism by which this occurs varies with each type of cancer. For example, physical activity reduces intestinal transit time, shrinking the amount of time dietary carcinogens reside in the intestinal tract, possibly reducing the chances of developing colon cancer. One study reported a 50 percent reduction in colon cancer in those with the highest levels of physical activity.[132] Exercise also favorably affects hormone metabolism and reduces body fat.

Foods and Drinks that Promote Weight Gain Limit consumption of energy-dense foods. Avoid sugary drinks. Consume processed energy-dense foods sparingly. (This advice doesn't refer to unprocessed foods, such as nuts and seeds, which haven't been shown to contribute to weight gain.) Avoid drinks with added sugar; the panel also recommends limiting fruit juices. Eat fast foods sparingly, if at all.

Consuming energy-dense foods and sugary drinks is associated with overconsumption and weight gain, which increase cancer risk. Generally, processed foods with added fat and sugar have the highest energy density. While sugary beverages aren't as energy dense (due to their water content), they fail to induce satiety the way solid foods do, and thus, are often overconsumed.

Plant Foods Eat mostly foods of plant origin. Eat at least five servings (at least 14 ounces/400 g) of a variety of nonstarchy vegetables and fruits every day. Eat relatively unprocessed cereals (grains) and/or legumes (pulses) with every meal. Limit refined starchy foods. People who consume starchy roots or tubers as staples should also ensure intake of five servings of nonstarchy vegetables, fruits, and legumes (pulses).

Plant foods are protective throughout the body. Of the seventeen cancer sites included in this report, risk reduction with plant food intake was reported for fourteen sites. Plant-based foods tend to be relatively low in calories but high in nutrients (such as vitamins and minerals) per calorie, helping to reduce the risk of overweight and obesity and enhancing nutritional status. In addition, these foods are high in numerous protective compounds, including dietary fiber, antioxidants, and phytochemicals, which can help to protect the body from cell damage that can lead to cancer.

Today, the WCRF/AICR's recommendation for a plant-based diet—including fiber-containing foods, such as whole grains, fruits, vegetables, and beans—is stronger than it was in 2007. A recent meta-analysis reported that for people with low fiber intakes, every 10 grams of added dietary fiber was associated with a 10 percent reduced risk of colorectal cancer.[133] In 2011, CUP stated that research published since 2007 has further strengthened the judgment from "probable" to "convincing" that fiber-containing foods protect against bowel cancer.[134]

Animal Foods Limit intake of red meat and avoid processed meat. People who eat red meat (beef, pork, lamb, and goat) should restrict their consumption to fewer than 18 ounces (500 g) per week. Very little of this intake, if any, should be processed (meat preserved by smoking, curing, or salting, such as bacon, salami, pastrami, corned beef, and ham).

The evidence linking red and processed meat to colorectal cancer was convincing at the time of the 2007 report. There was also limited evidence suggesting that red meat causes cancers of the esophagus, lung, pancreas, and endometrium; that processed meat causes cancers of the esophagus, lung, stomach, and prostate; and that grilled, barbecued, or smoked meat causes stomach cancer.

In 2011, CUP issued a press release noting that ten new studies conducted since the 2007 report had further strengthened the evidence linking both red and processed meat to bowel cancer. According to this review, the risk of bowel cancer increases 17 percent when a person eats 3.5 ounces (100 g) of red meat per day and 36 percent when one eats 3.5 ounces (100 g) of processed meat per day.[134]

Although scientists aren't certain why red meat increases cancer risk, it's known that cancer-causing compounds can be generated by heme iron, which is present in all these meats; by nitrates, nitrites, and N-nitroso compounds present in processed meats; and by high-temperature cooking, which can produce known carcinogens, such as heterocyclic amines.

Alcoholic Drinks Limit alcoholic drinks. If alcoholic drinks are consumed, limit consumption to no more than two drinks a day for men and one drink a day for women. There is convincing evidence that alcohol increases the risk of mouth,

How Much Is Okay?

When epidemiologist Walter Willet, chair of the department of nutrition, Harvard School of Public Health, was asked, "How much red meat is okay?" he replied, "Like almost everything, it's frequency and amount that influence our risk. There's no sharp cut-off. It's like radiation. We can't say that there's any safe amount."[135]

pharynx, larynx, esophageal, bowel (men), and breast cancers. Alcohol also probably increases the risk of liver cancer and bowel cancer in women. The evidence suggests that *all* types of alcoholic beverages are implicated and that there's no safe level of intake. Based solely on cancer data, alcohol should be completely avoided.

With its ability to act as a solvent, alcohol has the potential to ease the entrance of carcinogens into cells. Alcohol also produces reactive metabolites, such as acetaldehyde, and generates free radicals. Worse, alcohol and tobacco act synergistically to increase cancer risk. The body's ability to repair genetic mutations caused by tobacco is blunted by alcohol.

Preservation, Processing, Preparation Limit consumption of salt. Avoid moldy cereals (grains) or legumes (pulses). Avoid salt-preserved, salted, or salty foods; preserve foods without using salt. Limit consumption of processed foods with added salt to ensure an intake of less than 6 grams (2.4 g) of sodium a day. Note that only 11 percent of salt eaten is added at the table or during cooking; most is in processed foods. (For more on sodium, see pages 201 to 203.) Don't eat moldy cereals (grains) or legumes (pulses).

Some techniques of food preservation, processing, and preparation are associated with increased cancer risk. Examining consumption of processed meats, salted foods, and foods preserved by salting, smoking, and pickling provides the most compelling evidence for increased risk. Salt has been deemed a probable cause of stomach cancer, and the expert panel estimated that 14 percent of stomach cancers could be prevented if intake were limited to less than 6 grams (2.4 g) of sodium per day.

Dietary Supplements Aim to meet nutritional needs through diet alone. Dietary supplements aren't recommended for cancer prevention. Although several excellent indications for supplement use exist, such as vitamin B_{12} for vegans and vitamin D for people at northern latitudes, studies generally haven't found that supplements are effective for cancer risk reduction. Some evidence suggests that high-dose supplements could even increase cancer risk.

Supplements rarely contain the complete mix of protective compounds naturally found in foods. For example, vitamin A pills are no substitute for health-supportive carotenoids in orange, yellow, and red vegetables and fruits. For this reason, the panel recommended relying on a wide variety of vegetables, fruits, and other plant-based foods for cancer protection, rather than supplements.

The Vegan Verdict

Judging from the findings and recommendations of the WCRF/AICR Panel, one would expect that well-planned vegan diets would provide impressive protection against cancer, especially forms of cancer closely tied to dietary choices. Vegans are leaner; they eat more fiber, more nonstarchy vegetables, more fruits, and more legumes; and they consume greater amounts of folate and antioxidant vitamins from foods. Vegans don't eat meat or animal fat; they avoid dairy products and eat less total fat.

Cancer Rates among Vegans and Vegetarians

So, how do vegans fare when it comes to cancer? Evidence suggests that cancer risk is affected by choices throughout life, even choices in childhood. Although some information exists about cancer rates in vegetarian populations, it will likely be many years before reliable data on lifelong vegans is available. On the other hand, almost all studies on cancer among vegetarian populations show reduced cancer rates compared to the general population. Some, but not all, studies also report reduced cancer rates in vegetarians, compared to the cancer rates in similar health-conscious nonvegetarians.

A handful of studies have reported cancer rates in various dietary groups, including vegans. Although much of this data combines results for vegans with results for other vegetarians, AHS-2 recently provided data that separated vegan participants from other types of vegetarians.

In 2012, AHS-2 released a report examining cancer incidence in more than 69,000 people, with almost 3,000 incident cases of cancer. Vegans had a 16 percent reduced risk of developing cancer compared to meat-eating Adventists, and a 34 percent lower risk for female-specific cancers. This compares to the study's lacto-ovo vegetarians, who experienced an 8 percent reduced risk of developing cancer and a 24 percent lower risk for cancers of the gastrointestinal tract.[136] A second AHS-2 study reported an 8 percent risk reduction in deaths due to cancer for vegans compared to nonvegetarians, and a 10 percent risk reduction for lacto-ovo vegetarians. Vegan men had a 19 percent risk reduction in deaths from cancer compared to nonvegetarians.[23]

In 2014, the EPIC-Oxford group released findings of cancer rates in 61,647 British men and women after an average follow-up of almost fifteen years and 4,998 incident cancer cases. Compared to health-conscious meat eaters, total cancer risk was 19 percent lower in vegans, 11 percent lower in vegetarians, and 12 percent lower in fish eaters.

Among vegetarians and vegans (grouped together), risk was reduced by 63 percent for stomach cancer, 77 percent for multiple myeloma, 36 percent for lymphatic/hematopoietic tissue cancer, and 38 percent for bladder cancer. Rates of prostate cancer, breast cancer, and colon cancer for vegetarians and vegans were looked at separately. Although the findings were not statistically significant, prostate cancer rates were 38 percent lower among vegans, 13 percent lower among vegetarians, and 24 percent lower among fish eaters relative to health-conscious meat eaters. Female breast cancer was 13 percent lower among vegans, 6 percent lower among vegetarians, and 7 percent higher among fish eaters than among meat eaters. One surprising finding was higher colon cancer rates among vegans, although there were only 19 incident cases and the results were not statistically significant.[137]

Vegan Diets in the Treatment of Cancer

Numerous testimonies and anecdotes report excellent responses in cancer patients who consume largely or completely plant-based diets. While such evidence is interesting, it doesn't prove cause and effect, nor does it hold up to scientific scrutiny.

Well-constructed research on the effects of vegan diets on cancer is rare; however, one such study deserves mention. In a 2005 US prostate cancer study, the effects of lifestyle intervention (vegan diet, exercise, stress management, group therapy) were measured in men with early-stage prostate cancer who had opted against conventional therapy.[138] Participants were randomized to either a control group or the lifestyle-intervention group.

After one year, six of the men in the control group began conventional therapy based on the progression of their disease and/or increasing prostate specific antigen (PSA) levels; no one in the lifestyle-intervention group had to do so. PSA increased 6 percent in the control group and decreased 4 percent in the lifestyle-intervention group. In addition, prostate cancer cell growth was inhibited nearly eight times more in the lifestyle-intervention group than in the control group. This study provided compelling evidence that lifestyle intervention (including a vegan diet) effectively reduces cancer progression in early-stage prostate cancer. Further research is needed to see if similar benefits could be produced in patients with other forms of cancer.

Metabolic Markers of Cancer in Vegans and Vegetarians

Several studies have examined metabolic markers of cancer in vegans or in subjects fed a vegan diet. While metabolic markers of cancer are less clear-cut than those of heart disease or diabetes, they do provide some worthwhile information. One study compared metabolic markers for cancer in three groups: vegans (who ate predominantly raw diets), endurance athletes, and people consuming a non-vegetarian Western diet.[139] Insulin-like growth factor 1 (IGF-1), a known tumor promoter, was much lower in the vegan group than in the Western-diet group and also significantly lower than in the endurance runners (even when the percentage of body fat was controlled for). Test results for several other metabolic markers of cancer risk were all more favorable in the vegans and endurance athletes than in the Western-diet group, with the vegans enjoying the greatest advantage.

A second study examined the IGF-1 levels of 292 vegan, vegetarian, and meat-eating women. Higher IGF-1 levels have been associated with increased breast cancer risk. The mean serum IGF-1 concentration was 13 percent lower in vegans compared to meat eaters or vegetarians. In addition, levels of IGF-binding proteins were higher in vegan women. This suggests the amount of available IGF-1 would be reduced among vegans, again reducing cancer risk for the vegans.[140]

A small Finnish study compared several laboratory markers of cancer prevention in 40 women; 20 consumed a vegan diet (mostly raw foods) and 20 consumed a nonvegetarian diet.[73] Compared to the nonvegetarians, the vegan participants had less damage to DNA and/or better protection against DNA damage.

A second Finnish study assessed changes in metabolic markers of cancer in participants who consumed a vegan diet (mostly raw foods) for one month, followed by a conventional nonvegetarian diet for one month. The test participants were compared with controls who consumed a conventional nonvegetarian diet for the duration of the study.[141] The researchers measured the activity of four different fecal enzymes, each of which is known to generate toxic compounds associated with increased cancer risk. Within one week after participants began the vegan diet, the activity of all four enzymes in their bodies declined significantly to a 33 to 66 percent lower rate. Two other toxic metabolites declined from 30 to 60 percent within two weeks after participants began the vegan diet. All these favorable changes quickly disappeared when participants resumed the conventional diet. No changes in fecal enzymes and metabolites were observed in members of the control group, who did not change their diets.

Several studies have confirmed the positive effects of vegan diets (mostly raw foods) on gut microflora.[142–146] In addition, a number of metabolic changes that occur with vegetarian and vegan diets may provide additional protection against cancer:

- **Lower lifetime estrogen exposure.** Lower levels and reduced lifetime estrogen exposure are associated with a reduced risk of breast cancer.[147–151]

- **Lower concentrations of potentially carcinogenic bile acids.** There are fewer bacteria converting bile acids into more-carcinogenic secondary bile acids. A lower colonic pH also reduces the activity of the enzymes responsible for this unfavorable conversion process.[152–157]

- **Larger, heavier, softer stools resulting in more-frequent bowel movements.** Potential carcinogens have less time to harm the intestinal lining.[149, 152, 158, 159]

- **Lower levels of fecal mutagens (substances that damage DNA).** Fecal mutagens have less opportunity to damage DNA, reducing risk of colon cancer.[160–164]

- **Reduced oxidative stress.** Fewer products of oxidation and increased antioxidant status can protect against DNA damage, possibly decreasing cancer risk.[40, 43, 165–169]

Do Raw Plant Foods Provide Better Protection?

It isn't known for sure what type of plant-based diet provides the greatest protection against cancer, but we do know that whole plant foods are an important part of the answer and that raw vegetables appear to have an advantage over cooked vegetables.

More than two dozen studies have examined the relationship between raw and cooked vegetables and cancer risk. These studies were not done on people who consumed raw vegan diets; rather, they focused on the possible advantages of specific foods or components of foods. While most studies have shown that as vegetable intake increases, cancer risk decreases, the findings have been more consistent for raw vegetables than for cooked vegetables.[170]

The 2007 WCRF/AICR diet and cancer report cited twenty-three studies that provided separate cancer risk estimates for raw vegetable consumption.[131] Of these reports, sixteen showed statistically significant reductions in cancer risk with raw vegetable intake and with increasing rates of consumption. A comprehensive literature review by researchers from Columbia University in New York and the Fred Hutchinson Cancer Research Center in Seattle suggested several reasons why raw vegetables provide even greater protection against cancer than cooked vegetables.[170]

- Cooking vegetables decreases protective substances, such as vitamin C and phytochemicals, which are watersoluble and heatsensitive.

- Cooking foods disables the enzymes responsible for converting certain phytochemicals to active forms that have powerful anticancer effects (for more on phytochemicals and enzymes, see pages 260 to 263).

- Cooking foods produces changes in the foods' physical structure and its physiologic effects. For example, cooking may reduce insoluble fiber, decreasing the foods' ability to bind to cancer-causing substances.

- Cooking foods at high temperatures can cause the formation of compounds that damage DNA, such as acrylamide, heterocyclic amines, polycyclic aromatic hydrocarbons, and advanced glycation end-products (for more on these compounds, see pages 268 to 269).

We also know that raw diets can favorably alter gut microflora, reducing toxic metabolites associated with increased cancer risk. Raw-food preparation techniques can enhance the content of protective substances in foods or the availability of these compounds. For example, juicing removes plant cell walls and phytate that can inhibit absorption of nutrients and phytochemicals, and sprouting increases the nutrient and phytochemical content of foods. (For more on this, see pages 260 and 261.) However, it must be noted that cooking can kill potentially harmful organisms, improve the bioavailability of some nutrients (e.g., carotenoids), reduce antinutrients, and improve the digestibility of some foods, such as protein-rich legumes. Moist methods of cooking, such as steaming, are preferable, because these methods keep products of oxidation to a minimum and keep temperatures at or below 212 degrees F (100 degrees C).

For further information, see *Becoming Raw: The Essential Guide to Raw Vegan Diets* by Brenda Davis and Vesanto Melina (Book Publishing Company, 2010).

Does Soy Increase or Decrease the Risk of Breast Cancer?

There's been ongoing debate regarding the effects of soy products on cancer risk, particularly on breast cancer. Soybeans are unique among legumes because they contain phytoestrogens (plant estrogens) called isoflavones that can bind to estrogen-receptor sites. However, plant estrogens aren't the same as human estrogens and have generally much weaker activity. Plant estrogens are also more selective in the receptors to which they bind; thus, they're called selective estrogen-receptor modulators. The type of estrogen receptors in different tissues determines whether the isoflavones have weak estrogen-like effects or antiestrogen effects.[171]

For years, physicians warned patients with estrogen-positive breast cancer to avoid soy products due to concerns that soy phytoestrogens would act like human estrogen and increase cancer cell growth. However, recent research suggests that in reproductive cells (e.g., breast and uterus tissue), isoflavones act more as antiestrogens, while in osteoblasts (bone-forming cells), they behave as weak estrogens—with beneficial effects in both cases.[171, 172]

The evidence to date suggests lifetime soy consumption may actually help protect against breast cancer and improve breast cancer prognosis.[173, 22] The following is a brief summary of the findings on soy and breast cancer:

- Soy consumption during childhood and adolescence reduces lifetime breast cancer risk.[174–178]

- A significant inverse association exists between breast cancer risk and soy isoflavone intake in Asian populations—less breast cancer with more soy—although no association has been found in Western populations.[178–182]

- The inverse association between soy and Asian breast cancer risk is stronger in postmenopausal women than in premenopausal women.[180, 183]

- The soy isoflavone daidzein can be metabolized by bacteria into a compound called S-equol, which may provide added protection, although research is limited. Asian populations have more equol-producing bacteria in their intestines than Western populations. Interestingly, one study reported that vegetarians were 4.25 times more likely to be S-equol producers than nonvegetarians.[184, 185]

- Most studies show the risk of breast cancer recurrence or death from breast cancer is either reduced or unaffected by intake of soy isoflavones, even with estrogen-positive breast cancer and tamoxifen use.[186–192] However, one small Korean study found high intake of soy isoflavones (mostly from black soybeans) increased the risk of cancer recurrence in HER2-positive breast cancer patients, although it quite strongly reduced the risk in HER2-negative breast cancer patients.[193]

- A pooled analysis of both Chinese and American women found that those with the highest intakes (≥ 10 mg isoflavones) were 17 percent less likely to die from breast cancer and 25 percent less likely to have a recurrence of breast cancer.[194]

- A meta-analysis of Chinese and American studies showed the highest soy food intakes were associated with 16 percent reduced mortality and 26 percent reduction in cancer recurrence, compared with the lowest soy intakes. In postmenopausal women, high soy intake reduced recurrence by 36 percent in ER- cancers and 35 percent in ER+ cancers.[195]

- Any protective effect soy foods have against cancer appears to be due to their isoflavone content.[22, 173]

- The highest quartile of soy product intake was associated with a 61 percent reduced risk of breast cancer in BRCA1 and BRCA2 carriers (carriers of an inherited mutation that increases breast cancer risk); carriers with the highest quartile of meat intake had almost double the risk of breast cancer.[196]

The Bottom Line: Soy intake is either protective against breast cancer, or it doesn't affect risk either way. The risk of breast cancer recurrence and breast cancer death appears to be reduced with soy intake. The evidence of potentially beneficial effects is strongest for moderate intake (two servings a day) of traditional soy foods, such as tofu and soy milk.

Note that soy intake has also been associated with a reduced risk of prostate cancer and reduced prostate cancer cell growth.[171, 197–199]

The Vegan Advantage against Cancer

Based on the evidence currently available, vegans are at an advantage where cancer risk is concerned. There are many steps vegans can take to maximize the benefits of their diet. While it's still too early to estimate the potential of vegan diets in cancer treatment, consuming a well-planned vegan diet seems a reasonable addition to any treatment program. The following tips help to design a vegan diet that provides the greatest possible protection:

TOP 10 ANTICANCER DIET TIPS FOR VEGANS

1. Eat mostly whole plant foods. Opt for local organic foods whenever possible.
2. Include at least nine servings of vegetables and fruits daily, emphasizing all the colors of the rainbow and plenty of dark leafy greens.
3. Aim for at least 35 grams of fiber each day from a variety of plant foods.
4. Minimize processed foods, especially those containing refined carbohydrates.
5. Eliminate products containing trans-fatty acids.
6. Rely on whole foods (such as nuts, seeds, and avocados) for most fat intake, ensuring sufficient essential fatty acids. (For more on essential fatty acids, see page 117.)
7. Eat raw foods daily. Sprout foods more often.
8. If cooking, stick mainly to wet cooking methods, such as steaming and stewing.
9. Flavor foods with immune-boosting herbs and spices, such as turmeric, ginger, garlic, basil, oregano, rosemary, and coriander.
10. Make pure, clean water the beverage of choice. Other healthful beverages include fresh vegetable juices and antioxidant-rich teas, such as green tea.

TYPE 2 DIABETES

The rate of diabetes occurrence in the United States has increased more than 900 percent in fifty years, from 0.9 percent in the late 1950s to 9.3 percent in 2012, according to the Centers for Disease Control and Prevention (CDC). If current trends continue, the CDC estimates that as many as one in three American adults will have diabetes by 2050.[200, 201]

Diabetes Statistics in the United States 2012

Diabetes rate among the entire population: 9.3%

Diabetes rate among Americans more than 20 years old: 12.3%

Diabetes rate among Americans more than 65 years old: 25.9%

Estimated prediabetes rate among Americans more than 20 years old: 37%

Estimated prediabetes rate among Americans more than 65 years old: 51%

Source:[201]

Statistically, diabetes is the seventh leading cause of death in the United States. However, this figure belies the fact that most people *with* diabetes don't die *of* diabetes; instead, they die of heart disease, kidney failure, and other complications associated with diabetes. But the United States isn't the only nation experiencing this surge. Globally, diabetes has become the twenty-first-century plague, crippling rich and poor nations alike.

Who Gets Type 2 Diabetes?

Some people believe that type 2 diabetes is more a matter of bad genes than bad habits. Although some populations do have greater susceptibility to the disease, genes serve primarily as a loaded gun; it's almost always diet and lifestyle that pull the trigger.

The people of the Marshall Islands provide a poignant example. The Marshall Islands lie about 2,300 miles southwest of Hawaii and have a population of about 60,000. Sadly, an estimated 28 percent of Marshallese older than 15—and 50 percent of those older than 35—have type 2 diabetes.

Seventy years ago, diabetes was virtually unheard of there. Although changes in the population's genes have been negligible since then, dietary and lifestyle changes have been profound. In the 1940s, the Marshallese were slim and physically active and lived off the land and the sea. Their diet included fish and other seafood, as well as edible plants, such as coconut, breadfruit, taro, pandanus, and leafy greens. All of these foods were acquired through physical work, helping the people burn calories and maintain fitness.

Today, the Marshallese people have become largely sedentary, and their diet consists primarily of imported processed foods. It would be difficult to design a diet that could more efficiently induce type 2 diabetes than the diet adopted by the Marshallese. A typical adult's breakfast consists of cake donuts or sweet pancakes and coffee, while children often start the day with popsicles, chips, soda pop, or dry ramen noodles sprinkled with Kool-Aid. Lunch and dinner feature sticky white rice with meat or fish. Favorite meats are Spam, canned corned beef, chicken, and variety meats, such as turkey tails. Meals are often washed down with a sweetened beverage.

In a laudable effort to reverse the Marshallese diabetes epidemic, Canvasback Missions Inc. (a Christian nonprofit organization that specializes in medical missions to remote South Pacific islands) partnered with Loma Linda University and the Marshall Islands Ministry of Health to launch a lifestyle-based diabetes research study in 2006. Coauthor Brenda Davis served as lead dietitian to design and implement the diet portion of the treatment program.

For each intervention period, approximately half the qualified participants were assigned to an intervention group and half to a control group. Intervention participants received diet and lifestyle instruction over a three- to six-month period, while the control group received standard care (advice from a physician and/or other health care worker to exercise, eat more healthfully, and take the appropriate medication). Control group participants were guaranteed a place in the intervention group once their six-month control period had been completed (although from that point on, their data couldn't be used in the analysis).

The two key elements of the lifestyle intervention were diet and exercise. The treatment's primary objective was to overcome insulin resistance and to restore insulin sensitivity as much as physiologically possible. The diet was designed to support blood-glucose control, reduce inflammation, reduce oxidative stress, and restore nutritional status. (For information on the practical implementation of these parameters, see pages 259 to 265). To accomplish this task, these dietary parameters were set:

- whole-foods, plant-based diet
- minimal refined carbohydrates
- minimal ground grains, such as flour
- controlled portions of intact (whole) grains
- very high fiber (40 to 50 grams or more per day)
- emphasis on foods rich in viscous fiber (flaxseeds, oats, barley, beans, guar gum, psyllium seeds)
- moderate fat from healthful sources, such as nuts, seeds, and coconut (20 to 25 percent of total calories from fat)
- low saturated fat (less than 7 percent of total calories)
- zero trans-fatty acids
- sufficient omega-3 fatty acids (fish was permitted)
- high-phytochemical and high-antioxidant foods
- low dietary oxidants
- low glycemic load
- moderate sodium (less than 2,300 mg per day)

The program results were remarkable during the first two to four weeks. Average reductions in fasting blood glucose were more than 70 mg/dL (4 mmol/L), and weight loss averaged approximately 2 pounds (1 kg) per week. Total and LDL cholesterol, triglycerides, and blood pressure plummeted. By twelve weeks,

HbA1c (also called A1C or hemoglobin A1c, a measure of glucose control over two to three months) dropped by 2 points and hs-CRP by 1.2 points. Participants consistently reported dramatic reductions or complete disappearance of pain in the legs, arms, and joints. Many noted increased energy, improved mental clarity, fewer nightly trips to the bathroom, and rapid relief of chronic constipation. The majority of participants stopped taking diabetes medications.

After twelve weeks, progress varied according to the participant's commitment to the program. Those who stuck to the program continued to see improvements. Some completely reversed their disease, eliminating the need for medication and experiencing blood glucose levels well within the normal range. The Marshallese results prove the value of lifestyle interventions based on plant-strong, near-vegan diets.

Diabetes and Dietary Patterns

Plant-based diets have shown positive results in numerous studies. In 2011, researchers undertook an extensive review of epidemiologic and clinical trial evidence worldwide that related dietary patterns, nutrients, and foods to diabetes risk.[202] The study authors concluded

> "Together with the maintenance of ideal body weight, the promotion of the so-called prudent diet (characterized by a higher intake of food groups that are generally recommended for health promotion, particularly plant-based foods, and a lower intake of red meat, meat products, sweets, high-fat dairy, and refined grains) or a Mediterranean dietary pattern rich in olive oil, fruits, and vegetables, including whole grains, pulses, and nuts, low-fat dairy, and moderate alcohol consumption (mainly red wine) appears as the best strategy to decrease diabetes risk."[202]

The observational studies reviewed in this report are briefly summarized in table 2.5. Studies are listed according to publication date, beginning with the most recent. The studies show that the dietary factors most clearly associated with increased risk come almost exclusively from two food categories—animal products and processed foods—and they include red meat, processed meat, high-fat dairy products, trans fats, fried foods, soft drinks, and refined-carbohydrate foods (white flour and sugar-laden products). The dietary factors most strongly associated with decreased risk were plant-based foods or food components, such as vegetables, fruits, whole grains, and fiber.

Diabetes Rates in Vegan and Near-Vegan Populations

Although one might expect the occurrence of diabetes to be lower in vegan and near-vegan populations, data was completely lacking until 2009, when the AHS-2 released findings on diabetes rates in various dietary groups.[4] Participants in AHS-2 were all Seventh-day Adventists, a group that avoids smoking, uses little alcohol, and is generally health conscious. This means that all the study's dietary groups share certain health-promoting characteristics.

In this study, more than 60,000 participants had completed fifty-page questionnaires regarding their health status and lifestyle choices at baseline (data

TABLE 2.5. Observational studies on dietary intake and diabetes risk

STUDY, LEAD AUTHOR, YEAR	NUMBER OF SUBJECTS (YEARS OF FOLLOW-UP)	DIETARY FACTORS ASSOCIATED WITH HIGHER RISK	DIETARY FACTORS ASSOCIATED WITH LOWER RISK
Insulin Resistance Atherosclerosis, Liese, 2009	880 men and women (5 years)	Red meat, refined grains, beans (as in chili, burritos, refried), fried potatoes, eggs, cheese, tomatoes (as with pasta, pizza)	
Multiethnic Study of Atherosclerosis, Nettleton, 2008	5,011 men and women (5 years)	Red meat, high-fat dairy, refined grains, beans, tomatoes (grouped)	Green leafy vegetables, fruits, whole grains, nuts, seeds, low-fat dairy
Whitehall II, Brunner, 2008	7,731 men and women (15 years)		Vegetables, fruits, whole-meal bread, PUFA-rich* margarine
Melbourne, Hodge, 2007	31,641 men and women (4 years)	Red meats, processed meats, fried fish, fat-cooked potatoes	Salads, cooked vegetables, whole grains
EPIC-Potsdam, Heidemann, 2005	192 cases and 382 controls (NA)	Red meats, processed meats, poultry, refined breads, soft drinks, beer	Fresh fruits
Finnish Mobile, Montonen, 2005	4,304 men and women (23 years)	Red and processed meats, butter, high-fat milk, potatoes	Fruits and vegetables
Nurses' Health Study, Fung, 2004	69,554 women (14 years)	Red and processed meats, sweets and desserts, French fries, refined grains	Vegetables, fruits, whole grains, fish, poultry, low-fat dairy
Health Professionals, van Dam, 2002	42,504 men (12 years)	Red and processed meats, sweets, desserts, French fries, refined grains, high-fat dairy products	

Source:[202]

*PUFA = polyunsaturated fatty acids

collected between 2002 and 2006). One question asked whether the respondent had been diagnosed with diabetes. In the initial 2009 findings, only 2.9 percent of the vegans had been diagnosed with diabetes compared to 7.6 percent of the nonvegetarians (see table 2.6 on page 60).

A second AHS-2 report followed in 2011, showing the results of a follow-up questionnaire administered to more than 41,000 participants two years after the first questionnaire. It elicited information on the development of diabetes in participants who had had no previous diabetes diagnosis.[203] Only 0.54 percent of the vegans developed diabetes during this two-year period, compared to 2.12 percent of the nonvegetarians (see table 2.6).

TABLE 2.6. Rates of diabetes among various diet groups

2009 AHS-2 DATA AT BASELINE (DATA COLLECTED 2002–2006)—INITIAL DIABETES RATES					
	VEGAN	LACTO-OVO VEGETARIAN	PESCO-VEGETARIAN*	SEMIVEGETARIAN*	NONVEGETARIAN
Participants	2,731	20,408	5,617	3,386	28,761
2009 diabetes rates	2.9%	3.2%	4.8%	6.1%	7.6%
BMI	23.6	25.7	26.3	27.3	28.8
Odds ratio** adjusted for all factors	0.51	0.54	0.7	0.76	1
Odds ratio adjusted for all factors except BMI	0.32	0.43	0.56	0.69	1

2011 AHS-2 DATA (FOLLOW-UP AT 2 YEARS)—RATES OF DIABETES DEVELOPED IN SUBJECTS DISEASE-FREE AT BASELINE					
	VEGAN	LACTO-OVO VEGETARIAN	PESCO-VEGETARIAN*	SEMIVEGETARIAN*	NONVEGETARIAN
Participants	3,545	14,099	3,644	2,404	17,695
Developed diabetes since baseline	0.54%	1.08%	1.29%	0.92%	2.12%
Odds ratio adjusted for all factors	0.381	0.618	0.79	0.486	1
Odds ratio adjusted for age	0.228	0.461	0.597	0.38	1

Sources:[4, 203]

*The terms "pescovegetarian" and "semivegetarian" describe those who aren't actually vegetarians, but who eat a predominantly vegetarian diet; pesco-vegetarians are those who eat a vegetarian diet plus fish; semivegetarians are those who eat meat, poultry, or fish less than once a week but more than once a month.

**Odds ratio (OR): "All factors" is adjusted for age, sex, BMI, ethnicity, education, income, physical activity, television watching, sleep habits, and alcohol use. OR compares the probability that one group will develop diabetes versus the probability that another group will develop diabetes. If a group's OR is 1.0, then its odds would be the same as the control group (in this case, the nonvegetarians). If a group's OR is less than 1.0, then its odds of developing diabetes would be lower than the control group.

The data include figures with adjustments for lifestyle factors that can influence results. For example, some of the data is adjusted for multiple factors ("all factors"), including age, sex, BMI, ethnicity, education, income, physical activity, television watching, sleep habits, and alcohol use. These factors are all taken into account to isolate the difference in diabetes incidence most likely due to diet alone. When adjusted for all factors, vegans were 49 percent less likely (OR = 0.51) to develop diabetes compared to nonvegetarians in the 2009 report, and 62 percent less likely (OR = .381) in the 2011 report. Some data is adjusted for all factors except BMI, so both diet and body fat could account for the difference in diabetes incidence. For example, in the 2009 report, when the data was adjusted for all factors except BMI, vegans had a 68 percent lower risk (OR = 0.32) of developing diabetes than nonvegetarians.

Finally, a 2014 study compared diabetes rates in similar health-conscious Taiwanese Buddhist volunteers who consumed vegetarian (near-vegan) and omnivorous diets. After adjustments for age, BMI, education, family history of diabetes, physical activity, smoking, and alcohol consumption, vegetarian (near-vegan) diets were associated with a 51 percent lower risk in men (OR = 0.49), a 74 percent lower risk in premenopausal women (OR = 0.26), and a 75 percent lower risk in postmenopausal women (OR = 0.25).[204]

Based on the results of these studies, vegan and near-vegan diets provide significant protection against diabetes. Differences in risk remain strong even when BMI and other lifestyle factors are accounted for.

Red and processed meats have been associated with increased risk of diabetes, possibly due to the saturated fat and heme iron in meat or the nitrite and nitrate content of processed meats.[203] The advantages enjoyed by vegans and near-vegans are likely due to the combination of higher intakes of whole plant foods and the avoidance of meat.

Metabolic Markers of Diabetes in Vegan Populations

When the effects of a vegan diet are measured using metabolic markers, its advantages are further clarified. A 2005 US study assessed dietary intakes, insulin sensitivity, and the intramyocellular lipid (IMCL) concentration in vegans (on no special vegan diet) and in matched nonvegetarian controls.[205] IMCL is fat that accumulates inside cells, which interferes with the action of insulin and increases insulin resistance. The vegans had significantly lower IMCL in soleus muscle fibers (a primary site of glucose metabolism). The researchers also reported significantly better beta-cell function in vegans, meaning that the insulin-producing beta-cells of the pancreas were doing their job more effectively in vegans than in nonvegetarians. These results suggest metabolic advantages in vegans compared to matched nonvegetarians.

A vegan diet also can provide a distinct advantage for overweight postmenopausal women. A 2005 study by the Physicians Committee for Responsible Medicine (PCRM) randomly assigned 64 overweight postmenopausal nondiabetic women to a low-fat vegan diet or a National Cholesterol Education Program Step II Guidelines diet (NCEP II).[206] After fourteen weeks of diet therapy, weight loss was more than 50 percent greater in the vegan group—5.8 kg (12.8 lb)—compared to 3.8 kg (8.4 lb) in the NCEP II group. Fasting glucose dropped by 6.5 mg/dl (0.36 mmol/L) in the vegan group, compared to 1.8 mg/dl (0.1mmol/L) in the NCEP II group. Insulin sensitivity increased 1.1 points in the vegan group compared to 0.3 point in the NCEP II group.

In 2007, a German research team measured the impact of vegan diets on blood glucose levels (glycemic index [GI] and glycemic load [GL]).[207] (For more on GI and GL, see pages 172 and 173.) The vegans had very high intakes of dietary fiber, averaging close to 57 grams per day; the average GI of the vegan diets in this population was 51. By comparison, four large studies reported that

20 percent of the general population with the lowest GIs had levels ranging from 64 to 72; the rest had higher GIs.

In addition, the average GL in this vegan population was 144, which is considered low to moderate when compared with observational studies in omnivores. For example, in the Nurses' Health Study, GLs ranged from 117 to 206. The authors concluded that a vegan diet, including large amounts of fruit, vegetables, whole grains, legumes, and nuts, is characterized by a low GI and GL, relative to nonvegetarian diets. Evidence suggests that this difference could provide an advantage in terms of risk for diabetes, as well as CVD.[207]

In 2007, another US study reported significantly reduced fasting glucose, fasting insulin, insulin resistance, and inflammation (measured by hs-CRP levels) in participants who ate a raw vegan diet, compared to endurance athletes and those who ate standard Western diets.[67]

Vegan Diets in the Treatment of Diabetes

Reports abound of complete reversal of type 2 diabetes using plant-based or vegan diets. Lifestyle programs—such as those offered by the Weimar Center, TrueNorth Health Center, Dr. Joel Fuhrman, Lifestyle Center of America, Tree of Life, Dr. McDougall's Health and Medical Center, Newstart in Guam, and the Diabetes Wellness Center in the Marshall Islands—have all documented successful reversal in committed participants. Although the program designs vary in their starch, fat, and raw-food content, they share a common foundation of unprocessed, whole plant foods. The diets are consistently rich in fiber, phytochemicals, and antioxidants low in saturated fat and free of trans-fatty acids and cholesterol.

The first report of successful use of a vegan diet for the treatment of diabetes in the United States was published in 1994. Twenty-one patients with known type 2 diabetes and diabetic neuropathy (nerve damage) received treatment for twenty-five days in a residential program; they exercised and ate a low-fat (10 to 15 percent of calories from fat), high-fiber, unrefined vegan diet.

Within four to sixteen days, pain associated with their diabetic neuropathy was completely eliminated in 17 of the 21 patients; although numbness persisted, it improved significantly. Weight loss averaged close to 5 kg (11 lb) during the twenty-five days. Fasting blood glucose dropped, and insulin needs were cut in half. Five participants were taken off their hypoglycemic agents. Follow-up of 17 of the 21 participants indicated that 71 percent remained on the program, and in all but one, relief from diabetic neuropathy continued or further improved.[208]

Since this time, several trials have been conducted by PCRM researchers and their colleagues to test the effectiveness of low-fat vegan diets (with no caloric restriction) in type 2 diabetes treatment. One study from the Czech Republic compared the effects of a calorie-restricted near-vegan diet (vegan plus no more than one portion of low-fat yogurt per day).[209]

These randomized controlled clinical trials showed that vegan diets were more effective in treating type 2 diabetes than conventional treatment diets. The initial pilot study (1999) by a PCRM research team found that compared to a prudent conventional treatment diet, the low-fat vegan diet was associated with reductions in body weight, blood lipids, fasting glucose, and HbA1c.[210] These results were notable because reductions in oral diabetes medications were greater among the vegans, even though they had no restrictions on calories, carbohydrates, or portions, and their carbohydrate intakes increased.

A second PCRM study, initiated in 2004, followed 99 participants with type 2 diabetes for seventy-four weeks. Forty-nine of the participants were randomized to a vegan diet group and 50 to an American Diabetes Association (ADA) diet group, following the ADA's 2003 Guidelines. Results of the clinical findings from the first twenty-two weeks of the study were released in 2006.[211] Although both groups improved significantly, all markers of diabetes improved to a greater extent in the vegan group than in the control group during this period.

In 2009, the seventy-four-week results were released.[212] Although the diet effects were reduced for most clinical markers in both dietary groups compared to the initial findings at twenty-two weeks, generally, the differences between the vegan group and the ADA group were greater at seventy-four weeks. Questions often arise about the acceptability of a vegan diet, so it's also worth noting that PCRM study participants rated the vegan and ADA diets as being equally acceptable.[213]

A 2011 report compared the PCRM study group's GI and GL at twenty-two weeks.[214] While GI was lower in the vegan group, suggesting food choices that had a lower overall GI, its GL was higher. GL reflects total carbohydrate intake, and the vegan group had eaten an average of 245 grams per day at twenty-two weeks. In contrast, the ADA group ate an average of only 170 grams of carbohydrate per day. Although in this study, GL was not linked to weight loss or changes in HbA1c, GI was predictive of weight loss—for every point decrease in GI, participants lost about 0.2 kg (0.44 lb). In turn, weight loss was predictive of decreasing HbA1c.

Much of the published literature has emphasized very low-fat vegan diets, but there's little to support the notion that higher-fat whole plant foods are detrimental for prevention and/or reversal of type 2 diabetes. On the contrary, considerable evidence exists that higher-fat plant foods, especially nuts, may be beneficial. In the Nurses' Health Study, both nut and peanut butter consumption were inversely associated with diabetes risk, even after adjustments for other risk factors.[215] The relative risk of developing diabetes dropped 27 percent for those who ate five or more servings of nuts per week and by 21 percent for those who ate five or more servings of peanut butter per week, compared to those who never or almost never ate nuts.

The Nurses' Health Study also reported on a subgroup of women with type 2 diabetes and found that those who consumed nuts or peanut butter five or more times a week had a 44 percent reduction in CVD risk and the risk of myocardial infarction (heart attack) compared to those who never or almost never ate nuts or peanut butter.[216] It's thought that the protection provided by nuts is due to their favorable impact on blood cholesterol levels,[217] oxidative stress,[218, 219] markers of inflammation,[215, 220] and glycemic control.[219, 221–224]

Nuts and other high-fat plant foods have a very low GI and GL, and recent evidence suggests that consuming them attenuates postprandial (after-meal) blood glucose concentrations and insulin response.[223, 224] Eating nuts with a meal that includes high-carbohydrate foods (potatoes, pasta, rice, or bread) reduces glycemic response—despite an increase in carbohydrate intake (nuts provide small amounts of carbohydrate)—probably because nuts slow the flow of food into the small intestine.[223, 224]

Although most of the research has focused on nuts, seeds would likely provide at least equal, if not greater, benefits. Seeds are higher in protein (12 to 30 percent of calories from protein, compared to 4 to 15 percent in nuts), slightly lower in fat, and generally higher in vitamin E. Seeds also are much higher in essential fatty acids than are nuts (with the exception of walnuts).

Suboptimal Vegan Diets

Although vegan diets are clearly protective against diabetes, inadequate intakes of vitamins D and B_{12}, which are sometimes at suboptimal levels in vegan diets, may accelerate the progression of diabetes. Recent evidence suggests that many people with diabetes or prediabetes have a reduced vitamin D status, and that a lack of this nutrient can increase the severity of the disease.[225]

Popular medications used to treat diabetes, such as metformin, may reduce vitamin B_{12} absorption, further contributing to reduced B_{12} status and, in turn, increasing homocysteine levels and peripheral neuropathy (nerve damage that causes pain and numbness in hands and feet).[226] In scientific review articles, vitamin B_{12} was found to be an effective treatment for diabetic peripheral neuropathy[227] and was perhaps even more effective than standard medications.[228]

Long-chain omega-3 fatty acids seem to be most effective in preventing depression. Omega-3 fatty acids have also been shown to effectively reduce hypertriglyceridemia, although they appear to have marginal effects on insulin sensitivity and metabolic control.[230]

The Vegan Advantage against Diabetes

Type 2 diabetes is the plague of the twenty-first century. It isn't spread by viruses or bacteria, but by shifting cultural paradigms that encourage overconsumption and underactivity. Although research that suggests support for vegan diets in the treatment of diabetes is in its early stages, the published data to date offer evidence that whole-foods vegan diets appear somewhat more effective than conventional therapy. Efforts in the Marshall Islands and lifestyle-oriented medical centers suggest that intensive, well-designed vegan diets can reverse the disease in some individuals.

To maximize the potential benefits of a vegan diet in the treatment or prevention of type 2 diabetes, the diet must be based on whole plant foods, such as vegetables, fruits, legumes, nuts, seeds, and whole grains. It's also important that the diet be designed with care to ensure adequate intakes of all nutrients, especially vitamins B_{12} and D, and essential fatty acids.

OSTEOPOROSIS

If you ask the average person which food is best for bones, chances are they'll say milk or dairy products. To most consumers, the popular advertising slogan "Got Milk?" is essentially synonymous with "Got Bones?" People of every age assume it's risky to shun milk. As it turns out, consumers who eat the most calcium (also the most dairy products) aren't immune to osteoporosis—in fact, they have higher, not lower, rates of osteoporosis than some populations with far lower calcium intakes.

Although some people consider this proof that dairy products contribute to osteoporosis, the evidence doesn't bear this out either. There are plenty of studies within populations of consumers who have similar diets and lifestyles but varying dairy intakes. In such cases, dairy consumers tend to have better bone density than nondairy consumers. So what's going on?

To put it simply, osteoporosis isn't a "dairy deficiency" disease; it's not even a "calcium deficiency" disease—it's a disease that features an impressive interplay of factors. Calcium is important to bone health, but its impact can be augmented by other diet and lifestyle choices, none of which include milk of animal origin.

No one would disagree that cow's milk is a rich source of calcium (it provides about 300 mg of calcium per cup/250 ml). But that doesn't make it any more essential for people than moose or deer milk—which, incidentally, have about twice as much calcium as cow's milk.[231] It's estimated that during the Paleolithic era, when humans had no access to the milk of other species, calcium intakes averaged 2,000 mg per day or more. This calcium came predominantly from wild leafy greens, and some came from other plant foods; none came from animal milk.[232]

Bones: Where Do Vegans Stand?

A vegan diet doesn't guarantee strong bones, but neither does it preclude them. It's possible to maintain excellent bone health without a single drop of cow's milk when a diet is well planned. However, research on vegan bone health is somewhat limited to date, and the existing data isn't particularly encouraging.

Fifteen original studies have examined the bone health of vegans or near-vegans.[233–247] Twelve studies assessed the bone mineral density (BMD), bone mineral content, and/or bone width of vegans, compared with measures from lacto-ovo vegetarians and/or nonvegetarian controls.[233–244] Two studies reported on both BMD and fracture rates or fracture risk.[245, 246] One group of researchers reported on the fracture rates in vegans compared to other dietary groups.[247]

Of the fourteen studies assessing BMD, eight reported significantly reduced indicators of bone health among vegans compared to lacto-ovo vegetarians or nonvegetarians.[233–239, 246] On average, these studies found that vegan BMDs were 10 to 20 percent lower than those of lacto-ovo vegetarians or nonvegetarians. Six studies found little or no significant difference in the bone health of vegans compared to that of other dietary groups.[234, 241–245]

Of the three studies assessing fracture risk or fracture rates,[245–247] one showed increased fracture risk in vegans,[246] and the other showed increased fracture rates.[247] The first, a study of Taiwanese vegetarians and vegans, estimated the risk of lumbar spine fracture to be 2.5 times higher in long-term vegans (who had been vegan for at least fifteen years) than in other vegetarians and vegans.[246] The second, a large UK study that examined fracture rates among various dietary groups, reported 30 percent more fractures in vegans than in other dietary groups.[247] The third, a Vietnamese study, found no difference in fracture rates in vegans compared to nonvegetarians.[245]

No studies have reported significantly better bone health in vegans compared with lacto-ovo vegetarians or nonvegetarians. It's worth noting, however, that the vegan diets consumed by the participants in these studies generally included few foods fortified with calcium or vitamin D. Today, nondairy beverages are often fortified with calcium and vitamin D; this has been standard practice in North America since the late 1990s. Fortification can be expected to favorably impact vegans' bone health, and the results of future studies.

When current evidence is examined, it's clear that vegan diets offer no special protection against bone disease. However, there's reasonable evidence to suggest that vegans can achieve and maintain excellent bone health. The bone health of older adults reflects lifelong habits not only of diet but also of sun exposure and exercise. When we consider the dietary factors that affect bone health and how these factors are impacted by vegan dietary choices, we can establish ground rules for vegans to build and preserve bone mass throughout life.

Bone Buddies and Bullies

Two categories of factors increase the risk of osteoporosis. The first can't be changed: genetics, family history, advanced age, female gender, and Caucasian or Asian ancestry. The second category comprises behaviors that can change: smoking, heavy alcohol use, physical inactivity, sun exposure, and eating poorly planned diets. Low estrogen or testosterone levels can also increase osteoporosis risk, although these conditions can be treated.

Lifestyle choices have a profound impact on both the quality and quantity of the bones produced and maintained by the body. For example, physical activity—particularly weight-bearing exercise—sends a message to bones to intensify their bone-building efforts, helping to increase bone density during childhood and adolescence[248] and to maintain bone density as the body ages.[249]

The association between food choices and bone health is more complex, and current research findings are inconsistent. Dietary factors known to contribute positively to bone health include appropriate intakes of calcium, iron, zinc, copper, boron, fluoride, magnesium, manganese, and vitamins D, K, and C. Of course, good vitamin D status can also be achieved through adequate exposure to warm sunshine (page 69). Higher consumption of fruits, vegetables,[250] and soy may provide protection by inhibiting bone breakdown.[251, 252]

Phosphorus is an important structural mineral for bones; however, diets very high in phosphorus (i.e., more than 3 to 4 grams per day) and low in calcium may upset the calcium balance and weaken bones.[253, 254] And, although protein has generally been found to be protective, very high protein intakes may be detrimental, particularly when calcium intakes are low.[255] Excess protein—especially animal protein—increases metabolic acid load and calcium excretion. If calcium intakes aren't sufficient to compensate for these losses, a negative calcium balance can result (page 68). Vegan diets tend to produce a lower metabolic acid load, reducing urinary calcium excretion.[256] However, vegan diets often are lower in calcium, which can also have negative consequences for bones.

Dietary Factors that Adversely Affect Bone Health Vegans generally don't consume preformed vitamin A because it's not present in plants, and they often have lower intakes of sodium, alcohol, and caffeine. As a result, they may be protected from the adverse effects these dietary factors can have:

- **Sodium.** Sodium and salt increase calcium excretion through urine and perspiration.
- **Caffeine.** Caffeine appears to reduce the absorption of calcium; however, the effect is completely mitigated by a small increase in calcium intake. For example, adding milk to coffee compensates for the modest reduction in calcium absorption caused by the caffeine content.[232] (Fortified soy milk might be expected to do the same.)
- **Alcohol.** Chronic excessive alcohol consumption reduces calcium and vitamin D absorption and can injure the liver, impairing the body's ability to activate vitamin D. Alcohol also can decrease estrogen production, eroding a woman's bone-building capacity.[257, 258]
- **Vitamin A.** Preformed vitamin A or retinol (the type available in animal products and some supplements) is necessary for bone growth. However, very high intakes can increase bone breakdown and interfere with vitamin D's role in enhancing calcium absorption. Provitamin A from plants (e.g., beta-carotene) doesn't have this effect.[258, 259]

Excess preformed vitamin A can have adverse effects at various stages of the life cycle. Because excess vitamin A can be harmful to their babies, it's recommended that pregnant women avoid very rich sources of vitamin A, such as animal liver and other organ meats.[260] The Tolerable Upper Intake Level (UL) for vitamin A is set at 3,000 mg retinol equivalents (RE) per day; a single 3.5-ounce (100 g) serving of beef liver contains nearly 9,600 RE vitamin A. For postmenopausal women at risk for bone fracture, the Institute of Medicine (IOM) advises restricting intake of preformed vitamin A even further, to 1,500 mg RE per day, because excessive intakes can further compromise bone strength.[260, 261]

Numerous dietary factors positively affect bone health, and vegans generally have higher intakes of a long list of these, including potassium, vitamin K, vitamin C, folate, fruits, vegetables, and possibly soy foods. On the other hand, they tend to have lower intakes of calcium, vitamin D, and protein. These nutrients are all critical to the maintenance of bone homeostasis. The three nutrients of concern to vegan bone health (calcium, vitamin D, and protein) have been the source of major controversy among vegan advocates.

The Calcium Conundrum

There's no question regarding the importance of calcium for bone health. The facts are clear: calcium is the predominant structural mineral in bones, and it's necessary for both building and maintaining bone tissue. Calcium also is critical to the body's proper functioning and is tightly controlled in the blood. If dietary calcium isn't available in a sufficient quantity to maintain blood calcium levels, additional calcium is quickly mobilized from bones to avert disaster. However, this mobilization can lead to osteoporosis if bones transfer excessive amounts of calcium to the bloodstream.

Should vegans be concerned? When existing data on the bone health of vegans is examined, about two-thirds of the studies suggest a positive association between calcium intake and bone mineral density; the remainder don't report a significant benefit from higher calcium intake. Of two studies examining fracture rates, one study on Asian participants found calcium intakes in nonvegetarians were almost double that of vegans, but differences in fracture rates were insignificant (5.7 percent in vegans and 5.4 percent in nonvegans). In this study, the rate of bone loss was actually lower in the vegans (-0.86 percent per year in vegans compared to -1.91 percent per year in nonvegans).[245]

The second study, EPIC-Oxford, reported a 30 percent increase in fracture rates in UK vegans compared to other dietary groups in the United Kingdom.[247] However, about 45 percent of the vegans had calcium intakes below 525 mg per day, while less than 6 percent of those in other dietary groups (lacto-ovo vegetarian, fish eaters, and nonvegetarians) had intakes that low. When only participants who averaged more than 525 mg of calcium per day were compared, the vegans had about the same rate of fractures as other dietary groups (fracture rates were the same as those of meat eaters and slightly lower than those of lacto-ovo vegetarians and fish eaters).

Based on comparisons of this limited data, it's possible that Caucasian vegans may need more dietary calcium than Asian vegans. This could be related to genetics or bone structure, dietary practices, or lifestyle factors, such as sun exposure or weight-bearing activities.

This somewhat ambiguous and unpredictable relationship between calcium and bone health isn't unique to vegan populations. Some nonvegetarian populations whose average intake is less than 400 mg of calcium per day have lower rates of osteoporosis than populations who average more than 1,000 mg of calcium per day.

Two meta-analyses (one on premenopausal women[262] and one on postmenopausal women[263, 264]) reported a weak positive correlation between calcium intake and bone mineral density. The meta-analysis on thirty-three studies of premenopausal women reported a 13 percent increase in bone mineral density in those with higher calcium intakes.[262] The authors suggested that calcium supplementation of approximately 1,000 mg per day would prevent a loss of 1 percent of bone per year at most bone sites in premenopausal women. The meta-analysis on postmenopausal women found that supplementation with 500 to 2,000 mg of calcium per day provided a 2.05 percent increase in total-body bone density.[263, 264]

Two additional meta-analyses examined the relationship between calcium intake and fracture rates, and found no significant benefit conferred by increased calcium intake. The first analysis found no obvious reductions in hip fracture risk after the addition of 300 mg increments of daily calcium in more than 28,511 postmenopausal women.[265] The second analysis found that dietary calcium intake wasn't significantly associated with a lower hip fracture risk in men or women (although there was a small but insignificant benefit with higher intakes in men).[266] Surprisingly, in this meta-analysis, calcium supplements weren't associated with risk reduction for nonvertebral fractures and instead were actually associated with a 64 percent increase in risk of hip fractures.[266]

The calcium conundrum begins to unravel when we recognize that calcium intake isn't the only determinant of calcium balance (the net of calcium absorption and calcium excretion)—and it's not even the most important. One research team reported that only 11 percent of calcium balance is determined by calcium intake and 15 percent by calcium absorption; 74 percent is determined by calcium excretion (51 percent urinary excretion and 23 percent fecal excretion) and 15 percent by calcium absorption.[22] If a diet compromises calcium absorption and enhances calcium excretion, calcium intakes need to be high enough to compensate for these losses. On the other hand, if the diet maximizes absorption and minimizes excretion, dietary calcium requirements would be considerably lower.

Vegan diets can be carefully constructed to support calcium balance, but many vegans tend to fall short in calcium intake. When all other dietary factors are equal, higher calcium intake appears to provide protection to vegans. How much calcium do vegans need? It all depends on how well designed the diet is and on other lifestyle factors, such as physical activity. As noted above, there's good evidence that calcium intakes below 525 mg daily can jeopardize bone health in vegans. Until more-definitive research is released, it's wise for vegans to meet recommended calcium intakes. (For more information on calcium, see pages 182 to 186).

The Vitamin D Debacle

Vitamin D is no minor player in contributing to bone health. When blood levels of calcium begin to drop, the body converts vitamin D into its active form to enhance calcium absorption and utilization and reduce calcium losses. Considering the contribution made by calcium absorption and excretion to overall calcium balance, it's easy to understand why vitamin D is every bit as relevant to bone health as calcium.

Unfortunately, vegans consistently consume less vitamin D than nonvegetarians. In addition, people who live in cool climates or who don't get enough exposure to sunshine frequently fall short of ideal vitamin D levels. Historically, humans derived vitamin D from sunshine because, apart from fatty fish, very few foods were reliable vitamin D sources. As humans migrated further from the equator, clothed themselves, protected themselves from the elements by staying indoors, and later, lived in smog-filled cities, vitamin D deficiency became widespread. Health authorities responded by adding vitamin D to a basic staple—cow's milk.

Although many types of nondairy milk are now fortified with similar amounts of vitamin D, total intakes from these sources generally aren't sufficient for vegans to meet their dietary requirements for vitamin D.

As a result of extensive evidence of health benefits associated with higher intakes, in 2010 the IOM issued new dietary reference intakes (DRI) for vitamin D. The Recommended Dietary Allowance (RDA) was increased by 50 percent to 15 mg (600 IU) for everyone from ages 1 to 70 and 20 mg (800 IU) for people older than 70.

In spite of this significant increase in DRI, many experts believe that a higher intake—25 to 50 mcg (1,000 to 2,000 IU) per day—is required to minimize the risk of vitamin D-related diseases and disorders. It seems reasonable for vegans to aim for this target, particularly if their exposure to warm sunshine is limited. (For more on vitamin D, see pages 222 to 230).

The Protein Paradox

For many years, a common belief among vegans was that eliminating animal protein protected against osteoporosis. Epidemiological evidence added weight to this argument because osteoporosis rates were higher in developed nations with high animal protein consumption, even when calcium intakes were high.

The standard theory was that animal protein is rich in amino acids that raise the acidity of blood. Since blood pH is tightly maintained, such acids must be neutralized. The body has a huge alkaline reserve to do this job—the calcium in bones. Once this calcium neutralizes excess blood acid, it's excreted in urine. As a result, it was thought that over time, high intake of animal protein leads to bone loss and osteoporosis.

Given this association between animal protein and calcium loss, it follows that vegans should enjoy protection against osteoporosis and likely require less dietary calcium than meat eaters. Although logical, this theory hasn't been supported by scientific research. As it turns out, the connection between protein and bone health is a little more complicated. In addition, the data on vegans' bone health isn't as favorable as would be expected if the animal protein hypothesis were accurate.

Although some studies have linked high protein intakes with negative calcium balance,[268] lower bone mineral density,[269] and increased fracture rates,[270] others have reported better bone density[271] and reduced fracture risk.[272, 273] Additional systematic reviews and meta-analyses have either found no clear association between protein intake and fracture risk or found a slightly favorable protein effect.[274, 275] There is, however, some evidence that acid-forming diets may have an adverse effect by suppressing bone-building activity and stimulating bone breakdown.[1]

It appears as though protein promotes some metabolic activities detrimental to bone health while simultaneously supporting others that benefit bone health. How can this rather confusing and contradictory relationship be explained? We know that high protein intakes induce urinary calcium losses. However, these losses are less significant when protein is consumed as part of a whole food, rather than as an isolated or concentrated protein supplement. Although urinary calcium losses were long thought to be due to the metabolic acid load induced by dietary protein, more-recent evidence suggests that other mechanisms may be involved.[276]

Dietary protein has been shown to increase calcium absorption as well as enhance bone-building activities. When the positive and negative impacts of protein are weighed, it appears that protein generally provides modest protection for bones, particularly when calcium intake is adequate and fruit and vegetable consumption is sufficiently high.[277]

For vegans, getting sufficient protein appears to be an important piece of the bone-health puzzle. This message was strongly supported by a recent research study that reported the risk of wrist fractures in a group of 1,865 women followed for twenty-five years. Among the 40 percent of study participants who were vegetarian, those with the highest intakes of protein-rich plant foods (e.g., legumes, meat analogs, and nuts) had the lowest risk of wrist fracture. Those who ate fewer than three servings of protein-rich plant foods per week had the highest risk of wrist fracture.[278]

Building a Vegan Advantage

The weight of the evidence suggests that vegans need to be as concerned about long-term bone health as people of other dietary persuasions. This means a vegan diet needs to be designed with attention to the myriad factors that work for or against bone health.

Vegan diets can offer a number of advantages over omnivorous diets where bone health is concerned. The features of vegan diets that appear most protective are:

- **Higher in fruits and vegetables.** Vegans have higher intakes of vegetables and fruits than nonvegetarians.
- **Lower in sodium.** Vegans tend to eat more whole foods and use fewer processed foods (77 percent of dietary sodium comes from processed foods), thus their total sodium intakes may be reduced.
- **Lower in alcohol and caffeine.** Vegans tend to consume less alcohol and caffeine, both of which can contribute to bone loss.
- **Higher in bone-friendly vitamins,** such as vitamin K, vitamin C, and folate.
- **Higher in bone-building minerals,** including potassium, magnesium, and boron.
- **Higher in soy foods** and the potentially protective isoflavones they contain.
- **Adequate in protein,** without being excessive.
- **More alkali-forming** than nonvegetarian diets.

Conversely, poorly planned vegan diets can undermine bone health. Vegans must recognize and avoid common pitfalls:

- **Very low calcium intakes (less than 525 mg per day).** While some populations appear to maintain reasonable bone health despite relatively low calcium intakes, the average Western vegan seems to require higher amounts of calcium.

- **Insufficient vitamin D** from sun exposure or fortified foods.
- **Too little protein.** Protein intakes at lower-than-recommended levels can be detrimental. Protein is an essential bone component; it boosts calcium absorption and increases bone formation.
- **Inadequate energy intakes.** A lack of calories can lead to underweight (more common among vegans), a risk factor for osteoporosis.

With a well-designed diet, however, vegans can enjoy excellent bone health throughout their life cycle. Meeting nutritional requirements, not smoking, and moderating alcohol and caffeine intake also are invaluable contributors to life-long bone health. In addition, regular weight-bearing exercise sends a powerful signal to bones to build osteoblasts and strengthen the skeleton. For practical tips on building and maintaining strong, healthy vegan bones, see "Solid Solutions for Better Bones" on page 185.

OTHER DISEASES

Researchers have examined the relationship between specific dietary patterns and risk for developing a variety of other diseases. In these studies, people who eat vegan and other types of vegetarian diets are compared to similar health-conscious nonvegetarians, or in some cases, to people who eat standard Western fare. Although the evidence is currently limited, vegan diets have been associated with risk reduction and/or effective treatment of cataracts, gallstones, fibromyalgia, kidney disease, diverticular disease, hypothyroidism, and rheumatoid arthritis. The risk of developing dementia may increase or decrease with vegan diets, depending on several factors.

Cataracts

Globally, cataracts are the leading cause of blindness, and the risk of developing cataracts increases with age. In 2011, EPIC-Oxford reported a strong correlation between meat intake and cataract risk; risks decreased progressively from high meat eaters to low meat eaters, fish eaters, vegetarians, and vegans.[279] This study examined data on 27,670 participants (all over 40 years of age) followed for at least fifteen years. After adjustments for many variables, the study showed that compared to high meat eaters, vegans had a 40 percent reduction in the risk of developing cataracts. Although this study doesn't prove that eating meat causes cataracts, it certainly suggests an association that warrants further investigation.

Dementia

Based on headlines in the popular press several years ago, rumors about tofu began to circulate, alleging that tofu caused dementia and that a vegan diet could be detrimental to brain health. As evidence emerged, it became clear that the risk of developing dementia may indeed be greater for vegans who have suboptimal B_{12} status, but actually lower for vegans who have good B_{12} status.

In 1993, findings from AHS-1 suggested that dementia increased with meat consumption.[280] In this study, two separate cohorts were examined. In one investigation, vegans and lacto-ovo vegetarians were matched for age, gender, and zip code with people who consumed generous amounts of meat. The subjects who ate meat, poultry, and fish were more than twice as likely to develop dementia as their vegetarian or vegan counterparts.

The second investigation didn't match subjects. Results showed no significant difference among the vegans, vegetarians, and nonvegetarians in the incidence of dementia, although there was a trend toward delayed onset in the vegetarians and vegans.

In 2013, AHS-2 released its initial findings on neurologic disorders (e.g., Alzheimer's and Parkinson's disease). Vegetarians (including vegans) had a 7 percent risk reduction compared to nonvegetarians; there was a 14 percent lower risk for men, although the findings weren't statistically significant.

There are many reasons why these findings showed vegetarians and vegans could be protected from developing dementia. People who eat plant-based diets are less obese, have lower blood cholesterol levels, and are less likely to have hypertension, all factors that may help to protect the brain. In addition, plant-based diets often contain higher levels of the phytochemicals and antioxidants shown to benefit the brain.

However, less favorable results were reported in UK vegetarians in the Oxford Vegetarian Study.[281] Although there were only thirty-six deaths from mental and neurological diseases, the study reported vegetarians had 2.2 times more deaths from such dementia-related illnesses than nonvegetarians. Although the reason for this difference isn't known, suboptimal B_{12} status in the vegetarians is the most likely explanation.

It's well recognized that poor vitamin B_{12} status can contribute to memory loss and brain dysfunction. Four literature reviews from 2000 to 2011 reported significant positive associations between suboptimal B_{12} status, elevated homocysteine, and rates of dementia and Alzheimer's disease.[282–285] A fifth meta-analysis in 2008 found that vitamin B_{12} supplementation improved cognition in elderly individuals who had elevated homocysteine but no diagnosed dementia. Unfortunately, vitamin B_{12} supplementation provided no benefit to those who already suffered from dementia or Alzheimer's disease.[286]

In 2000, a study that followed more than 3,000 Japanese adults living in Hawaii reported that those who ate the most tofu during the period between their mid-40s and mid-60s were 2.4 times more likely to experience a decline in cognition during their 70s to 90s.[287] The results sent shock waves through the vegan world.

Unfortunately, the headlines didn't mention that the data on food intake was collected only twice—during the participants' mid-60s (baseline) and their early 70s—and for a limited number of foods. Cognitive function wasn't measured until about twenty years later. It's possible that food choices made during this period of twenty years played a larger role than the tofu eaten decades before. There was also some suggestion that those with higher midlife tofu intake came from poor immigrant families that were less able to provide adequate nutrition during the early years of childhood. Regardless, the findings generated interest within the scientific community, as well as further research.

In a study of Japanese-American seniors (65 and older) released the same year, tofu intake was very weakly linked to lower cognition scores, but only among women using estrogen replacement therapy, and only at baseline.[288] After two years of follow-up, it turned out that tofu consumption wasn't associated with cognitive decline in men or women (regardless of the use of hormone replacements).

In 2008, a study from Indonesia reported that tempeh consumption was associated with slightly improved memory scores, while tofu consumption yielded slightly reduced scores. The authors suggested that the most plausible explanation for the difference was due to production methods used in Indonesia; formaldehyde was commonly added to tofu but not to tempeh.[289] In 2010, the same investigators revisited the tofu/cognition relationship in participants between the ages of 56 and 97. They found that eating both tofu and tempeh improved immediate recall in relatively younger participants with an average age of 67, but that the association was no longer significant in older participants who averaged 80 years of age.[290]

Although these later studies allayed the fears of some consumers, other studies have provided additional reassurance. To date, approximately thirteen clinical studies have tested the link between soy and cognition. Of these, ten studies found soy consumption beneficial[291–300] and three reported that soy consumption is neither beneficial nor detrimental.[301–303] None of the clinical trials confirmed a causative effect between soy consumption and cognitive decline.

The message is that becoming vegan could either impair or enhance memory—it all depends on diet and lifestyle choices. Ensuring a daily reliable source of vitamin B_{12} is crucial to optimal brain function. Vegan seniors who take B_{12} supplements could actually be at an advantage in this regard, because animal products are unreliable B_{12} sources in people older than 50 (for more on vitamin B_{12}, see pages 214 and 222.

Folate and vitamin B_6 also are important; however, these nutrients are generously available in most vegan diets. As an added bonus, vegans tend to have high intakes of antioxidants and phytochemicals, which appear to protect brain health. Of course, vegans who are physically active, get sufficient rest, avoid smoking and excessive alcohol, and keep their brains active and challenged further reduce their risk of cognitive decline.

Diverticular Disease

Diverticular disease is an umbrella term that includes two diseases of the colon—diverticulosis (small pockets or pouches in the colon) and diverticulitis (inflamed or infected pockets or pouches). Often, diverticulosis goes unnoticed or causes fairly minor symptoms, while diverticulitis is generally more severe, with symptoms ranging from mild bloating and gas to debilitating abdominal pain, vomiting, diarrhea, and fever.

Although diverticular disease is rare in rural Africa and other areas where high-fiber unprocessed diets are standard fare, this painful condition is endemic in the Western world. Risk increases with age, and some studies suggest that as many as 60 percent of those older than 70 are afflicted.[304] In 1971, a research team released a seminal report suggesting that diverticular disease is essentially a result of fiber deficiency.[305]

An impressive body of evidence lends support to that theory.[306–308] In 1979, a British study reported that the risk of diverticulitis in vegetarians was only about half that of nonvegetarians. Interestingly, the vegetarians in this study consumed about twice as much fiber as the nonvegetarians.[309]

In 2011, results released from the EPIC-Oxford study compared the rates of diverticular disease among various dietary groups. The study cohort included 47,033 men and women, 15,459 of whom were vegetarian or vegan (about one-third of the cohort). Of these participants, 812 developed diverticular disease during follow-up. Compared with the meat eaters, when all confounding factors were adjusted for, the risk of developing diverticular disease was 27 percent lower among the lacto-ovo vegetarians and 72 percent lower among the vegans (it's important to note that only four vegans developed the disease). In this study, the risk of diverticular disease also was inversely associated with dietary fiber intake. Compared with the lowest-fiber consumers (men and women who ate less than 14 grams daily), the highest-fiber consumers (more than 25.5 grams daily for women and 26.1 grams daily for men) had a 42 percent lower risk for diverticular disease.[310] (For more on vegans' fiber intake, see pages 152 to 161.)

Although some studies have found a positive association between meat intake and diverticular disease,[306, 307, 311] the EPIC-Oxford study failed to show a significant association between the amount of meat consumed and the incidence of diverticular disease among the meat eaters. The authors suggested that meat intake in this relatively health-conscious group was too low to influence the risk of disease (they averaged about 3 ounces/90 grams per day), or that the range of intake was too small to detect a significant association. Although high meat intake is often associated with low fiber intake, meat consumption also negatively affects fecal flora. This can reduce the integrity of the colon wall, causing it to weaken and become more prone to developing the pouches or pockets associated with diverticular disease.[310]

Gallstones

Gallstone formation is one more condition commonly regarded as the product of Western dietary habits. To date, no studies have examined the rate of gallstone formation in vegans; however, there's good evidence to suggest that a vegan diet may provide some degree of protection.

In 1985, a study of 800 women ranging in age from 40 to 69 reported that nonvegetarians had more than double the risk of developing gallstones than vegetarians,[312] even after controlling for confounding variables. A research team from Germany also reported in three small studies a significantly reduced incidence of gallstones among vegetarians compared with nonvegetarians,[313–315] although a fourth study showed no significant difference.[316]

A twenty-year study of 80,898 women (the Nurses' Health Study) reported that higher long-term intake of vegetable protein was associated with a reduced risk of cholecystectomy (surgical removal of the gallbladder).[317] A separate evaluation of the same group of women noted a favorable effect of fruit and vegetable consumption on the risk of gallstone formation.[318] A third study with the same women[319] found significant risk reductions in women who ate 5 ounces or more of nuts per week compared with participants who ate no nuts. The same team of investigators reported similar benefits in a large cohort of men.[320]

Although questions remain, a number of dietary factors are known to influence the risk of gallstone formation. Overeating (leading to overweight or obesity) is strongly linked to increased risk.[321] High intake of saturated fat, trans-fatty acids, cholesterol,[322–324] and refined carbohydrates[325] also is thought to increase risk. Conversely, dietary fiber intake,[326, 327] fruit and vegetable consumption,[318] vegetable protein intake,[317] and unsaturated fat intake[328] are all associated with decreased risk.

Of all dietary patterns, a vegan diet has the lowest risk of overweight and obesity; the lowest intake of saturated fat and cholesterol; and the highest intake of fiber, vegetable protein, fruits, and vegetables. Thus, although definitive data is currently lacking, it's reasonable to assume that vegans' risk of developing gallstones would be even lower than that of lacto-ovo vegetarians.

Kidney (Renal) Disease

In 2013, AHS-2 released the first report to compare rates of renal disease in vegetarians (including vegans) relative to nonvegetarians. The vegetarians had a 52 percent lower risk of renal disease than similar health-conscious nonvegetarians, and the findings were statistically significant.[23]

High-protein diets are known to accelerate renal function decline in people with chronic kidney disease (CKD).[329] Traditionally, patients with advanced CKD have been advised to consume low-protein diets (no more than 0.6 grams per kilogram of body weight), and that what little protein they're allowed should come mostly from animal products that contain high-quality protein, such as eggs, meat, poultry, and fish. The general rule of thumb was that at least three-quarters of CKD patients' limited protein intake come from animal sources and no more than one-quarter from plant sources. In addition, sodium, potassium, phosphorus, and fluids are restricted in an effort to reduce the buildup in blood of toxic waste products that occur when kidney function is compromised.

Vegan diets were considered highly inappropriate for people afflicted with kidney disease. However, interest in plant-based diets began to grow with the recognition that vegan diets—which are low in saturated fat, cholesterol-free, and high in fiber—produced significant improvements in blood lipids, blood pressure, and atherosclerosis, all of which can worsen kidney disease.

The preponderance of evidence suggests that diets rich in vegetable protein don't promote renal decline to the same extent as diets rich in animal protein (specifically meat-based protein).[329] Although both animal and vegetable protein sources can cause renal injury and accelerate CKD, plant-based diets provide more moderate, though adequate, amounts of protein.

One research team reporting on two clinical trials found that consuming protein from plant sources resulted in less protein in the urine and less renal damage than eating animal protein, and that these changes were independent of total protein intake.[330, 331] The authors concluded, "Protein-modified, rather than protein-restricted, diets may prove advantageous in the long-term treatment of chronic renal failure."

A second team investigated the impact of shifting patients who had mild renal failure from an unrestricted-protein or conventional low-protein diet to a special vegan diet that included added essential amino acids.[332] The authors suggested that the vegan diet would be a suitable replacement for the conventional low-protein diet in patients with mild chronic renal failure. Subjects on the vegan diet showed benefits similar to those provided by the conventional low-protein diet—lowered glomerular filtration rate, improved acid-base balance, and a slower progression of the disease. However, the vegan diet had additional positive features, including less saturated fat, no cholesterol, and lower net acid production when compared to a nonvegetarian low-protein diet. Study participants also considered the vegan diet more economical and palatable than the conventional low-protein diet.

Finally, a 2014 study reported that pregnant women with stages 3–5 CKD who followed vegan or vegetarian low-protein diets and used supplements reduced their risk of having a baby that was small for its gestational age—without detrimental effects on kidney function or proteinuria in the mother.[333]

Controlling excess dietary phosphorus intake also is a key strategy in CKD management; protein-rich foods are the main source of phosphorus. Investigators of a short-term study that compared diets containing equal phosphorus concentrations from plant versus animal foods reported that plant sources of phosphorus have fewer adverse effects on phosphorus levels in CKD patients than those from animal sources.[333] The study authors stated, "These results, if confirmed in longer studies, provide rationale for recommending a predominance of grain-based vegetarian sources of protein to patients with CKD. This will allow increased protein intake without adversely affecting phosphorus levels."[334]

The interesting advantage of plant-based diets concerns the form of phosphorus consumed. Organic phosphorus comes from whole foods (both animal and plant foods), while inorganic phosphorus is found in processed foods. Inorganic phosphorus (such as phosphorus added to soft drinks and processed cheese) is essentially fully absorbed by the body. However, the body must convert organic phosphorus to inorganic phosphorus before it can be absorbed. As a result, 40 to 60 percent of the total phosphorus in protein-rich animal products is absorbed.[335] In contrast, the phosphorus in plant foods—some of which is in a form called phytate—may be absorbed at a rate of only 20 to 50 percent,[335] allowing better control of phosphorus intake. (For more on phytate, see page 181.)

Finally, it's been suggested that plant-based diets provide an additional advantage to overweight or obese CKD patients. These diets tend to be less energy dense and higher in fiber, and have been associated with more healthful body weights. As stated in the ADA position on vegetarian diets, "Soy-based vegan diets appear to be nutritionally adequate for people with chronic kidney disease and may slow progression of kidney disease."[1]

Hypothyroidism

In 2013, the AHS-2 released findings on the risk of hypothyroidism among various dietary groups. Prevalence among vegans was 11 percent lower than among nonvegetarians, although it was 9 percent higher among lacto-ovo vegetarians (statistical significance was not attained). In addition, vegans had a 22 percent lower risk of developing hypothyroidism compared to nonvegetarians. Incident hypothyroidism was positively associated with female gender, white ethnicity, higher BMI, and higher education.[336]

Although vegan diets are associated with reduced BMI, which is protective, the advantage for vegans was present even after controlling for BMI and other confounding variables. These findings were somewhat surprising, because vegan diets tend to be higher in goitrogens (such as cruciferous vegetables and soy products) and may also be lower in iodine. However, little evidence exists to suggest that goitrogenic foods are a problem when iodine intakes are adequate, so it's possible that this population has a sufficient, reliable source of iodine in the daily diet (possibly iodized salt or kelp).

Rheumatoid Arthritis

Rheumatoid arthritis (RA) is an autoimmune disease that causes chronic inflammation of the joints, the tissues around joints, and the vital organs. Autoimmune diseases occur when the body mistakes its own tissues for foreign intruders and produces antibodies to attack and destroy them. RA can result in severe pain in, damage to, and degeneration of muscles, joints, cartilage, and internal organs. As the disease advances, bones also can erode, resulting in significant deformity. Although research suggests that dietary intervention may serve as an effective treatment option for some RA patients, most trials to date have been small and of short duration, reducing the value or statistical significance of their findings. Still, the results are encouraging.

Seven studies conducted by research teams in Finland have reported the favorable effects of living-food vegan diets (raw diets rich in probiotics and enzymes) on RA patients.[337–343] Study participants reported significant reductions in pain, morning stiffness, swelling of joints, and other RA symptoms. More-modest benefits were observed in laboratory markers of the disease (blood tests, urine tests, and X-rays). A variety of additional positive health outcomes were noted in study participants, including favorable changes in fecal flora, reduced blood cholesterol levels, and increased concentrations of protective antioxidants.

Two studies by a team of Swedish investigators examined the impact on RA patients of a gluten-free vegan diet compared to a well-balanced nonvegetarian diet.[344, 345] In the first study, after one year of treatment, 40.5 percent of those in the vegan group had marked improvement in their disease (fulfilling a standard measure called the ACR20 improvement criteria); only 4 percent of those in the nonvegan group showed improvement.[344] The second study focused on changes in blood lipids in RA patients. In the vegan group, total cholesterol, LDL cholesterol, and oxidized-LDL cholesterol declined (as did BMI); levels of triglycerides and HDL cholesterol didn't change. Markers of inflammation also improved substantially in the vegan group. For these RA patients, the gluten-free vegan diet proved both cardioprotective and anti-inflammatory.[345]

One US team investigated the effects of a very low-fat vegan diet on participants with RA. Although this study lacked a control group, measures of RA symptoms in participants significantly decreased, with the exception of the duration of morning stiffness. Body weight and C-reactive protein (a measure of inflammation) were also reduced.[346]

A number of studies have tested variations of plant-based diets, with some including periods of fasting before introduction of the plant-based regimen.[347–359] Although the outcomes were variable, favorable changes in fecal flora, reduced pain and stiffness, and improvements in measurable RA indicators were reported.

Vegan diets have many mechanisms that could produce improvements in RA symptoms. The vegetables, fruits, and other whole plant foods that form the basis of vegan diets are key sources of protective anti-inflammatory and antioxidant compounds.[360] These diets are free of animal products, including red and processed meats, and are typically low in processed foods, all of which have been associated with inflammatory compounds.[361, 362] (There's evidence that animal products increase some individuals' risk of developing RA,[363, 364] although a recent study refutes these findings.[365])

One study noted that intakes of anti-inflammatory phytochemicals, such as quercetin (found in onions and apples), kaempferol (found in tea and broccoli), and myricetin (found in walnuts and grapes), were more than ten times higher in vegan diets compared to nonvegetarian control diets. Blood carotenoids also measured two to six times greater in living-food vegans than in nonvegetarian controls.[338]

Another study reported a significant drop of markers of inflammation present in feces.[341] The greatly increased fiber intake associated with vegan diets promotes regularity and reduces the time available for harmful compounds to be absorbed from the gut into the bloodstream.[338] These advantages disappear when participants resume their usual diets.

Researchers have also observed that when a vegan diet is adopted, it favorably alters the balance of microflora or bacteria that live in intestines.[338–341, 343] It's been noted that fecal flora in RA patients are significantly altered compared to controls.[366] The mechanism by which intestinal flora are thought to impact RA progression is that some of their harmful breakdown products can pass from the intestine to the bloodstream, behaving like foreign invaders. The body responds by manufacturing antibodies to attack these "foreign invaders," but in some cases, these antibodies also attack healthy tissue.[338]

Another popular theory regarding the success of all types of plant-based diets in reducing symptoms of RA is that such diets generally result in weight loss, causing less stress on painful joints. A team of investigators tested the support for this theory by pooling the results of three studies, each using a different type of plant-based diet (vegan, lacto-ovo vegetarian, and a Mediterranean diet) in RA treatment.[367] For all the diets, the average weight loss was 2.4 kg (5.3 lb) per person during a trial period of three to four months. When investigators analyzed changes in body weight versus changes in RA symptoms, no significant correlation was observed between weight loss and improvements in RA. Although this doesn't rule out the possibility that weight reduction is helpful in decreasing RA symptoms, it suggests that the diets provide positive effects outside of weight loss.

For example, some experts argue that benefits conferred by vegan diets are due to removal of food items that produce allergies and aggravate sensitivities in RA patients.[368] Common triggers, such as dairy products, eggs, and fish, are eliminated, and many vegan diets eliminate wheat and other gluten-containing grains, nightshades, and citrus fruits, as well. Any diet that excludes these triggers may prove advantageous for people who are sensitive to those particular foods. However, many individuals with RA also appear to benefit from vegan diets, even when gluten-containing grains and nightshade vegetables are included.

Regardless of the mechanisms of their action, for some RA sufferers, vegan diets appear to offer significant benefits. Limited evidence suggests that raw or living-food diets can be especially effective. However, larger longer-term studies are needed before these findings can be confirmed.

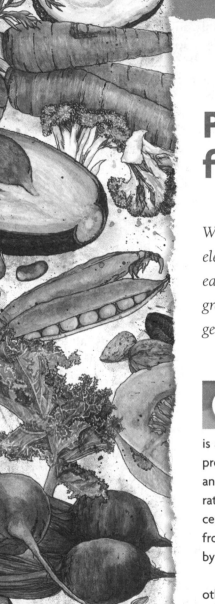

3

Protein Power from Plants

*When you think of the biggest animals on the planet—
elephants, buffalo, giraffes, huge, huge mammals—they don't
eat meat—where do they get their protein? It grows out of the
ground. Plants are full of protein. That's where these animals
get it, and that's where we can get it as well.*

MICHAEL KLAPER, PHYSICIAN, AUTHOR, AND SPEAKER

G iven the typical dietary patterns of North Americans, Australians, Europeans, and those with similar Western-style diets, it's not surprising that, in the minds of so many, protein is associated only with animal products. Currently, two-thirds of the protein intake in these parts of the world comes from animal sources and just one-third from plants. However, in the rest of the world, the ratio is reversed: 65 percent of the protein comes from plants (47 percent from grains; 8 percent from legumes, nuts, and seeds; 9 percent from vegetables; and 1 percent from fruits), with the balance provided by a more-sparing use of animal products.[1, 2]

Many people equate protein only with meat, eggs, cheese, and other animal products and assume that protein intake must be insufficient on a vegan diet. The first question vegans are often asked is, "Where do you get your protein?" On the other hand, many vegans take for granted that protein intake is automatically sufficient on any vegan diet. After all, every plant and every plant cell contains some amount of protein.

Neither position fully represents the actual situation. It's true that all grains, legumes, nuts, seeds, and vegetables are protein sources, and that even fruits contain a little protein. So vegans can easily meet their recommended protein intake, regardless of gender, size, or activity level. Yet a vegan diet can be short of protein if it's centered on fruit (as in some raw vegan diets); it also can be low in calories (being used for weight loss), can incorporate too many vegan junk foods (such as chips, fats, refined foods, and sweets), or can be lacking in legumes (such as beans, peas, lentils, soy foods, and peanuts).

The building blocks of proteins are amino acids (molecules of carbon, hydrogen, oxygen, and nitrogen). Some of these are called indispensable amino acids (IAAs) or essential amino acids because the human body can't manufacture them, and they must be supplied by diet. Every one of the IAAs is available in plant foods and also in animal products. Others are termed dispensable amino acids because the body can synthesize them from the IAAs.

As a component of muscle and bone, protein is essential for the body's structure and movement. Various proteins protect health (in the form of antibodies and other immune system constituents), accomplish reactions (as enzymes), coordinate activities (as hormones), and work as carriers (moving oxygen and electrons). Adults require protein for cell maintenance and replacement; infants and children need extra protein to build new cells.

During the early and mid-twentieth century, findings from many animal studies led to the undervaluation of plant protein for human diets. Such research typically involved baby rats, whose protein requirements differ significantly from those of humans. Rats double their birth weight in four days, grow to maturity in a few weeks, and have significant physiological differences, such as the growth and maintenance of fur (composed of specific proteins and amino acids) all over their bodies. As a result, they need the highly concentrated protein sources found in rat milk, cow milk, and other animal products; baby rats die on a diet of human breast milk (though obviously, breast milk is suitable for human infants). In experiments, lab rats were given a single food (such as cheese or wheat) as their sole protein source, a situation quite different from humans' preferred and usual choice of a varied diet. The diet composed of a single plant food didn't sustain the very fast growth of young rats.

At the time, scientists didn't take into consideration the dissimilarities between rat and human physiology—or between laboratory conditions and typical human eating patterns. Perspectives from that era led scientists to label most plant proteins as "incomplete." In fact, plant proteins are not incomplete; all the IAAs needed by humans are present (although not in the ratios and concentrated amounts needed by baby rats), and a vegan diet of mixed plant foods easily supplies complete protein, meaning the necessary mix of IAAs.[3-6]

Although plants can provide all the protein needed for human nutrition, the misconception persists that plant proteins are inferior to animal proteins. Unfortunately, complex social and cultural attitudes toward meat, as well as early scientific evaluation of relative protein quality based on animal studies, have conspired to support this mistaken belief.[1]

In more-prosperous parts of the world today, vegans can select a well-balanced plant-based diet that supports their health and that of the planet far better than does a meat-centered diet. In developing countries, some residents on vegan and near-vegan diets are among the healthiest people in the world, while others, whose meals are centered on one grain with very limited amounts of legumes or vegetables, consume insufficient calories. The grain (typically rice or wheat) that provides most of their calories can furnish only limited amounts of the amino acid lysine, a limitation that can have an impact on growth and some aspects of health.[1, 4, 7]

Experiments funded by the beef industry have shown, not surprisingly, that adding meat to these limited diets can improve nutritional status. Yet, scientists have established beyond a doubt that a mix of plant proteins will support optimal human growth and health. Excellent results can be achieved in developing nations by adding nutrient-rich legumes and vegetables, which are more affordable than beef.[8, 9] For example, peanuts, pigeon peas, and soybeans were introduced as crops for villagers in Malawi, with good results.[8, 10]

Putting Plant Protein in Proper Perspective

Although plant protein has sometimes been dismissed as being "incomplete" relative to animal protein, this term is inaccurate. In fact, the IAAs present in animal products are all derived from plants—whether the animals consumed the plants directly or indirectly (by eating other animals that have eaten plants). The point is that IAAs are manufactured by plants, so it makes little sense to assume that people must eat animals to get them. Well-balanced vegan diets consist of a variety of foods, which differ in the relative amounts of IAAs provided by each. When a diet consists of an assortment of plant foods with complementary strengths and weaknesses in their ratios of amino acids, it supplies the correct mix of amino acids needed to build and maintain healthy, strong bodies.

Another somewhat misleading phrase used in relation to plant protein when comparing it to animal products or to refined plant products (such as soy protein isolate) is "poorer protein quality." This refers to the amino acid mix and to digestibility. It's true that the proteins in whole plant foods may be less digestible, but the difference in digestibility can be offset by a slight increase in the recommended protein intake, which is easily achieved. As a bonus, whole grains, beans, and vegetables offer an abundance of healthful components: fiber, vitamins, trace minerals, and phytochemicals. (The latter are not present in animal products and are removed in significant amounts from refined plant foods).

COMPLEMENTARY PROTEINS AT A MEAL: NO LONGER A RULE

More than forty years ago, a popular theory based on the concept that plant proteins were "incomplete" stated that a person *must* eat complementary plant proteins at the same meal to obtain the full range of IAAs. This theory and the assumption that certain plant foods must be combined at the same meal has proved to be unnecessary and has been discarded. Research has established that people can easily get the full range of IAAs by consuming an appealing assortment of plant foods over the course of a day—so an overall mix is important.

It's true that proteins in various food groups differ in their proportions of amino acids. For example, most seeds and legumes provide abundant lysine but are somewhat short in methionine. In contrast, grains tend to be good sources of methionine but are low in lysine. When adults eat beans and whole grains within the same twenty-four-hour period, the body pools the amino acids and draws on this pool all day to build top-quality protein. Children *may* benefit by eating grains and legumes together—particularly if total protein intake is marginal; however, research hasn't shown this combination to be essential at each meal.[1, 11] A mix of 76 percent grains and 24 percent beans as part of the overall diet has been shown to satisfy the protein needs of preschoolers very well.[12]

Whatever the theory, in practice consumers mix food groups at plant-based meals all over the world unless they're restricted by severe poverty. For people who can afford to supplement a grain-centered diet, combining legumes and whole grains provides an optimum mix of amino acids, often with vegetables and nuts or seeds.[13] In Southeast Asia, meals are centered on tofu and rice. Ethiopians savor lentils and teff. In Egypt, menus feature fava beans and millet. The Scots have long relied on white bean soup and oat cakes. The French and French Canadians appreciate beautifully seasoned pea soup along with freshly baked bread. The Nepalese, who carry heavy packs through mountain passes, maintain their body protein with lentil dhal and millet. South Americans and Mexicans enjoy colorful meals of black or pinto beans along with quinoa, rice, or taco shells made from wheat or corn. Boston is known for baked beans and brown bread. In the southern United States, a favorite combination is black-eyed peas and cornbread, while the peanut butter sandwich is an easy-to-make North American staple.

Protein Quantity

How much protein is necessary for good health? Actual protein requirements vary somewhat from one individual to another, even when body weights are identical. The Recommended Dietary Allowance (RDA) is a generous amount; it includes a built-in margin of safety above average requirements to meet the needs of 97.5 percent of the healthy population, including those near the high end of the spectrum. More protein usually is needed to maintain a large body than a small body; this fact is reflected in the RDA, which is stated in grams of protein per kilogram of body weight per day (g/kg/d). (Note that 1 kilogram is equivalent to 2.2 pounds.) The extra fat tissue in overweight or obese people requires relatively little protein for maintenance. Thus, the body weight on which intakes are based is commonly interpreted to mean ideal or healthy body weight, although the RDA doesn't specify this. The RDA is based on diets that provide good-quality protein. In vegan diets, meeting the RDA for protein can easily be achieved with a mix of grains, legumes, nuts, seeds, and vegetables. (For more on protein quality in vegan diets, see page 87).

In the quickly evolving science of nutrition, recommended intakes for various nutrients are being continually revisited and gradually revised. Although the

Suggested Protein Intake for Vegan Adults based on 0.9 g/kg/day

TABLE 3.1. Ideal or healthy body weight with recommended protein intake

BODY WEIGHT (lb)	BODY WEIGHT (kg)	RECOMMENDED PROTEIN (g, rounded)
120	54	49
135	61	55
150	68	61
165	75	68
180	82	74
195	88.5	80

CALCULATING RECOMMENDED PROTEIN INTAKE FOR ADULT VEGANS

For a person whose healthy or ideal weight is 135 pounds (61 kg), multiply 61 x 0.9 = 55 g protein.

For a person whose healthy or ideal weight is 165 pounds (75 kg), multiply 75 x 0.9 = 68 g protein.

For yourself:

a) divide your healthy or ideal weight in pounds ___ by 2.2 lb/kg for weight in kilograms = ____kg

b) multiply ____kg x 0.9 = ___g to get your recommended protein intake for the day

RDA for protein has long been set at 0.8 g/kg/day, recent studies suggest that a slight increase may provide health advantages.[14–17] As a result, the World Health Organization (WHO) and a number of experts have set a "safe" protein recommendation of 0.83 g/kg/day.[12, 17]

The Food and Nutrition Board states that "available evidence does not support recommending a separate protein requirement for vegetarians" and assumes that vegetarians eat a variety of plant-based protein sources during the day (and for lacto-ovo vegetarians, eggs and dairy products, as well).[15] To compensate for the decreased digestibility of the protein in many plant foods, several small studies and a number of experts in vegan nutrition support a slightly higher recommended minimum protein intake for vegan adults of at least 0.9 g/kg/day (equivalent to 0.4 grams per pound) as seen in table 3.1.[18, 19] Some suggest a little more (such as 1 g/kg/day); these levels of intakes aren't difficult to achieve on plant-based diets.[20, 21]

PROTEIN FOR YOUNG AND OLD

During periods of growth, the body requires plenty of protein to build new bone, muscle, and other tissues. As a result, the recommended protein intakes of children are relatively high *per kilogram of body weight* compared with those of adults. During the first year of life, infants require almost twice as much protein per kilogram as do adults. Fortunately, the protein quality of breast milk is excellent, and infant formula comes in at a close second. Infants thrive on breast milk, although only 5 percent of its calories come from protein. This leads to occasional claims that adult protein requirements must be similarly low. However, the protein in human breast milk is highly digestible compared to that in other foods, and its balance of amino acids is superbly fitted to infant requirements. In addition, babies require *far* more calories relative to body weight than adults do, so the percentage of calories needed to meet protein needs is lower.

Yet because a child's body is small, the actual amount of protein needed also is small. Typically, a 6- to 12-month-old infant requires about 11 grams of protein per day; 4- to 8-year-old children need about 19 grams per day. The recommended (safe) level of protein is gradually reduced from a daily intake of about 1.14 grams per kilogram of body weight at age 1 to about 0.83 g/kg/day for adults.[15, 17] Of course, protein requirements during pregnancy and lactation are higher than those of nonpregnant women (for more on these requirements, see chapter 9).

Past the age of 60, the adult body's ability to utilize protein may become less efficient, so it's particularly important for older adults to aim for a daily protein intake of at least 0.9 grams per kilogram of healthy body weight, and 1 g/kg may be better (page 346).[22–25]

PROTEIN FOR ATHLETES

To have the energy to participate in most sports activities, athletes need extra calories. However, their ideal fuel is carbohydrate, not protein. Experts note that, despite the lack of supportive evidence, there's a broad misconception that *all* athletes need more protein.[27] In their joint position paper, "Nutrition and Athletic Performance," the Academy of Nutrition and Dietetics, Dietitians of Canada, and the American College of Sports Medicine make the point: "Because there is not a strong body of evidence documenting that additional dietary protein is needed by healthy adults who undertake endurance or resistance exercise, the current Dietary Reference Intakes for protein and amino acids does not specifically recognize the unique needs of routinely active individuals and competitive athletes."[27] So, for most vegans who keep fit with regular exercise, daily consumption of 0.9 grams of protein per kilogram of body weight is plenty.

Although it's true that strength athletes on any diet require extra protein, vegans are advised to consume 1.3 to 1.9 g/kg/day, particularly during the stage when they're adding muscle tissue.[27, 28] Vegan endurance athletes also need somewhat more protein while in training; typical recommendations range from 1.3 to 1.5 g/kg/day.[27, 28] These protein intakes aren't difficult to achieve, because people who exercise a great deal also have big appetites.

Finding simple and practical ways to prepare or obtain protein-rich vegan foods can pose a challenge. Combinations of grains, legumes, soy foods, and nuts and seeds (or their butters) supply sufficient protein for competitive athletes. For those who want to stay light and lean, beans, peas, and lentils provide a special benefit, because they're high in protein but not loaded with fat. (See table 3.5 on pages 97 to 103.) Cooked or canned lentils can be easily stirred into spaghetti sauce, tofu added to a stir-fry, and chickpeas or other beans heaped onto a salad. For an extra boost, vegan protein powders based on peas, rice, seeds, or soy can be added to smoothies. (For more on sports nutrition, see chapter 13; for menus that provide several levels of caloric and protein intake, see pages 439 to 442.)

Away from home, it takes planning, and sometimes ingenuity, to find or create protein-rich meals and snacks. A simple peanut butter sandwich can easily provide as much protein as a hamburger patty, and vegetables, seeds, and nuts add significantly to daily protein intake. A little more than half the world's protein comes from grains, so cereals, breads, and pasta shouldn't be discounted.[2] (Protein provides about 10 to 15 percent of the calories in grains.) Finally, ethnic restaurants often save the day for travelers; use Resources on page 450 to find vegan-friendly dining options.

Protein Quality

ecommendations for protein intake take into account protein quality, an attribute determined by two factors: digestibility and amino acid content.

DIGESTIBILITY

Digestibility refers to bioavailability, or the extent to which a protein is absorbed, a factor affected by the amount of fiber in the plants' cell walls. Most of this fiber isn't digested; it passes through the body's intestinal tract intact, carrying with it a small percentage of the protein. If the plant cell walls are removed by refining—as occurs when soy protein isolate (isolated soy protein) is extracted from soybeans—the fiber-free refined protein is as digestible as animal protein.

Considerable controversy exists about how to rate protein digestibility. Generally, if a body absorbs 96 percent of the nitrogen from a protein source and excretes 4 percent, the digestibility of that protein is rated as 96 percent. Depending on the specific food, its preparation, and the method of analysis used, the digestibility rating may vary from one source to another. Overall, the protein in American and Chinese diets has been rated as 96 percent digestible; proteins in the Brazilian diet and the Indian diet of rice and beans are rated as 78 percent digestible.[17]

At a glance, it might appear that white bread is a better source of protein than whole wheat bread. Or one might consider that due to its high digestibility, soy protein isolate would be a better choice than tofu or cooked beans. Yet the choice isn't so simple. Although processing plant foods increases the digestibility of their protein by removing fiber and other materials in cell walls, it strips the foods of valuable vitamins, minerals, and phytochemicals. On the other hand, including some processed or refined plant foods can help balance a diet that may otherwise be too bulky for small children or for those who have particularly

TABLE 3.2. Digestibility of protein in various foods

PLANT FOODS	DIGESTIBILITY (%)
White (refined) flour or bread	96
Soy protein isolate	95
Peanut butter	95
Tofu	93
Whole wheat flour or bread	92
Oatmeal	86
Lentils	84
Black, kidney, and pinto beans and chickpeas	72–89
ANIMAL PRODUCTS	
Eggs	97
Milk, cheese	95
Beef, fish	94

Sources: [2, 13, 17, 29, 20]

high energy or protein needs. (Dense foods, such as purées and nut butters, also help meet such needs.)

Food preparation techniques also can affect digestibility. For example, the process of cooking beans and lentils or sprouting buckwheat and peas starts the breakdown of their proteins, resulting in better absorption by the body.[31–34] When legumes and grains are soaked or sprouted, their proteins split into shorter chains of constituent amino acids, essentially beginning the digestion process.[31, 32]

Vegans may choose to soak and sprout plant foods before cooking, when possible. The digestibility of the protein in raw peas was shown to increase by 8 percent after six hours of soaking, and as much as 31 percent after eighteen hours of soaking. Soaking and cooking increased digestibility by 25 to 30 percent. Soaking followed by pressure cooking resulted in an increase of 30 to 33 percent, doubling the change in protein digestibility that occurred in dried peas that were cooked without soaking. In legumes, such changes are thought to be linked with the activation of plant enzymes that begin protein breakdown and with the destruction of phytate and of trypsin inhibitors that can limit digestion.[31, 35–37]

Allowing raw peas to sprout for forty-eight hours led to increases of 25 to 28 percent in protein digestibility. As a further benefit, sprouting beans for six days was shown to remove most (70 to 100 percent) of the oligosaccharides that sometimes cause flatulence.[36–39] Sprouting can further improve protein quality by slightly increasing the amount of IAAs, such as lysine, that may be in short supply (page 89).[40]

Protein Digestibility Corrected Amino Acid Score (PDCAAS)

A scoring system known as the PDCAAS has been developed to indicate the quality of a particular food protein. The PDCAAS is based on a food's digestibility and on its IAA profile. This profile is compared to the estimated or measured pattern of IAAs required by a person in good health. Proteins given the highest score (1.00 or 100 percent) are easily digested and have an amino acid content similar to the pattern required for health. The PDCAAS is a subject of lively debate among nutritional scientists, and the tool continues to be refined.[3]

Soy protein isolate is given a PDCAAS of 1.00 because it contains excellent proportions of IAAs and its digestibility has been increased by the removal of fiber. Eggs and the milk protein casein also have been assigned a PDCAAS of 1.00. Tofu and beef are given a PDCAAS of 0.9 or higher based on their digestibility (listed in table 3.2) and IAA content. Other legumes have lower scores due to somewhat lower amounts of the amino acid methionine and the presence in their plant cell walls of fiber that affects digestibility.[15] As an example of changing perspectives, recent research indicates that adaptation may occur with long-term use of a particular protein intake. Thus, once the body has had time to adapt to a vegan diet, plant protein may be better utilized and more well digested than was formerly believed.[3, 6, 17, 42]

AMINO ACID CONTENT

When a food's protein quality is rated, its pattern or profile of IAAs must be compared with the overall pattern of IAAs needed by the human body. In the body, an individual protein molecule is an intricate structure consisting of numerous amino acids arranged in specific sequences and folded into varying spatial arrangements. Depending on the sequence and three-dimensional placement of the amino acids, the resulting protein molecule can function as an enzyme, hemoglobin, or muscle protein, or can perform other tasks.

Human bodies need approximately twenty different amino acids to build these protein molecules.[15] This number includes the nine IAAs—isoleucine, leucine, lysine, methionine, phenylalanine, threonine, tryptophan, valine, and (for infants) histidine—that must be present in the diet. From these and other components available in cells, the remaining amino acids can be built.[15, 29, 43, 44] Every one of these IAAs is present in all plant foods; however, the content of each varies from one plant protein to another. Several other amino acids also present in plant foods are termed "conditionally indispensable" because they can be synthesized; however, such amino-acid synthesis may be limited under certain disease conditions.[44]

LYSINE AND TRYPTOPHAN IN PLANT FOODS

Two IAAs of particular interest to vegans are lysine and tryptophan. Lysine is required for growth and protein building. Low lysine intakes are in part responsible for the small stature of some impoverished people whose dietary options were limited during childhood.[3] This IAA is in relatively short supply where wheat, rice, or other grains with low lysine contents provide most of the calories. At the same time, recent research indicates that the lysine present in cooked white rice is better utilized by the body than was formerly believed and that the bodies of people whose habitual diets are somewhat low in lysine may adapt to low intakes by more efficiently using the available lysine and improving its conservation.[45] Browning rice before cooking reduces lysine content.[46]

Adult requirements are a subject of debate, because the body has some ability to recycle lysine.[3] Lysine requirements for adults have been set by the World Health Organization (WHO) at 30 mg per kilogram of body weight per day; the RDA set by the Institute of Medicine (IOM) is 38 mg/kg/day.[3, 5, 17] The challenge of getting enough lysine can be met by including sufficient amounts of plant foods that are good sources, such as peas, beans, and lentils. Legume-based protein supplements also can give a boost to protein and lysine intakes. Three servings of legumes are likely to provide about half the recommended intake of protein and two-thirds of the lysine for the day. (See The Vegan Plate on page 434 for examples of serving sizes; also see menus on pages 439 to 442.)

Raw vegan diets can be low in legumes or lack this food group entirely. Fresh green peas or sprouted lentils, peas, and mung beans are raw legume sources of protein, lysine, and tryptophan. Small increases in lysine and other IAAs have been reported when legumes are sprouted.[47, 48] Larger beans, such as chickpeas, can be sprouted, but it's best to then cook these sprouts to destroy the antinutritional factors present, such as trypsin inhibitors and hemagglutinins.[49]

Table 3.3 shows that cashews, pistachios, pumpkin seeds, buckwheat, quinoa, and edamame and other soy foods also are good sources of lysine. Soy foods in particular contribute stellar amounts of protein and lysine. With regard to vegetarian meat analogs, those with soy as the primary ingredient are likely to be higher in lysine content than those made primarily from wheat gluten. Pseudograins (botanically different from grains), such as buckwheat, corn, and quinoa, that are used as grains provide more lysine per serving than wheat and rice.

TABLE 3.3. Protein, lysine, and tryptophan content in foods

FOOD	PROTEIN (g)	LYSINE (mg)	TRYPTOPHAN (mg)
LEGUMES (COOKED UNLESS STATED)	**AVERAGE: 9.7**	**AVERAGE: 594**	**AVERAGE: 111**
Beans (adzuki, white), ½ c (125 ml)	9.1–9.2	630–690	90–110
Beans (black, black-eyed peas, chickpeas, cranberry, great Northern, kidney, lima, mung, navy, pink, pinto), ½ c (125 ml)	7–8.7	450–600	90–100
Lentils, ½ c (125 ml)	8.9	620	80
Peanut butter, 2 T (30 ml)	8.1	220	70
Peanuts, ¼ c (60 ml)	9.4	340	84
Peas, green, raw, 1 c (250 ml)	7.9	460	54

FOOD	PROTEIN (g)	LYSINE (mg)	TRYPTOPHAN (mg)
Peas, split, ½ c (125 ml)	8.6	620	100
Soybeans, ½ c (125 ml)	15.1	953	210
Soy milk, ½ c (125 ml)	6.3–11	180–710	50–120
Tempeh, firm, ½ c (125 ml)	16.3	800	170
Tofu, firm or extra-firm, ½ c (125 ml)	10.9–21.1	550–1,380	130–330
NUTS, SEEDS, AND THEIR BUTTERS	**AVERAGE: 5.4**	**AVERAGE: 219**	**AVERAGE: 85**
Almonds, ¼ c (60 ml)	7.7	190	70
Cashews, ¼ c (60 ml)	6.2	290	90
Flaxseeds, ground, ¼ c (60 ml)	5.1	241	124
Hazelnuts/filberts, ¼ c (60 ml)	5.1	140	60
Pecans, ¼ c (60 ml)	2.3	70	20
Pine nuts/pignolia nuts, ¼ c (60 ml)	4.7	170	41
Pistachios, ¼ c (60 ml)	6.3	350	80
Pumpkin seeds, ¼ c (60 ml)	9.9	370	186
Sunflower seeds, ¼ c (60 ml)	7.4	304	103
Tahini, 2 T (30 ml)	5.2	167	116
Walnuts, ¼ c (60 ml)	4.4	120	50
GRAINS (COOKED UNLESS STATED)	**AVERAGE: 3.5**	**AVERAGE: 119**	**AVERAGE: 40**
Bread, white, slice, 1 oz (30 g)	2.8	60	30
Bread, whole wheat, slice, 1 oz (30 g)	3.9	50	30
Buckwheat groats, dry, ¼ c (60 ml)	5.6	286	82
Cornmeal, dry, ¼ c (60 ml)	2.5	70	20
Millet, ½ c (125 ml)	3	60	33
Oatmeal, ½ c (125 ml)	3.1	150	40
Quinoa, ½ c (125 ml)	4.3	230	50
Rice, brown, ½ c (125 ml)	2.7	100	32
Rice, white, ½ c (125 ml)	2.2	80	20
Spaghetti, ½ c (125 ml)	4.3	100	56
Spaghetti, whole wheat, ½ c (125 ml)	3.9	90	48
Wild rice, ½ c (125 ml)	3.5	150	40
VEGETABLES (RAW UNLESS STATED)	**AVERAGE: 1.6**	**AVERAGE: 80**	**AVERAGE: 19**
Avocado, ½ c (125 ml)	1.5	100	20
Broccoli, chopped, cooked, ½ c (125 ml)	2	120	30

FOOD	PROTEIN (g)	LYSINE (mg)	TRYPTOPHAN (mg)
Carrot, medium, 2 oz (60 g)	0.6	30	0
Cauliflower, chopped, cooked, ½ c (125 ml)	1.2	60	20
Corn, yellow, ½ c (125 ml)	2.5	100	20
Eggplant, chopped, cooked, ½ c (125 ml)	0.4	19	0
Kale, 1 c (250 ml)	2.3	140	30
Lettuce, romaine, 1 c (250 ml)	0.6	30	0
Potato, medium, baked, 6 oz (180 g)	4.3	220	40
Potato, cooked, ½ c (125 ml)	1.4	89	23
Spinach, raw, 1 c (250 ml)	0.9	52	12
Sweet potato, dark orange, baked, ½ c (125 ml)	2.4	100	50
Tomato, medium, 4 oz (120 g)	1.1	33	9
Turnip, cooked, mashed, ½ c (125 ml)	0.9	32	11
FRUIT (RAW UNLESS STATED)	**AVERAGE: 0.8**	**AVERAGE: 40**	**AVERAGE: 10**
Apple, medium, 6 oz (180 g)	0.5	22	2
Banana, medium, 4 oz (120 g)	1.3	59	11
Dates, ¼ c (60 ml)	0.9	24	5
Mango, chopped, ½ c (125 ml)	0.7	50	21
Orange, 4.5 oz (135 g)	1.2	62	12
Strawberries, ½ c (125 ml)	0.5	20	12
SPECIAL SUPPLEMENTS (AS EXAMPLES)			
Naturade Soy Protein, ⅓ c (28 g)	24	1,552	305
Naturade Soy-Free Protein, ⅓ c (28 g)	22	1,455	228
Spirulina, dried, 1 T (9 g)	4	212	65
Vega Sport Performance Protein, 1 serving (36 g)	25	1,780	240
ANIMAL PRODUCTS (COOKED UNLESS STATED)	**AVERAGE: 11.1**	**AVERAGE: 955**	**AVERAGE: 108**
Beef hamburger, 2 oz (60 g)	15.2	1,250	70
Egg, large, 2.7 oz (50 g)	6.3	456	80
Milk, liquid, 2% fat, 1 c (250 ml)	8.5	670	100
Salmon, 2 oz (60 g)	15.3	1,450	180
Turkey breast, 2 oz (60 g)	10.2	950	110

Sources:[53–57]

In raw vegan diets, sprouted seeds and grains are moderately good sources of lysine. When seeds and grains (oats, millet, and rice) are sprouted, their lysine content has been shown to increase.[40, 41, 50–52] The percentage of lysine has been shown to double when corn was sprouted for five days and to increase by 65 percent when wheat was sprouted for ten days.[40]

Whereas extra lysine is essential for the growth spurt of early childhood, by adulthood, tryptophan is particularly important for maintenance of body tissues. Tryptophan is the sole precursor for the amino acid that's transformed into the neurotransmitter serotonin, an important compound used by the brain to regulate mood, behavior, and cognition. The body needs just a small amount of tryptophan, about 4 mg/kg/day, bringing the recommended daily intake of tryptophan to roughly 200 to 400 mg for most adults.[3, 17, 53]

Legumes, especially soy foods, and seeds, especially pumpkin seeds, have abundant tryptophan. In vegan and raw vegan diets, some good tryptophan sources are spinach, green peas, nuts (such as cashews, walnuts, almonds, pine nuts, pistachios, and macadamia nuts), and chocolate. The pseudograins buckwheat and millet provide significantly more tryptophan than corn or rice; wheat provides moderate amounts.[54]

Table 3.4 shows the average amounts of protein, lysine, and tryptophan for the food groups shown on The Vegan Plate (page 434); the totals are an average of the items listed in table 3.3. Table 3.4 is based on the minimum number of servings; note that many servings are relatively small amounts. One-half cup (125 ml)

TABLE 3.4. Protein, lysine, and tryptophan contributions by food group

FOOD GROUP	AVERAGE PROTEIN PER SERVING (g)	AVERAGE LYSINE PER SERVING (mg)	AVERAGE TRYPTO-PHAN PER SERVING (mg)	MINIMUM SERVINGS FOR GROUPS ON THE VEGAN PLATE (page 434)	MINIMUM INTAKE PER DAY BASED ON MINIMUMS ON THE VEGAN PLATE (page 434)		
					PROTEIN (g)	LYSINE (mg)	TRYPTOPHAN (mg)
Legumes	9.7	594	111	3	29.1	1,782	333
Nuts and seeds	5.4	219	85	1	5.4	219	85
Grains	3.5	119	40	3	10.5	363	357
Vegetables	1.6	80	19	5	8	400	95
Fruits	0.8	40	10	4	3.2	160	40
Total					56.2	2,924	910
Target intakes per kilogram of body weight					0.9	38	4
Example: target intakes for a 60 kg (132 lb) person					54	2,280	240

Sources: [53–57]

of cooked cereal, rice, or pasta plus two slices of bread add up to three servings from the Grain food group. Very active people are likely to eat more than three servings of these foods. It becomes apparent that fruitarian or raw diets that lack grains and legumes can be low in these amino acids, as can corn- or rice-based vegan diets without legumes.

CARNITINE

Before leaving the topic of amino acids, a discussion of carnitine (and taurine, covered in the next section) is warranted. Carnitine helps to convert fat into energy by carrying fatty acids into cell mitochondria (the body's energy-production centers) and by removing waste products. The body synthesizes carnitine in the liver and kidneys from lysine (legumes are good sources) and methionine (abundant in grains and vegetables) and typically makes sufficient amounts to meet the needs of most people. Carnitine synthesis is dependent on vitamin C, niacin, vitamin B_6, and iron,[58] all of which are abundant in balanced vegan diets. (For mineral and vitamin sources, see table 6.2 on page 204 and table 7.3 on page 252.)

Carnitine itself is found in beef and in lesser amounts in other animal products. Only miniscule amounts are present in a few vegan foods, such as asparagus or a peanut butter sandwich;[59-63] carnitine also is produced by yeast. As a result, research shows, vegans' plasma carnitine levels are somewhat lower than those of nonvegetarians, though within normal ranges. The ability of vegans to maintain adequate carnitine levels is believed to be due to adequate production and efficient reabsorption of losses through the kidneys.[58, 61, 64-67]

Carnitine is promoted as a weight-loss supplement and for improved sports performance, although the American College of Sports Medicine, the Academy of Nutrition and Dietetics, and the Dietitians of Canada list carnitine as a supplement that "does not perform as claimed."[27] However, supplementary carnitine is required by preterm infants, who aren't yet able to manufacture it, and by people (such as alcoholics) whose protein-deficient diets lack the amino acids from which they could build carnitine. A small proportion of people also have found that supplemental carnitine can help to reduce migraine headaches, hypoglycemia, or muscle weakness; for those with type 2 diabetes, carnitine can improve LDL cholesterol levels.[68, 69]

Over-the-counter acetyl-L-carnitine supplements—which are vegan and in veggie caps—are available in the United States (in Canada, they're only available by prescription). However, intakes of supplemental carnitine in the range of 2 to 4 grams per day can have undesirable side effects, such as nausea, diarrhea, and production of a fishy body odor.[70] In addition, carnitine is not to be taken during pregnancy or by those with thyroid problems or a history of seizures.

Intakes of dietary carnitine are linked with heart disease and prostate cancer, so vegans' lower intakes may turn out to be a considerable health advantage. Recent research has shown that intestinal bacteria in nonvegetarians convert the carnitine from animal products or supplements into a toxic compound known as TMAO (trimethylamine N-oxide), which may raise the risk of atherosclerosis and lead to strokes or heart attacks. Animal products other than meat can also contribute to TMAO levels.[71]

TAURINE

Animal products such as beef contain the amino acid taurine (hence the name, which is related to the Latin word for bull). Taurine isn't generally found in plant foods, although amounts from 1 to 26 mg of taurine per gram dry weight have been found in raw and sprouted lentils.[72] Cats need taurine, which for them is an essential amino acid; as a result, they require a meat-based diet or one supplemented with taurine.

Unlike cats, however, humans past infancy can synthesize taurine in their bodies from the amino acids methionine and cysteine.[73-75] Infants—especially preterm infants—do require dietary taurine; however, it's present in breast milk and in infant formula.[76] Research doesn't indicate that supplementary taurine is required past infancy, except in specific medical conditions.

Percentage by Weight versus Percentage of Calories in Foods

T o show the amounts or proportions of calorie-containing nutrients, foods are described in one of two ways. The first is in terms of the *percentage by weight* of fat, protein, and carbohydrate they contain. For example, the "reduced fat" beverage known as "2 percent milk" contains 2 grams of fat per 100 grams of milk; the remaining weight consists of 3 grams of protein and 6 grams of carbohydrate (lactose sugar), plus 89 grams of water.

Foods also may be described in terms of the *percentage of calories* derived from fat, protein, and carbohydrate—and this yields quite a different picture of their nutrient content. When the body converts fat, protein, and carbohydrate to calories, it derives approximately 9 calories from each gram of fat, 4 calories from each gram of protein or carbohydrate, and no calories from water. So, in "2 percent milk," protein provides 27 percent of the calories, 38 percent comes from carbohydrate, and 35 percent from fat. From this perspective, the beverage could effectively be called "35 percent milk" rather than "2 percent milk."

For comparison, in "original" soy milk, which is modeled on 2 percent milk, 32 percent of calories are derived from protein, 33 percent from carbohydrate, and 35 percent from fat. (Even when the quantity of fat in a nondairy milk is similar to that of cow's milk, the former contains far less saturated fat and is cholesterol-free.) In rice milk, protein provides about 3 percent of the calories, carbohydrate 82 percent, and fat 15 percent.

Recommended Ranges of Calories: Protein, Carbohydrate, and Fat

F or overall balance in a diet, aim for 10 to 20 percent of calories from protein, 50 to 75 percent of calories from carbohydrate, and 15 to 30 percent of calories from fat. This guideline is a blend of the recommendations from the two leading health organizations, WHO and IOM, regarding the optimal distribution of the calorie-providing nutrients in diets that supply sufficient calories.[15, 17, 75]

- **Protein.** Ideally, 10 to 20 percent of calories should come from protein. For most people, 10 to 15 percent of calories from protein is adequate. Those whose total caloric intakes are low (such as the elderly or dieters) should aim toward the upper end of this range. When people consume insufficient calories, as they intentionally do on a weight-loss plan, the percentage of calories from protein should be about 15 to 20 percent. Otherwise, they'll lose not only weight but also body protein and muscle mass.

Research from a nationally representative American study, the National Health and Nutrition Examination Survey III (NHANES III) indicates that those aged 50 to 65 whose intakes were greater than 20 percent protein had a 75 percent increase in overall mortality, a fourfold increase in cancer death, and a fivefold increase in death from type 2 diabetes over the next eighteen years (though these statistics didn't hold if the proteins were plant derived).[108]

- **Carbohydrate.** Carbohydrate should provide 50 to 75 percent of calories, though raw vegan diets may provide a little less carbohydrate and still support health.

- **Fat.** In most diets, fat should provide 15 to 30 percent of calories. Some raw vegan diets with abundant nuts, seeds, and avocados have a higher proportion of calories from fat, such as 35 percent, and still are healthful.[49] (For more details, see "Recommended Fat Intakes" on page 111.) At the other end of the spectrum, people whose goal is to reverse cardiovascular disease or other chronic disease can benefit from therapeutic diets with as little as 10 percent of calories from fat.[78–80] Surprisingly, as shown in table 3.5 (page 97), lettuce and other leafy greens provide 8 to 13 percent of calories from fat without a drop of salad dressing.

As table 3.5 shows, meat, eggs, and cheese are significant sources of protein, with 24 to 36 percent of total calories coming from protein. Yet meat, eggs, and cheese might well be viewed primarily as fat sources instead of protein sources, because about 60 to 75 percent of their calories are provided by fat. Fortunately, every whole (unrefined) plant food contains small or moderate amounts of protein; many provide 25 to 35 percent of calories from protein—but without all the fat and cholesterol of animal products. The percentage of calories from protein in green vegetables and legumes is in the range of 10 to 37 percent. Tofu is somewhat higher in protein, and vegan meat substitutes higher still. The percentage of calories from protein in nuts, seeds, and grains is in the range of 9 to 17 percent. At the low end of the spectrum are fruits, with just 2 to 10 percent of calories from protein.

Table 3.5 shows the calories, grams of protein, and the distribution of calories among a food's macronutrients. Note that nutrient content can differ from one variety or crop to another, so don't be surprised by differences from one database to another. For certain packaged items, the data in table 3.5 are typical; for variations among brands, check labels.

TABLE 3.5. Calories, protein, and percentage of calories from protein, carbohydrate, and fat in selected foods

FOOD	CALORIES PER UNIT	PROTEIN PER UNIT (g)	CALORIES FROM PROTEIN (%)	CALORIES FROM CARBO-HYDRATE (%)	CALORIES FROM FAT (%)
LEGUMES (COOKED UNLESS STATED)					
Adzuki beans, ½ c (125 ml)	147	9	23	76	1
Black beans, ½ c (125 ml)	114	8	26	70	4
Black-eyed peas, ½ c (125 ml)	105	7	26	70	4
Chickpeas, ½ c (125 ml)	134	7	21	65	14
Cranberry beans, ½ c (125 ml)	120	8	27	70	3
Edamame, ½ c (125 ml)	100	10	41	37	22
Falafels, three, 1.7 oz (51 g)	170	7	16	37	47
Great Northern beans, ½ c (125 ml)	104	7	27	69	3
Kidney beans, ½ c (125 ml)	112	7	27	70	3
Lentils, ½ c (125 ml)	115	9	30	67	3
Lentil sprouts, raw, 1 c (250 ml)	82	7	28	68	4
Lima beans, ½ c (125 ml)	115	7	25	72	3
Mung beans, ½ c (125 ml)	94	7	28	68	4
Mung bean sprouts, raw, 1 c (250 ml)	31	3	32	64	4
Navy beans, ½ c (125 ml)	127	7	23	73	4
Peanuts, ¼ c (60 ml)	207	9	17	11	72
Peanut butter, 2 T (30 ml)	192	8	16	12	72
Pea sprouts, raw, 1 c (250 ml)	154	11	23	73	4
Pinto beans, ½ c (125 ml)	122	8	25	71	4
Soybeans, ½ c (125 ml)	157	15	36	21	43
Soy milk, original, 1 c (250 ml)*	80–140	6–11	21–33	33–53	20–35
Split peas, ½ c (125 ml)	116	8	27	70	3
Tempeh, ½ c (125 ml)*	160	15	35	18	47
Tofu, firm, ½ c (125 ml)*	183	20	40	11	49
Vegan burger, selected, 2.5–3 oz (75–90 g)*	70–95	10–14	45–61	27–55	0–24
Vegan deli slices, 2 oz (60 g)*	77	13	85	14	1
Vegan hot dog, 1.5–2.5 oz (42–70 g)*	45–163	7–14	26–92	5–13	0–67
Vegan ground round, 2 oz (60 g)*	65–85	10–14	53–71	27–47	0–7
White beans, ½ c (125 ml)	124–127	8–9	25–27	70–71	2–4
NUTS AND SEEDS (RAW UNLESS STATED)					
Almonds, ¼ c (60 ml)	207–213	7–8	13	13	74
Almond butter, 2 T (30 ml)	203	5	9	13	78

FOOD	CALORIES PER UNIT	PROTEIN PER UNIT (g)	CALORIES FROM PROTEIN (%)	CALORIES FROM CARBO-HYDRATE (%)	CALORIES FROM FAT (%)
Almond milk, original, 1 c (250 ml)*	60	1	7	55	38
Brazil nuts, ¼ c (60 ml)	230	5	8	7	85
Brazil nut, large	31	0.7	8	6	86
Cashews, ¼ c (60 ml)	188	6	12	21	67
Cashew butter, 2 T (30 ml)	188	6	11	18	71
Chia seeds, ¼ c (60 ml)	196	6	12	34	54
Flaxseeds, ground, ¼ c (60 ml)	144	7	14	23	63
Hazelnuts/filberts, ¼ c (60 ml)	212	5	9	10	81
Hempseeds, ¼ c (60 ml)*	227	13	27	28	55
Hempseed milk, 1 c (250 ml)*	130	4	13	65	22
Pecans, ¼ c (60 ml)	187	2	5	7	88
Pine nuts/pignolia nuts, ¼ c (60 ml)	227–229	5–10	8–16	7–9	75–85
Pistachio nuts, ¼ c (60 ml)	178	7	14	19	67
Poppy seeds, ¼ c (60 ml)	179	6	13	17	70
Pumpkin seeds, ¼ c (60 ml)	180	10	17	12	71
Sesame seed kernels, ¼ c (60 ml)	237	8	12	7	81
Sesame seeds, whole, ¼ c (60 ml)	206	6	12	15	73
Sesame tahini, 2 T (30 ml)	178	5	11	14	75
Sunflower seed kernels, ¼ c (60 ml)	210	7	13	13	74
Sunflower seed butter, 2 T (30 ml)	185	6	13	18	69
Walnuts, black, ¼ c (60 ml)	190	8	15	7	78
Walnuts, English, ¼ c (60 ml)	194	5	9	8	83
Water chestnuts, Chinese, ¼ c (60 ml)	30	0.4	5	94	1
GRAINS (COOKED UNLESS STATED)					
Amaranth, ½ c (125 ml)	133	5	15	72	13
Barley, pearl, ½ c (125 ml)	102	2	7	81	6
Bread, rye, slice, 1 oz (30 g)	78	3	13	75	12
Bread, white, slice, 1 oz (30 g)*	80	3	14	75	11
Bread, whole wheat, slice, 1 oz (30 g)*	74	4	21	67	12
Buckwheat, ½ c (125 ml)	82	3	14	81	5
Buckwheat sprouts, raw, 1 c (250 ml)	65	2	14	80	6
Cornmeal, dry, ¼ c (60 ml)	110	2	9	82	9
Corn tortilla, 6 in (15 cm)*	65	2	10	79	11
Kamut, ½ c (125 ml)	133	6	17	78	5
Millet, ½ c (125 ml)	109	3	12	80	8

FOOD	CALORIES PER UNIT	PROTEIN PER UNIT (g)	CALORIES FROM PROTEIN (%)	CALORIES FROM CARBO-HYDRATE (%)	CALORIES FROM FAT (%)
Oatmeal, ½ c (125 ml)	88	3	14	67	19
Quinoa, dry, ¼ c (60 ml)	159	6	15	71	14
Quinoa, ½ c (125 ml)	117	4	15	71	14
Rice, brown, medium grain, ½ c (125 ml)	115	2	8	85	7
Rice, white, medium grain, ½ c (125 ml)	128	2	8	91	1
Rice milk, original, 1 c (250 ml)*	66	0.6	3	84	13
Spaghetti, ½ c (125 ml)	117	4	15	80	5
Spaghetti, whole wheat, ½ c (125 ml)	92	4	16	80	4
Spelt, ½ c (125 ml)	130	6	16	78	6
Wheat sprouts, raw, 1 c (250 ml)	226	9	14	81	5
Whole wheat tortilla, 1 oz (30 g)*	89	3	12	67	21
Wild rice, ½ c (125 ml)	88	3	15	82	3
VEGETABLES (RAW UNLESS STATED)					
Asparagus, cooked, ½ c (125 ml)	21	2	34	59	7
Avocado, all types, 7 oz (201 g)	324	4	5	17	78
Avocado, California, 4.5 oz (136 g)	227	3	4	19	77
Avocado, Florida, 10 oz (304 g)	365	7	7	24	69
Avocados, all types, chopped, ½ c (125 ml)	123	2	5	17	79
Basil, fresh, chopped, ½ c (125 ml)	10	1	44	37	19
Beans, snap green/wax, ½ c (125 ml)	17	1	20	77	3
Beet greens, 1 c (250 ml)	9	1	33	63	4
Beet juice, ½ c (125 ml)	41	1	12	88	0
Beets, chopped, cooked, ½ c (125 ml)	29	1	14	83	3
Bok choy, chopped, 1 c (250 ml)	10	1	36	53	11
Broccoli, cooked, ½ c (125 ml)	29	2	23–34	57–68	9
Brussels sprouts, ½ c (125 ml)	28	2	24	66	10
Cabbage, green, chopped, 1 c (250 ml)	22	1	18	79	3
Cabbage, napa, chopped, 1 c (250 ml)	15	1	29–33	67–71	0
Cabbage, red, chopped, 1 c (250 ml)	28	1	16	80	4
Carrot, 7½ in (19 cm)	30	1	8	87	5
Carrot, chopped, cooked, ½ c (125 ml)	42	1	9	88	3
Carrot juice, ½ c (125 ml)	48	1	9	88	3
Cauliflower, cooked, ½ c (125 ml)	14	1	26	59	15
Celery, chopped, 1 c (250 ml)	9	0.4	17	74	9
Celery rib, 11–12 in (28–30 cm)	10	0.4	17	74	9

FOOD	CALORIES PER UNIT	PROTEIN PER UNIT (g)	CALORIES FROM PROTEIN (%)	CALORIES FROM CARBO-HYDRATE (%)	CALORIES FROM FAT (%)
Celery root, chopped, 1 c (250 ml)	66	2	13	81	6
Cilantro, 1 c (250 ml)	19	2	27	58	15
Collard greens, chopped, 1 c (250 ml)	11	0.9	27	63	10
Corn, yellow/white, ½ c (125 ml)	66	2	13	76	11
Cucumber, chopped, ½ c (125 ml)	8	0.4	18	74	8
Dandelion greens, 1 c (250 ml)	26	2	20	68	12
Eggplant, cubed, cooked, ½ c (125 ml)	14	0.4	11	83	6
Endive greens, 1 c (250 ml)	9	0.7	25	66	9
Garlic clove, 0.1 oz (3 g)	3	0.2	16	81	3
Garlic cloves, ½ c (125 ml)	101	4	16	81	3
Green Giant Juice, 1 c (250 ml)**	36	3	35	58	7
Horseradish, ½ c (125 ml)	72	3	18	78	4
Jerusalem artichokes, ½ c (125 ml)	55	1	10	90	0
Kale, chopped, 1 c (250 ml)	35	2	22	67	11
Kale juice, 1 c (250 ml)**	64	6	39	50	11
Kelp, raw, ½ c (125 ml)	18	1	14	76	10
Leeks, chopped, 1 c (250 ml)	57	1	9	87	4
Lettuce, butterhead, chopped, 1 c (250 ml)	7	0.7	33	55	12
Lettuce, iceberg, chopped, 1 c (250 ml)	11	0.6	22	71	8
Lettuce, leaf, chopped, 1 c (250 ml)	6	0.5	30	62	8
Lettuce, red leaf, chopped, 1 c (250 ml)	5	0.4	33	55	12
Lettuce, romaine, chopped, 1 c (250 ml)	8	0.6	24	63	13
Mushrooms, ½ c (125 ml)	11	1	37	60	3
Mushrooms, shiitake, dried, ¼ c (60 ml)	122	10	31	62	7
Mustard greens, 1 c (250 ml)	15	2	34	60	6
Okra, cooked, ½ c (125 ml)	18	2	27	66	7
Olives, ½ c (125 ml)	77	0.6	4	7	89
Onion, green, 0.2 oz (5 g)	5	0.3	19	77	4
Onions, green, chopped, 1 c (250 ml)	32	2	19	77	4
Onions, red/yellow/white, ½ c (125 ml)	34	1	10	88	2
Parsley, chopped, 1 c (64 g)	23	2	27	57	16
Parsnips, chopped, cooked, ½ c (125 ml)	63	1	6	91	3
Peas, ½ c (125 ml)	62	4	26	70	4
Pea pods, snow/edible pod, ½ c (125 ml)	22	1	26	70	4
Pepper, bell, medium, 4.2 oz (119 g)	24	1	14	79	7

FOOD	CALORIES PER UNIT	PROTEIN PER UNIT (g)	CALORIES FROM PROTEIN (%)	CALORIES FROM CARBO-HYDRATE (%)	CALORIES FROM FAT (%)
Peppers, bell, chopped, ½ c (125 ml)	16–24	1	14	79	7
Peppers, hot chile, ½ c (125 ml)	32	2	17	79	4
Potato, baked, medium, 3 in (173 g)	189	4	8	91	1
Potato, cooked, ½ c (125 ml)	52	1	10	89	1
Radish, medium, ¾-1 in (2–3 cm)	0.8	0	16	79	5
Radish sprouts, 1 c (250 ml)	17	2	29	28	43
Radishes, chopped, ½ c (125 ml)	9	0.4	16	79	5
Radishes, Oriental, 7 in (18 cm)	61	2	12	83	5
Radishes, Oriental, dried, ½ c (125 ml)	157	5	11	87	2
Rutabaga, chopped, cooked, ½ c (125 ml)	33	1	12	83	5
Spinach, chopped, 1 c (250 ml)	7	1	39	49	12
Spirulina seaweed, dried, 1 T (15 ml)	22	4	58	24	18
Squash, acorn, cooked, ½ c (125 ml)	57	1	7	91	2
Squash, butternut, cooked, ½ c (125 ml)	41	1	8	90	2
Squash, crookneck and other summer, cooked, ½ c (125 ml)	18	1	15	73	12
Squash, Hubbard, cooked, ½ c (125 ml)	60	3	17	74	9
Sweet potato, cooked, ½ c (125 ml)	125	2	7	91	2
Tomato, cherry, 0.5 oz (17 g)	3	0.2	17	74	9
Tomato, Italian/plum, 2 oz (62 g)	11	0.6	17	74	9
Tomato, medium, 4 oz (120 g)	22	1	17	74	9
Tomatoes, chopped, ½ c (125 ml)	17	1	17	74	9
Tomatoes, sun-dried, ½ c (125 ml)	70	4	18	73	9
Turnip, cooked, ½ c (125 ml)	27	1	12	85	3
Turnip greens, chopped, 1 c (250 ml)	19	1	16	77	7
Watercress greens, chopped, 1 c (250 ml)	4	1	60	34	6
Yam, baked, ½ c (125 ml)	90	2	9	90	1
Zucchini, baby, 0.4 oz (12 g)	2	0.3	40	47	13
Zucchini, chopped, 1 c (250 ml)	20	2	25	67	8
FRUITS (RAW UNLESS STATED)					
Apple, chopped, ½ c (125 ml)	32	0.2	2	95	3
Apple, medium, 6 oz (180 g)	95	0.5	2	95	3
Apples, dried, ¼ c (60 ml)	110	1	4	96	0
Apricot (35 g)	17	0.5	10	83	7
Apricots, chopped, ½ c (125 ml)	40	1	10	83	7

FOOD	CALORIES PER UNIT	PROTEIN PER UNIT (g)	CALORIES FROM PROTEIN (%)	CALORIES FROM CARBO-HYDRATE (%)	CALORIES FROM FAT (%)
Apricots, dried, ¼ c (60 ml)	77	1	5	93	2
Banana, dried, ¼ c (60 ml)	86	1	4	92	4
Banana, medium (118 g)	105	1	4	93	3
Banana slices, ½ c (125 ml)	71	0.9	4	93	3
Blackberries, ½ c (125 ml)	31	1	11	80	9
Blueberries, ½ c (125 ml)	45	0.6	5	90	5
Blueberries, dried, ¼ c (60 ml)	140	1	3	97	0
Cantaloupe, chopped, ½ c (125 ml)	28	0.7	9	87	4
Cherimoya fruit, ½ c (125 ml)	73	1	5	92	3
Coconut, dried, ¼ c (60 ml)	122	1	4	13	83
Coconut milk, fresh, ½ c (125 ml)	292	3	4	9	87
Crab apple slices, ½ c (125 ml)	42	0.2	2	95	3
Currants, fresh, ½ c (125 ml)	31–35	0.8	8–9	87–88	3–5
Currants, Zante, dried, ¼ c (60 ml)	103	1	5	94	1
Dates, pitted, chopped, ¼ c (60 ml)	104	0.9	3	96	1
Durian, chopped, ½ c (125 ml)	179	2	4	66	30
Fig, medium, fresh, 2¼ in (6 cm)	37	0.4	4	93	3
Figs, dried, ¼ c (60 ml)	129	2	4	92	4
Gooseberries, ½ c (125 ml)	33	0.7	7	82	11
Grape juice, bottled, ½ c (125 ml)	77	0.7	4	95	1
Grapefruit, 8.5 oz (246 g)	103	2	7	90	3
Grapefruit juice, ½ c (125 ml)	51	0.7	5	93	2
Grapefruit sections, ½ c (125 ml)	37	0.7	7	90	3
Grapes, ½ c (125 ml)	31	0.3	3	93	4
Guava, fresh, ½ c (125 ml)	56	2	13	75	11
Honeydew melon, chopped, ½ c (125 ml)	31	0.5	5	92	3
Kiwifruit, chopped, ½ c (125 ml)	57	2	7	86	7
Kiwifruit, medium, 2.3 oz (69 g)	42	0.8	4	86	10
Loganberries, ½ c (125 ml)	31	1	11	80	9
Mango, 7 oz (207 g)	135	1	3	94	3
Mango, chopped, ½ c (125 ml)	54	0.4	3	94	3
Mango, dried, ¼ c (60 ml)	106	0	0	100	0
Orange, medium (131 g)	62	1	7	91	2
Orange juice, ½ c (125 ml)	56	0.9	6	90	4

FOOD	CALORIES PER UNIT	PROTEIN PER UNIT (g)	CALORIES FROM PROTEIN (%)	CALORIES FROM CARBO-HYDRATE (%)	CALORIES FROM FAT (%)
Orange sections, ½ c (125 ml)	45	0.9	7	91	2
Papaya, cubes, ½ c (125 ml)	27	0.4	6	91	3
Peach, chopped, ½ c (125 ml)	30	0.7	8	87	5
Peach, dried, 0.5 oz (15 g)	37	0.7	7	93	0
Peach, medium, 5 oz (150 g)	58	1	6	88	6
Pear, chopped, ½ c (125 ml)	41	0.3	2	96	2
Pear, medium (178 g)	103	0.7	2	96	2
Pear halves, dried, 2 halves (35 g)	92	0.7	3	95	2
Pineapple, chopped, ½ c (125 ml)	41	0.4	4	94	2
Plum (76 g)	35	0.5	5	86	0
Plum, chopped, ½ c (125 ml)	45	0.7	5	86	9
Prunes, ¼ c (60 ml)	104	1	4	95	1
Raisins, ¼ c (60 ml)	123	1	4	95	1
Raspberries, ½ c (125 ml)	30	0.6	7	84	9
Strawberries, ½ c (125 ml)	24	0.5	7	86	7
Strawberries, dried, ¼ c (60 ml)	75	0.5	3	97	0
Watermelon, ½ c (125 ml)	23	0.5	7	89	4
OILS AND SWEETENERS					
Flaxseed oil, 1 T (15 ml)	122	0	0	0	100
Granulated cane sugar, 1 T (15 ml)	48	0	0	100	0
Maple syrup, 1 T (15 ml)	52	0	0	99	1
Olive oil, 1 T (15 ml)	119	0	0	0	100
ANIMAL PRODUCTS					
Beef, ground round, broiled or baked, 2 oz (60 g)	152	15	39	0	61
Cheddar cheese, medium, 1 oz (30 g)*	118	8	24	4	72
Chicken breast, roasted, 2 oz (60 g)	118	18	63	0	37
Egg, large, 2.7 oz (50 g)	72	6	33	3	64
Milk, 2%, 1 c (250 ml)	121	8	27	39	35
Salmon, sockeye, baked, 2 oz (60 g)	101	15	63	0	37

Sources:[54, 55]

*Also see package label.

**Laboratory analyses by Cantest Lab. Green Giant Juice ingredients: kale, romaine lettuce, lemon juice, cucumber, apple, celery, lemon; recipe from *Becoming Raw* by B. Davis and V. Melina.

Vegan Protein and Caloric Intakes

Do vegans typically get enough dietary protein? Studies conducted since 1982 on vegans who live in the United States, Australia, France, Germany, Italy, and the United Kingdom show average protein intakes to be in the range of 10 to 14 percent of calories, well within the recommendations.[11, 81, 82]

The North American, Australian, and European studies show average caloric intakes of 1,982 calories per day for vegan men and 1,668 calories per day for vegan women. In contrast, a study of Vietnamese vegan women showed very low average intakes of 1,130 calories per day.[11] Somewhat lower caloric intakes, compared with the general population, are likely to be a factor in the relatively low BMIs of vegans.

Also, intakes on Western raw diets can be lower. A study conducted in Germany on 43 people who consumed raw vegan diets showed quite a different picture; their diets provided only 8.2 percent of calories from protein. The men and women on these raw vegan diets averaged caloric intakes of 1,888 calories per day.[11, 83]

For comparison, national surveys across the United States and Canada, which included men and women on all types of diets, show that protein provides about 15 percent of total calories for adults under 60 and 16 percent for those 60 and older and that caloric intakes are higher than vegan intakes.[15] The NHANES 1999–2000 Survey showed mean caloric intakes for American men to be 2,419 calories at ages 20 to 39; 2,196 calories at ages 40 to 59; and 1,772 calories at 60 years and older. This survey showed mean caloric intakes for American women to be 2,028 calories at ages 20 to 39; 1,828 calories at ages 40 to 59; and 1,534 calories at 60 years and older. Data show Canadian intakes to be similar.[84, 85]

Acid-Base Balance, Protein, and Diet

In past decades, a hypothesis that was popular among vegans and others linked diets high in protein (particularly animal protein) with osteoporosis. The theory was based on the premise that meat and other animal products are acid forming in the body. In addition, two grains prominent in American diets, wheat and rice, also can be acid forming. It had been presumed that calcium, which has an alkaline effect, is drawn from bones to neutralize the acid and is then excreted in urine. Epidemiological studies lent further support to the theory, because osteoporosis rates are elevated in countries with the highest intakes of animal protein. It seemed to be a closed case. However, recent evidence suggests that the urinary calcium excretion induced by protein is offset by the positive effects of protein, both on calcium absorption from foods and on bone formation. In other words, protein can help a body to absorb more calcium, and then the body loses some calcium in urine.[86]

The subject is complex, because bone health is a function of so many interacting factors, including numerous minerals and vitamins, and exercise. It's true that excessive animal protein can be acid forming and that roots, tubers, leaves, other vegetables, and fruits are alkali forming. Bone health is supported by diets centered on vegetables, fruits, and legumes, all rich in the mineral potassium, which can balance acid-forming dietary factors. Research also confirms that healthy bones require adequate intakes of protein, which is a key part of the bone matrix; clearly, legumes and vegetables have a lot to offer.[49, 87–95]

Soy and Health

Though soy isn't essential in vegan diets, including some soy foods provides an excellent and often easy way for children and adults to reach recommended intakes of protein and of the amino acids lysine and tryptophan. Soy is well-known for its top-quality protein; solid research also shows it offers protection against certain chronic diseases. At the same time, considerable controversy surrounds soy.[96] The roots of the controversy lie in good science and bad—and perhaps in the fact that soy foods pose a threat to the animal products industry.

THE RELIABLE SCIENCE ON SOY

Research has established that soy foods can have the following effects:

- Soy can affect the thyroid gland in the small number of people who are hypothyroid or who are deficient in iodine. For these individuals, it makes sense to limit soy consumption until the problem is corrected.[11, 96–98] Solutions involve adjusting the dosage of thyroid hormone for those with hypothyroidism, and where iodine intakes are insufficient, that problem is easily fixed. (For more on iodine and other foods that affect the thyroid, see page 192.)

- Soy's isoflavones can bind to the body's estrogen receptors (ER), and have a particular affinity for ER beta-receptors. This means isoflavones have some of the beneficial effects of estrogen, without having all this hormone's influences.[97–99] Considerable research has explored the impact of soy's affinity for these receptors on women's health. It turns out that moderate consumption of soy—meaning one to three servings per day—protects women against breast cancer, and that this protective effect may be particularly linked to soy consumption during childhood. For those who have had breast cancer, soy and its isoflavones reduce the risk of recurrence and death from the disease. Soy also may reduce hot flashes and wrinkles.[96, 98–101]

There's significant evidence that eating one or two servings per day of soy foods, such as tofu, soy milk, or tempeh, can lower LDL cholesterol. Intakes of about one serving per day of soy also have been shown to reduce the risk of prostate cancer by 26 to 30 percent.[96, 98, 100]

THE MISAPPLIED SCIENCE

Some of the science on soy has been distorted by people who misunderstood or sensationalized the research when scientific articles have been published—and then misinterpreted—leading to rumors that spiraled out of control. Some of this misinformation resulted from studies concerning two men who regularly consumed fourteen to twenty servings of soy daily (one derived almost all of his calories from soy) and subsequently developed health problems, such as enlarged breast tissue and loss of libido. In both cases, when soy intake was reduced, their health and libido reverted to normal.[103, 105, 106]

It's not surprising that such an unbalanced diet led to problems. These two situations shouldn't be construed to show that moderate intakes of soy foods are unsuitable for men and for other family members. It's been well established that two or three servings of soy foods daily is an appropriate, healthful intake.[96, 98, 100, 102, 103] However, soy shouldn't crowd out other health-supportive plant foods.

Some of the antisoy propaganda has been based on studies involving raw soybeans (which can be toxic to many species in their raw form due to the presence of trypsin inhibitors) and involving subjects such as rats or parrots—which are particularly unsuited to diets of raw soy. The health of parrots or rats forced to eat a diet of raw soybeans can't be compared to that of humans, who can thrive on several daily servings of soy foods prepared by traditional cooking methods.

SOY IN ITS VARIOUS FORMS

The different forms of soy have a variety of benefits.[96, 98, 103] Tofu and soy milk are versatile soy foods with proven nutritional features and health benefits established during centuries of use across Asia. The soaking and cooking that occur when soybeans are prepared for use in soy milk and tofu improve digestibility and mineral availability. The same can be said for tempeh, and its fermentation process further supports healthy gut flora and the body's absorption of minerals. Edamame, or young soybeans from the garden, are whole foods that can be steamed and eaten out of the shell. Soy protein isolate (also known as isolated soy protein) is highly rated in terms of protein quality. For occasions when convenience is a priority, soy-based meat substitutes or protein powders may come in handy. In general though, it's best to eat traditional forms of soy to benefit from the broad range of nutrients and to keep sodium in check. Rather than judging one form of soy as better than another, it makes sense to regard them as variations that suit one or another dietary preference or occasion, with organic and GMO-free products emphasized as much as possible.[15, 54, 96, 98, 107]

THE BOTTOM LINE

Unless someone chooses a "chips and soda" style of eating or a fruitarian diet, getting enough protein is easily accomplished with a vegan diet that provides sufficient calories. Menu planning may present a few challenges until people learn simple, tasty ways to include beans, peas, lentils, and soy foods in their diets. These high-protein ingredients deliver iron, zinc, lysine, tryptophan, and plenty of other nutrients; they also help to stabilize blood glucose. For these reasons, this book emphasizes the use of legumes. Its companion volume, *Cooking Vegan* by Vesanto Melina and Joseph Forest (Book Publishing Company, 2012), provides recipes for delicious protein-rich dips, spreads, soups, entrées, and desserts.[108] Beyond legumes, vegetables, seeds, nuts, and grains provide a healthy boost of protein (in addition to many other nutrients).

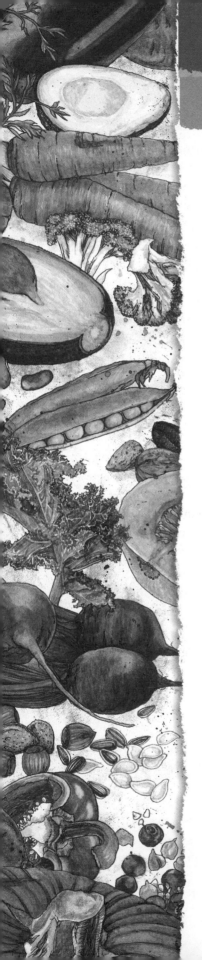

4

Balancing Fats

The best way to choose the best fats is to choose the best foods in the right proportions. If you are expecting to find your way to better eating and health by selecting a single villain or savior, well—fat chance.

DAVID KATZ, MD, FOUNDING DIRECTOR OF YALE UNIVERSITY'S PREVENTION RESEARCH CENTER

Consumers have questioned the relative health value of fats (or lack thereof) for decades. Many vegans consider the complete absence of animal fats and cholesterol as the nutritional trump card of plant-based diets. However, becoming vegan doesn't guarantee healthful fat intakes. Although vegan diets generally keep saturated fat, trans-fatty acids, and cholesterol in check, there are concerns that they could fall short where essential fatty acids are concerned. In fact, some experts maintain that fish-free diets can't provide optimal omega-3 fatty acid intakes. They advocate direct sources of long-chain omega-3 fatty acids for vegans and others who avoid fish.

Heated debates about the optimal amount of dietary fat rage on. Discussions surrounding the best sources of fat are no less intense, leaving vegan consumers with many unanswered questions. What are the differences among various fats, and which are the most valuable sources for vegans? Is coconut oil healthful or harmful? Should everyone heed the "no oil" message? Do vegans need to reduce their consumption of foods rich in omega-6 fatty acids when relying solely on plant sources of omega-3 fatty acids? What's the optimal intake for vegans at every stage of life?

A Primer on Fats

Lipids. Lipids are a family of organic compounds, most of which don't dissolve in water. The most widely recognized lipids include fatty acids, solid fats and liquid oils (triglycerides), sterols (such as cholesterol), phospholipids (such as lecithin), fat-soluble vitamins and phytochemicals, and waxes. Although fats are only one type of lipid, the words *fat* and *lipid* are commonly used interchangeably.

Fatty acids. Fatty acids are basic components of fats and oils, as well as emulsifiers. Triglycerides have three fatty acid chains; mono- and diglycerides have one or two fatty acid chains, respectively. These chains of varying lengths are built of carbon atoms to which hydrogen and oxygen atoms are attached. Each fatty acid chain can be saturated, monounsaturated, or polyunsaturated, depending on the number of carbon atoms in the chain that could accommodate a hydrogen atom. A fatty acid chain with one open carbon atom is monounsaturated, while two or more open carbon atoms make the fatty acid polyunsaturated. A fatty acid chain with no open carbon atoms is saturated. Foods can contain varying amounts of saturated, monounsaturated, and polyunsaturated fatty acids, depending on the type of fat, oil, or emulsifier in that food.

Saturated fatty acids. The carbon chain of a saturated fatty acid can't accept any more hydrogen atoms; all the carbon atoms have two hydrogen atoms attached. Saturated fatty acids occur naturally, although hydrogenation can turn a mono- or polyunsaturated fat into a saturated fat. Triglycerides that contain primarily saturated fatty acids are generally solid at room temperature.

A high intake of saturated fat has been linked to an increased risk of coronary artery disease (CAD) and insulin resistance, although this is a topic of considerable controversy.[1-4] Animal products contribute a large percentage of saturated fat in Western diets. Approximately 20 to 30 percent of the fat in fish is saturated, as well as 33 percent in poultry, 40 to 44 percent in red meat, and 62 percent in dairy products. In most high-fat plant foods, only 5 to 20 percent of the fat is saturated. The exceptions are tropical oils. Coconut oil comprises about 87 percent saturated fatty acids, palm kernel oil about 85 percent, and palm oil about 50 percent.

Monounsaturated fatty acids (MUFA). Monounsaturated fatty acids have one spot in the carbon chain where hydrogen is missing (one point of unsaturation). Oils rich in monounsaturated fatty acids are generally liquid at room temperature but become cloudy and thick when refrigerated, as occurs with olive oil.

Monounsaturated fatty acids have been shown to have neutral or slightly beneficial effects on health, with modest effects on blood cholesterol levels. Replacing saturated fats, trans-fatty acids, or refined carbohydrates with monounsaturated fatty acids reduces total and LDL cholesterol and slightly increases HDL cholesterol.[5, 6] The richest dietary sources of monounsaturated fatty acids are olives, olive oil, canola oil, avocados, and nuts (except walnuts, butternuts, and pine nuts).

Polyunsaturated fatty acids (PUFA). Polyunsaturated fatty acids have more than one spot in the carbon chain where hydrogen is missing (more than one point of unsaturation). Oils high in polyunsaturated fatty acids are liquid both at room temperature and when refrigerated. There are two distinct families of polyunsaturated fatty acids—the omega-6s and omega-3s.

Polyunsaturated fatty acids generally have favorable effects on health. When they replace saturated fats, trans-fatty acids, or refined carbohydrates in the diet, total and LDL cholesterol levels decrease and HDL levels may slightly increase.[7] The main dietary sources of polyunsaturated fatty acids are vegetable oils, seeds, nuts, grains, legumes, and other plant foods.

Essential fatty acids (EFA). Most fatty acids needed for survival can be produced in the body. However, two—known as essential fatty acids—can't be synthesized and must be obtained from food: linoleic acid (LA) from the omega-6 family and alpha-linolenic acid (ALA) from the omega-3 family. The body uses LA and ALA to make highly unsaturated fatty acids (HUFA), critical building blocks for the brain, nervous system, and cell membranes. The balance between LA and ALA can have significant consequences for health, particularly for people who don't consume direct sources of long-chain omega-3 fatty acids.

Cholesterol. Part of cell membranes, cholesterol is present in every body cell. Because the human body makes about 800 to 1,000 mg of this sterol each day, there's no need for any dietary cholesterol. Although trace amounts are found in plants, dietary cholesterol mostly comes from animal products and is concentrated in eggs and organ meats. High intakes may increase the risk for chronic diseases, especially those of the heart and blood vessels.

Phytosterols. Phytosterols are sterols naturally present in plants. By competing with cholesterol during digestion, plant sterols help to block cholesterol absorption in the gut. All whole plant foods contain small amounts of these compounds, although vegetable oils, seeds, nuts, avocados, wheat germ, legumes, and sprouts are the most concentrated sources. Plant-based diets are naturally higher in phytosterols than omnivorous diets.

Hydrogenation. The process of hydrogenation adds hydrogen atoms to oils with polyunsaturated fatty acid chains; the hydrogen atoms attach themselves to the unsaturated carbon atoms. Hydrogenation converts the liquid oil to a semisolid or solid fat, such as margarine. The process is controlled to yield the melting point and other physical properties desired; most oils are only partially hydrogenated because complete hydrogenation would result in a saturated fat. Partially hydrogenated fats extend the shelf life of foods, increase the melting point of cooking fats (allowing higher-temperature cooking), and improve the texture and mouthfeel of products in which they are used.

Trans-fatty acids. Trans-fatty acids are created when the position of one hydrogen atom—added to an unsaturated carbon chain during hydrogenation—changes the original curved fatty acid molecule to a straighter molecule, which has a negative impact on cell membrane function. Approximately 90 percent of trans-fatty acids are formed during partial hydrogenation, which turns liquid oils into solid fats. (The other 10 percent naturally occur through the biohydrogenation of fats in the forestomach of ruminant animals.)

Vegetable oils were originally partially hydrogenated to serve as healthier substitutes for the animal fats they replaced, such as lard and butter. However, they've since been found to be even more damaging to human health than animal fats.[8] Trans-fatty acids produced by hydrogenation strongly increase the risk of cardio-vascular disease (CVD) by adversely affecting a multitude of risk factors.[9–12] As a result, efforts are currently under way in North America to remove artificially produced trans-fatty acids from the food supply.

Trans-fatty acids found naturally in animal products don't appear to be as damaging as those produced during industrial hydrogenation.[11] However, evidence does suggest that these natural trans-fatty acids can impair insulin sensitivity in insulin-resistant individuals to a greater extent than manufactured trans-fatty acids.[13] In addition, natural trans-fatty acids reduce HDL cholesterol and markedly increase both lipid per-oxidation and the creation of free radicals.[14] As a result, trans-fatty acids, both natural and artificial, should be avoided when possible.

Optimal Quantities of Fat for Vegans

Fat intakes vary a great deal among healthy populations around the world. The traditional diets of rural Asians commonly provide about 10 to 15 percent of calories from fat, while those of Mediterranean populations frequently exceed 35 percent of calories from fat.[15, 16] This variation holds true even among the five so-called "Blue Zones," where large segments of the population remain healthy and active into their 90s and beyond. In Okinawa, Japan, traditional diets are very low in fat; in Loma Linda, California, and the Nicoya Peninsula of Costa Rica, fat intakes are moderate; in Sardinia, Italy, and Ikaria, Greece, diets are higher in fat. Although there's no question that overall diet matters, the percentage of calories obtained from fat is clearly not a critical factor for health and longevity.[1, 17]

So what do the diets of these protected people have in common? Residents of all the Blue Zones eat mostly plants. Highly processed fast foods and convenience foods are rarely used. Meat is reserved mainly for special occasions and isn't consumed at all by the vegetarian Adventists in Loma Linda. Blue-Zone researcher and author, Dan Buettner states, "Beans, whole grains, and garden vegetables are the cornerstone of all these longevity diets."[18] In addition, residents of one or more of these areas include nuts, soy foods, antioxidant-rich spices, and dark wines in their diets. Figure 4.1 features a diagram of the lifestyle factors shared by three Blue-Zone populations (Okinawa, Loma Linda, and Sardinia). In Ikaria, Greece, the dietary cornerstones are vegetables (including potatoes and wild greens) and beans; meat and sugar intakes are low. In the Nicoya Peninsula of Costa Rica, corn tortillas, beans, and tropical fruits serve as the dietary staples.

FIGURE 4.1. Lifestyle factors of three Blue Zones

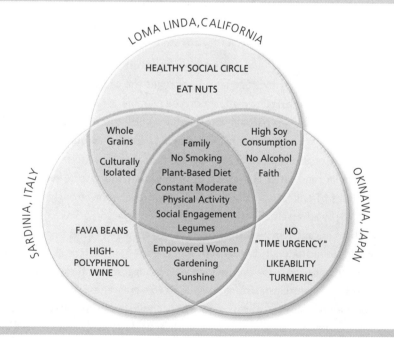

The large variation in the percentage of calories from fat consumed by Blue-Zone populations and other healthy populations throughout the world is mirrored within vegan populations. At one end of the spectrum are the no-oil, super-low-fat followers, and at the other are the raw, no-grain, no-legume, avocado aficionados. Somehow, diets at both ends of the spectrum appear to do a reasonable job of promoting health, as long as the fat is of high quality and caloric intakes aren't excessive.

RECOMMENDED FAT INTAKES

Most major health organizations agree that fat intake should range from a low of 15 to 20 percent of total calories to a high of 35 percent. They also agree that saturated fats, trans-fatty acids, and cholesterol should be restricted.[1, 2, 19]

The World Health Organization (WHO) has set the population dietary intake goal for fat at 15 to 30 percent of calories. A slightly more generous upper limit of 35 percent of calories applies to highly active groups who consume diets rich in vegetables, legumes, fruits, and whole-grain cereals.[19] In addition, a lower limit of 20 percent of total calories from fat is recommended for women of reproductive age. WHO also recommends that saturated fat intakes be less than 10 percent of calories (7 percent for high-risk populations) and trans-fatty acid intakes be less than 1 percent of calories.

In North America, the Institute of Medicine (IOM) hasn't set a Recommended Dietary Allowance (RDA), Adequate Intake (AI), or Tolerable Upper Intake Level for total fat except during the first year of life. Instead, the Acceptable Macronutrient Distribution Range (AMDR) is applied.[1] Based on evidence related to disease risk, the AMDR for fat varies by age and is indicated as a percentage of total calories:

- adults: 20 to 35 percent
- children (4 to 18): 25 to 35 percent
- children (1 to 3): 30 to 40 percent
- babies (6 to 12 months): 40 percent
- infants (birth to 6 months): 55 percent

The IOM report doesn't set maximum levels for saturated fat, cholesterol, or trans-fatty acids, because disease risks caused by these factors increase no matter how much is consumed. However, the report does suggest eating as little of these compounds as possible, while consuming a diet adequate in other important essential nutrients.

The American Heart Association strongly advises that all Americans over the age of 2 limit fat to less than 25 to 35 percent of daily calories, saturated fat to less than 7 percent of daily calories, trans-fatty acids to less than 1 percent of daily calories, and cholesterol to less than 300 mg daily for most people (200 mg per day for people with CAD).[2] Although the American Diabetes Association doesn't suggest a range for total fat intake, it does recommend that people with diabetes keep saturated fat to less than 7 percent of total calories, minimize trans-fatty acids, and keep cholesterol intake under 200 mg per day.[20]

RECOMMENDATIONS ON FAT INTAKE FOR VEGANS

The IOM makes no separate recommendations for total fat intake for vegans—but there's no reason to assume that the need for fats would be different from that of nonvegans. Limited evidence from studies on raw vegans suggests that higher total fat intakes can be consistent with health when the fat is derived from whole plant foods, such as nuts, seeds, and avocados.[21–23] Fat intakes below 15 percent of total calories have proved safe and effective in Asian populations and in the treatment and reversal of chronic disease; however, this low level is generally not advised for healthy individuals and isn't suitable for children or adolescents.

Table 4.1 provides target intakes for saturated, monounsaturated, and polyunsaturated fats at the various levels of fat intake. This guideline can easily be adjusted for higher or lower caloric intakes.

ACTUAL FAT INTAKES OF VEGANS

In conventional vegan diets, total fat intakes range from 18 to 36 percent of calories, averaging about 30 percent of calories.[24] This compares to 36 percent of calories from fat in the average standard American diet.[25] Although the average vegan's 6 percent lower total fat intake is significant, the differences in the sources of fat in vegan diets, compared to omnivorous diets, are even more noteworthy.

Vegans consume no cholesterol and only about one-half the saturated fat that omnivores do. Trans-fatty acid intakes vary according to the inclusion of convenience foods, fast foods, and other highly processed foods that contain partially hydrogenated vegetable oils. Limited research comparing the trans-fatty acid intakes of omnivores, vegetarians, and vegans suggests that vegetarians consume slightly smaller amounts than omnivores, with vegans who eat whole-foods diets consuming negligible amounts.[26]

The total fat intakes of raw vegans average about 36 percent of calories, because these diets feature nuts and seeds as prominent sources of protein. Also, raw-food eaters tend to consume fewer starchy foods (e.g., grains, legumes, and starchy vegetables), so the proportion of calories from fat is higher.

TABLE 4.1. Approximate fat targets at differing fat intakes (2,000-calorie diet)

CALORIES FROM FAT (TOTAL %)	APPROXIMATE FAT TARGET (g)	SATURATED FAT (g)	MONO-UNSATURATED FAT (g)	OMEGA-6 POLYUNSATU-RATED FAT (g)	OMEGA-3 POLYUNSATU-RATED FAT (g)
10	22.5	5	5	10	2.5
15	33	8	10	12	3
20	44.5	11	16	14	3.5
25	56	12	24	16	4
30	66.5	14	30	18	4.5
35	77	14	40	18	5

THE PROS AND CONS OF VERY LOW-FAT DIETS

Some of the most well-respected vegetarian and vegan health authorities recommend limiting fat to no more than 10 percent of total calories.[27–30] Their primary argument for very low-fat diets is that fat increases the risk of developing diseases, particularly chronic diseases, such as heart disease, type 2 diabetes, and certain cancers. Researchers have clearly demonstrated that, by reducing calories from fat to not more than 10 percent and also dramatically reducing harmful fats, heart disease can be successfully treated and, in many cases, significantly reversed.[27, 29, 31] One study reported that low-fat vegan diets provide more effective therapy for people with type 2 diabetes than the conventional American Diabetes Association diet.[30]

Unfortunately, no studies exist that compare the effectiveness of very low-fat vegan diets to vegan diets with more-generous intakes of whole-foods fats. However, very low-fat diets have provided effective therapeutic intervention to thousands of people with life-threatening chronic diseases. Considering the extent to which these diseases have afflicted the population, the value of very low-fat diets can't be overlooked.

Low-fat proponents strongly advise against the use of fats and oils. These foods aren't necessary in a healthful diet, and eliminating them generally increases the nutrient density (amount of nutrients per calorie) of the diet. Note, however, that all Blue-Zone populations use some oil; Okinawans eat very small amounts, while Mediterranean populations consume more-generous quantities.

Advocates of very low-fat vegan diets also suggest minimizing the role of higher-fat plant foods. However, studies examining the health effects of eating higher-fat whole plant foods yield results that are overwhelmingly positive. In fact, eliminating or severely restricting high-fat plant foods may put some individuals at a disadvantage, so a lower limit of 15 percent of calories from fat is suggested for healthy vegan adults, with higher minimum intakes suggested for children. Other potential disadvantages of very low-fat diets should also be considered:

- Very low-fat vegan diets (10 percent or fewer total calories from fat) that exclude higher-fat plant foods and oils may not provide sufficient EFA quantities for optimal health. With the exclusive use of vegetables, fruits, grains, and legumes as fat sources, the EFA content (both omega-6s and omega-3s) of a very low-fat vegan diet is typically about half the IOM's recommendations. Including higher-fat choices, such as soy products (e.g., tofu and soy milk), increases intakes, but EFA amounts may still fall short of the acceptable intakes (AI).

Although the implications of this shortfall are uncertain, it seems prudent for vegans to meet the AI for these nutrients. Adding approximately 1 ounce of seeds and/or walnuts to a diet with 10 percent fat would increase total fat to about 15 percent of calories in a 2,000-calorie diet. To meet the AI for both omega-6 and omega-3 EFAs, vegans should select seeds or nuts that provide a balance of both types of EFAs, (e.g., hempseeds or walnuts) or a combination of omega-3- and omega-6-rich products (e.g., flaxseeds plus pumpkin seeds, or chia seeds plus sunflower seeds).

• Absorption of fat-soluble vitamins (vitamins A, D, E, and K) and fat-soluble phytochemicals can be significantly reduced in very low-fat diets compared to diets with moderate amounts of dietary fat.[1, 32-35] Fat-soluble vitamins and phytochemicals are essential for health and play key roles in protecting against numerous diseases and health conditions. Including a small amount of fat in meals to maximize absorption of these protective elements ensures a truly optimal diet.

Low fat intakes also are associated with low intakes of zinc and some B vitamins, according to the IOM.[1] Because zinc is a nutrient of concern in vegan diets—especially for children—it's a good idea to include zinc-rich, higher-fat plant foods, such as nuts and seeds, in the diet.

• Very low-fat, high-carbohydrate diets can cause a decline in HDL cholesterol and a rise in triglyceride levels, particularly when the carbohydrates are refined. Low HDL cholesterol and high triglyceride levels are associated with an increased risk for CAD, metabolic syndrome, and type 2 diabetes.[1, 36]

Increased triglyceride levels can be averted by avoiding refined carbohydrates and relying on carbohydrates from whole plant foods, such as legumes, vegetables, and whole grains. In vegans and other populations that consume low-fat plant-based diets, HDL levels are typically slightly lower than in the general population, yet risk for CAD is also low. Although very low-fat, whole-foods vegan diets can cause a further drop in HDL cholesterol, this is a natural consequence of total cholesterol reduction and may not result in increased health risk. Removing excess cholesterol from the bloodstream is HDL's primary function; when there's less cholesterol to remove, less HDL is needed, so less is produced.

• Very low-fat, high-fiber diets may provide insufficient energy, particularly for infants and children;[1] adults with high energy needs may also find it challenging to eat enough calories on very low-fat diets.

The minimum level of fat necessary to support adequate growth and development in children is unknown. However, studies on omnivorous populations have found that in diets with adequate overall calories, as little as 21 percent of calories from fat is sufficient. It's also unknown whether higher fat intakes would be needed in vegan children's diets, which are higher in fiber and bulk. Studies of malnutrition in vegetarian and vegan populations have reported that highly fat-restrictive diets don't adequately support children's growth and development.[37, 38] One study of malnourished vegan infants noted that, by 14 to 16 months of age, their total calorie intake from fat was 17 percent.[37]

There's also some evidence that a low-fat diet could cause chronic diarrhea in children.[1] As a result, until additional research proves otherwise, it's advisable for vegan children to stay within the AMDR for fat.

• Higher-fat plant foods provide valuable nutrients, including a variety of antioxidants (such as vitamin E and selenium), trace minerals, and a host of protective phytochemicals. But when consumers make avoiding fat their highest priority for food selection, their diets' overall nutritional value may be reduced. By faithfully adhering to no-fat rules, they may choose less healthful products simply because they're fat-free.

For example, pretzels and red licorice would be fair game, while fermented raw almond cheese and flax crackers would be off limits. A fat-free, sugar-based commercial salad dressing would be permissible, while homemade lemon-tahini dressing would not. Such trade-offs can diminish the value of a very low-fat diet.

THE PROS AND CONS OF HIGH-FAT DIETS

High-fat diets (35 percent or more of total calories from fat) have long been thought to contribute to obesity and a variety of chronic diseases. However, some healthy populations have traditionally consumed diets that provide more than 35 percent of calories from fat. Good examples include Mediterranean populations and many raw-food adherents.[39, 40] Some leading health authorities promote Mediterranean-style diets as being optimal for health and encourage the liberal use of higher-fat foods, especially olive oil.[39]

In 1980, Ancel Keys's classic Seven Countries Study reported a strong connection between subjects' intakes of total fat and saturated fat and CAD.[41, 42] The link was unmistakable: as fat intake increased, so did rates of CAD. However, one group was an important exception—residents of the Greek island of Crete. In Crete, people averaged 37 percent of calories from fat, yet they had the lowest CAD rates among residents of all the nations studied—even lower than the Japanese, whose average fat intake was only 11 percent.

What separates the people of Crete (and other healthy Mediterranean populations) from less healthy populations that consume high-fat diets are their fat sources. The traditional Cretan diet includes abundant plant foods and olive oil; meanwhile, intakes of meat, poultry, and fish average less than 2 ounces per person per day. Religious practices also play a part in their diet. An estimated 60 percent of the study participants fasted during the 40 days of Lent; an unknown number also followed the Greek Orthodox Church's dietary doctrines, which prescribe almost 180 days of abstention from meat, fish, dairy products, eggs, and cheese, as well as from olive oil on certain Wednesdays and Fridays.[43] These practices weren't mentioned or factored into the results of Keys's study. However, leading experts from the University of Crete Faculty of Medicine believe that the regular restriction of certain foods—notably those of animal origin—had significant, positive health effects.[43]

Such Mediterranean-style diets provide a compelling argument that fat quality trumps quantity as a predictor of health outcomes when calories aren't overconsumed. However, even when the fats consumed are predominantly mono- and polyunsaturated fats, excessive intakes may increase health risk. Some of the primary criticisms of high-fat diets include:

- Fats and oils, such as shortenings and vegetable oils, contribute significant calories but few nutrients or other protective components, such as fiber and phytochemicals. As a result, high-fat diets can dilute nutrient density, making it a challenge to meet recommended intakes for nutrients, especially those already marginal in the diet. Of particular concern are sources of trans-fatty acids, such as hydrogenated vegetable oils and foods prepared or manufactured with these fats.

- Some evidence exists that diets very high in fat (42 to 50 percent of calories from fat) may increase several markers of blood coagulation and thrombosis, potentially increasing the risk of heart disease.[44, 45] Other high-fat diets have been linked to chronic medical conditions, such as CVD, metabolic syndrome, type 2 diabetes, gallbladder disease, and some cancers. The weight of the evidence linking fat intake to these diseases is specific to diets rich in saturated fats and/or trans-fatty acids.[1, 19, 46] However, intakes of these fats tend to be lower in vegan diets, and raw vegan diets completely avoid trans-fatty acids.

- The consumption of high-fat diets can increase overall energy intakes and induce weight gain.[1] Fat has more than twice the concentration of calories as protein or carbohydrate, so more calories are easily consumed despite a smaller volume of food. For populations and individuals at high risk for overweight and obesity, more-moderate fat intakes are advised.

- Some evidence suggests that in consumers of high-fat diets, the body converts fewer EFAs to the more biologically active HUFAs, compared to lower-fat diets.[47]

- High-fat diets may result in increased oxidative damage to body tissues. Free radicals are more likely to react with the relatively unstable molecules in polyunsaturated fats,[48] so people who consume greater amounts of these fats could be at increased risk. Oxidative stress has been linked to heart disease, cancer, type 2 diabetes, arthritis, age-related diseases, neurological disorders, and other illnesses.[48, 49]

THE BOTTOM LINE

The science is crystal clear: a broad spectrum of fat intake can support and promote excellent health, but there are two important caveats. First, consumers must achieve energy balance, and second, they must select healthful sources of fat. If most of their dietary fat comes from whole or minimally processed plant foods, they can maintain excellent health even when fat intake is relatively high. On the other hand, when fats are derived from highly processed foods, fast foods, or convenience foods, negative health consequences can occur even with low fat intakes.

Strong evidence supports the use of very low-fat, plant-based diets as therapeutic treatment for chronic disease, particularly CVD. However, it's not a foregone conclusion that all diets need to be so low in fat, that such diets set the gold standard for all vegans, or that very low-fat diets are suitable for all vegans.

Many factors need to be considered before establishing appropriate guidelines for fat intake in healthy vegan populations, because needs vary with the individual and change throughout the life cycle. Optimal fat intakes must support excellent health at every stage of life—including periods of rapid growth and development, such as pregnancy, infancy, and childhood—and must ensure excellent EFA status, adequate absorption of fat-soluble nutrients and phytochemicals, and smooth functioning of all body systems.

High-fat whole foods, such as nuts, seeds, avocados, and olives, aren't responsible for the epidemic of chronic disease that plagues modern societies. In fact, higher-fat plant-based diets can promote health if these healthful sources of fats are chosen instead of processed fats and oils. Still, overly generous use of oil can dilute the nutritional quality of a plant-based diet; if used, intakes should be moderate.

In practical terms, to treat CVD, the very low-fat vegan diet is worth exploring, but a source of EFAs must be included (see pages 117 to 125). To combat overweight or obesity, a diet should minimize the concentrated sources of calories that provide few nutrients, including fats and oils. However, a moderate intake of nuts and seeds (e.g., 1 to 2 ounces per day) is consistent with healthy weight loss.

Vegans with a healthy body weight should focus on eating a variety of nourishing plant foods, including higher-fat plant foods. Small amounts of fresh-pressed oils can be included, but they're not necessary for a healthful diet.

Maximizing Essential Fatty Acid Status

Necessary to survival are two essential fatty acids (EFA) that can't be made in the body and must be obtained from food: linoleic acid (LA) and alpha-linolenic acid (ALA). The body then constructs other complex fatty acids from LA, parent of the omega-6 (n-6) family, and ALA, parent of the omega-3 (n-3) family. LA and ALA are called parent fatty acids because it's from them that the body produces highly unsaturated fatty acids (HUFA)—also known as long-chain polyunsaturated fatty acids (LCPUFA)—that make up each family. HUFA can be synthesized in the body by a series of elongation and desaturation reactions, or they can be obtained directly from food. (See figure 4.2 on page 118 for synthesis reactions and table 4.2 on page 119 for dietary sources of EFA and HUFA.)

For example, in the omega-6 family, LA can be converted to gamma-linolenic acid (GLA), dihommogamma-linolenic acid (DGLA), and arachidonic acid (AA). Or we can consume GLA directly from primrose, borage, or black currant seed oil, and AA directly from animal-based foods, such as meat and dairy products.

In the omega-3 family, ALA can be converted to stearidonic acid (SDA), eicosapentaenoic acid (EPA), and docosahexaenoic acid (DHA). SDA can also be obtained directly from echium oil, black currant seed oil, hempseeds and hempseed oil, or fish. EPA and DHA can be consumed directly from fish (which contains both EPA and DHA), eggs (which contain only DHA), sea vegetables (which have small amounts of EPA), or microalgae (single-celled organisms that provide both EPA and DHA).

LA and ALA undergo a series of reactions that make these fatty acids more unsaturated (desaturation) and longer (elongation), which produces HUFA (see figure 4.2). The two fatty acids compete for the same desaturation enzymes, so an excess of one can reduce conversion of the other. ALA is usually favored in this process; however, there's a point where an overabundance of LA relative to ALA can cause the conversion enzymes to become more occupied with omega-6 fatty acids, reducing ALA conversion to EPA and DHA.[50–53]

FIGURE 4.2. Metabolism of essential fatty acids

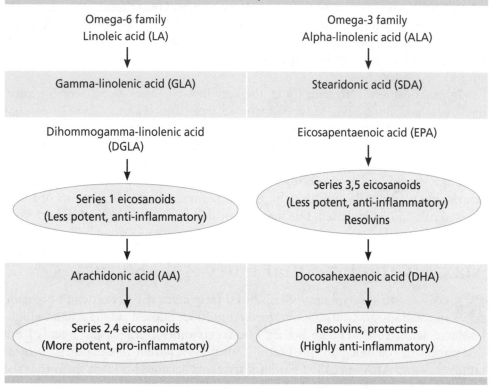

HUFA are more biologically active than EFA. They're metabolized to produce a wide variety of hormone-like compounds that have a significant impact on multiple body functions, including blood clotting, blood pressure control, immune response, cell division, pain control, and inflammation response. The body produces dozens of different compounds from HUFA, including eicosanoids (prostaglandins, prostacyclins, thromboxanes, and leukotrienes), protectins, and resolvins.

Although the body needs eicosanoids from both families of fats, having a balance of the two is helpful, particularly in diets that don't include direct sources of EPA and DHA. The eicosanoids formed within each family have somewhat opposing effects:

- Eicosanoids formed from the omega-3 derivative EPA tend to *reduce* platelet aggregation (stickiness of blood cells), *improve* blood flow, *decrease* cell division, and *enhance* immune function.

- Eicosanoids formed from the omega-6 derivative AA tend to *increase* platelet aggregation, *decrease* blood flow, *increase* cell division, and *suppress* immune function.

Protectins and resolvins are potent anti-inflammatory mediators; their names reflect their actions, because they protect against and resolve inflammation. They're derived mainly from DHA, although a series of resolvins is also derived from EPA.[54, 55]

Sources of Essential Fatty Acids and Highly Unsaturated Fatty Acids

The primary source of the two essential fatty acids, linoleic acid (LA) and alpha-linolenic acid (ALA), are plants from the land and sea. The richest sources are seeds and walnuts.

The most common dietary sources of highly unsaturated fatty acids (HUFA)—arachidonic acid (AA), eicosapentaenoic acid (EPA), and docosahexaenoic acid (DHA)—are animal products (although DHA and EPA are also available from micro- and macroalgae). Table 4.2 provides a list of food sources of HUFA and table 4.6 (pages 131 and 132) lists specific amounts of these fatty acids in a variety of foods.

TABLE 4.2. Sources of polyunsaturated fatty acids

OMEGA-6 FATTY ACIDS	OMEGA-3 FATTY ACIDS
LINOLEIC ACID (LA)	**ALPHA-LINOLENIC ACID (ALA)**
Corn kernels, corn oil	Camelina oil
Grapeseed oil	Canola oil
Hempseeds and hempseed oil*	Chia seeds, chia oil
Pine nuts/pignolia nuts	Flaxseeds, flaxseed oil
Pumpkin seed oil	Green leafy land and sea vegetables
Safflower seeds, safflower oil	Hempseeds, hempseed oil*
Sesame seeds, sesame seed oil	Soybeans, soybean oil*
Soybeans, soybean oil*	Walnuts, walnut oil*
Sunflower seeds, sunflower oil	Wheat germ, wheat germ oil*
Walnuts, walnut oil*	
Wheat germ, wheat germ oil*	**STEARIDONIC ACID (SDA)**
	Black currant seed oil
GAMMA-LINOLENIC ACID (GLA)	Echium oil
Black currant seed oil	Hempseeds, hempseed oil
Borage oil	Seafood and fish
Hempseeds, hempseed oil	
Primrose oil	**EICOSAPENTAENOIC ACID (EPA) AND**
Spirulina	**DOCOSAHEXAENOIC ACID (DHA)**
	Breast milk
ARACHIDONIC ACID (AA)	Eggs**
Dairy products	Fish and seafood, particularly
Eggs	cold-water oily fish
Fish	Microalgae (plant DHA/EPA), but not
Meat	blue-green algae
Poultry	Sea vegetables (less-concentrated EPA)

*Hempseeds, soybeans, walnuts, and wheat germ are significant sources of both LA and ALA.

**Most eggs contain small amounts of DHA; eggs from chickens given feed rich in omega-3s contain greater amounts.

Where EFAs are concerned, vegan diets appear to offer no advantages over omnivorous eating patterns. Vegans could actually be at a disadvantage, because plant sources of omega-3 fatty acids are limited, and vegan diets are generally lacking in direct sources of omega-3 HUFA.[56, 57]

Omega-3 fatty acids provide raw materials for building brains, nervous systems, and cell membranes (DHA is especially abundant in the retina, brain, and semen). They favorably affect the composition and functioning of cell membranes, enhancing intracellular signaling processes, gene expression, and the production of eicosanoids and cell mediators. There's strong evidence that these fatty acids play key roles in the prevention and modulation of numerous disease processes, including CVD, hypertension, rheumatoid arthritis, autoimmune diseases, and several types of cancer. They may also protect against dementia, diabetes, and asthma, although the evidence for these conditions is weaker.[55, 58–62]

CONVERSION OF ALA TO EPA AND DHA

Dietary ALA has a variety of possible fates once it's absorbed into the bloodstream. Approximately 15 to 35 percent is rapidly converted to energy.[63] ALA can also be incorporated into cell membranes, stored in fat tissue for later use, or converted into ketone bodies; the carbon fragments can be recycled to make saturated and monounsaturated fatty acids.

The balance is converted into omega-3 long-chain polyunsaturated fatty acids (HUFA). Conversion efficiency is unpredictable, varying among individuals, with stages of life, and in different body tissues.[1, 61, 64] An estimated average of 5 percent of ALA converts to EPA and less than 0.5 percent to DHA, although several studies have suggested higher conversion rates.[61, 65] ALA's rate of conversion to EPA can range from about 0.3 percent to as much as 21 percent, while the rate of conversion to DHA ranges from zero to about 9 percent.[66, 67]

Consuming direct sources of DHA, such as fish or eggs, depresses the final step in conversion from EPA to DHA by 70 percent or more.[66, 68] (In other words, not consuming direct sources of DHA is known to enhance the rate of conversion. This is the body's way of maintaining sufficient HUFA in the absence of direct dietary sources.) DHA itself can be converted back to EPA at a rate of up to 12 percent.[69, 70]

The body's conversion of ALA is limited by multiple factors, some of which are unrelated to diet. The most significant nondietary factors—gender and genetics—are outside of our control. Being female appears to provide an advantage in ALA conversion, particularly during the childbearing years. There's considerable evidence that estrogen boosts DHA synthesis in preparation for pregnancy or lactation.[71] During this stage of life, the rate of ALA conversion to both EPA and DHA is at the upper end of the conversion range. One study found young women converted a remarkable 36 percent of ALA to HUFA (21 percent to EPA, 9 percent to DHA, and 6 percent to an intermediary highly unsaturated fat called DPA).[67] The same study group reported that conversion rates in young men averaged 16 percent (8 percent to EPA, 8 percent to DPA, and zero to DHA).[66] However, genetic variations in desaturase enzymes can slow conversion in some individuals.[64, 72, 73] Other nondietary factors that adversely affect ALA conversion include smoking, advancing age, and chronic disease (e.g., diabetes, metabolic syndrome, hypertension, and hyperlipidemia).[74–76]

Dietary factors can have a profound influence on ALA conversion (see table 4.3). The most potent factor—high intakes of omega-6 fatty acids—can reduce conversion by as much as 40 to 60 percent.[77–79] Trans-fatty acids can also inhibit conversion, as can excessive intake of alcohol and caffeine.[80] Nutritional inadequacies, such as protein deficiency or a lack of vitamins and minerals—especially zinc, magnesium, niacin, pyridoxine, and vitamin C—can diminish the activity of conversion enzymes.[75, 81, 82]

Although fasting may reduce ALA conversion, low-fat or calorie-restricted diets appear to enhance conversion.[75] One study compared two similar controlled diets, equal in calories and having similar omega-6 to omega-3 ratios, but differing in fat and carbohydrate content. The principal difference between the diets was that one was relatively low in fat (about 20 percent of calories from fat) while the other was high in fat (45 percent of calories from fat).[47] Study investigators found that the lower-fat diet produced much more favorable ALA conversion than the high-fat diet. (See table 4.3 for a summary of the factors most strongly affecting n-3 conversion).

Direct sources of SDA have been shown to raise both EPA and DHA concentrations more effectively than ALA consumption.[80, 83] Although SDA isn't abundant in the food supply, it accounts for about 12 to 14 percent of the fatty acids in echium oil, 3 percent in black currant seed oil, and 2 percent in hempseed oil.[84–86] Echium oil comes from a plant called Purple Viper's Bugloss, which is native in parts of Europe but invasive in America and Australia.

TABLE 4.3. Factors affecting ALA conversion

NONDIET FACTORS	EFFECTS
Genetics	Genetic variations in desaturase enzymes can reduce conversion.
Gender	Women of childbearing age are more-efficient converters than men, possibly due to differences in sex hormones.
Age	Conversion is reduced with advancing age.
Smoking	Smoking depresses desaturase enzymes, slowing conversion.
Chronic disease	Diabetes, metabolic syndrome, hypertension, and hyperlipidemia (elevated blood lipids) can adversely affect conversion.
DIET-RELATED FACTORS	
Omega-6 fatty acids	High intake can reduce conversion by 40 to 60%.
Poor nutrition	Protein deficiency and suboptimal intakes of vitamins (niacin, pyridoxine, and vitamin C) and minerals (zinc and magnesium) can reduce conversion.
Very high-fat diets	Diets very high in fat (45% fat) appear to diminish conversion relative to lower-fat diets (20% fat).
Direct sources of SDA	Direct sources of SDA enhance conversion relative to ALA.

RATIO OF OMEGA-6 TO OMEGA-3 FATTY ACIDS

Changes in the human diet during the last century have affected intakes of the two essential fatty acids, LA and ALA, altering the natural balance that previously existed. Experts estimate that until about 100 to 150 years ago, most diets provided omega-6 and omega-3 fatty acids in a ratio of approximately 1:1.[60] Research suggests that, at this ratio, conversion to long-chain polyunsaturated fatty acids (HUFA) would be significantly higher. This makes sense. If the body couldn't convert ALA to EPA and DHA, humans wouldn't be able to survive without fish, seaweed, and other foods rich in these fatty acids. A century ago or more, inland residents may not have had regular access to these foods, so conversion must have been adequate and appears to be related to the balance of EFA in their diets.

Since then, enormous changes in the food supply have pushed the ratio of omega-6s to omega-3s to 10:1 and higher.[24, 71, 87] In vegan diets, the balance is even more precarious, ranging from 8:1 to 18:1,[24] due to increased LA intakes commonly associated with today's plant-based diets. These intake levels can adversely impact growth and development, cell membrane function, inflammatory reactions, and numerous disease processes.[60, 62]

There's still considerable debate about whether the ratio of omega-6s to omega 3s should be a matter of concern. However, conversion efficiency has been shown to be significantly affected by this ratio.[88] As a result, awareness of the ratio is useful for vegans and others who don't consume sufficient EPA and DHA from direct sources, and who rely solely on conversion of ALA to meet their need for EPA, DHA, and other omega-3 HUFA. The ratio is less relevant for nonvegetarians, who consume direct sources of HUFA, such as fish.[89]

Although the optimal ratio of LA to ALA for efficient conversion is uncertain, international recommendations—which assume some direct intake of long-chain fatty acids—range from a low of 2:1 to a high of 10:1.[56] Although vegans are well-advised to keep intakes within this range, there's convincing evidence that conversion is more efficient at the lower end of the range.[60, 87, 90]

A recent Canadian study found that, in a diet providing 1 percent of energy from ALA, an LA to ALA ratio of 4:1 resulted in higher amounts of EPA and lower amounts of AA than a diet with an LA to ALA ratio of 10:1.[90] An earlier study also found that a ratio of 4:1 allows for adequate conversion in healthy vegetarians.[91] Two additional research groups reported that optimal conversion was achieved with ratios of 2.3:1 and 2:1, respectively.[92, 93] Finally, a Japanese research team reported significant improvements in conversion with a shift from soy oil to a high-ALA oil called perilla oil.[94] This change reduced the omega-6 to omega-3 ratio from 4:1 to 1:1 and increased EPA by 44 percent and DHA by 21 percent. A few other studies have shown significant increases in DHA with increased ALA intake; however, most of the studies have been of short duration and few have used diets with such a low omega-6 to omega-3 ratio. Other experts have also suggested that a ratio of 1:1 maximizes conversion,[75, 87] but modern diets make it challenging to achieve this ratio. Based on the evidence to date, ratios ranging from 2:1 to 4:1 seem a reasonable target for vegans.[56]

Although it's not common, it *is* possible for vegans to overconsume omega-3 fatty acids. If individuals avoid nuts, seeds, avocados, and other high-fat plant foods but eat large amounts of flaxseeds, flaxseed oil, or chia seeds, the reduced proportion of omega-6s to omega-3s could result in an unfavorable ratio of 1:2 or more. (For example, flaxseed oil has a remarkable omega-6 to omega-3 ratio of 0.28:1 and averages about 57 percent alpha-linolenic acid.) This would reduce the conversion of LA to AA, potentially leading to omega-6 deficiency. Symptoms include dry hair, scaly skin, dry eyes, joint pain, brittle nails, and increased risk of chronic disease.

ESSENTIAL FATTY ACID INTAKE AND STATUS OF VEGANS

Intakes of LA tend to be somewhat higher among vegans than nonvegetarians, while total ALA intakes are similar for vegans, vegetarians, and nonvegetarians (less than 1 to 3 grams per day).[52, 56, 61, 95] Not surprisingly, intakes of long-chain omega-3 fatty acids vary widely: vegans consume negligible amounts, lacto-ovo vegetarians consume small amounts, and omnivores consume higher amounts, as determined by their level of fish intake. The average intake of EPA and DHA in the United States is approximately 100 mg per day.[57]

The majority of scientific studies that assess vegan EFA status have reported lower levels of EPA and DHA in blood, plasma, and platelets. However, vegan DHA status appears not to diminish as people age, suggesting an ongoing, constant level of conversion, however low.[62] Among nine studies reporting reduced levels in vegans compared to omnivorous controls, EPA ranged from 12 to 79 percent that of the controls, while DHA ranged from 32 to 67 percent. On average, EPA and DHA levels in vegans were about half that found in omnivores.[52, 62, 95–101] It's interesting to note that levels of EPA and DHA in vegans were significantly lower in older studies (1978 to 1992) than newer studies (1994 to the present). It's unclear whether this is due to changes in analytic methods for measuring omega-3 status or recent improvements in dietary intakes of EFA.

However, one study found omega-3 fatty acid status wasn't reduced in vegans.[61] The UK EPIC-Norfolk study assessed the EFA intake and status of almost 5,000 men and women from different dietary groups, including meat eaters, fish eaters, lacto-ovo vegetarians, and vegans. Unfortunately, there were only 10 vegans in the study (after supplement consumers were excluded). It's possible that results derived from this small group aren't a true reflection of the status of the wider vegan population or that the vegans in this study weren't completely vegan (they were assigned to their dietary group based on a seven-day food record).

Although the vegans in this study had lower intakes of all omega-3 fatty acids compared to the nonvegans, differences in the plasma levels of EPA and DHA between the two groups were not as great. In male vegans, plasma levels of EPA and DHA were 113 and 81 percent that of fish eaters, respectively. In female vegans, plasma levels of EPA and DHA were 77 and 106 percent that of fish eaters, respectively. The investigators suggested that vegan conversion rates from ALA to EPA and DHA were approximately twice that of other dietary

Are Fish Eaters Healthier than Vegans?

To reduce CVD risk, the 2010 *Report of the Dietary Guidelines Advisory Committee on the Dietary Guidelines for Americans* recommends eating 8 ounces (240 g) or more of seafood each week. There's no question that fish eaters have much higher intakes of EPA and DHA than vegans, because fish is the most concentrated dietary source of these HUFA. Vegans normally consume almost no EPA or DHA unless they eat fortified foods or use supplements.

However, the evidence to date isn't terribly convincing that a diet that includes fish yields a distinct advantage over a vegan diet. Although observational studies do suggest that diets rich in omega-3 fatty acids (especially EPA and DHA) reduce cardiovascular events, the results of clinical trials are less clear.[103] Although adding EPA and DHA to vegan diets may provide cardiovascular benefits, evidence comparing heart disease rates of fish eaters and vegans is very limited.

In a 1999 meta-analysis comparing vegans, lacto-ovo vegetarians, fish eaters, and meat eaters, vegans had the lowest body fat, blood pressure, and blood cholesterol levels of all the dietary groups. However, mortality rates from heart disease were lower among lacto-ovo vegetarians and fish eaters than vegans. (Compared with meat eaters, mortality rates were 34 percent lower among lacto-ovo vegetarians and fish eaters, and 26 percent lower among vegans.)[104]

More recently, EPIC-Oxford investigators reported that vegetarians (including vegans) had a 32 percent lower risk of heart disease than other dietary groups when results were adjusted for all confounding variables except BMI, and a 28 percent lower risk when BMI was factored in. In this study, fish eaters had the same rates of heart disease as meat eaters.[105]

The reputed cardioprotective effects of fish are tied to its EPA/DHA content. Vegans and others who avoid fish have the option of getting EPA and DHA from cultured microalgae supplements. Unlike fish, cultured microalgae are free of heavy metals, such as lead, mercury, and cadmium, and industrial pollutants, such as polychlorinated biphenyls, DDT, and dioxin. Considering the increasing demands for EPA and DHA, and the rapid decline in fish species and stocks, consuming alternative sources of long-chain omega-3 fatty acids makes good sense. (See pages 15 to 18.)

groups (for example, 209 percent higher in vegan men and 184 percent higher in vegan women than in fish eaters).

Although this study is encouraging, a larger study showed different results. EPIC-Oxford, a UK cohort with a larger number of vegan participants, reported on the EFA status of 659 men, including 232 vegans.[62] In these vegans, plasma EPA was 47 percent and plasma DHA was 41 percent that of meat eaters. Although the vegan men's plasma EPA and DHA concentrations were low, they were quite stable over time (anywhere from one year to twenty years).[62] As a result, further investigation is needed about EFA conversion rates in vegan populations.

Finally, a group of investigators from the United Kingdom found that vegans' breast milk contained about 38 percent of the DHA found in the breast milk of omnivores. In this study, the omega-6 to omega-3 ratio was about 18:1 in the vegans compared to about 10:1 for the omnivores.[102]

RECOMMENDED INTAKES FOR EFA

The IOM hasn't set an RDA for EFA because of a lack of evidence for determining actual requirements.[1] However, the IOM has set the Adequate Intake (AI) for LA at 12 grams a day for women and 17 grams a day for men. The AI for ALA is 1.1 grams a day for women and 1.6 grams a day for men.[1] These AIs aren't designated as optimal intakes but are simply a reflection of median intakes in a population in which EFA deficiencies are considered essentially nonexistent. The IOM has also set an AMDR of 5 to 10 percent of energy from LA and 0.6 to 1.2 percent of energy from ALA.[1, 106–109]

The WHO recommends that 5 to 8 percent of calories come from omega-6 fatty acids and 1 to 2 percent of calories from omega-3 fatty acids[106] (this corresponds to an ALA intake of 2.2 to 4.4 grams per day in a diet that provides 2,000 calories). Meanwhile, many health authorities recommend direct intakes of EPA and DHA in the range of 250 to 550 mg per day.[107–109] For example, the European Food Safety Authority proposed dietary reference values of 10 grams of LA and 2 grams of ALA *plus* 250 mg of EPA and 250 mg of DHA for adults, 100 mg of DHA for infants 7 to 24 months of age, and an additional 100 to 200 mg of DHA for pregnant and lactating women (above the 250 mg of DHA already suggested for adults).[110] Although the IOM hasn't set AIs for EPA and DHA, a panel of experts convened in 2008 to reassess this position recommended that the AI for EPA and DHA be set between 250 and 500 mg per day.[107]

SUITABLE RECOMMENDATIONS FOR VEGANS

No separate official EFA recommendations exist for vegans, vegetarians, or other consumers who don't eat fish. Although many national health authorities have recommended intakes for EPA and DHA, vegans can't meet these levels without using supplements. But, would vegans benefit by taking DHA and EPA supplements? Unfortunately, we don't yet know the answer.

Considering that men and postmenopausal women convert ALA less efficiently, it's possible their needs for omega-3 fatty acids are modest and serve mainly to support cell membrane turnover. In addition, DHA is the most highly unsaturated fat in the diet and also the most easily oxidized by free radicals in the blood. Because oxidized fats can contribute to disease processes, it's possible that the body avoids making DHA when it's not needed. On the other hand, conversion is enhanced in women of childbearing age, particularly those who are pregnant or lactating, because more DHA is needed—the developing fetus requires at least 400 mg of DHA per week during the last trimester.[71]

So, although conversion to EPA and DHA is generally slow and incomplete in vegans, it appears to be sufficient to meet the needs of most healthy people if their ALA intake is adequate and their diet is well balanced.[62, 87, 88] Yet, it's possible that vegan health outcomes could be improved by adding direct sources of long-chain omega-3 fatty acids. More research is required to help clarify this issue.

Although it's unknown if vegans would benefit by adding supplemental DHA (and possibly EPA), there's a clear inverse association between direct EPA and DHA intake and CVD risk. There's more limited evidence for an inverse association between direct EPA and DHA intake and depression, cognitive decline, and age-related macular degeneration[107, 111–115]

Some evidence exists for improvements in infants' visual acuity, growth, development, and cognition with higher maternal DHA intakes during pregnancy and lactation, and during the first two years of life.[116–118] (These benefits are more pronounced in poorly nourished children.[118]) Nonetheless, research on the growth and development of vegan children has failed to reveal any demonstrated deficiencies in visual or mental development when care has been taken to ensure they eat sufficient calories and get adequate amounts of vitamin B_{12}.[88] In addition, although there's limited data on cognitive function in vegan adults, one study reported an average IQ of 119 in 118 vegan men.

Because moderate increases in omega-3 fatty acid intake are generally considered safe and potentially beneficial, it seems prudent for vegans to take steps to optimize omega-3 fatty acid status. (See pages 117 to 125.)

Consuming sufficient omega-3 fatty acids can be ensured by increasing intakes of ALA relative to LA or by adding a direct source of DHA, and possibly EPA, to the diet. Increasing ALA intake can be an effective strategy for boosting conversion to EPA and DHA, but the body's capacity for conversion is limited, and genetic variations in metabolism can compromise conversion in some people.[72, 119] Instead, adding direct sources of DHA or DHA plus EPA effectively increases omega-3 status.[69, 88, 120–123]

One small trial showed that taking 200 mg of DHA for three months increased DHA in the plasma of male vegans by 50 percent.[122] However, the primary vegan sources—DHA- and EPA-rich microalgae supplements or fortified foods—may not be affordable or available to everyone, so there are limitations to both these options (in addition to wildly differing opinions as to which option is preferable for vegans). Considering the uncertainty and the need for further research, the decision is a personal one.

The following suggestions for increasing EFA intake can be regarded as informed guesses based on a careful examination of the literature and discussions with leading international experts. Some authorities suggest a minimum 1.5 grams of ALA per day for optimal health, which exceeds the current AI for women.[124, 125] When relying almost exclusively on ALA for omega-3 fatty acids, vegans should base the intake amount on double the current AI.[56] Using North American AIs, vegan men should consume 3.2 grams of ALA per day, while vegan women should obtain 2.2 grams per day. (See table 4.4 for suggested intakes for all age groups.) Doubling the AI would require a parallel increase in the AMDR for ALA to 1.2 to 2.4 percent of calories. The AMDR for LA would remain unchanged at 5 to 10 percent of calories.

Of course, augmenting ALA intake doesn't guarantee optimal EFA status, although it helps to ensure that sufficient raw materials are available for conversion to long-chain polyunsaturated fatty acids (HUFA). Alternatively, vegans could include direct sources of DHA, and possibly EPA, aiming for about 10 per-

TABLE 4.4. Adequate Intake (AI) of omega-3 fatty acids and suggested intakes for vegans

AGE GROUP	ADEQUATE INTAKE ALA (OMEGA-3)	SUGGESTED INTAKE ALA WITHOUT EPA/DHA SOURCES	SUGGESTED INTAKE ALA WITH EPA/DHA SOURCES
Infants newborn–12 months	0.5 g/day	N/A*	N/A*—n-3 adequate from breast milk; if using formula, select one with DHA
Children 1–3 years	0.7 g/day	1.4 g/day	Breast milk or 0.7 g ALA + 70 mg DHA
Children 4–8 years	0.9 g/day	1.8 g/day	0.9 g ALA + 90 mg DHA/EPA
Boys 9–13 years	1.2 g/day	2.4 g/day	1.2 g ALA + 120 mg DHA/EPA
Girls 9–13 years	1 g/day	2 g/day	1 g ALA + 100 mg DHA/EPA
Males 14 years or older	1.6 g/day	3.2 g/day	1.6 g ALA + 160 mg DHA/EPA
Females 14 years or older	1.1 g/day	2.2 g/day	1.1 g ALA + 110 mg DHA/EPA
Pregnancy	1.4 g/day	2.8 g/day	1.4 g ALA + 200–300 mg DHA (or DHA/EPA with ≥ 200 mg DHA)
Lactation	1.3 g/day	2.6 g/day	1.3 g ALA + 200–300 mg DHA (or DHA/EPA with ≥ 200 mg DHA)

Source: 1

*Not applicable; infants will get DHA from breast milk (or appropriate commercial formula).

cent of the AI for ALA (see table 4.4). Individuals who regularly consume a direct source of DHA wouldn't need to increase ALA over the current AI. A more affordable option would be to add a 200 to 300 mg DHA (and possibly EPA) supplement two to three times a week.

To ensure the availability of sufficient long-chain omega-3 fatty acids for infants, it's wise to breast-feed for two years and beyond. If breast-feeding stops before the baby is 12 months old or if formula is used as the primary milk, select a milk or formula with added DHA. Once the baby begins consuming fortified full-fat soy milk (sometime after 1 year of age), a supplement providing 70 mg of DHA per day could be introduced, if desired. For pregnant and lactating women, several expert panels and health authorities have recommended DHA intakes of at least 200 to 300 mg per day,[126–128] so this level seems reasonable for vegans as well.

POSSIBLE RISKS OF HIGH ALA INTAKES

A bit of a buzz surrounds the possible link between ALA and the risk for prostate cancer and degenerative eye diseases. This has raised concerns because vegans rely on ALA-rich foods (such as walnuts, flaxseeds, hempseeds, and chia seeds) as primary sources of omega-3 fatty acids. However, there's likely no cause for concern among vegans who get their ALA from whole plant foods or from oils that have been stored and used in ways that minimize damage to ALA.

Of twenty-three studies assessing the relationship between ALA and prostate cancer risk, eleven reported that higher intakes and/or higher tissue or blood levels of ALA are positively associated with prostate cancer.[129–139] The remaining twelve studies found either no association or an inverse association between intake, tissue or blood levels of ALA, and prostate cancer.[140–151]

In addition, six meta-analyses reviewed the evidence on ALA and prostate cancer risk.[152–157] Of these, one study reported no significant association between ALA and prostate cancer risk;[152] three studies found a weak protective effect of ALA;[154–156] and two studies found ALA was associated with increased prostate cancer risk, although the association wasn't significant in one study, and after adjustment for publication bias, the positive association was eliminated in the other study.[153, 157]

Three reports have assessed the risk for degenerative eye diseases, such as cataracts and age-related macular degeneration, in participants of the Nurses' Health Study. These studies all found positive associations between ALA intake and risk for eye diseases. A 2005 study found that those with the highest ALA intakes (1.26 grams of ALA per day) had slightly more than double the risk of cataracts compared to those with the lowest ALA intakes (0.86 grams per day).[158] A 2007 report on the same cohort found a 16 percent increase in lens nuclear density (a risk factor for cataracts) in those who consumed the greatest amounts of ALA compared to those with the lowest intakes.[159] Finally, another 2007 study of participants older than 50 found that the highest ALA consumers had a 41 percent increased risk of age-related macular degeneration compared to those with the lowest intakes.[160]

Why do some reports show an increased risk of prostate cancer and degenerative eye diseases in people who consume greater amounts of ALA? Experts suggest that the answer may lie in the dietary sources of the ALA. In the United States and many other Western countries, the primary dietary sources of ALA are meat and other animal products. Other sources include processed foods made with ALA-containing oils, such as soybean oil and canola oil (e.g., mayonnaise and margarine), and foods fried or cooked using these oils. Considering these sources of ALA, it's quite possible that ALA itself is not the issue, but rather ALA damaged by heat, light, oxygen from food processing, and high-temperature cooking. Researchers have also suggested that ALA may simply be a marker for high meat and fat intakes, as well as unhealthful eating patterns.[152]

Conversely, walnuts, ground flaxseeds, hempseeds, and chia seeds weren't major sources of ALA in these studies, raising confidence that vegans have no cause for concern. In fact, a small handful of studies by one research team in the United States found that adding 3 tablespoons (45 ml/30 g) of ground flaxseeds per day consistently decreased prostate cancer cell proliferation in men with prostate cancer, compared to men who didn't consume ground flaxseeds.[161–163]

In addition, the high ratio of omega-6 to omega-3 fatty acids diminishes the conversion of ALA to EPA and DHA, both of which may protect against degenerative eye diseases.[164] In this case, improving the ratio by reducing omega-6 fatty acids and increasing omega-3 fatty acids would help to solve the problem. A final possible explanation is that those who consumed the highest amounts of ALA may not also have consumed sufficient quantities of antioxidants to preserve and protect these fragile fatty acids. Western-style diets centered on animal products and processed foods are notoriously low in antioxidants. A variety of whole plant foods, such as leafy greens and other colorful vegetables and fruits, is needed to obtain these protective dietary compounds.

The Bottom Line: Based on the science to date, the evidence doesn't warrant any adjustment in suggested ALA intakes for vegans (see table 4.4 on page 127 for suggested intakes for all age groups). It's also very important that ALA sources are of high quality and are protected from damage in storage and during cooking.

ACHIEVING OPTIMAL EFA STATUS

To improve EFA status, vegans should take the necessary steps to achieve an omega-6 to omega-3 ratio that maximizes conversion of ALA to EPA and DHA. They also may wish to consider adding a direct source of DHA (and possibly EPA). To reach the suggested ratio of 2:1 to 4:1, the goal is approximately 5 to 10 percent of calories from LA and 1.2 to 2.4 percent from omega-3 fatty acids. In a 2,000-calorie diet, this would be 11 to 22 grams of LA and 2.7 to 5.3 grams of ALA. (See table 4.5.) Individuals with increased needs or decreased capacity for conversion may need to boost intake of ALA to the upper end of this range

TABLE 4.5. Essential fatty acid content of selected plant foods

FOOD	SERVING SIZE	ALA (% OF FATTY ACIDS)	LA (% OF FATTY ACIDS)	OMEGA-6 TO OMEGA-3 RATIO	ALA (g/SERVING)
Canola oil	1 T (15 ml/14 g)	9	19	2:1	1.3
Chia seeds	2 T (30 ml/22 g)	58	20	0.34:1	4
Flaxseeds, ground	2 T (30 ml/14 g)	54	14	0.26:1	3.2
Flaxseeds, whole	2 T (30 ml/20.6 g)	54	14	0.26:1	4.7
Flaxseed oil	1 T (15 ml/14 g)	54	14	0.26:1	7.3
Hempseeds	2 T (30 ml/20 g)	18	57	3:1	1.7
Hempseed oil	1 T (15 ml/14 g)	18	57	3:1	2.5
Spinach, raw	1 c (250 ml/50–60 g)	58	11	0.19:1	0.041
Walnuts (English)	¼ c (60 ml/28 g)	14	58	4:1	2.6

Sources:[165, 166]

(2 to 2.4 percent of calories) and keep LA near the lower end of this range (5 to 8 percent of calories). In a 2,000-calorie diet, this would be 11 to 18 grams of omega-6 fatty acids and 4.4 to 5.3 grams of omega-3 fatty acids.

Finding the right balance between getting 5 to 10 percent of calories from polyunsaturated fats and achieving a desirable ratio of omega-6s to omega-3s of 2:1 to 4:1 can be relatively simple. A very low-fat diet should include enough seeds to meet minimum EFA needs. A diet that includes more liberal amounts of fat should focus on foods rich in monounsaturated fatty acids, such as avocados and nuts, with the addition of some more-concentrated omega-3-rich foods. (A higher-fat diet also can include fresh or dried coconut, which is almost exclusively saturated fat with few omega-6 and no omega-3 fatty acids.)

Vegans can ensure adequate EFA intakes with a diet based on whole foods, provided that a rich source of omega-3 fatty acids to balance the omega-6s in these foods is included. (See table 4.6.) Avocados, olives, and nuts (except for walnuts, butternuts, and pine nuts) are concentrated sources of monounsaturated fatty acids, although they contain saturated fatty acids and LA as well. Each ounce of nuts provides an average of 1 to 3 grams of omega-6 fatty acids.

Seeds, seed oils, and soybeans are principal sources of polyunsaturated fatty acids, both omega-6s and omega-3s. Both walnuts and hempseeds provide a good balance of omega-6 to omega-3 fatty acids, but hempseeds also provide small amounts of SDA, which converts more readily to longer-chain omega-3 fatty acids than ALA. Flaxseeds are a rich and economical source of ALA. (Because whole flaxseeds tend to go undigested through the gastrointestinal tract, they should be ground before being eaten.) Chia seeds also are an excellent source of ALA, though they can be pricey.

Oils rich in omega-3 fatty acids are unstable and have a low smoke point, so they shouldn't be used for cooking. Instead, they should be eaten or served uncooked (for example, in salad dressings). Good choices are cold-pressed flaxseed oil, hempseed oil, or balanced oils that include plenty of omega-3 fatty acids (often these oils have a 1:1 or 2:1 ratio of omega-6 to omega-3 fatty acids). Liquid Gold Salad Dressing (page 219) provides a delicious way to boost omega-3 fatty acid intake.

Grains, legumes, vegetables, and fruits are generally very low in fat, so they make fairly minor contributions to fatty acid intake. One exception is soy foods, such as tofu and soybeans, which derive more than 40 percent of their calories from fat. The fat in grains is predominantly omega-6 fatty acids, although the ratio of omega-6 to omega-3 fatty acids varies considerably. For example, oats have a ratio of 22:1, while it's 13:1 for wheat, 10:1 for brown rice, 9:1 for barley and quinoa, 4:1 for rye, and only 1.25:1 for wild rice. Greens provide more omega-3s than omega-6s. Legumes and fruits contain mainly polyunsaturated fatty acids, with some being higher in omega-6 fatty acids and others higher in omega-3 fatty acids. Legumes average a ratio of about 1:1 with a few notable exceptions, such as chickpeas with a ratio of 26:1 and lentils with a ratio of about 4:1. The average ratio for fruit rests somewhere between 1:1 and 2:1, with apples at about 5:1 and papayas at about 1:5.

TABLE 4.6. Fatty acid composition of selected foods

FOOD (ALTERNATIVE SERVING SIZE)	TOTAL CALORIES	TOTAL FAT (g)	SATURATED FAT (g)	MONOUN-SATURATED FAT (g)	OMEGA-6 FATTY ACIDS LA (g)	OMEGA-3 FATTY ACIDS		
						ALA (g)	EPA (mg)	DHA (mg)
NUTS, SEEDS, PEANUTS,* AND WHEAT GERM; SERVING SIZE: 1 OZ (30 G), ABOUT 3.2 T (48 ML), UNLESS OTHERWISE NOTED								
Almonds	163	14	1.06	8.8	3.4	0	0	0
Butternuts	174	16	0.37	3	9.5	2.5	0	0
Cashews	157	12.4	2.2	6.7	2.2	0.018	0	0
Chia seeds, 2 T (30 ml)	109	6.9	0.75	0.52	1.3	4	0	0
Flaxseeds, ground, 2 T (30 ml)	75	5.9	0.51	1.05	0.8	3.2	0	0
Flaxseeds, whole, 2 T (30 ml)	110	8.7	0.76	1.6	1.2	4.7	0	0
Hazelnuts/filberts	178	17.2	1.3	12.9	2.2	0.025	0	0
Hempseeds, 2 T (30 ml)	113	8.7	1	1	5.3	1.7	0	0
Macadamia nuts	204	21.5	3.4	16.7	0.37	0.06	0	0
Peanuts*	161	14	1.9	6.9	4.4	0.001	0	0
Pecans	196	20.4	1.7	11.6	5.8	0.3	0	0
Pine nuts/pignolia nuts	191	19.4	1.4	5.3	9.4	0.05	0	0
Pistachios	159	12.9	1.6	6.8	3.8	0.073	0	0
Pumpkin seeds	158	13.9	2.5	4.6	5.9	0.034	0	0
Sesame seeds	165	14.3	2	5.4	6.2	0.1	0	0
Sunflower seeds	172	15.1	1.3	5.4	6.8	0	0	0
Walnuts	185	18.5	1.7	2.5	10.8	2.6	0	0
Wheat germ: 2 T (30 ml)	52	1.4	0.24	0.2	0.76	0.1	0	0
OILS; SERVING SIZE: 1 T (15 ML)								
Canola oil	124	14	1	8.9	2.7	1.3	0	0
Coconut oil	117	13.6	11.8	0.8	0.25	0	0	0
Corn oil	120	13.6	1.7	3.8	7.3	0.16	0	0
Cottonseed oil	120	13.6	3.5	2.4	7	0.03	0	0
Flaxseed oil	120	13.6	1.2	2.5	1.9	7.3	0	0
Grapeseed oil	120	13.6	1.3	2.2	9.5	0.014	0	0
Hempseed oil	126	14	1.5	2	8	2.5	0	0
Olive oil	119	13.5	1.9	9.9	1.3	0.1	0	0
Palm oil	120	13.6	6.7	5	1.2	0.03	0	0
Palm kernel oil	117	13.6	11.1	1.6	0.2	0	0	0
Peanut oil	119	13.5	2.3	6.2	4.3	0	0	0

FOOD (ALTERNATIVE SERVING SIZE)	TOTAL CALORIES	TOTAL FAT (g)	SATURATED FAT (g)	MONOUN- SATURATED FAT (g)	OMEGA-6 FATTY ACIDS LA (g)	OMEGA-3 FATTY ACIDS ALA (g)	EPA (mg)	DHA (mg)
Safflower oil	120	13.6	0.8	2	10.1	0	0	0
Safflower oil, high-oleic	120	13.6	1	10.2	1.7	0.01	0	0
Sesame oil	120	13.6	1.9	5.4	5.6	0.04	0	0
Soybean oil	120	13.6	2.1	3.1	6.9	0.9	0	0
Sunflower oil	120	13.6	1.4	2.7	8.9	0	0	0
Sunflower oil, high-oleic	124	14	1.4	11.7	0.5	0.03	0	0
Walnut oil	120	13.6	1.2	3.1	7.2	1.4	0	0
SEAWEEDS; SERVING SIZE: 3.5 OZ (100 G) RAW								
Irish moss	49	0.16	0.033	0.015	.002	.001	46	0
Kelp	43	0.36	0.25	0.1	.02	.004	4	0
Spirulina	26	0.39	0.14	0.03	0.064	0.042	0	0
Wakame	45	0.64	0.13	0.06	0.01	0.002	186	0
VEGETABLES								
Avocado, medium, 7.4 oz (210 g)	322	29.5	4.3	19.7	3.4	0.25	0	0
Olives, 10 large	51	4.7	0.623	3.5	0.37	0.03	0	0
Spinach, raw, 1 c (250 ml)	29	0.12	0.019	0.003	.008	0.041	0	0
ANIMAL PRODUCTS (FOR COMPARISON)								
Cod, 3 oz (90 g)	89	0.73	0.14	0.11	0.005	0.001	30	131
Egg, large, 2.7 oz (50 g)	72	4.8	1.6	1.8	0.8	.024	0	26
Wild Atlantic salmon, 3 oz (90 g)	155	6.9	1.1	2.3	0.19	0.321	349	1,215

Sources:[165, 168]

*For convenience, peanuts are included in the nuts and seeds category; peanuts are a legume.

The following guidelines are useful in putting together a diet that ensures an excellent intake and balance of essential fatty acids:

• **Follow the guidelines in chapter 14 to ensure a healthful, nutritionally adequate diet.** Eating sufficient protein, vitamins, and minerals maximizes the body's ability to convert ALA to long-chain polyunsaturated fatty acids (LCPUFA). Avoid trans-fatty acids and excess consumption of alcohol or caffeine; these can reduce conversion efficiency.

• **Include good sources of ALA daily.** The richest plant sources of ALA are seeds (chia seeds, flaxseeds, flaxseed oil, hempseeds, and hempseed oil) and walnuts.

(Although most of the fatty acids in leafy greens are omega-3 fatty acids, the total fat content in raw greens is so low that 10 cups provide just 1 gram of ALA.) Individuals who don't use DHA/EPA supplements should aim for 1.2 to 2.4 percent of calories from ALA (about 3.2 grams of ALA for men and 2.2 grams for women). Using DHA/EPA supplements lowers the need for dietary ALA to 0.6 to 1.2 percent of calories (1.6 grams of ALA for men and 1.1 grams for women). (See table 4.4 on page 127 for suggested intakes for various age groups.)

- **Reduce intake of omega-6 fatty acids, if excessive.** Regular use of cooking oils rich in omega-6 fatty acids, such as sunflower, safflower, corn, grapeseed, or sesame oil, can result in excessive consumption of these fatty acids. Also, many processed foods, such as salad dressings, margarines, crackers, cookies, and other high-fat foods, rely on omega-6-rich oils. Substitute oils that are mainly monounsaturated, such as extra-virgin olive oil, organic canola oil, or high-oleic sunflower oil, or oils with a high monounsaturated fatty acid content, such as safflower oil. Although these oils still provide omega-6 fatty acids, the omega-6s are present in much smaller quantities. For example, 1 tablespoon of omega-6-rich oil has about 7 to 10 grams of LA, compared to about 1 gram in 1 tablespoon of olive oil and 2.7 grams in 1 tablespoon of canola oil (the canola oil also provides about 1.3 grams of omega-3 fatty acids, for an excellent ratio of 2:1).

Eating large quantities of seeds or nuts that are low in omega-3 fatty acids (e.g., sunflower seeds, pumpkin seeds, sesame seeds, and pine nuts) could also push omega-6 intake above recommended levels. To keep omega-6 fatty acids under control, minimize the use of omega-6-rich oils and limit consumption of omega-6-rich seeds and pine nuts to about 1 ounce per day in a 2,000-calorie diet. Balance larger quantities of omega-6-rich foods with increased omega-3s accordingly.

Although the fatty acids in most nuts and avocados are mainly monounsaturated, these foods do contribute to omega-6 intakes. Most nuts contain about 1 to 3 grams of omega-6 fatty acids per ounce (pecans have almost 6 grams), while an avocado half provides less than 2 grams. Most grains are also far higher in omega-6 than omega-3 fatty acids. So, including some concentrated omega-3 sources when consuming these foods can help to bring omega-6 fatty acids into balance.

- **Consider a direct source of DHA, and possibly EPA.** Although it's not essential to use supplements or fortified foods that provide direct DHA (and possibly EPA), there's good evidence that doing so effectively boosts omega-3 fatty acid status. As noted previously, adequate DHA levels may be especially important during pregnancy and lactation and for individuals who have difficulty with ALA conversion (e.g., those with hypertension or diabetes). (See table 4.4 on page 127 for suggested intakes.)

The most common sources of EPA and DHA are fish and seafood; the only plant sources are plants from the sea—microalgae and seaweed. Seaweed doesn't contribute significantly to EPA intakes in the West but is a significant source in nations where people use large quantities of seaweed daily (e.g., Japan and other parts of Asia). Although seaweed does contain small amounts of highly unsaturated omega-3 fatty acids, it's even lower in fat than most vegetables. A 100-gram serving provides about 100 mg of EPA, but little DHA. In addition, some varieties of seaweed may provide excessive iodine if consumed in large quantities (See table 6.1 on page 194.)

Blue-green algae (spirulina and *Aphanizomenon flos-aquae* [AFA]) are low in highly unsaturated omega-3 fatty acids. Spirulina is rich in GLA—a beneficial omega-6 fatty acid—while about 40 to 50 percent of the fat in AFA is the omega-3 fatty acid ALA. Although neither type of blue-green algae is a significant source of EPA or DHA, some research indicates that they may promote more-efficient omega-3 conversion than plants grown on land.[167]

Microalgae-based vegan supplements are the most promising source of ecologically sustainable long-chain omega-3 fatty acids. These supplements, which provide DHA or DHA plus EPA, are widely available but are relatively expensive. For most people, an intake of 100 to 300 mg per day (or just two to three times a week) is reasonable. Microalgae-based DHA is also being added to some soy milks, cold-pressed oils, juices, cereals, and other foods, although the amounts are relatively small.

Many people aren't sure whether to stick to straight DHA or opt for combination DHA/EPA supplements. DHA is necessary for the development and maintenance of brain and eye function and is most important during pregnancy, lactation, and infancy. Because conversion from ALA to DHA can be limited, adequate intake of DHA appears more critical during these life stages. However, there may be further benefits to consuming supplements that combine DHA and EPA. EPA plays an important role in reducing chronic inflammation and may protect against some mental disorders. Both EPA and DHA appear to support heart health. As a result, a combination supplement may be most appropriate.

Fat Sources—The Quest for Quality

A s the Roman philosopher Seneca noted, "It is quality rather than quantity that matters." With regard to fat, the evidence that quality is more important than quantity has become increasingly convincing, particularly when energy intakes aren't excessive.

All fats in nature (whether from plants or animals) contain a mixture of saturated, monounsaturated, and polyunsaturated fatty acids; the relative amounts depend—at least in part—on climate. In plants, both fluidity and stability are critical. Generally speaking, in plants found closer to the equator, a greater proportion of their fat is saturated. For example, coconuts and palm fruits are high in saturated fatty acids to help protect and preserve the plants. Avocados and olives grow in more moderate climates and contain relatively stable monounsaturated fatty acids. In plants that grow in cold climates, polyunsaturated fatty acids often predominate to retain fluidity; a good example is flaxseeds. We see this in animals, as well. For example, warm-water fish are generally higher in saturated fat compared to cold-water fish, which contain much greater amounts of the highly unsaturated fatty acids, EPA and DHA.

Although the relative amounts of saturated, monounsaturated, and poly-unsaturated fatty acids in foods have implications for human health, we're beginning to discover that other factors (such as how people process, store, and prepare foods, and how much they eat relative to their energy needs) may weigh more heavily. Although fat was once regarded as a dietary villain, it's now viewed as a valuable part of the whole food package.

The highest-quality fat is present in fresh, whole, and minimally processed plant foods. All plant foods contain some fat, although nuts, seeds, avocados, coconuts, and olives are the most concentrated fat sources in any plant-based diet. One of the reasons that the fat in these foods is so beneficial is that it's unaltered and is protected from rancidity by naturally present antioxidants. In addition, whole plant foods are neatly packaged with protective components, such as proteins, unrefined carbohydrates, fiber, phytochemicals, plant sterols, and a variety of vitamins and minerals.

Plant-food fats are largely unsaturated, with the exception of coconut and palm fruits, whose fats are predominantly saturated. Although excessive con-sumption of saturated fats has been linked to increased disease risk, there's little evidence that suggests adverse effects when moderate amounts are consumed as part of a whole-foods, plant-based diet.

Conversely, meat and dairy products are rich in the type of saturated fats most strongly linked to increased blood cholesterol levels and insulin resis-tance.[274, 275] The presence of cholesterol in these foods is thought to exaggerate the impact of their fats. Evidence also suggests that eating animal fats increases the risk of colorectal cancer.[169]

Clean fish is widely considered one of the best fat sources, due to the signifi-cant content of the long-chain omega-3 fatty acids, EFA and DHA, in the fat. However, high-fat fish—especially those at the top of the food chain, such as King mackerel, tuna, swordfish, and shark—also can be a key source of environmental contaminants, including mercury, which diminishes their overall value.

Regardless of whether they're derived from plant or animal sources, fats that have been chemically altered by food-processing techniques or exposed to high temperatures pose particular concern. Among the most damaging to health are fats that have been chemically altered and solidified via partial hydrogenation, resulting in the creation of harmful trans-fatty acids. These fats are implicated in many disease processes; they raise blood cholesterol levels, trigger inflammation, increase insulin resistance, and compete with essential fatty acids for incorpora-tion into cell membranes.

Unfortunately, based on a belief that partially hydrogenated vegetable oils were more healthy than animal fats, food manufacturers liberally used partially hydrogenated fats—with their trans-fatty acids—for several decades before re-search revealed their dark side. Governments are now actively trying to reduce and, in some cases, eliminate trans-fatty acids from food supplies.

When any fats or oils are heated to temperatures of 350 to 400 degrees F (177 to 204 degrees C), their smoke points often are exceeded, allowing mutagenic products of oxidation to form. It's safest to avoid deep-fried foods and minimize the use of oils when cooking over high heat.

Generally, refined oils are more heat stable than unrefined oils, because they contain fewer of the solid particles that burn easily. However, the refining process itself can damage fat molecules, and it removes most of the protective components associated with the whole food. Unrefined oils (which can be a source of healthful fats when properly stored) have smoke points as low as 200 to 225 degrees F (93 to 107 degrees C); they're best reserved for salads and other unheated foods.

SATURATED FAT CONTROVERSIES: SEEING PAST THE HEADLINES

The longstanding view that saturated fats are "bad" has recently come under fire. At the core of the controversy are studies suggesting that saturated fat may not increase risk of heart disease.[170–171, 273] Two key reports sent shock waves throughout the scientific community. The first was a 2010 meta-analysis of twenty-one studies by Siri-Tarino and colleagues, which investigated the relationship between saturated fat intake and CVD in almost 350,000 people.[171] The second was a 2014 meta-analysis of seventy-six studies by Chowdhury and colleagues, which involved more than 510,000 people.[273] Contradicting decades of national and international dietary recommendations, no clear association between saturated fat intake and these diseases was found. A media frenzy ensued, leading consumers to believe that saturated fat had been vindicated and that beef, butter, bacon, and brie could be eaten with abandon.

Why did these large meta-analyses show no significant relationship between saturated fat and heart disease? First, many of the studies included in these meta-analyses compared similar populations that ate Western-style diets high in both fat and saturated fat (studies that examine a more diverse range of saturated fat intakes tend to show more significant disparity in disease risk); even the lowest intakes of saturated fat were above recommended intakes. Second, many of the studies used in these analyses relied on a single twenty-four-hour recall to determine dietary intakes; this method isn't reliable for ascertaining long-term dietary patterns. Third, several of the studies were adjusted for serum cholesterol levels. Because serum cholesterol concentrations increase with higher intakes of saturated fat, controlling for this variable obscures the results.

Since the mid-1990s, thirteen meta-analyses and scientific reviews have examined the relationship between saturated fats and CVD.[170–181, 273] Of these studies, ten reported that saturated fat increased CVD risk.[172–181] In 2010, the US Department of Agriculture Dietary Guidelines Advisory Committee summarized the evidence regarding the effects of saturated fat intake on risk of CVD and type 2 diabetes. They concluded that evidence supporting saturated fats' harmful effects is very high, and that replacing just 5 percent of saturated fats in a diet with polyunsaturated fats will decrease risk for CVD and type 2 diabetes and improve insulin response.[182] A 2011 consensus statement from an expert panel (convened to review the evidence regarding saturated fat and CVD) came to the following conclusion: "The evidence from epidemiological, clinical, and mechanistic studies is consistent in finding that the risk of coronary heart disease is reduced when saturated fatty acids (SFA) are replaced with polyunsaturated fatty acids (PUFA). In populations who consume a Western diet, the replacement of 1 percent of the energy from SFA with PUFA lowers LDL cholesterol and is likely to produce a reduction in coronary heart disease incidence of ≥ 2 to 3 percent."[274] (It's interesting to note that two of the coauthors of the Siri-Tarino meta-analysis were among the experts on this panel.) Finally, a 2012 Cochrane review reported that reducing saturated fat lowered the risk of cardiovascular events by 14 percent.[173]

Clearly, the media don't always tell the whole story. In the case of the Siri-Tarino analyses, the media reported that saturated fat had been vindicated. In fact, the study showed that when saturated fat is replaced by trans-fatty acids or refined carbohydrates, there's no improvement in cardiovascular risk—and, in the case of trans-fatty acids, risk is significantly heightened.

For many years, consumers were told that replacing saturated fats with carbohydrates would effectively reduce CVD risk because carbohydrates lower LDL cholesterol. More recently, however, research studies are suggesting that replacing saturated fat with refined carbohydrates (e.g., white flour products, white rice, and sugar-sweetened beverages and treats) provides no advantage and may actually increase CVD risk relative to saturated fat.[172, 174, 183, 274] Although refined carbohydrates reduce LDL cholesterol, they also reduce HDL cholesterol and increase triglyceride levels.

More research is required to determine the relative effectiveness of unrefined carbohydrates as a replacement for saturated fat,[183] although populations consuming diets low in saturated fat and high in unrefined carbohydrates are well protected against CAD. Evidence suggests that diets containing carbohydrate sources with a low GI are beneficial,[184] as are diets rich in unrefined carbohydrates.[186, 187]

We asked Dr. Francesca Crowe, one of the coauthors of the 2014 Chowdhury meta-analysis, about the weight of the evidence concerning saturated fat and CVD risk. She responded, "The best available evidence (from randomized controlled trials) shows that saturated fat intake affects blood cholesterol levels, which is an important risk factor for heart disease. Therefore, current guidelines should still recommend that people minimize their intake of saturated fat." The take-home message remains the same as it was thirty years ago: Western-style diets rich in animal products and processed foods increase CVD risk, while diets based on high-fiber, whole plant foods (such as vegetables, legumes, fruits, whole grains, nuts, and seeds) are protective.

HEALTHFUL HIGH-FAT PLANT FOODS

Some people take a hard-line view against all fat, including the fat found in whole plant foods. However, hundreds of scientific studies have confirmed that high-fat plant foods not only deserve a place in diets, but also that they deserve a place of honor. The research on these foods provides a powerful rebuttal to criticisms leveled against higher-fat plant foods in vegan diets.

Nuts

Although nuts are sometimes vilified for their high caloric content, they offer remarkably dietary and health benefits. Adding nuts to a diet enhances the quality of the diet, while improving intakes of multiple nutrients and protective dietary components.[188, 189]

Nutrient-dense nuts are brimming with beneficial vitamins and minerals. They're important sources of vitamin E and contribute to niacin, thiamin, riboflavin, pantothenic acid, vitamin B_6, and folate intakes. They're also valuable sources of trace minerals, such as iron, zinc, copper, calcium, selenium, magnesium, manganese, potassium, and phosphorus, and are very low in sodium (unless they're salted).

Nuts are among the most naturally antioxidant-rich foods (especially walnuts, pecans, hazelnuts, pistachios, and almonds) and also are rich in lignans, phytosterols, ellagic acid, and many other bioactive compounds. Due to their low carbohydrate content, nuts (as well as seeds) have the lowest glycemic index (GI) and glycemic load (GL) of any whole plant food. (For more on GI and GL, see pages 172 to 178.)

Most of the calories in nuts come from healthful fats, predominantly monounsaturated fatty acids (except for walnuts and pine nuts, which are high in polyunsaturated fatty acids), and nuts are low in saturated fats and free of trans-fatty acids and cholesterol. They're also are good sources of plant protein and particularly rich in L-arginine. This amino acid is a precursor of nitric oxide, which helps to preserve the elasticity and flexibility of blood vessels, enhancing blood flow.

As a result, nuts offer some protection from CVD and can enhance longevity. In several population groups, the frequency of nut consumption has been found to be inversely related to all causes of death;[190] regular nut-eating is estimated to increase longevity by about two years.[191] Moderate intakes of 1 to 2 ounces per day are associated with maximum benefits.

In 2011, a large research study compared a variety of metabolic markers for CVD, type 2 diabetes, and metabolic syndrome in nut consumers versus nonconsumers. The data was derived from the 1999–2004 National Health and Nutrition Examination Survey (NHANES), in which more than 13,000 American adults participated.[189] Results showed that, compared to nonconsumers, participants who ate nuts had a lower body mass index (BMI), lower body weight, smaller waist circumference, lower systolic blood pressure, reduced incidence of hypertension, higher HDL cholesterol levels, reduced fasting blood glucose, and lower rates of metabolic syndrome. This data supports the authors' conclusion that nut consumption decreases multiple risk factors associated with these diseases. Other studies have reported favorable effects of nuts on the risk of developing diabetes[192–194] and metabolic syndrome.[189, 193, 195]

In addition, nuts appear to protect against coronary heart disease (CHD). Two large review studies released in 2010 reported the wide-ranging cardiovascular and metabolic benefits of nut consumption, including significant risk reduction for CHD.[196, 197] Four major population studies (the Nurses' Health

Study, the Physicians' Health Study, the Iowa Women's Health Study, and the Adventist Health Study) also linked regular nut consumption to an extraordinary 35 to 50 percent risk reduction in CHD.[198–203] Of sixty-five food items examined in the Adventist Health Study-1, nuts provided the greatest protection against CHD, reducing deaths due to CHD by more than 50 percent in participants who consumed nuts five or more times a week, compared to those who ate nuts infrequently.[204]

Dozens of research studies have noted the beneficial effects of eating nuts on blood cholesterol levels.[188, 196, 205–209] Not only do nuts lower LDL cholesterol and raise HDL cholesterol, but they also appear to normalize the more-harmful, small, dense LDL particles that damage the cells lining blood vessels.[210] In addition, preliminary evidence suggests that compounds in nuts protect against inflammation and oxidized LDL and promote endothelial function.[211, 212]

According to data from the Nurses' Health Study, substituting calories in the form of the fat in 1 ounce of nuts for an equivalent amount of calories from carbohydrates would reduce coronary heart disease (CHD) risk by about 30 percent; replacing saturated fat with the equivalent amount of nut fat would reduce risk by about 45 percent.[180] These researchers estimated that people who eat nuts every day may gain an extra five to six years of life free of CHD.

Nuts may also be useful in the prevention and treatment of stroke,[213, 214] dementia,[215, 216] gallstones,[217] and advanced macular degeneration.[218]

An ongoing concern about nuts is that they might contribute to overweight and obesity. However, population studies have reported either no association or an inverse association between nut intake and BMI or body fat.[198, 219–222] Various clinical trials have recorded little or no weight change when various types of nuts are included in diets.[188, 195, 207, 208, 223–225]

A number of possible mechanisms may explain this unexpected phenomenon.[188, 226, 227] First, nuts appear to promote satiety, in turn reducing caloric intake from other foods. Second, some evidence indicates that nut consumption increases resting metabolic rate. Third, research suggests that bodies don't efficiently extract all the calories nuts provide, and that a considerable portion of nut fat is excreted in the feces. One research team suggested that, combined, these three mechanisms offset about 55 to 75 percent of the energy (calories) provided by nuts.[227]

A common question is whether raw or roasted nuts offer more nutritional benefits. Most population studies don't distinguish between raw and roasted nuts (or nut butters), and both types have been shown to afford protection. However, roasted nuts contain acrylamide and other products of oxidation that could potentially reduce their beneficial effects.[228] For example, acrylamide begins to form in almonds when their internal temperature reaches approximately 266 degrees F (130 degrees C),[229] and commercial nut-roasting temperatures are generally 285 to 300 degrees F (140 to 150 degrees C).[230] Of course, nut butters also can have added fats, sugar, and salt, so read the label.

Either roasting or soaking nuts results in reductions in phytate content. However, soaking and sprouting nuts increase the content and availability of their protective components, such as phytochemicals and antioxidants; the enzymes released by soaked nuts liberate these beneficial nutrients without forming acryl-amide. Soaked nuts are crunchy and delicious but are perishable and should be refrigerated and used within a few days (for more on storing nuts, see sidebar, page 145). Soaked nuts can also be dehydrated and used the same way as roasted nuts.

Seeds

Less research has been conducted on seeds than on nuts. Consequently, their value in human nutrition is often underestimated. Seeds vary in their protein content from about 12 percent of calories to more than 30 percent of calories; in contrast, the total protein in nuts ranges from about 4 to 15 percent of their calories. Seeds are among the richest sources of vitamin E and provide an impressive array of other vitamins, minerals, and phytochemicals, as well as fiber. This concentrated food also is the most plentiful source of healthy fatty acids. Pumpkin seeds, sunflower seeds, poppy seeds, hempseeds, sesame seeds, and tahini are rich in omega-6s, while flaxseeds, chia seeds, hempseeds, and canola seeds are high in omega-3s.

Flaxseeds are particularly high in ALA, so their consumption can go a long way toward correcting an imbalance between omega-3 and omega-6 fatty acids. Flaxseeds also provide a number of other nutrients. They're the richest known source of lignans (preliminary evidence suggests lignans may help to reduce growth of human cancer cells)[231, 232] and are also one of the best sources of boron. In addition, they're very high in soluble fiber. Studies show that eating flaxseeds can help to reduce blood cholesterol levels[233] and improve a number of other markers of CAD.[234–236]

Like other plant foods, flaxseeds contain a variety of antinutrients, such as phytic acid, oxalates, and cyanogenic glycosides. These compounds don't pose a health risk to most individuals, and consuming moderate amounts of raw flax-seeds (1 to 2 tablespoons per day) or larger amounts of cooked flaxseeds is safe for most people.[237] However, the body converts cyanogenic glycosides into substances that can block the uptake of iodine by the thyroid gland when iodine intake is inadequate (see pages 191 to 194).

Meanwhile, chia seeds, both whole and sprouted, are rapidly gaining popularity in raw-food cuisine. They're the only food higher in omega-3 fatty acids than flax-seeds; as much as 64 percent of chia oil comprises omega-3 fatty acids,[238] compared to an average of 57 percent in flaxseed oil. Chia seeds are packed with antioxidants and don't appear to contain the antinutritional factors found in flaxseeds.

The nutritional value of hempseeds is no less remarkable. About 20 percent of their calories come from easily digestible, high-quality protein,[239] and eating them provides an impressive array of trace minerals, vitamins, and phytochemicals. Hempseed oil has an excellent balance of omega-6 to omega-3 fatty acids and is one of the few foods that provide both SDA and GLA (page 117). (As a bonus, hemp may well be the most environment-friendly crop that can be grown. It takes only about one hundred days to mature, can be planted in the same fields year after year, and requires no pesticides or fertilizers. Besides providing nutri-tious seeds, the plant can be used to make more than 25,000 different products.)

Avocados

Most people know avocados are rich in monounsaturated fatty acids, but they may be surprised to learn about avocados' high levels of nutrients, fiber, and phytochemicals. Avocados contain more folate and potassium per ounce than any other fruit (60 percent more potassium than bananas) and are a good source of vitamins C and E. As a high-fiber food, the average avocado (about 200 grams) provides 13.5 grams of fiber—the equivalent of about three medium-sized apples.[165]

Avocados are rich in carotenoids and, of all commonly eaten fruits, have the highest concentration of lutein.[240] They also contain 76 mg of beta-sitosterol per 100 grams of fruit—more than four times that of other commonly eaten fruits, and double the amount in other whole foods.[241] (Plant sterols, such as beta-sitosterol, possibly inhibit tumor growth and can inhibit cholesterol absorption from the intestine, helping to reduce blood cholesterol levels.[241]) Avocados are also among the richest sources of glutathione, a powerful antioxidant.

Unfortunately, clinical data on the health effects of avocado consumption is limited. One study examined its effects on women's blood lipid levels, comparing an avocado-enriched diet (with avocados providing approximately 37 percent of the calories from fat and 20 to 35 percent of the total calories) with an American Heart Association-III (AHA-III) diet (approximately 20 percent of calories from fat, 100 to 150 mg of cholesterol, and high amounts of complex carbohydrates).[242] Participants consumed each of the diets for three weeks.

Participants' total cholesterol dropped an average of 4.9 percent while on the AHA-III diet and 8.2 percent on the avocado-enriched diet. There was no significant difference in their HDL cholesterol levels between the pre-entry diet and the avocado-enriched diet. However, HDL cholesterol dropped 13.9 percent when participants switched from the pre-entry diet to the AHA-III diet and 12.8 percent when they switched from the avocado diet to the AHA-III diet, suggesting that avocados contribute to maintaining HDL levels.

Studies also suggest that blends of bioactive compounds derived from avocados may provide benefits in cancer prevention and treatment and in reducing certain inflammatory diseases.[243] One study group reported that carotenoids and tocopherols in an extract of avocado inhibited the growth of human prostate cancer cells in vitro;[240, 243] lutein alone was unable to reproduce these effects. Investigators also showed that avocado extract selectively induced death in human oral cancer cells, specifically blocking two key components in the cancer pathway.[244, 245] Finally, a research team from India reported that the phytochemicals in avocados selectively inhibit growth and induce cell death in both precancerous and cancerous cell lines, and they show potential as chemoprotective agents to lower the side effects of certain chemotherapy drugs.[246]

Preliminary evidence exists that avocado extract acts against *Helicobacter pylori,* the bacteria associated with ulcers and stomach cancer.[247] Avocado extract also has been shown to provide anti-inflammatory effects, with some evidence suggesting reduction in the symptoms of knee and hip osteoarthritis.[248, 249]

Olives

Cultivated from antiquity, olives are a cherished part of the Mediterranean diet, and for good reason. They're a rich source of monounsaturated fat; a good source of iron, copper, and vitamin E; and rich in phytosterols as well as a host of beneficial phytochemicals, particularly polyphenolic compounds.[250, 251] For example, oleuropein, the major polyphenol in olives, is a potent free radical scavenger, inhibiting oxidative damage in body cells and protecting heart tissue.[252]

Both olives and olive oil contain bioactive compounds with known anticancer effects, including lignans, squalene, and terpenoids.[253] Extra-virgin olive oil is also rich in a polyphenol called oleocanthal, an anti-inflammatory agent.[254]

Are olives more nutritious than olive oil? Certainly; as a whole plant food, olives contain fiber and a variety of nutrients. Fermented olives also can be a good source of friendly bacteria. Olive oil does have the advantage of being much lower in sodium, although the sodium content of olives varies with the curing method. However, olive oil has 120 calories per tablespoon, while a serving of ten large olives contains only 50 calories.

The availability of olives has grown dramatically. A few decades ago, only two types of olives were commonly available—canned black olives and green olives (usually stuffed with pimiento) in a jar. Today, even mainstream supermarkets showcase a stunning variety of these little fruits arrayed in olive bars. Most bars don't provide nutritional information, preventing comparisons among the choices. However, green olives generally contain about double the sodium of black olives.

Given the increased availability of olives, it might be wise to avoid canned black olives, which have been reported to be high in acrylamide; however, most other olives contain no detectable amounts.[255] (Olive oil has not been found to contain acrylamide.)

Coconut Oil—Menace or Miracle?

Few foods have been at once as maligned and acclaimed as coconut oil. Because it's the most concentrated source of saturated fat in the food supply—even higher than lard or butter—some view it as a notorious health villain. Not surprisingly, it rests atop the "avoid" column in the list of mainstream heart-health foods.

Others view coconut oil as a fountain of youth and the greatest health discovery in decades. These advocates claim that coconut oil can provide therapeutic benefits for Alzheimer's disease, dementia, cancer, diabetes, digestive disturbances, heart disease, high blood pressure, HIV, kidney disease, osteoporosis, overweight, Parkinson's disease, and many other serious conditions. So what's the truth?

Based on the available science, coconut oil is neither a menace nor a miracle food. Coconut oil should be regarded like any other oil: a concentrated food that provides a lot of calories with limited nutrients. It certainly provides a vegan option for solid fat when preparing special-occasion treats, but as with other fats and oils, its use should be minimized. On the other hand, whole coconut (at varying stages of maturity) should be treated in much the same way as other high-fat plant foods—enjoyed in moderation, primarily as a whole food. As such, coconut is loaded with fiber, vitamin E, and healthful phytochemicals and has antimicrobial properties.

The relative health effects of coconut oil consumption remain somewhat uncertain. Some people believe that eating coconut oil does no harm because it's cholesterol-free; others claim it's harmful because it lacks essential fatty acids. But we can't ignore the fact that in many parts of the world where coconut and coconut oil are the principal sources of dietary fat, the rates of chronic disease, including CAD, are low.[256-258] There's one major caveat: the benefits seem to apply only when coconut products are consumed as part of a diet rich in high-fiber plant foods and lacking processed foods.

Recall the Marshallese (see pages 56 to 58), who had virtually no diabetes seventy years ago. The traditional Marshallese diet employed a wide variety of coconut products, which furnished an estimated 50 to 60 percent of total calories. When an indigenous diet gives way to a Western-style diet containing processed foods laden with white flour, sugar, and fatty animal products, disease rates escalate even when coconut products continue to be consumed. The Marshallese experience with increased rates of diabetes after such a dietary switch offers confirmation.

The main reason coconut oil is so often blacklisted by health care providers is because approximately 87 percent of its fat is saturated.[165] Many people imagine saturated fat as a single tyrant that clogs arteries, but different types of saturated fats exist. Depending on the length of the carbon chain, these fatty acids have very different effects on blood cholesterol levels and on health. Short-chain fatty acids contain 1 to 6 carbon atoms; these fats come largely from bacterial fermentation of indigestible carbohydrates. There's mounting evidence that short-chain fatty acids are highly beneficial to health, particularly colonic health. Medium-chain fatty acids contain 8 to 12 carbon atoms. These fatty acids have generated a great deal of interest among scientists and consumers, because they're quickly metabolized and used as energy (relative to longer-chain fatty acids, which are more likely to be stored in adipose tissue). Some evidence suggests that medium-chain fatty acids promote greater total energy expenditure, possibly aiding in weight control.[259] Long-chain fatty acids contain 13 to 21 carbon atoms, while very long-chain fatty acids contain 22 or more carbon atoms. Not all authorities agree on the chain length for each category. For example, 6-carbon fatty acids are sometimes considered medium-chain fatty acids, and 12-carbon fatty acids are sometimes classified as long-chain fatty acids.

The saturated fatty acids most abundant in the food supply are lauric acid, myristic acid, palmitic acid, and stearic acid. Their carbon-chain length and main food sources are:

- Lauric acid (12 carbon atoms): coconuts, coconut oil, palm kernel oil
- Myristic acid (14 carbon atoms): dairy products, coconuts, coconut oil, palm oil, palm kernel oil, nutmeg oil
- Palmitic acid (16 carbon atoms): palm oil, animal fats
- Stearic acid (18 carbon atoms): cocoa butter, mutton fat, beef fat, lard, butter

Saturated fatty acids with 12 to 16 carbon atoms increase LDL cholesterol levels, while 18-carbon stearic acid doesn't.[260] However, stearic acid isn't completely off the hook; some evidence shows high intakes could adversely affect other CVD risk factors, such as lipoprotein(a) and certain clotting factors.[180, 260]

As it happens, approximately 70 percent of the fat in coconut oil comprises saturated fatty acids known to raise blood cholesterol levels: about 45 percent is lauric acid, 17 percent is myristic acid, and 8 percent is palmitic acid. Another 15 percent is 6- to 10-carbon fatty acids, and about 3 percent is stearic acid.[165] Case closed?

Well, not exactly. The predominant fatty acid, lauric acid, does raise total cholesterol, but it appears to raise HDL cholesterol to an even greater extent than LDL cholesterol, favorably altering the ratio of HDL to total cholesterol.[261, 262] In addition, lauric acid is converted in the body into monolaurin, an antiviral, antifungal, and antiseptic compound—and coconut oil is among the richest food sources of lauric acid.[263–267] There's also evidence that coconut products have anti-inflammatory and antioxidant activity. Note that the compounds responsible for these benefits (which include a variety of phytochemicals, such as phenolic acids) are largely eliminated when coconut oil is refined.[263, 268, 269] The conclusion: Coconut products, including mature-coconut meat, young-coconut meat, and coconut water, can be part of a healthy vegan diet. Consumption of coconut oil, like other fats and oils, is best minimized.

CHOOSING FATS AND OILS

Including moderate amounts of high-fat plant foods can make eating more enjoyable and can add immensely to a diet's nutritional quality. One serving equals 1 ounce of nuts or seeds or half an avocado. For most people, two or three daily servings of such higher-fat plant foods is reasonable, while higher intakes are appropriate for athletes and others with increased caloric requirements.

The use of fats and oils alone is more controversial. At 9 calories per gram—about 120 calories per tablespoon—fats and oils are the most calorically dense foods. However, because they provide few nutrients per calorie, they have the lowest nutrient density of any food. As a result, direct consumption of fats and oils isn't necessary; nutrient-packed whole foods can provide all the fat needed by most individuals. On the other hand, added fats and oils can have a place in a healthful diet, as they do in the diets of many healthy populations throughout the world. Fats and oils add variety, flavor, and extra calories (without adding bulk) when needed. They also help to improve the absorption of fat-soluble vitamins and protective phytochemicals.

Oil-extraction methods can influence the quality and nutrition of the finished product. Most vegetable oil sold in mainstream grocery stores is refined oil; the solvent extraction process relies on hexane, a petroleum by-product. The oils then are degummed using acid, neutralized using caustic soda, bleached, deodorized, and dewaxed; the goal is to produce oils that are clear, colorless, and odorless. Finally, preservatives are commonly added to extend their shelf life.

Protecting Fat During Storage

To prevent deterioration of the unsaturated fats in high-fat plant foods, they're best kept refrigerated or frozen. Most nuts will keep four to six months in their shell at room temperature (although cooler temperatures will extend storage time). If stored in the refrigerator at 32 to 45 degrees F (0 to 7.2 degrees C), nuts and seeds will keep in their shells for a year or longer. Once their protective coating has been removed or is broken, nuts and seeds will keep for three to four months in the refrigerator and up to a year in the freezer. Because walnuts, chia seeds, ground flaxseeds, hempseeds, and wheat germ have higher levels of the more unstable omega-3 fatty acids, they're best kept frozen.

Oils, particularly the more nutritious expeller-pressed oils, will stay fresher when refrigerated or frozen. Although most oils will keep up to three months or longer in the refrigerator, oils high in omega-3 fatty acids, such as those extracted from flaxseeds and hempseeds, spoil very quickly and should be used within four to six weeks. (For sparing use, keep a small bottle in the refrigerator and freeze the rest.) Olive oil can be stored in a cool, dark place because it's more stable than most other mechanically pressed oils; however, it's still a good practice to keep it refrigerated. It becomes semisolid when cold but melts at room temperature.

Expeller pressing is an extraction technique that uses a screw or auger to squeeze oil from nuts, seeds, fruits, grains, or legumes. Although some heat is naturally produced from friction during this process, temperatures generally remain below 200 degrees F (93 degrees C). Some oils are truly cold-pressed, either because the oil is easily extracted and little heat is generated during the process, or because the pressing is conducted under temperature-controlled conditions to keep the materials cold. As a result, more valuable nutrients, antioxidants, phytosterols, and phytochemicals are retained in cold- and expeller-pressed oils than in conventionally refined vegetable oils. Also, the rich colors and flavors of the plants from which they were extracted are preserved, making expeller-pressed or mechanically pressed oils preferable to refined oils.

Virgin and extra-virgin olive oils are expeller pressed; today, they're widely available in stores. Most other expeller-pressed oils are sold in the supermarket's natural food section or in a natural food store. Those rich in omega-3 fatty acids are kept refrigerated.[270]

In any case, consumption of added fats and oils should be moderate. For salads and raw food preparation, oils rich in omega-3s (or with a good balance of essential fatty acids) are an excellent choice. (For more on essential fatty acids, see pages 117 to 134.) It's best not to expose these oils—especially good-quality unrefined oils—to direct heat, because they have a very low smoke point and are rapidly damaged.

For cooking, refined oils (such as pure olive oil or organic canola oil) are sensible choices, because they can withstand higher temperatures. People often mistakenly assume that coconut oil is the best cooking oil. However, virgin and extra-virgin coconut oils have smoke points closer to 350 degrees F (177 degrees C). Only refined coconut oil has a high smoke point of about 450 degrees F (232 degrees C).[271]

In general, vegetable margarine is a less healthy choice than refined oil, and its use should be minimized. (The most healthful spreads are nut and seed butters; they provide far greater nutritional value per calorie than any concentrated fats or oils.) Margarine is more highly processed, generally contains undesirable additives, and often is made with cheap oil or oils that are sourced unsustainably. Margarine may also contain trans-fatty acids.

Unfortunately, a claim that a product is free of trans fats is no guarantee that it actually is. A manufacturer can legally state on its nutrition label that a product has no trans-fatty acids if it contains less than 0.5 gram per serving in the United States and less than 0.2 gram per serving in Canada. The best way to be sure a product really is free of trans fats is to read the list of ingredients; if "partially hydrogenated oil" is present, the product contains trans-fatty acids.

Carbohydrates: The Whole Story

America is a constipated nation . . . If you pass small stools, you have to have large hospitals.

DENIS BURKITT, LIFESTYLE MEDICINE PIONEER, SURGEON, MEDICAL MISSIONARY

C arbohydrates are packages of solar energy, created by plants through photosynthesis and stored by them after conversion to sugar molecules that become linked in a variety of ways. The main source of energy (calories) for the body, carbohydrates are the preferred fuel for the brain, nervous system, and red blood cells.

Accordingly, carbohydrate-rich plant foods are the most valuable sources of food energy in the human diet. With the exception of dairy products, foods derived from animals contain few or no carbohydrates. Carbohydrate-rich whole plant foods reduce hunger, control blood glucose and insulin metabolism, and keep cholesterol and triglyceride levels in check. The nondigestible carbohydrates (or fiber) in these foods also help to maintain a healthy gastrointestinal tract by protecting against constipation and intestinal diseases and disorders. Conversely, carbohydrate-rich foods exhibit a far less flattering face when stripped of their protective components and consumed in a refined form.

The World Health Organization (WHO) recommends that 55 to 75 percent of calories come from carbohydrates, although a 2007 scientific update suggested that a lower limit of 50 percent could be acceptable.[1, 2] WHO adds that not more than 10 percent of calories should come from added sugars. Meanwhile, the Institute of Medicine (IOM) recommends somewhat lower intakes, ranging from 45 to 65 percent of calories from carbohydrates.[3] Both organizations agree that whole plant foods, such as vegetables, fruits, whole grains, legumes, nuts, and seeds, should provide most of these carbohydrates.

These health authorities set the lower end of the recommended carbohydrate range (45 to 55 percent of calories) to ensure that people eat enough carbohydrates to meet energy needs. The lower limits also ensure ample intakes of the beneficial compounds associated with carbohydrate-rich foods: fiber, minerals, vitamins, antioxidants, and phytochemicals. When carbohydrate intakes fall below 45 percent of energy, relative fat or protein intakes become excessive, potentially increasing the risk of chronic diseases.

Conversely, not exceeding the higher end of the recommended range (65 to 75 percent of calories) allows for adequate intakes of protein, fat, and their related essential nutrients. For example, intakes below 10 percent of calories from protein may be insufficient for vegans, particularly if the mix of plant foods is limited (for example, with few legumes); if the overall digestibility of the protein is poor (for example, with bulky, very high-fiber diets); or if protein requirements are high (for example, in children and athletes). In addition, fat intakes under 10 percent of calories can be too low to provide sufficient amounts of essential fatty acids, to ensure optimal absorption of fat-soluble nutrients and phytochemicals, or to supply sufficient energy, particularly for infants and children.[3]

Globally, carbohydrate intakes range from about 40 to 80 percent of calories, with those in developing countries tending toward the higher end of this range; Western dietary patterns fall near the lower end of the range.[4] In the United States, carbohydrate consumption averages about 50 percent of calories, which falls within IOM recommendations but below WHO recommendations.[3, 5] Vegan's carbohydrate intakes usually are higher, averaging closer to 60 percent of calories.[6] Low-fat vegan diets typically provide 75 to 80 percent of calories from carbohydrates; raw vegan and Mediterranean-style diets, which contain generous amounts of nuts, seeds, avocados, and oils, commonly supply closer to 50 percent of calories from carbohydrates.[7]

Based on the average minimum amount of glucose used by the brain, the recommended dietary allowance (RDA) for carbohydrate is set at 130 grams per day for adults and children. Most adults readily exceed this minimum, with average intakes ranging from 180 to 330 grams per day.[3] However, in obesity-ridden nations, advocates of low-carb diets have urged consumers to shun carbohydrates in favor of meat and other protein-rich foods, claiming that carbohydrates are at the root of all health problems. Although there's no question that diets rich in refined carbohydrates are detrimental to health, there's strong evidence of the protective effect of carbohydrates from whole plant foods. Long-lived populations throughout the world thrive on diets rich in unrefined carbohydrates.

In contrast, today's popular low-carb diets provide about 20 to 70 grams of carbohydrate per day—far below the RDA. Two recent systematic literature reviews reported increased all-cause mortality in those who consumed low-carbohydrate diets. The first, from Denmark, reported suggestive evidence for increased all-cause mortality with protein intakes of at least 20 to 23 percent of calories, and suggestive evidence for an inverse relationship between cardiovascular mortality and vegetable protein intake.[8] The second, from Japan, reported a 31 percent increase in all-cause mortality in those consuming low-carbohydrate, high-protein diets.[9]

Finally, a Harvard study that tracked almost 130,000 participants reported that low-carbohydrate diets were associated with a 12 percent increase in

Making Sense of Common Carbohydrate Terms

The term "simple carbohydrates" has long been used to identify potentially harmful carbohydrate sources, while the term "complex carbohydrates" has been used to distinguish the more healthful choices. Not only is this view an oversimplification, it's fundamentally inaccurate. Whether a carbohydrate is simple or complex is related to its molecular structure, not the healthfulness of the foods in which it's found.

Simple carbohydrates. Simple carbohydrates contain one or two molecules of sugar. They're found in whole foods, such as fruits and vegetables, or in refined sweeteners or products made with those sweeteners.

Complex carbohydrates. Starches that contain three or more molecules of sugar are known as complex carbohydrates. They're found in whole foods, such as whole grains, starchy vegetables, legumes, nuts, and seeds. They can also be found in flours, starches (e.g., cornstarch and potato starch), and products made from these foods.

Unrefined carbohydrates. Carbohydrates naturally present in whole plant foods are unrefined; they may be either simple or complex. Some of the unrefined simple-carbohydrate foods include fruit, dried fruit, and nonstarchy vegetables, such as broccoli, cucumbers, greens, peppers, and tomatoes. Examples of unrefined complex-carbohydrate foods are barley, quinoa, sweet potatoes, and beans.

Refined carbohydrates. Carbohydrate-rich foods made from processed grains (e.g., white flour), other processed starchy foods (e.g., cornstarch), and/or processed sweeteners (e.g., white or brown sugar) are called refined carbohydrates. They may contain either simple or complex carbohydrates. Soda, candy, jam, and jelly are refined simple-carbohydrate foods; bread and pasta made with white flour are refined complex-carbohydrate foods.

all-cause mortality. However, when the researchers separated the participants based on their protein sources, those consuming animal-rich, low-carbohydrate diets had a 23 percent higher all-cause mortality, a 14 percent higher cardiovascular mortality, and a 28 percent higher cancer mortality. In contrast, those consuming plant-rich, low-carbohydrate diets had a 20 percent lower all-cause mortality and a 23 percent lower cardiovascular mortality.[10] There's no question that low-carbohydrate, high-protein diets are effective for weight loss in the short term; however, this benefit becomes irrelevant when weighed against their long-term impact on all-cause mortality.

Healthful carbohydrates provide an efficient and safe source of energy for the entire body. The only other sources of energy—protein, fat, and alcohol—are less ideal. Protein can be used as a fuel, but it must first be deconstructed by the liver and kidneys to form glucose; if overconsumed, protein is converted to fat for storage. High protein intakes can place a burden on the liver and kidneys, especially in people with existing conditions.

Fat isn't a preferred energy source either. If the body uses fat instead of carbohydrates for energy on an ongoing basis, by-products called ketones can accumulate. In extreme cases, this can cause ketoacidosis, which drops the body's pH to dangerously low levels. Finally, in quantities large enough to act as a fuel, alcohol is highly toxic to the body, especially the brain, liver, and pancreas.[3, 4] That leaves carbohydrates, in all its various forms.

Scientific Carbohydrate Terminology

Photosynthesis enables plants to manufacture a variety of carbohydrates, from simple sugars (such as glucose and fructose) to complex carbohydrates (such as cellulose). Plants store energy for later use by stringing together the simple sugars to make the larger carbohydrates called starches (other complex carbohydrates, such as cellulose, are used to create the plants' cell walls). When young plants sprout and start to grow, they convert stored starches back into simple sugars to support their growth and metabolism. Humans use these carbohydrates in a similar fashion.

Carbohydrates, such as sugars, starches, and fibers, are categorized according to the number of basic sugar molecules ($C_n(H_2O)_n$) bound together in larger molecules of various arrangements:

- **Monosaccharides.** Monosaccharides, such as glucose, fructose, or galactose, are the smallest carbohydrate units and consist of a single molecule of sugar. Monosaccharides aren't further broken down in the intestinal tract, but rather are absorbed directly into the bloodstream.

- **Disaccharides.** Two chemically bonded sugar molecules are called disaccharides. The most common disaccharides are sucrose (table sugar), which combines a glucose and a fructose molecule; maltose (malt sugar), which combines two molecules of glucose; and lactose (milk sugar), which links one molecule each of glucose and galactose. Although monosaccharides and disaccharides are both considered simple sugars, the bond between the two component sugar molecules that make up the disaccharides must be broken through enzymatic action before the sugars can be absorbed and used for energy. The related enzymes are sucrase, maltase, and lactase, which break down sucrose, maltose, and lactose, respectively.

- **Oligosaccharides.** Relatively short carbohydrate chains that comprise three to nine molecules of sugar are called oligosaccharides. Many oligosaccharides are obtained by processing more-complex carbohydrates. For example, maltodextrin, a maltooligosaccharide used to thicken or bind processed foods, is produced from the breakdown of starch either through enzymatic action and/or acid hydrolysis, or both.

Other types of oligosaccharides aren't digested before they reach the large intestine; they serve as fuel for beneficial bacteria in the large intestine and may contribute to flatulence. Such oligosaccharides are also known as prebiotics. Examples include ciceritol, fructans (inulin and fructooligosaccharides), raffinose, starchyose, and verbacose. (For helpful tips, see "Dealing with Gas" on page 157.)

- **Polysaccharides.** Polysaccharides are glucose polymers that consist of at least 10 but often hundreds or thousands of glucose molecules. Polysaccharides are divided into two groups: starch and nonstarch polysaccharides (NSP). The distinction is based on whether the plant uses the polysaccharide for energy storage (starch) or structure (NSP, also known as fiber) and on their digestibility.

Starches are digestible polysaccharides that are broken down by enzymes into glucose molecules. Examples of starches include amylose, amylopectin, and modified starches, such as those used by the food industry as fat replacers or texture enhancers.

NSP are the components of plant cell walls and other indigestible parts of plants that can't be broken down by enzymes; they make up the bulk of the dietary components known as fiber. When NSP reach the colon, they're either fermented by colonic bacteria to yield many beneficial compounds and energy, or they're passed through the stool. Cellulose, hemicelluloses, mucilages, pectin, and plant gums are all examples of NSP found in food.

- **Polyols (sugar alcohols).** Neither a sugar nor an alcohol, polyols are nonsugar carbohydrates formed by the hydrogenation of either mono- or disaccharides. One part of their chemical structure resembles a sugar molecule and the other part resembles an alcohol molecule. Sugar alcohols are found in small amounts in fruits and vegetables; they're also manufactured in larger amounts from sugars or starches for use as sweeteners. Although they're slightly less sweet than sugar, polyols don't promote tooth cavities. Because they're poorly digested, they contribute fewer calories per gram than sugars or alcohol. But when consumed in excess, polyols can cause gastrointestinal distress. Examples include erythritol, isomalt, lactitol, maltitol, mannitol, polydextrose, sorbitol, xylitol, and hydrogenated starch hydrolysates.[3, 4, 11, 12]

Carbohydrate Digestion: Getting the Goods

C arbohydrates supply approximately 4 calories per gram, as does protein. (In practical terms, 1 tablespoon of either pure protein or carbohydrate provides about 50 calories.) When nutritional analyses are performed, all carbohydrates are calculated as providing 4 calories per gram, regardless of the degree to which they are digested.

The relative digestibility of plant carbohydrates depends on the plants' growth stage when consumed; the riper the plant, the more digestible its carbohydrates. As plants ripen, they convert their stored carbohydrates into the simpler sugars that sweeten fruits and vegetables. Then, when food preparation begins and the plants' cells are broken down by chopping, grating, blending, juicing, and cooking, starch-digesting enzymes in the plants are activated.

Once carbohydrates enter the mouth, amylase (a starch-splitting enzyme in saliva) begins to sever some of the bonds between the molecules in the starches. However, the greater part of starch digestion occurs in the small intestine, where additional enzymes break down the starches to allow monosaccharides to pass through intestinal walls and enter the blood.

Once in the bloodstream, glucose is either used for energy or removed by the liver and converted into a storage carbohydrate called glycogen. The body can store only limited amounts of glycogen, so excess glucose is converted into fatty acids for unlimited long-term storage as fat. Meanwhile, fructose and galactose are quickly taken up by the liver and converted to glucose to be used for immediate energy.

If there's already enough energy available, they too are converted to glycogen for short-term storage or fatty acids for long-term storage.

Fiber and nondigestible oligosaccharides aren't broken down in the small intestine but move on to the large intestine, where they either add bulk to the stool or are used as food by intestinal bacteria. Consequently, the usable calories in many high-fiber, high-carbohydrate foods may be overestimated. In other words, high-fiber foods may actually provide somewhat fewer calories than the amounts listed in nutrient databases. Some experts suggest that for carbohydrates that reach the large intestine intact (i.e., fiber), the calorie count should be 2 calories per gram.[4]

Fiber does provide some calories. When it reaches the large intestine, short-chain fatty acids are produced as a by-product of microbial fermentation; these fatty acids are absorbed into the blood stream, providing some energy in the process.[11]

Fiber: Just Passing Through?

Besides serving as a major source of calories, unrefined carbohydrate-rich whole plant foods can help to reduce hunger, control blood glucose and insulin metabolism, and keep cholesterol and triglyceride levels in check. These foods also help to maintain a healthy gastrointestinal tract by protecting against constipation and intestinal diseases and disorders. Most of these beneficial effects are the result of the nondigestible content of carbohydrates, better known as fiber.

Fiber has come to be viewed as nature's broom—the part of plants that keeps things moving smoothly and efficiently through the body's intestinal tract. Its benefits became universally recognized in the 1970s when researcher Denis Burkitt discovered that rural Africans were free of Western diseases, such as heart disease, diabetes, and obesity, as well as intestinal disorders, such as colon cancer and constipation. He determined that dietary fiber set Africans apart from Westerners and that size and frequency of bowel movements were excellent predictors of health.

Burkitt's message was enthusiastically embraced by the public. Wheat bran became the food fad of the decade and was added to everything from muffins to meat loaf. What consumers failed to realize was that spiking their diet with wheat bran didn't provide the same benefits as consuming a variety of high-fiber plant foods, as rural Africans do or as Burkitt advocated.

FIBER FUNDAMENTALS

Although technical differences exist throughout the world, most definitions of fiber include all nonstarch polysaccharides (NSP) with 10 or more sugar molecules, oligosaccharides (3 to 9 molecules), and lignin (a noncarbohydrate component of plant cell walls).[3, 11, 15] Dietary fiber can't be broken down by digestive enzymes in the small intestine of humans.

Another type of fiber—called functional, novel, or added fiber—consists of nondigestible carbohydrates that are extracted from plants or synthetically produced, and that have some health benefits. Most functional fibers are oligosaccharides (isolated from plants or synthetically produced) or manufactured NSP.

The IOM defines total fiber as "the sum of dietary fiber and functional fiber." The inclusion of functional fiber in this definition is controversial within the international scientific community, because there's concern that functional fiber may not provide the same physiological benefits as dietary fiber. For example, a manufacturer could add isolated or synthetic fiber to otherwise unhealthy food, declare its high fiber content, and mislead consumers into thinking that the food is nutritious. By contrast, whole plant foods are naturally good sources of fiber, are rich in dozens of nutrients and phytochemicals, and are beneficial to health in myriad ways.[11]

TYPES OF FIBER

Fiber has traditionally been divided into two categories: soluble and insoluble. Examples of soluble fibers are gums, mucilages, and pectins. Cellulose and lignin are examples of insoluble fiber. Hemicelluloses and beta-glucans vary in solubility, although hemicelluloses are usually insoluble and beta-glucans are usually soluble. All fiber-rich foods contain both soluble and insoluble fibers.[11, 16]

For many years, experts believed a fiber's solubility determined its physiological effects. It was thought that soluble fiber formed viscous gels and was fermentable, thus favorably impacting blood glucose and blood cholesterol. Insoluble fiber was associated with stool bulk and regularity.

However, more recent research suggests that the physiological benefits attributed to soluble and insoluble fiber are highly inconsistent. For example, some types of soluble fiber have little influence on blood glucose or cholesterol but do improve gut health and regularity. Likewise, some insoluble fiber is rapidly and completely fermented in the large intestine, and therefore wouldn't contribute to stool bulk as expected.

The research concludes solubility doesn't predict viscosity or fermentability. Many of the earlier studies were done using isolated fibers, rather than the plant foods in which these fibers coexist. So while the terms "soluble" and "insoluble" are useful when referring to specific, isolated types of fiber, they're less useful in relation to whole foods. Although these terms have long been used to classify fiber types in research papers, in nutrition education materials, and on food labels, scientific health authorities are attempting to phase them out and use viscosity and fermentability instead.[16]

- **Viscous and nonviscous fiber.** Viscous fiber becomes gel-like or thick and gummy when mixed with water. Nonviscous fiber may absorb water but doesn't become gluey. While fiber must be somewhat soluble to make water viscous or gel-like, not all soluble fiber has this property. Viscosity is thought to be responsible for some of fiber's greatest health advantages. Viscous fiber helps to delay stomach emptying and increases feelings of fullness after eating. It can stabilize blood glucose levels and reduce blood cholesterol. Guar gum, mucilages, and pectin are all examples of viscous fiber. Cellulose and lignin are examples of nonviscous fiber. Hemicelluloses and beta-glucans can fall into either category, although most hemicelluloses are nonviscous and most beta-glucans are highly viscous. [17]

- **More-fermentable and less-fermentable fiber.** Fiber feeds bacteria in the colon. These microorganisms extract energy from fiber by fermenting it, creating short-chain fatty acids and intestinal gases as by-products. The short-chain fatty acids can be absorbed into the bloodstream and used by the body for energy. Butyrate, a major short-chain fatty acid metabolite, is the preferred energy source for colonocytes (cells lining the colon); some evidence exists that a lack of butyrate may contribute to ulcerative colitis and colon cancer.[3]

The types of fiber most fermentable by bacteria include beta-glucans, guar gum, hemicelluloses, pectins, and nondigestible oligosaccharides. Gums and mucilages are the most slowly fermented, while oligosaccharides are the most rapidly fermented. Less-fermentable types of fiber, such as cellulose, resistant starch, and lignin, make an impressive contribution to stool bulk. Wheat bran is an excellent example of a food rich in these less-fermentable fibers. For various types of fiber and their food sources, see table 5.1.

FIBER FIGHTS DISEASE

While the benefits of fiber begin in the intestine, they extend to every part of the body. High-fiber diets positively contribute to gastrointestinal health, cardiovascular health, blood glucose control, and weight management:

- **Gastrointestinal health.** Fiber is important for preventing constipation, diverticulosis (small sacs in the wall of the intestines that press outward), and hemorrhoids (painful, swollen tissues in the anus and rectum). It may also protect

TABLE 5.1. Common sources of specific fibers

TYPE OF FIBER	COMMON SOURCES
Beta-glucans	Oats, barley, and mushrooms
Celluloses*	Grains, fruits, vegetables, legumes, nuts, and seeds
Gums and mucilages (used to thicken, stabilize, and add texture to foods)	Seeds, such as psyllium and guar seeds (guar gum), and sea vegetable extracts, such as carageenans and alginates
Hemicelluloses**	Fruits, grains (especially outer husks), legumes, nuts, seeds, and vegetables
Lignins	Stringy vegetables and the outer layer of cereal grains
Nondigestible oligosaccharides	Fruits, grains, legumes, and vegetables
Pectins	Berries and fruits (especially apples and citrus fruits)
Resistant starches	Legumes, raw potatoes, underripe bananas

Sources:[3, 11, 12, 18]

*Celluloses account for about 25 percent of the fiber in grains and fruits and 33 percent in vegetables and nuts.

**Hemicelluloses account for about 33 percent of the fiber in plants.

against intestinal cancers (especially colorectal cancers), gallstones, and inflammatory bowel diseases, such as ulcerative colitis. A high-fiber diet makes stools softer and heavier, helping them pass more easily and rapidly out of the colon. While the insoluble, nonviscous, less-fermentable fibers, such as cellulose and lignin, are particularly helpful in this regard, fiber fermented in the colon also contributes to stool softening and bulk. It's estimated that for every 3.5 ounces (100 g) of carbohydrate fermented in the colon, about 1 ounce (30 g) of bacteria is produced, contributing to fecal mass.[3, 11]

Many fermentable carbohydrates serve as prebiotics, stimulating the growth of friendly bacteria in the colon. These beneficial bacteria and the fermentation products they generate (carbon dioxide, hydrogen, methane, and short-chain fatty acids) reduce the pH of the colon and feces, inhibiting the growth of harmful yeast and bacteria. Friendly bacteria can also enhance mineral absorption, reduce food sensitivities and allergies, disable carcinogens, attack cancer cells, and favorably affect the metabolism of fat and sugar.[3, 11]

- **Cardiovascular health.** In numerous studies, fiber-rich diets have been associated with a reduced risk of cardiovascular disease.[19] One pooled analysis of ten prospective cohort studies reported that each additional 10 grams of dietary fiber was associated with a 14 percent decrease in risk of coronary events and a 27 percent decrease in coronary death.[19] (See table 5.2 on page 160 for the fiber content of common foods.) Another study of more than 40,000 male health professionals reported that participants who consumed the greatest amounts of fiber had a 40 percent reduction in the risk of developing coronary artery disease, compared to those consuming the smallest amount of fiber.[20]

It's difficult to determine whether these benefits are attributable only to fiber, to other healthful components in plant foods, or to reductions in saturated fat, trans-fatty acids, and cholesterol associated with plant-based diets. However, research suggests a variety of mechanisms by which fiber may exert protection. One popular theory is that soluble, viscous fiber binds with bile acids that contain cholesterol, carrying them out with the feces.[19] Other possibilities include reduced synthesis of fatty acids by the liver (because products of fermentation inhibit their production) and increased satiety leading to reduced caloric intake.[21] Fiber can also reduce blood pressure, improve enzymatic breakdown of fibrin that can help to remove blood clots, and enhance insulin sensitivity.[19]

- **Diabetes and metabolic syndrome.** Fiber intake has been associated with a reduced risk of metabolic syndrome and type 2 diabetes.[22–25] Fiber, particularly soluble viscous fiber, delays the absorption of fat and carbohydrates from the small intestine, favorably influencing insulin levels and blood glucose response. Delayed absorption of carbohydrate and fat helps to curb appetite, possibly reducing overeating and weight gain.[11]

- **Overweight and obesity.** High-fiber foods are associated with reduced overweight and obesity. Generally, high-fiber foods take more space on plates and in stomachs; they also require more chewing. Many high-fiber foods are less energy dense, meaning they have fewer calories for a specific volume of food. All these factors contribute to satiety or feelings of fullness.[11]

RECOMMENDED AND ACTUAL FIBER INTAKES

Populations that consume very high-fiber diets generally have low rates of chronic disease. As a result, WHO recommends at least 25 grams of dietary fiber per day for adults;[1] IOM recommends 14 grams of fiber per 1,000 calories for everyone older than 1 year.[3] Although an RDA hasn't been set for fiber, the Adequate Intake (AI) was established in accordance with this 14-gram figure. Based on average energy intakes for various ages and genders, the daily AI is 38 grams for men 19 to 50 years old (30 grams for older men), and 25 grams for women 19 to 50 years old (21 grams for older women). The International Life Sciences Institute suggests that an intake of 32 to 45 grams of fiber per day may be necessary to achieve the critical fecal mass of 160 to 200 grams per day (about 5.5 to 7 ounces) necessary for preventing constipation.[11]

Nutritional anthropologists estimate preagricultural fiber intakes at 70 to 150 grams per day.[26] Clearly, cavemen ate a lot of plant foods (for more on this topic, see pages 279 to 281). In contrast, Western-style diets provide about half the current recommended intakes, or approximately 15 to 17 grams of fiber per day.[27, 28] Among contemporary populations, high fiber intakes have been reported in rural Chinese (up to 77 grams of fiber per day) and rural Africans (60 to 120 grams of fiber per day).[26] Average vegan intakes consistently exceed the AI. Based on studies conducted between 1984 and 2005, vegan men average 45 to 50 grams of fiber per day and vegan women average 35 to 40 grams of fiber per day.[6]

NATURAL REGULARITY

Vegans are at a definite advantage when it comes to stool bulk and healthy laxation, and are the one dietary group in the Western world that typically exceeds current recommended fiber intakes. Switching to a vegan diet normally solves any problems with irregularity, but additional steps also may be taken:

• Eat at least one serving of legumes (½ to 1 cup/125 to 250 ml) per day. Add beans to soups, stews, loaves, and patties; top salads with them. Note that processed alternatives, such as tofu and vegan meat substitutes, are much lower in fiber.

• Aim for nine or more servings of vegetables and fruits each day. Wash but don't peel fruits and vegetables. Eat a good proportion of these foods raw. Enjoy a large raw salad every day. When cooking vegetables, minimize cooking time. Select higher-fiber options more often. (See table 5.2 on page 160.)

• Opt for intact whole grains most of the time. Grinding breaks down fiber, and smaller particles generally contribute less to stool bulk. While bran increases stool bulk greatly, it's best to rely on whole grains rather than isolated bran due to the latter's negative impact on mineral absorption.

• Sprinkle on seeds. Seeds can increase stool weight. Whole flaxseeds are especially effective, as are psyllium seeds, though even ground seeds are helpful.

Menus for Fiber

The menus on pages 439 to 442 provide between 48 and 88 grams of fiber. In addition, for excellent recipes that list fiber content and include a complete nutritional analysis, see *Cooking Vegan* by Vesanto Melina and Joseph Forest (Book Publishing Company, 2012) and *Becoming Raw* by Brenda Davis and Vesanto Melina (Book Publishing Company, 2011).

- Select whole-grain options when using processed grain products. Read labels. Aim for at least 2.5 grams of fiber in a serving of bread or pasta and 5 grams from a serving of breakfast cereal.

- Spike baked goods with high-fiber ingredients. Use or buy cookies, muffins, breads, or other baked goods that contain high-fiber ingredients. When baking from scratch, use dates, prunes, or bananas in place of sugar; nut or seed butters or applesauce in place of oil; coarsely ground whole-grain or sprouted-grain flours in place of refined flour; and ground flaxseeds in place of eggs.

- Choose high-fiber snacks. Raw fruits and vegetables, trail mixes, stuffed dates or other raw treats, and popcorn are excellent options.

- Keep well hydrated. Most people need at least 8 cups (2 L) of fluid each day.

- Exercise daily. Whether it's a brisk walk or jog, an aerobics or yoga class, a swim or game of tennis—any physical activity keeps intestines working well.

DEALING WITH GAS

On average, people pass gas twelve to twenty-five times a day. Gas production protects the colon against genetic damage that may lead to cancer; it dilutes carcinogens, stimulates beneficial bacterial growth, favorably alters the gut pH, and improves the function of the epithelial cells of the colon.[11, 29] Of course, there's a point at which passing gas becomes a social liability. The annoyance and embarrassment caused by flatulence provides grounds for some people to drastically limit or even avoid beans and high-fiber foods altogether.

However, a recent study found that only about 50 percent of participants who added ½ cup (125 ml) of pinto beans, black-eyed peas, or vegetarian baked beans to their daily diet experienced an increase in flatulence during the first week of their addition compared to those who added ½ cup (125 ml) of carrots. Of the participants who experienced increased flatulence with bean intake, 70 percent found that it dissipated by the second or third week of daily bean consumption.[30]

There are two main causes of gas: swallowing air and bacterial fermentation of carbohydrates that reach the large intestine. The following suggestions will help to keep gas production tolerable.

To reduce the amount of air swallowed:

- eat slowly and with the mouth closed
- chew food well
- avoid drinking carbonated beverages, chewing gum, and sucking on candies
- make sure dentures fit properly

To diminish the impact of undigested carbohydrates that reach the colon:

- **Reduce the oligosaccharides in beans.** Beans are among the most notorious flatulence producers. The offending compounds are raffinose, starchyose, and verbacose—oligosaccharides that can't be broken down before they reach the colon because humans don't produce alpha-galactosidase, the enzyme needed to break apart the bonds in the oligosaccharides found in beans. They arrive in the colon relatively undigested and are fermented by bacteria in the colon, resulting in intestinal gas. There are a number of ways to reduce oligosaccharide intake from beans:

1. Use fresh beans instead of dried beans because their oligosaccharide content is much lower.

2. Buy only as many dried beans as can be used within a few months. The longer beans are stored, the higher their oligosaccharide content becomes.

3. Soak beans for about twelve hours or overnight; discard the soaking water and rinse well before placing in fresh water and cooking. Plan ahead for a double soak, during which this procedure is completed twice before cooking. If there's no time to soak, boil the beans briefly, let them sit in the water for an hour or two, discard the soaking water, rinse well, and cook in fresh water. When boiling beans, remove any white foam that forms at the surface; this foam contains oligosaccharides.

4. Sprout legumes. Sprouting converts oligosaccharides into sugars.[31] Sprouted mung beans, lentils, and peas can be eaten raw. Other legumes should be cooked after sprouting. Soak beans for twelve to twenty-four hours, drain, and rinse well; then sprout for at least one to three days, or until small sprouts appear. Be sure to rinse and drain two or three times a day. Once the beans have a tiny sprout, they're ready to cook; sprouting cuts cooking time in half.

5. Start with small portions of beans and gradually increase the portion size. This will allow time for more formation of bacterial flora that can completely digest oligosaccharides.

6. Make sure beans are thoroughly cooked. Undercooked beans are more difficult to digest. Beans are sufficiently cooked when they can easily be crushed between the tongue and the roof of the mouth.

7. Rinse canned beans well before eating.

8. Select small legumes that are easier to digest. The least problematic are skinless, split legumes, such as mung dahl (split mung beans), red lentils, and split peas. Generally, smaller beans, such as adzuki and mung beans, are easier to digest than large beans, such as lima or kidney beans.

The Power of Legumes

In South America, Africa, China, the Middle East, and India, legumes have served as dietary staples for centuries. Per capita consumption of legumes is approximately 6.5 pounds (about 3 kg) per year in the United States;[33] intakes exceeding 88 pounds (40 kg) per year are common in countries that rely on legumes as dietary staples, and intakes of up to 145 lbs (66 kg) per year have been reported in some African countries (e.g., Kenya).[34]

Legumes provide many of the key nutrients found in meat (e.g., protein, iron, and zinc) along with protective compounds concentrated in plants and largely absent from meat (fiber, plant sterols, antioxidants, and phytochemicals). Recent evidence suggests that the nonheme ferritin iron in legumes is highly absorbable and may provide important advantages over heme iron or iron supplements.[35] (For more on iron, see pages 186 to 189.)

Researchers at the US Department of Agriculture Food Composition and Nutrient Data Laboratories assessed the total antioxidant capacity of more than one hundred foods and released a rather stunning result—legumes claimed three of the top five prizes. Another study reported that legumes were the only food group found to produce a significant reduction in mortality. For every 0.66-ounce (20 g) increase in daily bean intake, risk of death dropped 7 to 8 percent.[36] Legume consumption has also been shown to favorably alter the risk of developing cancer, cardiovascular disease, and diabetes and to provide benefits in weight loss.[37]

Although dried beans contain lectins (often associated with food allergies) and phytate (substances that reduce mineral absorption), common food preparation methods significantly reduce or eliminate these compounds, particularly lectins.

9. Include fermented bean products, such as tempeh and miso, and lower-fiber legume options, such as tofu.

• **Use seasonings that counteract the production of intestinal gas.** Spices prized for their ability to ward off gas production are cloves, cinnamon, garlic, turmeric, black pepper, asafetida (hing), and ginger.[32] The Mexican spice epazote and the Japanese seaweed kombu are commonly added to foods to neutralize the gas-producing compounds they contain.

• **Improve gut flora.** Take probiotics in supplement form or use in preparing fermented vegan cheeses, yogurts, and other dishes.

• **Avoid overeating.** Eat smaller meals; stop eating when 80 percent full.

• **Limit foods rich in added fructose or sugar alcohols.** The small intestine isn't equipped to handle large quantities of fructose or sugar alcohols, such as sorbitol, maltitol and xylitol; when these sugars aren't completely absorbed, they're fermented by bacteria in the colon. Even fructose from fresh or dried fruits can be a problem when consumed in excess.

• **Take activated charcoal.** Taking activated charcoal right before eating foods that trigger flatulence is reported to reduce both the amount and odor of intestinal gas.

• **Take an enzyme supplement with gas-producing food.** If all else fails, consider taking a supplement containing the oligosaccharide-digesting enzyme alpha-galactosidase, which humans do not produce.

SOURCES OF DIETARY FIBER

All whole plant foods provide fiber; it's what gives plants their structure. (Animal products don't contain fiber; bones give animals structure.) Table 5.2 provides a list of the fiber content of foods.

TABLE 5.2. Fiber content of selected whole plant foods

AMOUNT OF FIBER PER CUP OR SERVING	FOOD AND SERVING SIZE
Very high-fiber foods 10 to 19.9 g	Legumes (all varieties), cooked, 1 c (250 ml)
	Split peas, cooked, 1 c (250 ml)
	Avocado, medium, 6.7 oz (200 g)
	High-fiber bran cereals, ½ c (125 ml)
High-fiber foods 5 to 9.9 g	Berries (raspberries, blackberries), fresh, 1 c (250 ml)
	Fruit (Asian pears, papayas, pears), medium
	Dried fruit (apricots, figs, peaches, pears, prunes, raisins), ½ c (125 ml)
	Coconut, fresh, shredded, ½ c (125 ml)
	Flaxseeds, 2 T (30 ml)
	Grains (most whole grains), cooked, 1 c (250 ml)
	Potato, regular or sweet, baked, medium
	Pasta, whole wheat, 1 c (250 ml)
	Artichoke, medium
Moderate-fiber foods 2 to 4.9 g	Berries (blueberries, strawberries), fresh, 1 c (250 ml)
	Fruit (most varieties), 1 medium/2 small or 1 c (250 ml)
	Vegetables (most), raw: 2 c (500 ml); cooked: 1 c (250 ml)
	Nuts and seeds (most varieties), ¼ c (60 ml)
	Grains (brown rice, millet, oats), cooked, 1 c (250 ml)
	Whole-grain breads (read label), 2 slices
	Pasta, white, 1 c (250 ml)
	Popcorn, 3 c (750 ml)
Lower-fiber foods 1.9 g or less	Melon, 1 c (250 ml)
	Fruit or vegetable juice (all varieties), 1 c (250 ml)
	Sprouts* (grain, legume, or vegetable), 1 c (250 ml)
	Lettuce, all types, 2 c (500 ml)
	Cucumber, medium, 8 in (20 cm)
	Refined grains, most (white rice, Cream of Wheat), ½ c (125 ml)
	Refined cold cereals, 1 oz (30 g)

Source:[13]

*The fiber content in sprouts is far lower than the fiber in an equal volume of the unsprouted food, because it takes only a few tablespoons of the unsprouted food to produce a cup of sprouts (which are largely water). Furthermore, some of the fiber in seeds or legumes is converted to simple sugars during the sprouting process.

TOO MUCH FIBER?

Though possible, excessive fiber intake is unlikely if consumers eat whole plant foods and drink sufficient fluids. Excessive fiber is more of an issue for people who consume concentrated fiber sources, such as wheat bran, in large amounts. In small children, very high fiber intakes can make the diet too bulky, jeopardizing energy intake and potentially resulting in failure to thrive. This is seldom a concern in healthy adults.

Fiber can bind calcium, iron, and zinc and reduce their absorption, although these minerals are at least partly liberated during fermentation in the large bowel. Short-chain fatty acids (also products of fermentation) help to facilitate their absorption from the large bowel.[11] In addition, compared to refined foods, high-fiber whole foods generally provide enough extra minerals to compensate for any losses incurred. In contrast, concentrated fiber such as wheat bran, which is particularly high in phytate, can inhibit mineral absorption when routinely added to other foods. It's best to limit the use of wheat bran and avoid fiber supplements in fiber-rich plant-based diets. (For more on phytates, see page 181.)

Carbohydrate Content of Whole Foods

In plant foods, the percentage of calories from carbohydrates ranges from about 90 percent in fruits and starchy vegetables to about 12 percent in nuts and seeds. (See table 3.5 on page 97 and figure 5.1 for more-precise percentages of calories from carbohydrates in common foods. These figures are based on current nutrient analysis methodology; all carbohydrates are calculated as 4 calories per gram, regardless of fiber content.)

FIGURE 5.1. Average percentage of calories from carbohydrates in common foods

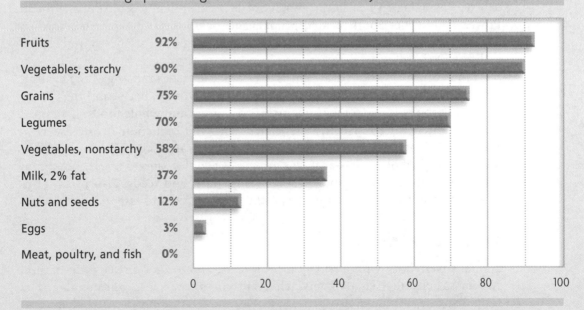

Food	%
Fruits	92%
Vegetables, starchy	90%
Grains	75%
Legumes	70%
Vegetables, nonstarchy	58%
Milk, 2% fat	37%
Nuts and seeds	12%
Eggs	3%
Meat, poultry, and fish	0%

Source:[13]

Refining Carbohydrates:
A Troubling Transformation

While most carbohydrates are derived from plant foods, relatively few are consumed as whole foods. Instead, nutritious plants are routinely transformed into fat-, sugar-, and salt-laden processed foods whose lure is undeniable.

When whole plant foods are processed or refined, many of their nutritious elements are destroyed or discarded. For example, the process of turning wheat berries into white flour causes the loss of approximately 80 percent of their vitamins, minerals, and fiber. In addition, a 200- to 300-fold loss in phytochemicals occurs.[14] When whole wheat grains are milled into white flour, the grains' bran and germ are removed, leaving behind only the endosperm. Bran, the outer husk of the grain, protects its contents. (Although bran provides nutrients and phytochemicals, its main claim to fame is fiber.) To support the life and growth of a new wheat plant, a grain's germ contains essential fatty acids, vitamins, minerals, and phytochemicals. The remainder of the grain, its endosperm, comprises mainly starch, some protein, and a miniscule amount of vitamins and minerals. The end-product—white flour—may have a long shelf life, but it has little remaining nutritional value with which to support human or other life.

The metabolic processes that transform starches and sugars into useable energy require many of the nutrients lost in refining. To compensate, food processors add back some of these nutrients. For example, after wheat is refined, it's commonly enriched with thiamin, riboflavin, niacin, folic acid, and iron. However, other vitamins and minerals lost during processing—vitamin B_6, vitamin E, pantothenic acid, zinc, boron, selenium, magnesium, potassium, and manganese—are not added back, nor are any of the fiber or phytochemicals.

Few health experts would dispute that processed or refined carbohydrates can be damaging to health. Promoters of low-carb diets (e.g., Atkins, Protein Power, The Zone, South Beach, primal, and paleo diets) go one step further, claiming that carbohydrates are responsible for rising rates of obesity and chronic disease, regardless of their origin.

However, anticarbohydrate gurus overlook the fact that many of the healthiest populations in the world consume high-carbohydrate diets—and that many of those carbohydrates come from unrefined sources and whole foods. Unrefined carbohydrates are consistently associated with the reduction of disease risk. What really matters is whether or not the carbohydrate is consumed in, or close to, its natural whole state—as it was grown. When the sources of carbohydrates are vegetables, fruits, legumes, whole grains, nuts, and seeds, also present are vitamins, minerals, antioxidants, phytochemicals, fiber, and essential fatty acids.

SWEET ATTRACTION

Humans were born with a soft spot for sweets, and for good reason. In nature, sweetness generally signals safety, while bitterness serves as a warning flag. The simple sugars in plants also provide a reasonable concentration of glucose to keep the human machine running smoothly. Normally, it's difficult to consume excessive sugar when eating a variety of vegetables, fruits, legumes, grains, nuts, and seeds.

Yet when sugars are extracted from whole foods and used to augment baked goods, beverages, and other sweet offerings, their increased availability exploits the human bias for sugar. The passion for sweet foods has steadily increased. In the United Kingdom, sugar consumption averaged 4 pounds in 1700 and 18 pounds in 1800.[38] By 1900, per capita added-sugar intakes in the United States were estimated at 64 pounds per year, which ranked among the highest in the world.[39] Between 1900 and 2005, this figure jumped to 142 pounds per person per year.

After factoring in losses (what goes down sinks and into the garbage), actual sugar intakes in the United States are estimated at 30 teaspoons of sugar per person per day—about 480 calories, or almost 25 percent of calories in a 2,000-calorie diet.[40] Soft drinks and other sugar-sweetened beverages account for close to half the added sugars consumed by Americans. Between 1970 and 2000, the consumption of sugary soft drinks increased by 70 percent, from 7.8 ounces to 13.4 ounces per person per day.[38]

Between 1970 and 1995, sugar intake increased by 19 percent. However, the most notable change wasn't the amount of sugar consumed, but the type. While consumption of sucrose (table sugar from cane and beet sugars) declined by 38 percent, the intake of corn sweeteners (mainly high-fructose corn syrup) increased by 387 percent.[40] By 2007, 45 percent of total added sugars came from sucrose, 41 percent came from high-fructose corn syrup (HFCS), and 14 percent came from glucose syrup, pure glucose, and honey.[41]

SWEET SORROW

Sugar itself, whether a monosaccharide (such as fructose) or disaccharide (such as sucrose), isn't inherently harmful. Simple sugars aren't poison—they're molecules that the human body prefers as a fuel source and can handle fairly well in reasonable doses. In fact, when it's part of a whole plant food, sugar is a valuable and healthful source of energy. Even adding small amounts of additional sugars to nutritious prepared foods doesn't appear to pose a health risk. It's excess sugar consumption that's the issue, particularly when it comes from refined sweeteners.

The detrimental effects of eating sugar are most pronounced with excess calorie consumption. Diets that obtain a high proportion of calories from added sugars (and, in most instances, other refined carbohydrates) are associated with adverse health consequences:

- **Reduced micronutrient intakes.** More-nutrient-dense foods may be crowded out.
- **Hypertension.** Excessive sugar intake may raise blood pressure.[38, 42]
- **Elevated triglycerides.** Sugar increases triglyceride levels, with fructose having the most significant impact. The effect appears to be even greater in men, in sedentary and overweight individuals, and in those with metabolic syndrome.[2, 3, 38, 41–43]

- **Decreased HDL cholesterol.** Fructose appears more potent than sucrose in reducing HDL cholesterol levels.[3]

- **Increased insulin secretion and insulin resistance.** Sugars increase blood sugar levels and insulin secretion; fructose is also associated with increased levels of visceral fat (fat in and around vital organs), further increasing insulin resistance.[41]

- **Increased cancer risk.** Limited evidence suggests that high intakes of sucrose increase the risk of colorectal cancer,[2, 44–46] and high intakes of lactose raise the risk of ovarian cancer.[2, 44] There's also limited evidence that high intakes of sugar increase insulin-like growth factor 1 (IGF-1), and that elevated IGF-1 boosts the risk for breast cancer.[47, 48]

- **Overconsumption.** Added sugars, especially from beverages, can result in excessively high total energy consumption, contributing to overweight and obesity.[2, 3, 49]

- **Poor dental health.** High sugar intakes are strongly associated with dental caries and reduced dental health.[3]

- **Nonalcoholic liver disease (NAFLD).** About 70 percent of people with metabolic syndrome are also afflicted with NAFLD. Excessive intake of simple sugars, particularly fructose in soft drinks, is thought to cause accumulation of fatty acids in the liver. People with NAFLD are at increased risk for atherosclerosis (plaque-filled arteries) and cardiovascular disease.[43]

- **Inflammation.** Proinflammatory molecules may increase with elevated blood glucose levels, especially in insulin-sensitive individuals.[50–53]

- **Impaired immunity.** Short- and long-term elevations in blood glucose may adversely affect immunity and increase susceptibility to infection, although research is very limited.[50–52, 54]

- **Increased formation of advanced glycation end-products (AGE).** Limited research suggests that fructose is linked to AGE formation within body cells and is approximately eight times more likely to form these compounds than glucose. AGE contribute to numerous disease processes and accelerate aging.[55]

DETERMINING A SAFE LEVEL OF SUGAR CONSUMPTION

Where sugar is concerned, it's the dose that makes the poison. The USDA Dietary Guidelines for Americans recommend that no more than 5 to 15 percent of calories come from added sugar and solid fat. While the guidelines don't specify a percentage for either, assuming equal amounts would mean allowing no more than 150 calories from sugar in a 2,000-calorie diet, or about 9 teaspoons (45 ml) of sugar per day.[56] The American Heart Association has more specific guidelines for added sugar—no more than 6 teaspoons (30 ml) per day for women and 9 teaspoons (45 ml) per day for men.

The big challenge in trying to follow these guidelines is determining the amount of sugar in processed foods. Food labels provide a clue. On the Nutrition

Facts panel, manufacturers must list the total amount of sugar in grams per serving (including sugars naturally present in foods plus any added sugar). There are approximately 4 grams of sugar in 1 teaspoon (5 ml), so 32 grams of sugar would equal roughly 8 teaspoons (40 ml). The serving size also matters; servings are often smaller than consumers expect.

In addition, food manufacturers aren't required to separately note added sugars, except in the ingredient listing. If the food had no natural sugars, then any sugar listed is all added sugar. (The exception to this rule is fruit juice concentrate, which is included as an added sugar.) If the food contains natural sugars from fruits, dried fruits, or even vegetables, such as tomatoes, the ingredient list needs further scrutiny. If sugar (sucrose or high-fructose corn syrup) is high on the list, the amount of added sugars likely is also high.

Some manufacturers try to push sugars lower down on the ingredient list by using several different sweeteners, some of which consumers might not recognize as sugar. These include:

- agave nectar
- barley malt syrup
- blackstrap molasses
- brown rice syrup
- brown sugar
- cane sugar
- corn syrup
- crystalline fructose
- dextrose
- dried cane juice
- evaporated cane juice
- fructose
- fruit juice concentrate
- glucose
- high-fructose corn syrup
- honey
- invert sugar
- lactose
- malt syrup
- maltodextrin
- maltose
- maple syrup
- molasses
- raw sugar
- rice syrup
- Sucanat
- sucrose
- syrup
- turbinado sugar

THE BANE OF SWEETENED BEVERAGES

In 2008, more than 20 billion gallons of soft drinks were sold in America.[57] That amounts to approximately two 12-ounce (180 ml) soft drinks per day for every man, woman, and child in the nation. Soft drinks include all beverages with added sugars: nondiet sodas, fruit drinks, energy drinks, sports drinks, lemonade, sweet powdered drinks, vitamin waters, and sweetened iced teas.

The average 12-ounce (180 ml) serving of soda or fruit drink provides about 150 calories from sugar; some sweetened beverages have even more. That's close to 10 teaspoons (50 ml) of sugar per serving. One 12-ounce (180 ml) serving, added to the daily diet, can cause a weight gain of about 15 pounds (6.8 kg) per year. While consumers might believe they can compensate for those calories by reducing intake elsewhere, the evidence suggests otherwise. When calories arrive in liquid form, the body fails to register those calories with the appetite-control center quite as precisely as it does solid food. If those calories aren't consciously offset, weight gain will result.

In fact, scientific studies consistently link consumption of soft drinks with weight gain.[58,59] A high intake of soft drinks has also been linked with osteoporosis and dental cavities.[60] Researchers also recently reported a surprising association between soda consumption and lung diseases, such as chronic obstructive pulmonary disorder and asthma.[61]

The basic message is simple: both adults and children should avoid sugar-sweetened beverages. Beverages that are naturally calorie-free, such as water, soda water (with a squeeze of lemon or lime), or herbal tea are best. Other healthful options are fresh-squeezed vegetable and fruit juices. (Fruit juices are higher in calories and natural sugars, so should be limited; when mixed with carbonated water, they're a great stand-in for sweet soda.)

THE MOST HEALTHFUL CALORIC SWEETENERS

Sweeteners fall in and out of favor with health-conscious consumers on a regular basis, but the differences between various simple sugars are of relatively minor consequence. Most sugars are essentially glucose, fructose, or some combination of the two.

Some people select sweeteners based on their effect on blood glucose levels or their glycemic index. (For more on the glycemic index, see pages 172 to 178.) Pure glucose raises blood glucose levels quite quickly; pure fructose doesn't. However, consuming more fructose isn't an advantage because it appears to be more damaging than glucose when consumed in excess.

Although a few sweeteners contain tiny amounts of nutrients, most make no significant contribution to nutritional needs when consumed in normal quantities. One notable exception is blackstrap molasses; 2 tablespoons (30 ml) can provide as much as 400 mg of calcium, 7 mg of iron, 1,200 mg of potassium, and 200 mg of magnesium (check labels).[13] That's more calcium than 1 cup (250 ml) of milk, more iron than an 8-ounce (240 g) steak, more potassium than two large bananas, and more magnesium than 1 cup (250 ml) of quinoa. (Choose organic molasses to avoid pesticides.)

Date sugar is made from dried and ground dates, so it's a whole-food sweetener and is more nutrient dense than most other sugars. However, it's expensive and not widely available. Other minimally refined sugars, such as maple syrup and coconut palm sugar (derived from the sap of the coconut palm tree), are slightly more nutrient dense than heavily refined products.

While intake of sugars should be minimized, judicious use is acceptable. The top vegan choice would be a sweetener that's organic, fair trade, and minimally refined. The most nutrient dense—and often the most economical—sweets are whole foods, including fruits and dried fruits, such as dates. Both are commonly used as a primary sweetener in creative vegan and raw vegan recipes.

Alternative Sweeteners

Sweeteners fall into two categories: nutritive or caloric sweeteners and nonnutritive or noncaloric sweeteners. Simple sugars, such as fructose and sucrose, are nutritive sweeteners. So are sugar alcohols.

Consumers often confuse sugar alcohols with noncaloric sweeteners and assume they're calorie-free. Although poorly digested, they do provide an average of about half the calories of other carbohydrates, or about 2 calories per gram. Common sugar alcohols include erythritol, isomalt, lactitol, maltitol, mannitol, sorbitol, polydextrose, xylitol, and hydrogenated starch hydrolysates.

Although sugar alcohols affect blood glucose, their impact is less than that of other carbohydrates.[64, 65] This quality makes them attractive to food manufacturers. Products that contain sugar alcohols are often labeled "sugar-free"; however, most experts recommend including half the grams of sugar alcohol in a total-carbohydrate count.

As an added bonus, sugar alcohols aren't as likely as simple sugars to attract molds or bacteria, making them very shelf stable. They also don't promote tooth decay, so they're the sweetener of choice in many dental hygiene products, such as toothpaste and mouth rinse. On the downside, sugar alcohols may have side effects, especially when large amounts are eaten at one time. The most common complaints include gastrointestinal disturbances, such as abdominal pain, gas, bloating, and diarrhea.

Nonnutritive or noncaloric sweeteners include products that are hundreds to thousands of times sweeter than sugar. As a result, they can be used in such tiny amounts to sweeten foods that they're essentially calorie-free. The safety of artificial sweeteners is highly controversial, although most health organizations, including the American Diabetes Association and the Academy of Nutrition and Dietetics, approve their use. In the United States, the Food and Drug Administration has approved the use of five artificial nonnutritive sweeteners—acesulfame K, aspartame, neotame, saccharin, and sucralose—in addition to one natural sweetener derived from the stevia plant, called rebaudioside A.[65]

Although rebaudioside A has been approved for use as a food additive (sweetener) in the United States, due to concerns about possible side effects, stevia itself has only been approved as a nutritional supplement. However, stevia is approved for use in several other nations and for several decades has been the principal nonnutritive sweetener used in Japan. Two recent scientific reviews found no health concerns associated with stevia.[66, 67] A third review reported that stevioside and related active compounds in stevia have antihyperglycemic, antihypertensive, anti-inflammatory, antitumor, antidiarrheal, diuretic, and immunomodulatory properties.[68] However, stevia's beneficial effects on blood glucose and blood pressure were observed only in participants whose markers for these conditions were elevated.

Opinion is somewhat mixed on the effectiveness of using nonnutritive sweeteners for weight loss, reducing carbohydrate intake, or controlling blood sugar. In reality, many people who consume foods and beverages that contain nonnutritive sweeteners make up for the missing calories by eating more. Although there's been conflicting research,[69] several large-scale studies have reported a positive correlation between artificial-sweetener use and weight gain.[70] Some experts believe that this may be at least partly because the intensity of artificial sweeteners causes people to become desensitized to sweetness. Naturally sweet whole foods, such as fruits, may become less appealing, compared to less nutritious foods that contain powerful artificial sweeteners. Finally, research suggests that the body may have sweetness receptors in fat tissues. Nonnutritive sweeteners may actually trigger weight gain by stimulating the development of new fat cells.

The Bottom Line: Artificial sweeteners appear to offer no clear advantages to consumers and may have negative health effects. If a noncaloric sweetener is desired, products containing rebaudioside A appear to be the safest choice. Another option would be to use stevia leaf products judiciously. Sugar alcohols seem safe when used in moderation.

THE SCOOP ON HIGH-FRUCTOSE CORN SYRUP

Although there's some evidence that HFCS may have slightly more-pronounced adverse effects than sucrose when consumed in excess, the differences between the two most widely used sweeteners are relatively small. Sucrose is 50 percent glucose and 50 percent fructose. HFCS is either 55 percent fructose and 42 percent glucose (HFCS-55) or 42 percent fructose and 53 percent glucose (HFCS-42). Compared to a sweetener such as agave syrup, HFCS isn't especially high in fructose; it's just higher in fructose than regular corn syrup, which is mostly glucose.

Fructose molecules are the same, whether they come from sucrose, HFCS, or fresh fruit. However, in sucrose, the fructose and glucose molecules are chemically bound and must be cleaved by an enzyme or acid before being absorbed.[62] In HFCS, both the fructose and glucose are present as free monosaccharides. Very preliminary evidence suggests that blood levels of fructose are higher when HFCS is consumed, compared to equal amounts of sucrose from beverages. Researchers also noted slightly higher uric acid and systolic blood pressures immediately following the consumption of beverages containing HFCS compared with those containing sucrose.[63] The metabolic consequences of these differences over the long term are unknown, but they appear to be relatively small.

However, fructose does have more-damaging effects on the body than glucose, based on the scientific research to date. Because fructose doesn't raise blood glucose levels significantly, consumers have been led to believe that fructose-rich sweeteners, such as agave syrup, are more-healthful choices, particularly for those with metabolic syndrome, prediabetes, or diabetes. However, fructose consumed in excess exceeds the body's capacity to handle it. When the liver is presented with large volumes of fructose to process, it rapidly converts the fructose to fatty acids. Some of the fatty acids take up residence in the liver, while the remainder find their way into the bloodstream (as triglycerides) and then into fat cells. Also, of the adverse health effects of added sweeteners, many are even more pronounced with fructose.[38, 41, 55]

The Goods on Grains

When consumers think of complex carbohydrates, grains often spring to mind. Grains, or cereal grains, are the edible seeds of grasses. Examples include wheat, oats, rye, corn, rice, barley, Kamut, spelt, millet, teff, and triticale. Although they're also commonly referred to as grains and used in similar ways, the pseudograins, or pseudocereals, such as amaranth, quinoa, and buckwheat, are the seeds of nongrass plants; wild rice, which is the seed or fruit of an aquatic grain, is also classified as a pseudograin. Grains and pseudograins are key sources of both calories and protein for the majority of humans, as well as significant sources of fiber, B vitamins, several trace minerals, plant sterols, and phytochemicals.

According to the USDA 2010 Dietary Guidelines for Americans, grains are an important part of a healthful diet. The guidelines specify that at least half the grains consumed should be whole grains, and that refined grains be limited. In sharp contrast, many promoters of raw and low-carb diets declare that grains have no place on plates. Some claim that grains are not only unnecessary, but also that they're inflammatory and acid forming, cause leaky-gut syndrome, impair mineral absorption, and are bad for joints, teeth, and skin. (It's believed that gluten, a protein common to many grains, wreaks much of the havoc.) So, whose advice should consumers—and, more specifically, vegans—follow?

One way of approaching grain consumption is to choose other plant foods first (e.g., vegetables, fruits, legumes, nuts, and seeds) and tweak grain intake based on additional calorie needs. Low energy requirements would result in a low allowance for grains. Consumers whose energy needs are moderate or high can afford a more generous grain intake.

For the most part, the choice should be whole grains. The majority of studies that examine the health consequences of grain consumption have reported favorable effects for whole grains and unfavorable effects for refined grains. Less is known about the differences in health, if any, between people who consume whole grains and those who consume no grains, because few populations eschew grains as dietary staples. Grains make a significant contribution to total nutrient intakes while providing little fat and no cholesterol; their attraction is also due to their affordability, versatility, shelf stability, and energy content.

However, the proponents of low-carb diets aren't completely misguided. Their advice likely springs from the fact that an estimated 90 percent of grains consumed by Americans are refined.[71] There's unanimous agreement that the rising consumption of refined grains has been an important contributing factor to overweight, obesity, and chronic diseases. Research suggests that diets rich in refined grains can result in a variety of adverse health consequences, similar to those associated with excess sugar consumption.[3, 4, 72–75]

On the other hand, although refined grains should be limited in the diet, eating a piece of pizza or dish of pasta—or making a batch of cookies with a little sugar—won't sabotage a healthy diet. Indeed, occasional departures from whole foods can make a vegan diet more interesting, enjoyable, and inviting for nonvegan friends. However, for daily fare and optimal health, it's best to choose whole grains over refined grains—and intact whole grains, such as barley or quinoa, instead of processed whole grains, such as bread or crackers made with whole-grain flour.

SEPARATING THE WHEAT FROM THE CHAFF

A diet may include flaked whole-grain cereal in the morning, whole-grain bread at lunch, whole wheat pasta at dinner, and brown rice cakes with almond butter as a snack. All are made from whole grains, but because they've been processed to varying degrees, they still aren't the best choices for a healthy diet. Intact whole grains that have been sprouted or cooked provide the greatest return on investment.

The more whole grains are processed, the more their nutritional value diminishes. As a grain's surface area increases, more of it is exposed to the air, increasing nutrient losses. Heat, light, and oxidation can destroy valuable vitamins, for example. Figure 5.2 (page 170) ranks processed grains from the most nutritious to the least. At the top are intact whole grains; their nutrient and phytochemical content can be further enhanced by soaking and sprouting them.[76] Next are cut whole

FIGURE 5.2. The whole-grain hierarchy

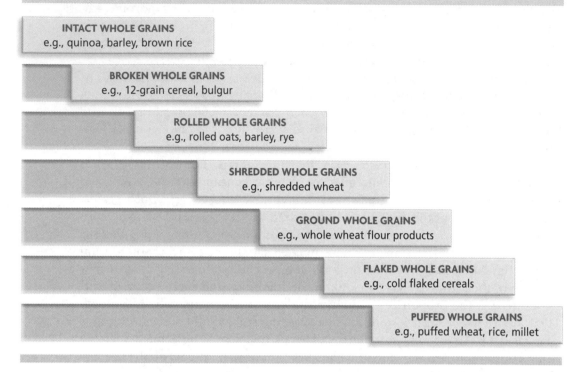

grains, followed by rolled and ground grains. At the bottom are flaked and puffed whole grains. Puffing makes grains so light and airy that they're broken down by the digestive system very quickly; puffed grains have the greatest impact on blood sugar.

Sometimes fractions of whole grains, such as oat bran, wheat germ, and wheat bran, can still play a useful role in the diet. For example, wheat germ can boost the content of B vitamins and vitamin E in baked goods made with whole wheat flour. Oat bran can provide extra viscous fiber to the diet and can be helpful in controlling blood glucose or reducing cholesterol levels.

GROWING ANXIETY OVER GLUTEN

Gluten is a protein composite present in wheat, spelt, Kamut, rye, barley, and triticale (a hybrid of wheat and rye). Approximately 1 percent of the population suffers from celiac disease, a severe autoimmune response to gluten. For many years, patients who experienced adverse reactions to gluten but tested negative on celiac tests (blood tests to detect presence of antibodies and/or microscopic examination of intestinal tissue) were told that gluten likely wasn't the cause of their symptoms. However, in 2011, a team of experts from the Center for Celiac Research at the University of Maryland School of Medicine released groundbreaking research suggesting that nonceliac gluten sensitivity is a distinct clinical entity, affecting roughly 10 percent of the population.[77]

In wheat, Kamut, and spelt, the proteins that combine to form gluten are gliadin and glutenin. Other proteins toxic to those with celiac disease are secalin in rye and hordein in barley. Oats don't contain gluten and are safe for most people with celiac disease if they're not contaminated by contact with wheat, rye, or barley. However, a small percentage of celiac patients is sensitive to a protein in oats called avenin and are unable to tolerate it. Although uncontaminated oats are becoming more widely available, most of the oats in North America are processed on the same machinery as other grains and, as a result, aren't suitable for people with celiac disease.[78-80]

Although gluten sensitivity can generate symptoms similar to those caused by celiac disease, the effects are less severe. People with celiac disease experience inflammation and general damage to the small intestine, which causes flattening of the villi (tiny hair-like appendages that line the small intestine) and malabsorption of nutrients; those with gluten sensitivity don't. Also, transglutaminase (tTG) autoantibodies show up in blood tests used to diagnose celiac disease; the bodies of people with gluten sensitivity don't produce tTG.

However, gluten sensitivity appears to be part of a spectrum of gluten-related disorders and creates a measureable immune response with significant health implications. The research team noted there may be damage to other tissues, organs, and body systems in people with gluten sensitivity.[77] As with celiac disease, symptoms often affect the gastrointestinal system (abdominal pain, cramping, bloating, diarrhea, and constipation), although they can cause problems in any body system. Behavior issues (depression, foggy mind, ADHD-like behavior, and autism), iron-deficiency anemia (fatigue, weakness, lack of concentration), joint pain, muscle disturbances, osteoporosis, leg numbness, migraines, and sinus problems are commonly reported.

When asked about what appears to be a sudden surge in gluten-related diseases, the study's lead investigator and world-renowned expert on celiac disease, Dr. Alessio Fasano, pointed out that human bodies don't have the enzymes to completely digest gluten, leaving undigested peptides that can be absorbed into the bloodstream with adverse health consequences for some individuals. Also, although controversial, he stated that grains have been bred to contain more gluten than in the past, and autoimmune diseases are on the rise, suggesting that it's difficult for human bodies to adapt to a rapidly changing environment.[81]

Must people with gluten sensitivity completely avoid every trace of gluten in foods (as people with celiac disease must do)? The answer is not black and white, because sensitivity is on a continuum. For individuals with more severe sensitivity, gluten is best avoided completely. For those who are mildly sensitive, the occasional gluten-containing foods may not be a problem. Others may find that they can only tolerate gluten-containing grains if they've been sprouted (e.g., sprouted flour-free breads or sprouted grains for cereals and salads). Although sprouting does reduce the gluten content of grains, it doesn't eliminate it. Gluten levels may also be lower in older varieties of wheat and in organic and fermented products (such as sourdough bread).

Even when gluten isn't much of an issue, it's wise to vary the grains eaten. Whole grains differ in their content of fiber, nutrients, and phytochemicals, so consuming a variety of grains, gluten-free grains (such as corn, job's tears, millet, oats, rice, sorghum, and teff), and pseudograins (such as amaranth, buckwheat, quinoa, and wild rice) will provide a better balance of protective factors.

Whole-Grain Guidelines

- Vary grain consumption. Include some pseudograins in the mix.

- Opt for gluten-free grains if gluten sensitivity is a factor. Use more squash, sweet potatoes, corn, and starchy vegetables for additional calories.

- Don't regularly add wheat bran to foods; because it's loaded with phytates (page 181), it can interfere with mineral absorption.

- Choose intact whole grains most of the time—sprout them for added nutrition.

- Use flaked and puffed whole grains sparingly.

- Limit intake of flour products, even whole-grain products.

The Glycemic Impact of Carbohydrates

When carbohydrate-containing foods are consumed, the body's digestive enzymes break them into monosaccharides so they can be absorbed into the bloodstream. Two pancreatic hormones (insulin and glucagon) are responsible for regulating blood glucose levels. As blood glucose levels rise, the pancreas releases sufficient insulin to shuttle excess glucose into cells so it can be used for energy or stored for later use. When blood glucose dips too low, the pancreas releases sufficient glucagon to attach to liver receptor cells, triggering the conversion of enough stored glycogen to glucose to restore blood glucose levels. The actions of these two important hormones keep blood sugar levels stable, ensuring a continuous supply of fuel for body tissues, particularly the brain.

Choosing the right foods helps the body maintain good blood glucose control. This is especially important when the regulatory system is challenged, as with diabetes. Chronically elevated blood glucose levels accelerate development of the disease's complications, including cardiovascular disease, blindness, neuropathy, kidney failure, and amputations. Foods with a lower glycemic impact can aid people with diabetes in controlling their disease, but they also provide advantages for healthy populations.

A recent meta-analysis of thirty-seven studies showed that diets with a high glycemic impact increased the risk of type 2 diabetes, heart disease, gallbladder disease, breast cancer, and all diseases combined.[82] This study used two tools to assess the glycemic impact of the diet: glycemic index and glycemic load.

The glycemic index (GI) is a measure of the effect of carbohydrate sources on blood glucose levels. Carbohydrates that are slowly digested and absorbed release sugar molecules gradually into the bloodstream; they have a low GI. Carbohydrates that are quickly digested and absorbed into the bloodstream have a high GI. Foods with a high GI usually trigger a correspondingly high insulin response, adversely affecting long-term blood glucose control, increasing triglycerides, and reducing protective HDL cholesterol.[83–85]

In order for researchers to determine a food's GI, a number of test subjects consume an amount of a food that provides 50 grams of carbohydrate. Changes in the subjects' blood glucose are compared to changes in their blood glucose after they've consumed a control food (usually pure glucose) and then averaged to obtain the food's GI. GI uses a scale of 0 to 100; 0 to 55 is low, 56 to 69 is medium, and 70 or more is high. Pure glucose has a GI of 100. White bread has a GI of 75, which means that the blood-sugar response to the carbohydrates in white bread is 75 percent of the blood-sugar response to pure glucose. By comparison, cooked barley has a GI of 28 relative to glucose.[84]

Sometimes these comparisons lead to interesting and surprising results. For example, sucrose has a GI of 65—lower than that of whole wheat bread, which has a GI of 74. The explanation lies in the types of sugar molecules that form the more-complex carbohydrates in bread; the starches in bread are chains of glucose molecules.

Monosaccharides (glucose, galactose, and fructose) don't impact blood glucose equally. Fructose and galactose must first be transported by the bloodstream to the liver to be converted into glucose, glycogen, or fatty acids. As a result, their impact on blood glucose is about one-fifth that of glucose. In sucrose, half the sugar molecules are fructose, which reduces sucrose's GI relative to pure glucose. On the other hand, although whole wheat bread may be more slowly digested and absorbed than sucrose, the glucose in bread causes a greater rise in blood glucose than the combination of glucose and fructose present in sucrose.

The GI figure produces a ballpark idea of how a serving of food that contains 50 grams of carbohydrate affects blood glucose. However, hardly any serving of food provides exactly 50 grams of carbohydrate, so a more practical tool, called the glycemic load (GL), was created to factor in the amount of carbohydrate actually eaten. A GL of 0 to 10 is low, 11 to 19 is medium, and 20 or more is high.

Foods that have a high GI don't always have a high GL. GL is calculated by multiplying a food's GI by the grams of carbohydrate provided in a serving and dividing the total by 100. For example, watermelon has a GI of 72; however, a 4-ounce (120 g) serving of watermelon provides only 6 grams of carbohydrate. Almost eight servings (2 pounds/960 g) of watermelon would be needed to yield 50 grams of carbohydrate.

That 4-ounce (120 g) serving of watermelon has a GL of 4 (GI of 72 times 6 grams of carbohydrate per serving divided by 100). When it comes to determining a food's actual impact on blood glucose, the total amount of carbohydrate is just as important as its GI. Table 5.3 (page 176) provides the GI and GL of several common foods.

LIMITATIONS OF GLYCEMIC INDEX AND GLYCEMIC LOAD

GI has frequently been used to judge the healthfulness of foods. Unfortunately, it conveys nothing about a food's total nutritional content or any harmful contaminants or products of oxidation that may be present. Foods that contain little, if any, carbohydrate have a very low GI and a negligible GL. For example, meat—even processed meat or deep-fried meat—has a small impact on blood sugar. However, it has the potential to significantly increase insulin resistance and have adverse effects on blood glucose control over time.[86–88]

Further, unhealthy choices of carbohydrate-rich foods also can result from overreliance on their GI. For example, because fat- and salt-laden potato chips have a lower GI than a healthy baked potato, the chips would be selected. Other unhealthful snacks, such as candy bars, cupcakes, and ice cream, may also be viewed as acceptable because they frequently fall within the low-GI range due to their high fat content. Consumers may mistakenly shun nutritious, higher-carbohydrate whole foods (such as some fruits, starchy vegetables, and whole grains) because they have a relatively high GI.

Generally, foods aren't eaten alone but in combinations; the choice of foods can have a profound effect on the meal's overall glycemic impact. For example, baked potatoes have a high GI and GL. However, when eaten with the skin and accompanied by a black bean–peanut sauce (or a lentil loaf) and kale salad, a potato's sugars are absorbed more gradually and the potato's GI is blunted. In addition, the body benefits from the many other nutrients potatoes contain.

Although relying on a food's GI and GL to make food choices has limitations, these indicators are helpful when appropriately used. For instance, compare the GI and GL of similar foods or foods of the same category: oatmeal versus cornflakes; the different intact grains, such as barley and millet; and rice milk versus soy milk (see table 5.3 on page 176).

GI AND GL OF VEGAN DIETS

Relative to the diets of nonvegetarians, vegan diets overall have a low GI and a low to moderate GL. One study that examined vegans' GI and GL reported an average GI of 51 and an average total GL of 144 (the combined GL of all the foods consumed during the day).

This compares very favorably to nonvegetarian populations. In four large studies of nonvegetarians, average GIs ranged from 64 to 72 for participants who were in the lowest quintile of the study groups. One study also reported total GLs ranging from 117 for the lowest quintile to 206 for the highest quintile of the group. The authors suggested that the vegan population's low GI and GL may be one factor that explains the lower risk of heart disease and type 2 diabetes in vegans compared to omnivores.[89]

FACTORS AFFECTING GLYCEMIC INDEX

Many foods are absent from the GI list because they're either essentially free of carbohydrates (e.g., meat, poultry, and fish) or they don't contain enough carbohydrates to make the GI test practical. Nonstarchy vegetables, such as leafy greens, broccoli, cauliflower, celery, peppers, and cucumbers, are good examples. To get 50 grams of carbohydrate from chopped broccoli, the test would require eating almost 9 cups.

As noted in the comparison between the GIs of sugar and bread, a food's GI sometimes appears to be counterintuitive. Some of these factors help to explain such discrepancies:[84, 85, 88, 90–93]

- **Type of monosaccharide present.** Glucose has a much greater impact on blood glucose than do fructose or galactose. Sweeteners with a lower GI contain more fructose, but this doesn't make them a more healthful choice.

- **Type of starch present.** The two principal starches in foods—amylose and amylopectin—are digested at very different rates. Amylopectin, which constitutes about 70 percent of the starch in foods, is rapidly absorbed into the bloodstream; amylose is digested more slowly. Foods rich in amylopectin tend to have a high GI relative to foods rich in amylose. The remarkable range in GI of rice, for example, is due to its widely divergent amylose and amylopectin content. This explains why some varieties of low-amylose brown rice have higher GIs than some varieties of high-amylose white rice.

- **Amount and type of fiber present.** Fiber generally reduces the GI of a meal. However, foods rich in viscous fiber (e.g., beans and barley) reduce the meal's overall GI to a greater extent than foods rich in nonviscous fiber, such as wheat bran. In addition, the GIs of high-fiber foods are generally lower than their refined counterparts. For example, if brown and white rice had the same amylose content, the brown rice would have a lower GI.

- **Physical barrier.** Beans and whole grains are surrounded by a fibrous coating that serves as a physical barrier to protect the seed. Because this barrier makes it more difficult for enzymes to digest them, these foods have a lower GI.

- **Ripeness.** As foods ripen, their starches turn into sugars, increasing their GI.

- **Exposure to heat.** Raw foods have a lower GI than the corresponding cooked foods. Cooking breaks down plant cell walls, increasing the rate at which their starches and sugars are absorbed by the body.

- **Particle size.** In smaller food particles, surface area is increased, allowing more-rapid digestion and absorption. For example, intact whole grains have a much lower GI than ground grains, whole fruits have a lower GI than fruit sauces or juices, and puréed beans have a higher GI than whole beans.

- **Density.** Foods that contain less air have a lower GI than light and fluffy foods. White bread has a higher GI than dense white pasta. Puffing grains also dramatically increases their GI.

- **Crystallinity.** Raw starch is crystalline—its molecules are organized in a sequence that repeats. Cooking disrupts this structure, making the starch more digestible and resulting in a higher GI. However, as the cooked starchy food cools, the starch recrystallizes to some extent, resulting in a lower GI. For example, red potatoes, cubed and boiled in their skin, have a GI of 89. Refrigerated overnight and eaten cold the next day, the same potatoes have a GI of 56.

- **Acidity.** Adding an acid, such as lemon juice or vinegar, to a food reduces its GI. Even small amounts of vinegar (less than an ounce) have been shown to reduce GI by about 30 percent. Fermentation produces acid, yielding foods with a lower GI. Yogurt has a lower GI than milk, and sourdough bread has a lower GI than regular bread.

TABLE 5.3. Glycemic index (GI) and glycemic load (GL) of selected foods

FOOD	GI	GL
GRAINS		
Barley, cooked, 5 oz (150 g)	28	12
Bread, white, 1 oz (30 g)	75	11
Bread, whole wheat, 1 oz (30 g)	74	9
Buckwheat groats, cooked, 5 oz (150 g)	45	13
Bulgur wheat, cooked, 5 oz (150 g)	47	12
Corn tortilla, 1.7 oz (50 g)	49	11
Cornflakes, 1 oz (30 g)	81	20
Millet porridge, cooked, 5 oz (150 g)	62	22
Oatmeal, instant, 8 oz (250 g)	79	21
Oatmeal, made from old-fashioned rolled oats, 8 oz (250 g)	55	13
Quinoa, cooked, 5 oz (150 g)	53	13
Rice, brown, cooked, 5 oz (150 g)	50–87	16–33
Rice, white, cooked, 5 oz (150 g)	38–109	14–46
Rice cakes, plain, 0.9 oz (25 g)	82	17
Rice crackers, plain, 1 oz (30 g)	91	23
Shredded wheat cereal, 1 oz (30 g)	67	13
Sourdough rye, 1 oz (30 g)	48	6
Spaghetti, white, cooked, 6 oz (180 g)	49	24
Spaghetti, whole wheat, cooked,* 6 oz (180 g)	44	18
LEGUMES		
Baked beans, canned,* 5 oz (150 g)	40	7
Chickpeas, cooked,* 5 oz (150 g)	29	7
Kidney beans, cooked, 5 oz (150 g)	22	6
Lentils, cooked,* 5 oz (150 g)	32	6
Mung beans, sprouted, raw, 5 oz (150 g)	25	4
Navy beans, cooked,* 5 oz (150 g)	31	9
Peanuts, crushed, 1.7 oz (50 g)	7	0

*average of all studies listed

KEY:

Low GI (≤ 55) or GL (≤ 10)
Medium GI (56–69) or GL (11–19)
High GI (≥ 70) or GL (≥ 20)
Range from low to high

FOOD	GI	GL
Peas, split, yellow, 5 oz (150 g)	25	3
Soybeans, cooked,* 5 oz (150 g)	16	1
NUTS		
Cashews, 1.7 oz (50 g)	22	3
Mixed nuts, 1.7 oz (50 g)	24	4
VEGETABLES		
Carrots, raw or boiled,* 2.7 oz (80 g)	39	2
Carrot juice, 1 c (250 ml)	43	10
Corn, boiled, 2.7 oz (80 g)	52	9
Parsnips, boiled, 2.7 oz (80 g)	52	4
Peas, frozen, boiled, 2.7 oz (80 g)	51	4
Potato, baked, 5 oz (150 g)	86	22
Potato, white, boiled, 5 oz (150 g)	82	21
Pumpkin, boiled, 2.7 oz (80 g)	64	6
Sweet potato, cooked, 5 oz (150 g)	70	22
Yam, 5 oz (150 g)	54	20
FRUITS		
Apple,* 4 oz (120 g)	36	5
Apple juice,* 8 oz (250 ml)	41	12
Apricot, 4 oz (120 g)	34	3
Apricots, dried, 2 oz (60 g)	31	7
Banana,* 4 oz (120 g)	60	14
Cantaloupe,* 4 oz (120 g)	68	4
Cherries, 4 oz (120 g)	63	9
Dates, 2 oz (60 g)	42	18
Grapes, black, 4 oz (120 g)	59	11
Kiwifruit, 4 oz (120 g)	58	7
Mango, 4 oz (120 g)	51	8
Orange,* 4 oz (120 g)	37	4
Orange juice, 8 oz (250 ml)	50	12
Papaya, 4 oz (120 g)	56	5
Peach, dried, 2 oz (60 g)	35	8
Pear, dried, 2 oz (60 g)	43	12
Pineapple, 4 oz (120 g)	66	6

FOOD	GI	GL
Plum, 4 oz (120 g)	39	5
Strawberries, 4 oz (120 g)	40	1
Watermelon, 4 oz (115 g)	76	4
MILKS		
Cow's milk, 1 c (250 ml)	31	4
Rice milk,* 1 c (250 ml)	86	23
Soy milk,* 1 c (250 ml)	32	5
SNACK FOODS		
Chocolate, dark, 1.7 oz (50 g)	23	6
Chocolate, milk, 1.7 oz (50 g)	43	12
Popcorn, 0.7 oz (20 g)	65	7
Potato chips, 1.7 oz (50 g)	56	12
Pretzels, 1 oz (30 g)	84	18
Skittles candy, 1.7 oz (50 g)	70	32
SUGARS		
Agave nectar, 0.3 oz (10 g)	13	1
Fructose, 0.3 oz (10 g)	15	2
Glucose, 0.3 oz (10 g)	103	10
Golden syrup, 0.9 oz (25 g)	63	13
Honey, 0.9 oz (25 g)	61	12
Lactose, 0.3 oz (10 g)	47	5
Maltose, 0.3 oz (10 g)	105	11
Maple syrup, 0.3 oz (10 g)	54	10
Sucrose, 0.3 oz (10 g)	65	7

Source:[84]

*average of all studies listed

KEY:

Low GI (≤ 55) or GL (≤ 10)
Medium GI (56–69) or GL (11–19)
High GI (≥ 70) or GL (≥ 20)
Range from low to high

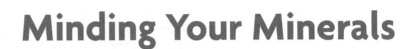

Minding Your Minerals

One farmer says to me, "You cannot live on vegetable food solely, for it furnishes nothing to make the bones with"; and so he religiously devotes a part of his day to supplying himself with the raw material of bones; walking all the while he talks behind his oxen, which, with vegetable-made bones, jerk him and his lumbering plow along in spite of every obstacle.

HENRY DAVID THOREAU, PHILOSOPHER, AUTHOR, AND PIONEER OF VEGAN LIVING

H uman bodies are never entirely at rest. During the day and throughout the night, the body remodels bones, builds enzymes and thyroid hormones, forms red blood cells, and maintains the precise acid-base balance in body fluids that sustains life. Minerals are a vital part of these dynamic systems, and food is the body's source of minerals.

But where do these minerals come from? As part of the cycle of nature (with the help of bacteria and fungi), decaying plant matter releases minerals into the soil; these minerals are then absorbed by newly growing plants. As a result, plant-based diets can provide optimal amounts of every essential mineral, without exception. Yet, both health professionals and the general public are inundated with messages that link calcium and strong bones with dairy products and that associate iron with meat consumption rather than with plant foods.

It's important to recognize that plants can provide all the necessary minerals—no need for animal products. Of particular interest to vegans are calcium, iron, zinc, and iodine. Following is a review of the functions of various minerals, including recommended intakes, vegan sources, and special issues.

Mineral Absorption

 he bioavailability of minerals (the ease with which they're absorbed from the intestine) is affected by numerous factors:

- Minerals can be bound (for example, as components of plant oxalates and phytates) and thus be unavailable.

- A person's nutrient status affects mineral absorption. For example, someone who has a low serum ferritin level will absorb iron from plant foods far more efficiently than someone with abundant iron stores.

- Age or life circumstances can be a factor. A woman's intestinal absorption of calcium might double during pregnancy, and an infant's ability to absorb calcium to accommodate rapidly growing bones is also high. In contrast, after people reach 40 years of age, the percentage of calcium absorbed declines.

- Calcium, copper, iron, magnesium, and zinc compete for absorption sites; taking a single-mineral supplement may lessen the absorption of other minerals. Thus, for example, calcium supplements should be taken between meals by people who want to maximize their absorption of iron, magnesium, and zinc from food.

- When a smaller quantity of calcium, iron, or zinc is consumed, the body absorbs a higher percentage of the dose, compared to its absorption from a large quantity. Thus, two 250 mg calcium supplements taken at different times during the day deliver more calcium than a single 500 mg dose.

- Foods or beverages that accompany mineral intakes can affect absorption negatively or positively. For example, the amount of iron absorbed can vary sixfold or more, depending on whether factors that inhibit absorption (such as cow's milk, black tea, and wheat bran) or factors that enhance absorption (such as vitamin C–rich foods) are part of a meal.

- Normal gastric acidity (hydrochloric acid) ionizes minerals, increasing their bioavailability. Low gastric acidity, which can occur with age or with frequent use of antacids, reduces mineral absorption.

The combination of so many possible influences on mineral bioavailability makes each individual's situation rather complex.[1–3]

MINERALS, FOOD PROCESSING, AND FOOD PREPARATION

Refining whole foods—particularly grains—significantly impacts their mineral content (for more information, see page 162). Minerals are soluble in water; if cooking water is discarded, they can be lost. Steaming leads to greater nutrient retention. Minerals can survive very high temperatures; for example, they form the ash that remains after a fire. When preparing corn dishes, the Hopi Indians, whose diets were mainly plant based, traditionally used the ash from burnt corn cobs, bean vines, juniper bushes, and other plants to fortify meals with calcium, copper, iron, phosphorus, and zinc.[4, 5]

PHYTATES

To put mineral requirements in perspective, it helps to consider their form within foods, because this can affect ease of absorption. In whole plant foods, calcium, iron, magnesium, and zinc can be bound with phosphorus in compounds called phytates. These bound minerals are less available for direct absorption. However, they're released by common food practices that are traditional among populations that rely on legumes, whole grains, nuts, and seeds.[6–10]

Vegans often soak, sprout, ferment, blend, or juice plant foods, which significantly increases mineral availability. In nature, sprouting releases minerals to support growing seedlings. When seeds, nuts, mung beans, lentils, and whole grains are soaked or sprouted for food, the naturally present phytases (phytate-splitting enzymes) become active, and the bound minerals are released. When plant foods are juiced or blended, their cell walls are broken, releasing phytases and increasing mineral bioavailability.[1, 6–9]

Phytases also are present in bacteria, yeast, and fungi. When plant foods are fermented, as when soy is made into tempeh or miso, more than half the phytates are broken down. Yeast has a similar effect on wheat; plus, with the acidity that results from sourdough fermentation, phytate breakdown increases to as much as 97 percent. These common food preparation processes release bound calcium, iron, magnesium, and zinc for absorption.[4, 6, 7, 10–12]

Diet also affects the population of microbes that are present in intestines to process phytate. Compared to nonvegetarians, vegetarians (whose diets are naturally high in phytates) have intestinal bacteria that are far more capable of breaking down phytate-mineral complexes.[13] There may be an impression that phytates themselves are harmful, yet their presence also brings benefits. These compounds are antioxidants that appear to provide protection against cancer, cardiovascular disease, and diabetes.[6, 11, 12] Vegans typically don't need added bran because they get enough fiber; bran is a concentrated source of phytates that can significantly impact mineral availability. (Wheat germ is low in phytates and isn't an issue.)

OXALATES

Oxalates are tightly bound combinations of oxalic acid and minerals (calcium, iron, magnesium, or zinc) that resist breakdown during food preparation and digestion. Amaranth, beets, beet greens, cassava, chives, chocolate soy milk, lamb's-quarters, miso, parsley, purslane, sorrel, spinach, star fruit, Swiss chard, and whole sesame seeds are among the most oxalate-dense plant foods. (For specific amounts, search online for the US Department of Agriculture list, "Oxalic Acid Content of Selected Vegetables.")[14]

Of the minerals mentioned above, calcium is most tightly bound by oxalic acid. For example, although spinach is calcium-rich, only about 5 percent of its calcium may be absorbed by the body; the rest is transported out in the feces, bound by oxalic acid. Much of the iron in spinach can still be absorbed, because the oxalate is primarily bound with calcium. Despite mineral binding, such greens are still valuable dietary additions because they provide abundant folate, vitamin K, beta-carotene, and numerous other protective nutrients and phytochemicals unaffected by oxalates.[15, 16]

Recommended Intakes

The Institute of Medicine (IOM) of the National Academy of Sciences has developed sets of recommended intakes—known as Dietary Reference Intakes—of the various nutrients for healthy people. These values include the Recommended Dietary Allowance (RDA), the Adequate Intake (AI), and the Tolerable Upper Intake Level (UL).

The RDA is the average daily intake that meets a nutrient requirement of 97 to 98 percent of healthy individuals. AI is a value listed when there's insufficient research to determine an RDA; it can be viewed as a sort of "best guess." UL is the highest level of intake that won't pose a risk of adverse effects for most healthy people when used indefinitely on a daily basis without medical supervision.

Finally, the Nutrition Facts panel required by the US Food and Drug Administration on food labels lists one Daily Value (DV) each for vitamins A and C, calcium, and iron, as well as other micronutrients the food may contain (for example, as a result of fortification or enrichment). DV is based on a 2,000-calorie diet and on past recommended intakes, some of which are similar to current RDAs and AIs.[98, 99]

To see RDAs and AIs for various age groups and for women during pregnancy and lactation, see page 445. For further information online, see Resources on page 449.[3, 20, 38, 81, 84, 89]

RDA—Recommended Dietary Allowance   UL—Tolerable Upper Intake Level

AI—Adequate Intake   DV—Daily Value

When foods are soaked and the soaking water discarded, some oxalates are disposed of along with bound minerals. Research has shown that boiling can reduce the total oxalate content in spinach by 60 percent and in lentils by 16 percent. Losses result from a combination of leaching into the cooking water plus some breakdown of the calcium-oxalate complex.[4, 7, 10, 15–18]

Oxalates are found in body fluids. However, when these stone-forming salts become too concentrated in urine and the urine pH is acidic, sediments can form prickly-surfaced calcium oxalate salts (the most common type of kidney stones). Limiting calcium intake hasn't proved effective in preventing such stones; on the contrary, calcium can bind oxalate in the intestine, preventing its absorption. Instead, eating alkali-forming foods (vegetables and fruits) to reduce urine acidity, avoiding animal protein, limiting high-oxalate foods, consuming calcium citrate supplements with meals, and drinking plenty of water provide more-successful solutions.[19]

Minerals

CALCIUM

Calcium in Perspective

Calcium is the most common mineral in the body. Humans acquire calcium from direct consumption of plant foods, through milk from a human or other mammal, or from other dietary sources, such as powdered lime used to process corn for tortillas.

Before the advent of animal husbandry, humans in many parts of the world had dairy-free diets that were calcium-rich (averaging 2,000 mg per day or more). However, many of the plants and plant parts they consumed aren't commonly eaten in modern times. Much of the produce in supermarkets has been bred for sweetness or ease of transport rather than for nutritional excellence. As a result, it's far lower in calcium than plant foods gathered by early humans.[21–23]

Meanwhile, nutrition-education campaigns and dairy advertisements lead the public to believe that humans require cow's milk to meet their calcium needs. Although the food guides of most Western countries might imply otherwise, the milk of other mammals, such as cows, has *not* been a cornerstone of the human diet throughout history. The practice of dairying appears to be a recent phenomenon, conducted only in specific areas of the world. In these regions, natural selection favored a genetic adaptation that allowed people to drink milk after the age of weaning. Normally, after the first few years of life, as much as 70 percent of the world's population shows diminished production of the enzyme lactase (a trait known as lactase nonpersistence) and lose the ability to digest lactose, the sugar in the milk of humans, cows, and other mammals. In South America, Africa, and Asia, more than 50 percent of the population has lactase nonpersistence after they've passed the age of weaning; these individuals can experience abdominal pain, bloating, flatulence, and diarrhea when cow's milk is consumed. In some Asian countries and among Native Americans, this rate is close to 100 percent.[22–24]

Function

Calcium is best known for its structural role: giving hardness to bones and teeth. Bone is a dynamic tissue that's continually formed and resorbed, with formation taking the lead during stages of growth and early adulthood, and resorption prevailing in the elderly. The body achieves peak bone mass by about age 28. A few decades of minimal change in total bone mass follow, and then a period of loss, estimated at 1 to 2 percent per year in women after menopause and in the elderly of both genders. Adequate calcium intakes during growth and adolescence help to avoid fractures in later life.[25]

Calcium also has crucial nonstructural functions, though these involve just 1 percent of the calcium in the body. These include roles in blood coagulation (required after injury), muscle relaxation (without calcium, muscles remain tight after contracting), nerve cell transmissions, and the regulation of cell metabolism (such as the storage of energy as glycogen). Maintaining calcium intakes at recommended levels also may help to prevent hypertension.

Calcium is vital for survival, and the body must keep the calcium levels in blood and in interstitial fluid within a specific and narrow range. A drop in calcium levels is registered by the parathyroid gland, which produces parathyroid hormone, activating vitamin D. This action quickly raises calcium levels by increasing the efficiency of intestinal absorption, decreasing urinary losses, and if necessary, breaking down bone to release this mineral.[3, 20] For more information on the role of calcium and other nutrients in building and maintaining bone, see page 68.

Recommended Intake

The calcium RDA for adults is 1,000 mg per day, and 1,200 mg per day for women over 50 and men over 70. The UL has been set at 2,500 mg per day to age 50 and 2,000 mg for those older than 50.[3, 20]

Vegan Intakes

Since 1954, worldwide studies have shown that average vegan intakes of calcium range from about 500 to 940 mg daily, providing about 50 to 94 percent of recommended levels for adults to age 50.[26–30] In many of these studies, fortified products weren't available to vegans; this situation is changing. Since the late 1990s, fortified nondairy beverages have been sold across North America, and these and other calcium-rich vegan foods can be obtained in many other regions, as well. (Interestingly, the average calcium intakes of nonvegetarians in the United States also were well below recommended intakes for every age and gender group, especially for females and for adults older than 50.[20, 31, 32])

A higher risk of bone fractures in vegans has been linked with relatively low calcium intakes, though overall, plant-based diets don't appear to increase risk of osteoporosis.[30] In addition to the dietary sources listed below, supplemental calcium can easily help vegans reach recommended intake levels.

Dietary Sources

Calcium is abundant in a wide assortment of vegetables, particularly low-oxalate greens (broccoli, bok choy, kale, napa cabbage, watercress, and mustard and turnip greens); from these, the body absorbs 40 to 60 percent of the calcium present.[29, 100] Collard and dandelion greens are considered medium-oxalate greens and thus are fair calcium sources. Absorption is poor—about 5 percent—from high-oxalate greens (beet greens, spinach, and Swiss chard).[29, 100]

This mineral is well absorbed (about 50 percent) from juices fortified with calcium citrate malate. It's added to fortified nondairy milks and tofu, making these good sources (check labels); the body absorbs 30 to 32 percent of the calcium in both (about the same rate as from cow's milk and some mineral waters).[33–35]

The fractional absorption of calcium from sesame tahini and from assorted beans is about 20 percent.[29, 100] From almonds, which contain phytates, the body absorbs 14 to 21 percent of the calcium; however, absorption is increased after almonds are soaked for eight to twelve hours.[100] Calcium is present in oranges, figs, organic blackstrap molasses, and (in smaller amounts) in many plant foods. The Vegan Plate (page 434) devotes a column to calcium-rich foods in all food groups. Also see table 6.2 (page 204).

Solid Solutions for Better Bones

- Follow The Vegan Plate guidelines (page 434). This healthful eating plan provides the whole team of bone-building nutrients, which includes protein; essential fatty acids; the minerals boron, calcium, copper, fluoride, magnesium, manganese, phosphorus, and zinc; and the vitamins B_{12}, B_6, C, D, folate, and K.

- Eat dark green vegetables daily. Include broccoli, kale, collard greens, bok choy, and napa (Chinese) cabbage on the shopping list. Find a nearby market with great produce, grow greens in the garden or on the balcony, or arrange for a weekly organic produce delivery. Learn delicious ways to prepare greens. Use the mineral-rich cooking water in soups or in grain preparation.

- Use calcium-set tofu. Tofu is versatile; it can be a main ingredient for tasty items from soup to dessert. Check the label for calcium content; the Daily Value (DV) is 1,000 mg. The protein and isoflavones in tofu, tempeh, and soy milk also benefit bone.[94]

- Drink calcium-fortified beverages. Fortified nondairy milks and juices can help bring total calcium intake to recommended levels. For good calcium suspension, shake the container well.

- Make almonds, almond butter, sesame tahini, and blackstrap molasses a part of meals and snacks. Replacing 2 tablespoons (30 ml) of peanut butter with an equal amount of almond butter boosts calcium intake by 73 mg. Replacing 1 tablespoon (15 ml) of jam with blackstrap molasses can add a surprising 80 to 200 mg of calcium (check labels).

- Monitor intakes of calcium thieves. Avoid high intakes of salt, alcohol, and caffeine—and don't smoke.

- Take some sun (or vitamin D). Walk outside in the sunshine during midday to allow the body to form the day's supply of vitamin D. (For more on this topic, see page 69.) When sunlight isn't available, take a vitamin D supplement to ensure adequate intake.

- Exercise. Walk, jog, dance, play ball, hike, and participate in aerobics classes or other weight-bearing exercise to strengthen bones.

- Top up dietary intakes with a supplement. If necessary to reach recommended levels, add a daily calcium supplement.

Supplements

Many vegan adults would benefit from a few hundred milligrams of supplementary calcium to top up daily intakes. Multivitamin-mineral supplements typically contain about 200 to 400 mg of calcium; much more would make the pill too large to swallow. Many calcium supplements are best absorbed in the presence of stomach acid, and thus are better assimilated when taken with a meal. However, calcium citrate and calcium citrate malate can be taken anytime. If taken between meals, these forms won't hinder iron and zinc absorption from food. Because vitamin D is essential for optimal calcium absorption, a calcium-vitamin D combination that includes at least 15 mcg (600 IU) of vitamin D would be beneficial.

Special Issues

High salt or sodium intakes result in increased calcium losses. Each teaspoon (6 g) of salt contains 2.3 grams of sodium. When excreted by the kidneys, this amount of sodium draws with it 24 to 40 mg of calcium. Over time, such urinary losses can markedly influence bone loss. It's been estimated that, in adult women, each gram of sodium beyond daily needs will result in an additional rate of bone loss of 1 percent per year if all the related calcium loss comes from the skeleton.[20]

IRON

Iron in Perspective

In the past, nutrition texts rated nonheme iron from plant foods as inferior to heme iron in meat, because the body generally absorbs a lower percentage of nonheme iron. We're now aware that relying on nonheme iron gives the body more control over absorption efficiency, by allowing it to adjust uptakes to suit its needs. If its iron reserves are low, the body absorbs more iron from plant foods; if iron reserves are abundant, the intestines can absorb a lower proportion of nonheme iron. (Food preparation and combinations also affect absorption of nonheme iron.)[2, 29, 36-40]

The heme form of iron found in meat and blood tends to be more readily absorbed—even when the body doesn't need any iron. Once iron has been absorbed, the body has limited mechanisms for ridding itself of any excess. Because iron is a prooxidant, too much in the body may damage DNA and other molecules. New research also indicates that high iron intakes and a burden of excess iron in the body have been associated with Alzheimer's and Parkinson's diseases, arthritis, type 2 diabetes, cardiovascular disease, and colorectal and other cancers. To avoid iron overload, consuming the nonheme form found in plants is recommended.[2, 29, 36-40]

Although the oxidative stress of excess iron is best avoided, the body does need enough for vital functions. Iron-deficiency anemia is no more prevalent among vegans and other vegetarians than among nonvegetarians. Yet iron deficiency is the primary nutritional deficiency worldwide for people on any diet, especially for women of childbearing age, infants, and teens. In the United States, the prevalence of iron-deficiency anemia among youths and adults is estimated at 2 to 5 percent among females and 1 to 2 percent among males.[2, 29, 38, 41]

Function and Losses

As a constituent of red blood cells, iron plays a central role in transporting oxygen throughout the body, releasing this life-giving substance where needed, and carrying away the metabolic waste product, carbon dioxide. In myoglobin, iron delivers oxygen to working muscles. As part of many enzyme systems, iron is a key element in the production of cellular energy, in immune system functioning, in detoxification, and in the mental processes surrounding learning and behavior.[20]

The body continuously breaks down red blood cells and builds new ones, efficiently recycling the iron reclaimed from spent red blood cells. However, each day tiny amounts of iron are lost in cells sloughed from the skin and from the inner lining of the intestine; these losses must be replaced from food or supplements.

Other causes can contribute to iron deficiency. Women of childbearing age have menstrual iron losses in the range of an extra 30 to 45 mg each month, making their dietary requirements higher than those of men. Growth and the building of new cells can deplete the small reserves of iron in infants and children. Teens experience the challenges of a powerful growth spurt and notoriously poor eating habits; in addition, girls have menstrual losses. Young obese women on poorly designed weight-loss diets are another group at risk for iron deficiency. People with blood loss for any reason (such as ulcers or blood donation) have an increased need for iron. Athletes have somewhat higher requirements due to increased oxygen demands and greater iron losses (see chapter 13).[38, 49]

Recommended Intake

The RDAs for men and postmenopausal women are set at 8 mg of iron per day and for women of childbearing age at 18 mg of iron per day. Although a separate RDA hasn't been set for vegetarians (including vegans), the Institute of Medicine (IOM) advises aiming for 1.8 times as much iron as nonvegetarians due to the lower bioavailability of nonheme iron from plant foods. Following this guide, vegetarian women of childbearing age are advised to get 32.4 mg of iron per day, and other adults are urged to get 14.4 mg of iron. For other ages, see page 447 and multiply recommended intakes for iron by 1.8.[29, 38, 42, 43, 49]

The higher recommendation for vegetarians is controversial, because it was based on a single poorly designed study. In this study, participants consumed vegetarian diets low in components known to enhance iron absorption (such as vitamin C and organic acids from fruits and vegetables) and high in substances known to interfere with iron absorption (such as tannins). In addition, the study wasn't conducted on vegetarians or vegans, who typically develop lower serum ferritin levels that optimize absorption. Vegans who include vitamin C–rich foods as part of their meals and who don't routinely include tea, coffee, or calcium supplements with meals are less likely to need this suggested level of iron intake. Still, there's widespread agreement that vegetarians, including vegans, should aim for more iron than nonvegetarians.[29, 38, 42, 43, 49]

Vegan Intakes and Iron Status

Research has shown vegans have average iron intakes that are similar to or higher than those of nonvegetarians and higher than the RDA, though they don't generally reach the higher levels of 32.4 mg iron per day suggested for vegetarian women of childbearing age. Studies have shown vegan women in the United States have average intakes of about 22 to 23 mg iron daily, higher than those of nonvegetarian controls; vegan women in Germany had average intakes of 20 mg iron daily. Average iron intakes of vegan men in the United States were significantly higher than those of nonvegetarians. For both genders, the average iron status of vegan groups—as shown by hemoglobin, hematocrit, and ferritin levels—was adequate and, where reported, compared favorably with nonvegan controls.[29, 30]

Laboratory Tests for Iron

A number of routine laboratory tests reflect iron status. These include hemoglobin (showing the amount of this iron-containing protein), hematocrit (indicating the concentration of red blood cells), and serum ferritin (a measure of the amount of stored iron). Vegetarians typically have lower serum ferritin levels than nonvegetarians. This common situation doesn't affect how a person feels and isn't an issue if a person's diet continues to replenish lost iron. Unless a period of starvation occurs, there's no apparent benefit to having more than minimal iron stores. In fact, lower levels of serum ferritin may be an advantage and are linked with better insulin sensitivity and reduced risk of type 2 diabetes.[2, 36, 36, 40, 44] Researchers also are exploring the possibility of links between lower serum ferritin and reduced risk of coronary artery disease, colon cancer, and inflammatory conditions.[2, 29, 45]

With iron depletion, however, there can be a decrease in other indicators of iron status. A tired feeling and sensitivity to cold may develop. Iron-deficiency anemia occurs when blood hemoglobin drops below the normal range. When the body's oxygen-delivery system is impaired, people are likely to feel exhausted, irritable, and lethargic and have headaches; the skin may appear pale. Iron deficiency is easily diagnosed; doubts can be resolved with a blood test, and progress can be tracked as the situation is remedied.[46]

Dietary Sources

Legumes are good plant sources of iron. They provide 3 to 6 mg of iron per 1 cup (250 ml) of beans or lentils or per ½ cup (125 ml) of soybeans or tofu (see table 6.2 on page 204). A serving of fortified breakfast cereal can supply as much as 18 mg of this mineral. Iron intake can quickly reach recommended levels with an assortment of vegetables, oatmeal or other whole grains, pumpkin seeds, and dried fruit. Dark chocolate or molasses (especially blackstrap) offer sweet ways to increase iron intake. Because molasses can also be a concentrated source of pesticides, organic brands should be chosen. Finally, when acidic foods (such as tomato sauce) are prepared in iron cookware, the sauce takes up some iron from the pan.[2]

Special Issues

The percentage of nonheme iron absorbed from plant foods varies, based on the body's needs, on food preparation methods, and on the food and beverage combinations eaten. Although iron (and zinc) deficiencies are associated with marginal plant-based diets of impoverished people in some parts of the world, this isn't the situation in regions where the food supply and variety are sufficient.[1, 2, 6, 8, 38, 47, 48]

As noted in the section on phytates (page 181), soaking, fermenting, yeasting, and sprouting plant foods increases the body's absorption of iron and other valuable minerals.[48] Oxalate appears to have a variable, and sometimes minimal, impact on iron availability from calcium- and iron-rich foods such as spinach, for example, because its calcium is preferentially bound.[15, 16]

Absorption from iron-rich plant foods increases markedly when foods high in vitamin C (such as red bell peppers or strawberries) are eaten at the same time because iron is converted from a ferric form to a more readily absorbed ferrous form. The citric acid in citrus fruits also enhances iron absorption. Obsolete food-combining rules that insist fruit must be eaten separately from other foods can be ignored, especially by consumers low in iron. The beta-carotene in yellow, red, and orange foods also aids iron absorption.[2, 6]

Vegans eat plenty of fruits and vegetables, and typically get more than one and a half times as much vitamin C as nonvegetarians—a clear advantage when it comes to iron absorption. For example, 5 ounces (150 ml) of orange juice containing 75 mg of vitamin C has been shown to increase the absorption of iron from foods eaten at the same time by a factor of four. Other studies show 50 mg of vitamin C to enhance iron absorption sixfold. Eating ¾ cup (185 ml) of any of the following provides 50 mg of vitamin C: broccoli, Brussels sprouts, cauliflower, collard greens, bell peppers, snow peas, cantaloupes, citrus fruits and juices, guavas, papayas, strawberries, and vitamin C–fortified juices; so does having a kiwifruit, ¼ cup (60 ml) of sweet red bell pepper, or a big salad.

Even after cooking, some vitamin C remains; for example, vegetables retain about 85 percent of their vitamin C when microwaved, 70 percent when steamed, and 50 percent when boiled. (Losses vary with cooking time and temperature.) A large baked potato retains 30 mg of vitamin C after baking.[2, 49–51]

Onions and garlic can increase the availability of iron (and zinc) from grains and legumes by 50 percent, further boosting iron intake.[52]

In contrast, absorption of dietary iron decreases in the presence of tannins and other polyphenols in black tea, coffee, cocoa, and red wine. Calcium supplements also inhibit iron absorption.[2, 6] To maximize iron absorption, it's wise to consume these inhibitors an hour apart from iron sources.

Supplements

For people whose blood tests show they're anemic, iron supplements or iron as part of a multivitamin-mineral supplement can be helpful. However, excessive amounts of this prooxidant mineral in supplements are best avoided. When the deficiency has been resolved, a diet that features good plant sources of iron—combined with vitamin C–rich foods—is a better choice for long-term maintenance.[46]

ZINC

Zinc in Perspective

Measures of iron status are readily available and commonly done; testing for zinc is less prevalent. Severe zinc deficiency is reflected in low zinc levels in plasma, red blood cells, hair, and urine; it also results in stunted growth, reduced immune defenses, diarrhea, poor appetite, and impaired ability to taste. Marginal zinc deficiency can be difficult to detect. With a shortage, the body may shift its available zinc to the most crucial areas of need, absorb zinc more efficiently, and recycle what it has.[2, 53, 93]

Zinc-deficient individuals may be smaller in stature through childhood and adolescence and into adulthood. Three decades ago in Iran and other parts of the Middle East, the effects of zinc deficiency were observed among poor people whose diets were high in phytates and low in overall variety. Whole wheat flatbreads with little or no yeast leavening provided 50 to 75 percent of the calories—and sometimes more—in their diets. Though the flour contained sufficient zinc, calcium, and magnesium, the bioavailability of these minerals was low. Even when yeast was used, the bread-making process was speedy, giving insufficient time for the yeast's phytase to break down the phytate-mineral complex.[54] The resultant zinc deficiency could have been alleviated if:

- a more extensive yeasting process were used
- zinc-rich legumes, seeds, or tahini were affordable
- onion or garlic were added to the meal, increasing zinc bioavailability[52, 54]

Impoverished people with limited diets in south and southeast Asia, sub-Saharan Africa, Central America, and the Andes have similar plights; in fact up to 20 percent of the world's population is lacking in adequate zinc intake or absorption.[53] The effects are particularly apparent during the stages of rapid growth from pregnancy through adolescence.

The fault can lie with limited diets composed mainly of either whole or refined grains. When grains are refined, they lose most of the phytates that limit zinc absorption, but they also lose most of the zinc. Diets centered on refined-grain products and sugar- and fat-laden foods and beverages also can be low in zinc.[55, 56] In North America, marginal, rather than severe, zinc deficiency is more likely to occur, particularly among pregnant women (sometimes resulting in pre-term delivery) and among children in low-income families.[55]

Function

Zinc is essential to cell division and plays key roles in growth during pregnancy and from infancy through adolescence. Zinc is important for the immune response and is necessary for wound healing. It's also a catalyst for about three hundred different enzyme systems and is critical for nerve development. The ability to taste is highly dependent on zinc. Certain tissues and fluids in the body contain relatively high concentrations of zinc, including the iris and retina of the eye, and also the prostate, sperm, and seminal fluid.[38, 57, 58] Zinc is also a factor in regulating men's serum testosterone levels.[59]

Recommended Intake

The RDA is 8 mg of zinc daily for women and 11 mg for men. Men's requirements are higher in part because they lose zinc in semen—0.6 mg per seminal emission.[38] (Ardent vegans might want to keep a bowl of cashews or pumpkin or sunflower seeds by their beds.)

The IOM has suggested that vegetarians with high intakes of unrefined grains and phytate may need 50 percent more zinc than recommended. However, due to the lack of sensitive clinical measures of marginal zinc status, this hasn't been confirmed.[38, 93]

Vegan Intakes

In seven studies conducted in the United States, the United Kingdom, Canada, Australia, and Germany, vegan women and men met or exceeded the standard recommended intakes for zinc, on average.[29, 30] In two studies in the United States and the United Kingdom, average zinc intakes fell about 10 percent short of recommended intakes.[29] Vegans with particularly low caloric intakes tend to have low intakes of this mineral. Some elderly people, regardless of diet, have low zinc intakes related to limited food consumption, insufficient variety, or a focus on refined foods.[60]

Dietary Sources

Typically, zinc is available from the same vegan foods as iron: seeds, nuts, legumes and tofu, and whole grains, including oatmeal and brown rice. One study determined that despite less-efficient absorption, participants gained 50 percent more zinc from whole wheat bread than from white bread because of the higher zinc content in the whole-grain product.[2] A glance at table 6.2 (page 204) will show that seeds and seed butters can be zinc superstars in vegan diets. Hummus and whole-grain bread or crackers make a zinc-rich snack for children and adults.

Special Issues

Food preparation methods, such as fermentation, leavening (of bread), soaking (of nuts, seeds, legumes, and whole grains), sprouting, and the use of sourdough can greatly improve zinc absorption. The acids present in foods or produced during fermentation break down phytates that bind zinc, increasing the bioavailability of zinc.[2, 7, 49] Adding garlic to hummus or rice enhances zinc uptake from the chickpeas, tahini, and grains.[52]

If the body is short of zinc, its ability to absorb this mineral becomes more efficient and body losses are reduced. Absorption efficiency and conservation of zinc also occurs in times of greater need, such as during pregnancy. Adaptation to somewhat lower intakes may also occur.[49, 58, 93]

IODINE

Iodine in Perspective

Iodine is required in miniscule amounts—but it's absolutely critical to life and health. Most of the world's iodine is found in the oceans. The soil content of this mineral varies greatly from one region to another; as a result, some crops are rich in iodine, while others contain very little.[38, 61]

Before the 1920s, iodine deficiency was common around the Great Lakes and in Appalachia and the northwestern United States. Since 1924, North American salt manufacturers have fortified salt with iodine to provide this essential nutrient to the general population and prevent the tragedies of iodine deficiency that were common in some regions.[61] This action has been powerfully effective. However, iodine deficiency remains an issue in some parts of Europe, Africa, and Asia and for some individuals whose diets lack either iodized salt or sea vegetables.

Function

Iodine is an essential component of thyroid hormones (triiodothyronine, or T3, and thyroxin, or T4), which influence most of the organ systems in the body. Iodine is essential for energy metabolism; iodine deficiency can result in depressed metabolic function (also known as hypothyroidism).

Iodine exerts its effects via the thyroid gland located in the lower part of the throat. Hypothyroidism can result in a growth called a goiter, in which the thyroid gland becomes greatly enlarged due to its efforts to trap iodine. Other symptoms of iodine deficiency are skin problems, weight gain, and increased cholesterol levels, all of which can be reversed in adults by increasing iodine intake. Insufficient iodine has been linked with fibrocystic breast disease.[38]

Iodine deficiency during pregnancy is a more tragic story, because the maternal thyroid hormones that depend on iodine for their production are essential for normal brain development in the fetus. Their lack causes the world's most important—and most easily preventable—cause of developmental disabilities, an irreversible condition known as cretinism. Even a mild deficit can impair cognitive ability.[38, 61–66]

Recommended Intake

The adult RDA is 150 mcg of iodine per day. Excess iodine can be toxic; the UL is set at 1,100 mcg of iodine per day (unless medically prescribed).

Vegan Intakes and Thyroid Status

Research has shown iodine intakes to be low in Swedish, German, and British vegans.[29] In a group of 62 vegans in the Boston area, just one in three used a supplement containing iodine (14 people) or consumed iodized salt (3 people) or kelp (1 person). Without such sources, iodine intake from a vegan diet may be about 10 percent of recommended levels. These people had been vegan for an average of 5.6 years and weren't showing iodine-deficiency symptoms at the time of the study.[67] (With high intakes of seaweeds, diets can provide amounts above the UL.[80])

Among nonvegans, dairy products can be significant sources because of contamination of milk with iodine-containing cleaning solutions; these are used to remove mastitis-related pathogens from milking equipment and cows' teats.[61] Bread has contained iodine due to dough conditioners, though this is decreasingly common.

Don't Overlook Iodine

Iodine intakes of people on vegan diets may be insufficient unless they use iodized salt, sea vegetables, or a supplement that contains iodine. Iodine deficiency is particularly risky during pregnancy.

Dietary Sources

In many nations, including Canada, iodization of table salt is mandatory. In the United States, where this is voluntary, about 70 percent of table salt is iodized. In both countries, standards decree that about ½ teaspoon (3 g) of iodized salt should deliver the day's recommended intake of 150 mcg of iodine. In practice, amounts may vary from one sample of iodized salt to another.[61, 68] In the United Kingdom, iodization is voluntary and less common, and iodized salt contains only about 25 percent as much iodine as that in North America.

Only a small proportion of sea salt is iodized (check labels), and tamari, soy sauce, Bragg Liquid Aminos, and miso are not. In addition, the vast majority of salt in Canada and the United States, which is used in food processing and in fast foods, isn't iodized—this represents more than two-thirds of the salt consumed in these nations.[61]

Plants grown in iodine-rich soil can be good sources; however, the iodine levels in produce aren't generally known, so it's difficult to determine intakes. Plant foods from the ocean (seaweeds) can be excellent sources; the challenge lies in knowing how much iodine they provide, because amounts can vary as much as eightfold from one batch to another. For example, quantities are higher in seaweed that grows near coral reefs. Amounts of iodine also can vary depending upon how the seaweeds were dried and stored. It can be difficult to find a supplier with accurate information about iodine content. To confirm amounts in salts and sea vegetables, check labels and contact manufacturers.[61, 69]

Kelp tablets may deliver stated amounts of iodine. Some people use a guideline of ¼ teaspoon (1.5 ml) of kelp every four days to meet their recommended intake of iodine (see table 6.1 on page 194). However, amounts of the mineral can vary greatly in kelp and regular, moderate intakes can easily exceed the UL. Though hijiki seaweed is rich in minerals, consumers are advised to avoid it because it commonly contains excessive amounts of arsenic. To meet recommendations, it's preferable to consume iodine in small but frequent amounts several times a week, rather than to consume a large dose less frequently.[29, 62–64, 69–71]

Special Issues

Soy foods, flaxseeds, and foods from the cabbage family (broccoli, Brussels sprouts, cabbage, cauliflower, collard greens, kale, and kohlrabi) tend to be nutritious staples in vegan diets. These foods can trigger thyroid problems *only if* a person is deficient in iodine. If iodine is in short supply, isoflavones in soy foods or thiocyanates in the other foods may interfere with thyroid metabolism.

TABLE 6.1. Iodine in salt and dried sea vegetables

IODINE SOURCE	AMOUNT SUPPLYING 150 MCG OF IODINE	AMOUNT SUPPLYING 1,100 MCG OF IODINE (TOLERABLE UPPER LIMIT)
Iodized sea salt or table salt	½ tsp (3 ml)	4 tsp (20 ml)
Noniodized sea salt or table salt	Not a source of iodine	Not a source of iodine
Arame	½ tsp (2 ml)	1⅕ T (18 ml)
Dulse granules	½ tsp (2 ml)	3⅓ tsp (16 ml)
Kelp	less than ¹⁄₁₆ tsp (0.3 ml)	0.4 tsp (2 ml)
Nori	1½ sheets	10½ sheets
Wakame	1⅛ tsp (6 ml)	2¾ T (40 ml)

Sources:[72–76]

The solution is not to avoid these foods but instead to solve the iodine deficiency by consuming a good source of the mineral.[29, 77, 78] In Asia, soy and seaweeds are viewed as complementary foods.[78] Fermentation (as in making kimchi) causes thiocyanates to disappear. In addition, the study of Boston vegans (page 182) showed that thiocyanate intakes weren't associated with thyroid problems in vegans.[67]

Perchlorates (solid-fuel by-products that cause water pollution) and various minerals from fertilizers and pesticides can amplify thyroid problems in people who are iodine deficient or whose intakes are low. Selenium deficiency also can worsen marginal iodine deficiency.[79]

The Bottom Line: Get enough iodine (but not too much). Supplements, such as multivitamin-mineral supplements that provide iodine, are most reliable in delivery of a known amount.[62]

CHROMIUM

Function

Chromium helps with carbohydrate metabolism by supporting the action of insulin.[38]

Recommended Intake

Because there's insufficient evidence to establish an RDA for chromium, an AI has been set instead. For those up to age 50, it's 35 mcg daily for men and 25 mcg daily for women; for older adults, the AI decreases by 5 mcg.[38]

Vegan Intakes

Vegan intakes of chromium have not been assessed.

Dietary Sources

The amount of chromium in foods seems to vary considerably from one sample to another. Also, no large databases quantify these amounts, in part because the presence of chromium in laboratory testing equipment has interfered with accurate testing.[81]

Whole grains, ready-to-eat bran cereals, green beans, broccoli, grape juice, and spices are relatively rich in chromium. Although the total amounts of chromium available may be inconsistent from one batch to another, 1½ cups (375 ml) of broccoli may supply a day's requirement of chromium, for example. Other vegetables and fruits supply small amounts that add up over the course of a day. Vitamin C–rich foods likely improve chromium absorption.[81]

Special Issues

Diets high in sugar (sucrose) have been found to promote chromium loss. Refined grains have lost their natural chromium content.[20, 29, 38, 81]

COPPER

Function

Copper plays a key role in energy metabolism as part of the enzyme cytochrome-c oxidase, which allows the body to store energy from food for bursts of activity. Other copper-containing enzymes can latch on to potentially damaging free radicals, preventing them from harming cells. This mineral also is part of specific enzymes essential to the normal function of the brain and nervous system, as well as other enzymes throughout the body. Copper aids in formation of connective tissue, bones, and red blood cells. As part of the pigment melanin, copper plays a key role in producing color in skin, hair, and eyes.[38]

Recommended Intake

Adults require 900 mcg daily.

Vegan Intakes

Studies show vegan intakes of copper to be higher than those of nonvegetarians and more than adequate.[29]

Dietary Sources

Rich sources of copper include asparagus, avocados, beans, coconuts, cucumbers, dried fruit, durians, guavas, kale, kiwifruit, lentils, parsnips, peas, potatoes, mangoes, mushrooms, nuts, seeds, spinach, spirulina, sun-dried tomatoes, water chestnuts, and whole-grain products. One ounce (30 g) of cashews, chocolate, hazelnuts, or seeds (pumpkin, sunflower, or sesame) or ½ cup (125 ml) of cooked lentils provides an entire day's supply, and then some.

Special Issues

Lively discussions about whether plant-based diets provide excessive amounts of copper have raised concern among vegan consumers. Although vegan protein sources are higher in copper than animal protein sources (especially relative to zinc content), research shows that copper absorption is significantly lower in vegetarian diets compared to nonvegetarian diets. Over time, plasma copper tends to decrease for those on vegetarian diets; fractional absorption is known to decrease with higher intakes, and also, adaptation may occur. Although such studies have been conducted on vegans, a similar—or even greater—reduction in copper absorption could be expected.[97]

Single-mineral zinc supplements above the RDA can interfere with the body's absorption of copper.[20, 29, 38] Because copper is a prooxidant, copper supplements are best avoided—and aren't needed in typical vegan diets.

MAGNESIUM

Function

Magnesium is present in bones, teeth, muscles, and cell membranes. Bones are less brittle when they contain sufficient magnesium. This mineral also performs an essential role in more than three hundred metabolic reactions in the body, more than any other nutrient. Magnesium affects muscle contraction and heart rhythms, helps transport minerals across cell membranes, and supports the transmission of nerve impulses. It's part of the team of minerals and vitamins responsible for energy production and has a role in building protein and DNA. Magnesium-rich diets (those rich in vegetables and fruit) are associated with lower blood pressure, and a reduced risk of type 2 diabetes, heart disease, and stroke.[20, 82, 83]

Recommended Intake

The RDA for young women is 310 mg of magnesium daily, increasing to 320 mg after age 30. The RDA for young men is 400 mg daily, increasing to 420 mg after 30.

Vegan Intakes

Studies show average vegan intakes of magnesium are significantly higher than those of nonvegetarians and are more than adequate.[29, 30]

Dietary Sources

Magnesium is abundant in vegetables, fruits, whole grains, and nuts. It's a central element in the chlorophyll molecules that provide the green pigment in plants and is fundamental to photosynthesis. It follows that green leafy vegetables are rich in magnesium. A varied diet that includes greens, whole grains, and other plant foods can easily meet recommended intakes. Magnesium is one of many nutrients that are lost in the refining process. (A slice of whole wheat bread contains 30 mg of magnesium, but a slice of white bread has only 5 mg.) The magnesium intakes of elderly people can fall short when they rely on refined foods or consume few calories. The amount of magnesium in drinking water varies from one region to another and is higher in hard water.

Special Issues

Magnesium absorption could be an issue in high-phytate diets. Leavening bread dough with yeast, as well as other food preparation practices, such as sprouting, soaking, and fermenting, increases the availability of this and other minerals.

Excess magnesium from food doesn't cause problems in healthy people because the kidneys simply excrete unneeded amounts. High intakes from supplements can result in diarrhea, sometimes with nausea and cramping; magnesium is a constituent of certain laxatives and antacids. Unless medically prescribed, adults shouldn't take amounts higher than 350 mg daily in the form of supplements; the UL for children from supplements is much lower. Larger amounts can result in more-serious side effects.[20, 29]

MANGANESE

Function

Manganese is part of the main antioxidant enzyme in mitochondria, the cells' energy factories. Manganese supports the activity of other enzymes and is required for the formation of bone and cartilage and for wound healing.[20, 38]

Recommended Intake

The RDA is 2.3 mg daily for men and 1.8 mg daily for women.

Vegan Intakes

Vegan diets easily meet and exceed the recommended intakes for manganese.[29]

Dietary Sources

Rich sources include leafy vegetables, nuts, teas, and whole grains. Any of the following provide approximately one day's supply: 1 cup (250 ml) of cooked brown rice or oatmeal, 20 pecans, 1½ cups (375 ml) of pineapple or cooked spinach, or 3 cups (750 ml) of green tea.

Special Issues

Manganese is potentially toxic in large amounts, though excessive intakes would occur from taking single-mineral supplements, not from consuming foods. Manganese is a prooxidant; supplemental manganese isn't needed or advisable in typical vegan diets.[20, 38]

PHOSPHORUS

Function

Next to calcium, phosphorus is the most abundant mineral in the body. About 85 percent of the body's phosphorus resides in bones, where it's a structural component along with calcium and protein. Every cell needs phosphorus to produce and store energy from food. It's part of cell membranes and genetic material and helps maintain the body's acid-base balance.[20]

Recommended Intake

The adult RDA is 700 mg of phosphorus per day.

Vegan Intakes

Studies in Canada, Finland, Germany, and the United States have consistently shown the average phosphorus intakes of vegans to be well above recommended levels.[29, 30]

Dietary Sources

Phosphorus is present in seeds and plays a structural role in plants in the form of phytates. In typical diets, about half the phosphorus is available for absorption and half is bound. When food preparation includes soaking, yeasting, fermenting, leavening, or sprouting, most of the phosphorus and bound minerals are released. Yeasts possess phytases; when whole grains are made into leavened (yeasted) breads, the available amount of phosphorus increases significantly. Between 100 to 200 mg of phosphorus is present in ½ cup (250 ml) of cooked lentils, two slices of whole wheat bread, or 2 ounces (60 g) of almonds or peanuts.

Special Issues

Excess phosphorus intake—especially in relation to calcium—is more common than insufficient dietary phosphorus; the two minerals must be kept in balance for good bone health. High intakes are often due to overconsumption of meat and poultry (which can have ten to twenty times as much phosphorus as calcium) and of colas (which can have 500 mg of phosphorus per serving). These excesses aren't typical of vegan diets; the fact that some phosphorus in plant foods is bound in phytates and is essentially unavailable may turn out to be an advantage.

Regular consumers of aluminum-containing antacids risk phosphorus deficiency, because the aluminum can bind phosphorus in the intestine and prevent its absorption.[20, 29]

POTASSIUM

Potassium in Perspective

Early humans consumed plenty of high-potassium plant foods, and they ate their meals without salt shakers. Thus, prehistoric cultures consumed potassium and sodium in a 7:1 ratio; conversely, modern Western diets provide these minerals in a 1:3 ratio. It's believed these altered proportions may contribute to many chronic diseases.[21, 23, 25, 90]

Potassium-rich foods (fruits and vegetables) have the ability to shift the body's acid-base balance in an alkaline direction. With adequate consumption of protein and calcium, a diet that emphasizes fruits and vegetables may reduce the risk of osteoporosis. Higher potassium intakes seem protective against strokes, hypertension, and kidney stones.[20, 84, 90]

Function

The body's transmission of nerve impulses, its muscle contractions, and the beating of the heart rely on potassium's presence and function inside cells. As a positive ion, potassium can conduct electricity, just as sodium can. In fact, life itself depends on the relative locations of potassium (primarily inside cells) and sodium (primarily outside). The maintenance of an electrical gradient or potential across cell membranes is based on the differing concentrations of these substances in the body.[20, 84]

Recommended Intake

The new AI (Adequate Intake) for potassium for adults is 3,400 mg for males and 2,600 for females.[20, 84]

Vegan Intakes

Surveys show typical American intakes of potassium to be low, averaging 2,300 mg per day for women and 3,100 mg for men; 97 percent of those surveyed failed to meet the recommended daily intake.[29, 60] Vegans do much better, though intakes aren't always above recommended levels. Potassium intakes average between 3,931 and 6,400 mg for various vegan groups studied in the United States; between 3,817 and 4,855 mg for vegan groups in Great Britain; 3,587 mg for Canadian vegans; and 4,460 to 5,460 mg for German vegan groups.[29, 30]

Dietary Sources

Plenty of fruits and vegetables are high in potassium, so a vegan diet can easily provide enough. Though the banana is often hailed as the queen of potassium-rich foods, in fact, Brussels sprouts, cantaloupes, grapefruits, green beans, strawberries, and tomatoes all have more potassium per calorie than bananas. Dried fruits, avocados, nuts, seeds, and legumes also are excellent sources.

To boost potassium intake:

- Start the day with a fruit smoothie, with or without added greens.
- Encourage children to drop fruit into the blender for a smoothie and to arrange cut vegetables or fruit pieces on a snack tray; they'll develop an early appreciation for these nourishing foods.
- Include a big salad at lunch, supper, or both. Shop for new varieties of produce at the supermarket.
- Add potassium-rich foods (see table 6.2 on page 204) to the shopping list.
- Use fruit to feed a sweet tooth and replace sugar with dried fruits in desserts.

- Eat the skin on baked potatoes and the edible skins of other vegetables and fruits.
- Add beans to soups, stews, and salads.
- Use nut or seed butters as spreads on bread or toast.
- Sprinkle nuts and seeds on cereal, salads, and main dishes.
- Feature avocado in salads, sandwiches, smoothies, and raw soups.

SELENIUM

Function

The body needs only miniscule amounts of selenium. It's used to build powerful antioxidant enzymes known as selenoproteins, which protect cells from damage by free radicals, reducing the risk of cancer and heart disease. Other selenoproteins help regulate thyroid function, synthesize DNA, and participate in fertilization.[20, 79, 85]

Recommended Intake

The adult RDA is 55 mcg of selenium per day.

Vegan Intakes

Studies of vegans in the United States, Britain, and New Zealand showed them to meet recommended selenium intakes. Among North Americans, there appears to be little difference between the average selenium status of those on plant-based diets and nonvegetarians; adequate intake from plant sources is thought to be due to efficient food distribution from regions with different soil levels.[29] European vegans in regions with low soil levels of selenium, such as Sweden, have relatively low intakes. Research has shown that German vegetarians and vegans have adequate levels of the protective selenoprotein glutathione peroxidase 3, while some indicators of selenium status were 70 to 80 percent of the maximal levels.[29, 86]

Dietary Sources

The Brazil nut (which is botanically a seed, not a nut, and more often comes from Bolivia rather than Brazil) has become known as the selenium superstar. If it's been grown in selenium-rich soil, just half a big Brazil nut provides a day's selenium supply; however, many nuts come from regions where soil has less of this mineral, so intake can vary. The daily recommended intake of selenium may also be obtained from 1½ cups (375 ml) of whole wheat spaghetti. Beans, grains, nuts, and seeds also can be good sources.[20, 87–89]

Special Issues

Plant foods provide selenium in amounts that vary with local soil content. For example, soils in Nebraska and the Dakotas are rich in selenium; other areas in the United States have much less. Many nations have soils that are low in selenium;

in fact, Finland includes selenium in its fertilizers. Eating foods sourced from different locations can help ensure adequate intake.[2, 85]

Selenium is toxic in excess; the UL is 400 mcg per day for adults. Avoid supplements at higher than recommended levels, and don't eat more than three or four Brazil nuts a day.[29, 85, 86, 88, 89]

SODIUM

Sodium in Perspective

The human body evolved on a diet far lower in sodium than today's fast-food fare.[22, 23, 90] Historically, salt wasn't always easy to come by and therefore was highly valued (hence the saying "the salt of the earth"). Although the body requires sodium to replenish that lost in perspiration, urine, tears, and other body fluids, getting too much sodium is more of an issue today. Even people who rarely add salt when preparing food or at the table may have significant salt intakes. Current research shows that 77 percent of the sodium consumed by North Americans comes from processed and restaurant foods, 5 percent is from salt added during cooking, 6 percent is sprinkled on at the table, and 12 percent is that which occurs naturally in foods.[84, 91]

Function

Due to its hygroscopic nature, sodium plays an important role in maintaining the proper amount of fluid between the body's cells. It's a central part of internal communication systems, because sodium is essential for the electrical current that allows transmission of nerve impulses. This mineral also is a part of digestive secretions from the pancreas.[84]

Although rarely a concern for most people, sodium deficiency—with symptoms of headache, nausea, vomiting, muscle cramps, fatigue, disorientation, and fainting—can occur when considerable salt is lost through perspiration during long hours of physical labor or endurance athletic events, particularly in hot environments.

Recommended Intake

The new AI (Adequate Intake) for sodium for males and females aged 14 years and older is 1,500 mg per day. [20, 84] The UL (Upper Limit) is 2,300 mg per day, although further reduction below the UL can reduce risk of chronic disease for many.[84, 91]

The minimum biologic requirement for survival is between 180 and 500 mg per day. It's estimated that Paleolithic humans managed on 660 to 770 mg of sodium per day, though of course intakes varied with their geographical region and whether it was inland or coastal.[22, 23] To cover routine sodium losses that may occur, such as in perspiration on warm days, the lower intake limit has been set at a level higher than necessary for survival. In contrast, individuals engaging in prolonged periods of physical activity in hot environments may need more sodium—in the short term—than the UL because of losses in sweat.

Tips for Recovering Saltoholics

Sodium is essential to the body; after hours of intense work or vigorous exercise, people do need to restore the sodium lost in perspiration. However, in the absence of these activities, follow these guidelines to prevent excessive sodium consumption:

- Use lemon juice and exotic vinegars to help beat salt cravings and bring out the flavor of foods.

- Use salt-free seasonings or prepare a mixture of herbs for use as seasoning.

- Use salty condiments sparingly. Buy low-sodium tamari, dilute it, and keep it in a spray bottle. Dilute Bragg Liquid Aminos with an equal amount of water and spray the mixture on food rather than pouring it.

- To stretch the flavor of added salt, sprinkle a little on food surfaces rather than mixing it in. This surface salt touches taste buds for maximum sensation without excess sodium.

- Buy fewer processed foods, because these contribute most to intakes of dietary sodium.

- Check the labels of soups or similar packaged items and choose those with less sodium. For example, the sodium content of a ½-cup (125 ml) serving of tomato sauce can vary from about 20 to 700 mg.

- Consumption of certain foods is best minimized or avoided: pickles (a single pickle can deliver 900 mg of sodium), olives, salty snack foods, and some canned goods. Check the labels of vegan meat substitutes, crackers, cereals, breads, and baked goods.

Excess sodium intakes (above 2,300 mg per day) are particularly problematic for older people with established hypertension. Among those with hypertension, about 50 percent of African-Americans and 25 percent of American Caucasians are salt sensitive; the rates increase with age or with reduced kidney function.[20, 29, 84, 91] People who want to determine whether they're salt sensitive should check their blood pressure, cut down on salt intake for four days, and then see if this results in a lower blood pressure. Some people can reduce the risk of developing hypertension by avoiding high salt intakes and consuming amounts within or at the lower end of the recommended ranges. High sodium chloride intakes and high sodium to potassium ratios also can be linked to calcium losses from bone and in the urine.[92]

Vegan Intakes

In vegan diets of the Americans, Canadians, and Germans studied, average sodium intakes are generally within the recommended range. These moderate sodium intakes may be due in part to many (though not all) vegans' preference to avoid processed foods. A favorable balance between relatively low sodium intakes and high potassium intakes is a positive feature of many vegan diets. However, average vegan sodium intakes of North Americans in the Adventist Health Study-2, British, and Vietnamese were somewhat high, ranging between 2,500 to 3,100 mg.[29, 30]

Three Simple Strategies for Maximizing Minerals

1. Eat whole plant foods, guided by The Vegan Plate (page 434). Minerals are found in all food groups, but in far smaller quantities in refined foods.

2. Make sure caloric intake is adequate. If on a weight-loss diet, consider using a multivitamin-mineral supplement.

3. Include some foods fortified with calcium, zinc, iron, and iodine. Although it's possible to meet recommended intakes without such foods, these can make it easier to reach the goal.

Still, the average sodium intakes of American nonvegetarians are significantly higher—about 3,400 mg per day, equivalent to 1½ teaspoons (7 ml) of salt—well above the UL and about five times the estimated intake from the Paleolithic diet.[84, 91]

Dietary Sources

Sodium is naturally present in celery, spinach and other leafy greens, carrots and carrot juice, sweet potatoes, and sun-dried tomatoes; sea vegetables are high in sodium. Salt is added to many vegan processed foods: canned tomatoes, soups, and beans; peanut butter; vegan meat substitutes, burgers, and hot dogs; bread and other baked goods; bottled sauces and dressings; vegetable bouillon and stock; olives; miso; snack foods, such as chips, crackers, and popcorn; vegan pizzas; and ready-to-eat entrées. The condiments tamari, Bragg Liquid Aminos, and nama shoyu each provide between 212 and 320 mg of sodium per teaspoon (5 ml). Check labels for exact amounts.

Special Issues

Many vegans choose sea salt rather than regular table salt, which has been refined and then enriched with iodine. Iodized table salt is a good source of the mineral iodine, but sea salt lacks this mineral; it's lost in the drying process and most sea salt isn't fortified. Although sea salts are advertised as containing trace minerals, these are usually present in miniscule amounts and also include tiny amounts of heavy metals, such as lead. Tamari, Bragg Liquid Aminos, and miso also are not enriched with iodine. Vegans who use noniodized salt should be sure to include a reliable source of iodine.

Ensuring Adequate Mineral Intakes

The amounts of minerals in vegan foods are shown in table 6.2 (page 204). For menu-planning purposes, compare these with the recommended mineral intakes for women and men shown at the top of each column.

TABLE 6.2. Minerals in vegan foods

FOOD	CAL-CIUM (mg)	COP-PER (mcg)	IRON* (mg)	MAG-NESIUM (mg)	PHOS-PHORUS (mg)	POTAS-SIUM (mg)	SELE-NIUM (mcg)	SO-DIUM (mg)	ZINC (mg)
Recommended intakes for women	1,000	900	8–18	310–320	700	2,600	55	1,500	8
Recommended intakes for men	1,000	900	8	400–420	700	3,400	55	1,500	11
FRUITS (RAW UNLESS STATED)									
Apple, chopped, ½ c (125 ml)	4	20	0.1	3	14	71	0	1	0
Apple, medium	11	50	0.2	9	20	195	0	2	0.1
Apricot, medium	5	27	0.1	4	8	91	0	0	0.1
Apricots, dried, ¼ c (60 ml)	18	110	0.9	11	23	383	1	3	0.1
Apricots, sliced, ½ c (125 ml)	11	70	0.3	9	20	226	0	1	0.2
Banana, dried, ¼ c (60 ml)	6	98	0.3	27	74	375	1	1	0.2
Banana, medium	6	90	0.3	32	26	422	1	1	0.2
Banana, sliced, ½ c (125 ml)	4	59	0.2	21	17	284	1	1	0.1
Blackberries, ½ c (125 ml)	22	130	0.5	15	17	123	0	1	0.4
Blueberries, ½ c (125 ml)	5	40	0.2	5	9	60	0	1	0.1
Cantaloupe, diced, ½ c (125 ml)	7	32	0.2	10	12	220	0	13	0.2
Cherimoya, ½ c (125 ml)	8	60	0.2	14	22	242	—	6	0.1
Coconut, dried, ¼ c (60 ml)	6	160	0.8	21	48	126	4	9	0.5
Crab apple, sliced, ½ c (125 ml)	10	40	0.2	4	9	113	—	1	—
Currants, black, ½ c (125 ml)	33	50	0.9	14	35	191	0	1	0.2
Currants, red/white, ½ c (125 ml)	20	60	0.6	8	26	163	0	1	0.1
Currants, Zante, dried, ¼ c (60 ml)	31	170	1.2	15	46	326	0	3	0.2
Dates, chopped, ¼ c (60 ml)	14	80	0.4	16	23	245	1	1	0.1
Durian, chopped, ½ c (125 ml)	8	270	0.6	39	50	560	—	3	0.4
Fig, medium	18	35	0.2	8	7	116	0	0	0.1
Figs, dried, ¼ c (60 ml)	61	110	0.8	26	25	257	0	4	0.2
Gooseberries, ½ c (125 ml)	20	60	0.2	8	21	157	0	1	0.1
Grape juice, unsweetened, ½ c (125 ml)	15	20	0.3	13	19	139	0	7	0.1
Grapefruit, pink	54	79	0.2	22	44	332	0	0	0.2
Grapefruit juice, ½ c (125 ml)	12	40	0.3	16	20	211	0	1	0.1
Grapefruit sections, ½ c (125 ml)	15	60	0.1	10	10	169	0	0	0.1
Grapes, ½ c (125 ml)	7	20	0.1	2	5	93	0	1	0
Guava, ½ c (125 ml)	16	200	0.2	19	35	363	1	2	0.2

FOOD	CAL-CIUM (mg)	COP-PER (mcg)	IRON* (mg)	MAG-NESIUM (mg)	PHOS-PHORUS (mg)	POTAS-SIUM (mg)	SELE-NIUM (mcg)	SO-DIUM (mg)	ZINC (mg)
Honeydew melon, diced, ½ c (125 ml)	5	20	0.2	9	10	205	1	16	0.1
Kiwifruit, diced, ½ c (125 ml)	32	120	0.3	16	32	297	0	3	0.1
Kiwifruit, medium	23	99	0.2	12	23	215	0	2	0.1
Loganberries, frozen, ½ c (125 ml)	20	90	0.5	16	20	113	0	1	0.2
Mango, dried, ¼ c (60 ml)	61	—	0.3	—	—	8	—	15	—
Mango, medium	37	370	0.5	34	47	564	2	3	0.3
Mango, sliced, ½ c (125 ml)	10	100	0.1	9	12	146	1	1	0.1
Orange, medium	52	59	0.1	13	18	237	1	0	0.1
Orange juice, ½ c (125 ml)	14	60	0.3	14	22	262	0	1	0.1
Orange sections, ½ c (125 ml)	38	40	0.1	10	13	172	0	0	0.1
Papaya, cubed, ½ c (125 ml)	15	30	0.2	16	8	139	0	6	0.1
Papaya, mashed, ½ c (125 ml)	24	50	0.3	26	12	221	1	10	0.1
Peach, medium	9	100	0.4	14	30	285	0	0	0.3
Peach slices, ½ c (125 ml)	5	60	0.2	7	16	155	0	0	0.1
Pear, medium	16	150	0.3	12	20	212	0	2	0.2
Pear halves, dried, ¼ c (60 ml)	15	170	1.0	15	30	243	0	3	0.2
Pear slices, ½ c (125 ml)	7	60	0.1	5	8	88	0	1	0.1
Pineapple, diced, ½ c (125 ml)	11	100	0.2	10	7	95	0	1	0.1
Plum slices, ½ c (125 ml)	5	50	0.2	6	14	137	0	0	0.1
Prunes, ¼ c (60 ml)	19	120	0.4	18	30	323	0	1	0.2
Raisins, seedless, ¼ c (60 ml)	21	130	0.8	13	42	313	1	5	0.1
Raspberries, ½ c (125 ml)	16	60	0.4	14	19	98	0	1	0.3
Strawberries, whole, ½ c (125 ml)	12	40	0.3	10	19	116	0	1	0.1
Watermelon, diced, ½ c (125 ml)	6	30	0.2	8	9	90	1	1	0.1
VEGETABLES (RAW UNLESS STATED)									
Arugula, chopped, 1 c (250 ml)	34	0	0.3	10	11	78	0	6	0.1
Asparagus, cooked, ½ c (125 ml)	22	160	0.9	13	51	213	6	13	0.6
Avocado, all varieties, medium	24	380	1.1	58	105	975	1	15	1.3
Avocado, all varieties, puréed, ½ c (125 ml)	15	230	0.7	35	63	589	0	9	0.8
Avocado, all varieties, sliced, ½ c (125 ml)	9	150	0.4	22	40	374	0	5	0.5
Avocado, California, medium	18	230	0.8	39	73	690	1	11	1.0

FOOD	CAL-CIUM (mg)	COP-PER (mcg)	IRON* (mg)	MAG-NESIUM (mg)	PHOS-PHORUS (mg)	POTAS-SIUM (mg)	SELE-NIUM (mcg)	SO-DIUM (mg)	ZINC (mg)
Avocado, California, puréed, ½ c (125 ml)	16	210	0.7	35	65	616	0	10	0.8
Avocado, Florida, medium	30	945	0.5	73	122	1,067	0	6	1.2
Avocado, Florida, puréed, ½ c (125 ml)	12	380	0.2	29	49	427	0	2	0.5
Basil, fresh, chopped, 1 c (250 ml)	79	170	1.4	29	25	132	0	2	0.4
Beans, green/yellow, ½ c (125 ml)	20	40	0.6	13	20	110	0	3	0.1
Beet greens, 1 c (250 ml)	46	80	1	28	16	305	0	91	0.2
Beets, sliced, ½ c (125 ml)	12	50	0.6	17	29	234	0	56	0.2
Bok choy, cooked, ½ c (125 ml)	84	20	0.9	10	26	333	0	31	0.2
Broccoli, cooked, ½ c (125 ml)	33	50	0.6	17	55	241	1	34	0.4
Brussels sprouts, cooked, ½ c (125 ml)	30	70	1.0	16	46	261	1	17	0.3
Cabbage, green, chopped, 1 c (250 ml)	38	20	0.4	11	24	160	0	17	0.2
Cabbage, red, chopped, 1 c (250 ml)	42	15	0.7	14	27	217	0	24	0.2
Carrot, chopped, ½ c (125 ml)	22	30	0.2	8	24	216	0	47	0.2
Carrot, medium	20	30	0.2	7	21	195	0	42	0.2
Carrot juice, ½ c (125 ml)	30	60	0.6	17	52	364	1	36	0.2
Cauliflower, cooked, ½ c (125 ml)	10	15	0.2	6	21	93	0	10	0.1
Celery, diced, ½ c (125 ml)	21	21	0.1	6	13	139	0	43	0.1
Celery rib, large	26	22	0.1	7	15	166	0	64	0.1
Celery root, ½ c (125 ml)	35	60	0.6	16	95	247	1	82	0.3
Collard greens, chopped, 1 c (250 ml)	55	14	0.1	3	4	64	0	8	0
Corn, yellow/white, ½ c (125 ml)	2	40	0.4	28	68	207	0	11	0.4
Cucumber, medium, peeled	28	142	0.4	24	42	273	0	4	0.2
Cucumber, peeled, sliced, ½ c (125 ml)	20	100	0.3	17	30	191	0	3	0.2
Cucumber, with peel, sliced, ½ c (125 ml)	18	50	0.3	14	26	162	0	2	0.2
Dandelion greens, 1 c (250 ml)	109	100	1.8	21	38	231	0	42	0.2
Eggplant, cooked, ½ c (125 ml)	3	30	0.1	6	8	64	0	1	0.1
Endive, chopped, 1 c (250 ml)	27	0	0.4	8	15	166	0	12	0.4
Garlic clove, medium	5	9	0	0.8	5	12	0	1	0

FOOD	CAL-CIUM (mg)	COP-PER (mcg)	IRON* (mg)	MAG-NESIUM (mg)	PHOS-PHORUS (mg)	POTAS-SIUM (mg)	SELE-NIUM (mcg)	SO-DIUM (mg)	ZINC (mg)
Garlic cloves, ½ c (125 ml)	130	210	1.2	18	110	288	10	12	0.8
Green Giant Juice, 1 c (250 ml)**	103	1	1.0	32	79	556	—	74	0.4
Jerusalem artichoke, ½ c (125 ml)	11	110	2.7	13	62	340	1	3	0.1
Kale, 1 c (250 ml)	100	210	1.2	24	40	316	1	30	0.3
Kale, Scotch, 1 c (250 ml)	145	170	2	62	44	319	1	50	0.3
Kelp, chopped, ½ c (125 ml)	71	50	1.2	51	18	38	0	98	1
Kelp, dried, 1 T (15 ml)	43	30	0.7	31	11	22	0	59	0.3
Leeks, chopped, ½ c (125 ml)	27	60	1.0	13	16	85	0	9	0.1
Lettuce, butterhead/Boston/Bibb, chopped, 1 c (250 ml)	20	10	0.7	8	19	138	0	3	0.1
Lettuce, iceberg, chopped, 1 c (250 ml)	14	20	0.3	5	15	107	0	8	0.1
Lettuce, looseleaf, chopped, 1 c (250 ml)	14	10	0.3	5	11	74	0	11	0.1
Lettuce, red leaf, chopped, 1 c (250 ml)	10	10	0.4	4	8	55	0	7	0.1
Lettuce, romaine, chopped, 1 c (250 ml)	16	20	0.5	7	15	123	0	4	0.1
Mushrooms, ½ c (125 ml)	2–8	160	0.2	5	44–52	195	5	3	0.3–0.5
Mustard greens, 1 c (250 ml)	61	90	0.9	19	25	209	1	15	0.1
Okra, cooked, ½ c (125 ml)	65	70	0.2	30	27	114	0	5	0.4
Olives, black, canned, ½ c (125 ml)	59	180	2.3	3	2	6	1	522	0.2
Onions, green, chopped, ½ c (125 ml)	38	40	0.8	11	20	146	0	8	0.2
Onion, green, medium	11	12	0.2	3	6	41	0	2	0.1
Onions, red/yellow/white, ½ c (125 ml)	19	30	0.2	8	25	123	0	3	0.1
Parsley, 1 c (250 ml)	89	100	4	32	37	356	0	36	0.7
Parsnips, cooked, ½ c (125 ml)	31	110	0.5	24	57	302	1	8	0.2
Peas, ½ c (125 ml)	19	130	1.1	25	83	187	1	4	1
Peas, cooked, ½ c (125 ml)	23	150	1.3	33	99	229	2	3	1
Pea pods, snow, ½ c (125 ml)	14	30	0.7	8	18	67	0	1	0.1
Pepper, bell, green, chopped, ½ c (125 ml)	8	50	0.3	8	16	138	0	2	0.1
Pepper, bell, green, medium	12	79	0.4	12	24	208	0	4	0.2

FOOD	CAL-CIUM (mg)	COP-PER (mcg)	IRON* (mg)	MAG-NESIUM (mg)	PHOS-PHORUS (mg)	POTAS-SIUM (mg)	SELE-NIUM (mcg)	SO-DIUM (mg)	ZINC (mg)
Pepper, bell, red, chopped, ½ c (125 ml)	6	10	0.3	9	20	166	0	3	0.2
Pepper, bell, red, medium	8	20	0.5	14	31	251	0	2	0.3
Peppers, hot green chile, ½ c (125 ml)	14	140	1.0	20	36	269	0	6	0.4
Peppers, hot red chile, ½ c (125 ml)	11	100	0.8	18	34	255	0	7	0.2
Potato, baked, medium	26	200	1.9	48	121	926	1	17	0.6
Potato, with skin, cooked, ½ c (125 ml)	7	140	0.3	16	33	270	0	4	0.2
Radish sprouts, ½ c (125 ml)	20	50	0.4	18	45	35	0	2	0.2
Radishes, daikon (Oriental), medium	91	389	1.4	54	78	767	2	71	0.5
Radishes, sliced, ½ c (125 ml)	15	30	0.2	6	12	143	0	24	0
Rutabaga, chopped, cooked, ½ c (125 ml)	43	40	0.5	21	50	293	1	18	0.3
Seaweed, spirulina, dried, 1 T (15 ml)	9	427	2	14	8	97	0	74	0.1
Spinach, chopped, 1 c (250 ml)	31	40	0.9	25	16	177	0	25	0.2
Spinach, cooked, ½ c (125 ml)	129	170	3.4	83	53	443	1	67	0.7
Squash, acorn, baked, ½ c (125 ml)	48	91	1	47	49	473	1	4	0.2
Squash, all varieties summer, cooked, ½ c (125 ml)	30	110	0.4	27	43	213	0	1	0.4
Squash, all varieties winter, baked, ½ c (125 ml)	24	90	0.5	14	21	261	0	1	0.2
Squash, butternut, baked, ½ c (125 ml)	44	70	0.6	31	29	308	1	4	0.1
Squash, crookneck, baked, ½ c (125 ml)	28	80	0.5	19	37	215	0	0	0.3
Squash, Hubbard, baked, ½ c (125 ml)	18	50	0.5	24	25	388	1	9	0.2
Sweet potato, cooked, ½ c (125 ml)	47	160	1.2	31	55	399	1	47	0.4
Tomato, cherry	2	10	0	2	4	40	0	1	0
Tomato, chopped, ½ c (125 ml)	10	60	0.3	10	23	225	0	5	0.2
Tomato, green, chopped, ½ c (125 ml)	12	90	0.5	10	27	194	0	12	0.1

FOOD	CAL-CIUM (mg)	COP-PER (mcg)	IRON* (mg)	MAG-NESIUM (mg)	PHOS-PHORUS (mg)	POTAS-SIUM (mg)	SELE-NIUM (mcg)	SO-DIUM (mg)	ZINC (mg)
Tomato, medium	12	70	0.3	14	30	292	0	6	0.2
Tomato, Roma, medium	6	37	0.2	7	15	147	0	3	0
Tomato, sun-dried, ¼ c (60 ml)	16	205	1.3	28	51	489	0.8	35	0.3
Tomato, yellow, chopped, ½ c (125 ml)	8	70	0.4	9	26	189	1	17	0.2
Turnip, cooked, ½ c (125 ml)	40	—	0.2	11	32	215	0	19	0.2
Turnip greens, chopped, 1 c (250 ml)	110	200	0.6	18	24	172	1	23	0.1
Water chestnuts, Chinese, sliced, ½ c (125 ml)	7	200	0	14	39	362	0	9	0.3
Watercress, chopped, 1 c (250 ml)	43	30	0.1	7	21	119	0	15	0
Yam, cooked, ½ c (125 ml)	40	170	0.7	29	57	502	0	38	0.3
Zucchini, chopped, ½ c (125 ml)	10	30	0.2	12	25	171	0	5	0.2
NUTS AND SEEDS									
Almond butter, 2 T (30 ml)	113	300	1.1	91	165	243	1	3	1.1
Almonds, ¼ c (60 ml)	96	360	1.4	97	176	256	1	0	1.1
Brazil nut, large	8	82	0.1	18	34	31	91	0	0.2
Brazil nuts, ¼ c (60 ml)	57	620	0.9	133	257	234	681	1	1.4
Cashew butter, 2 T (30 ml)	14	710	1.6	84	148	177	4	5	1.7
Cashews, roasted, ¼ c (60 ml)	16	770	2.1	90	170	196	4	6	2
Chia seeds, ¼ c (60 ml)	269	390	3.3	143	366	173	24	7	2
Flaxseeds, ground, ¼ c (60 ml)	81	230	3.2	114	211	243	—	15	0.6
Hazelnuts/filberts, ¼ c (60 ml)	39	590	1.6	56	99	233	1	0	0.8
Hempseeds, ¼ c (60 ml)	27	—	4.9	—	—	—		0	—
Pecans, ¼ c (60 ml)	18	300	0.6	30	70	103	1	0	1.1
Pine nuts/pignolia nuts, ¼ c (60 ml)	5	450	1.9	86	197	204	0	1	2.2
Pistachio nuts, ¼ c (60 ml)	33	410	1.2	38	153	320	2	0	0.7
Poppy seeds, ¼ c (60 ml)	490	550	3.3	118	297	245	4	9	2.7
Pumpkin seeds, ¼ c (60 ml)	15	440	2.9	194	403	265	3	2	2.6
Sesame seeds, hulled, ¼ c (60 ml)	23	530	2.4	131	254	141	13	18	2.6
Sesame seeds, whole, ¼ c (60 ml)	356	1,490	5.3	128	230	171	13	4	2.8
Sesame tahini, 2 T (30 ml)	43	490	1.4	29	240	140	10	11	1.4

FOOD	CAL-CIUM (mg)	COP-PER (mcg)	IRON* (mg)	MAG-NESIUM (mg)	PHOS-PHORUS (mg)	POTAS-SIUM (mg)	SELE-NIUM (mcg)	SO-DIUM (mg)	ZINC (mg)
Sunflower seed butter, 2 T (30 ml)	21	520	1.3	101	216	187	34	1	1.6
Sunflower seeds, hulled, ¼ c (60 ml)	28	640	1.9	115	234	229	19	3	1.8
Walnuts, black, ¼ c (60 ml)	19	430	1	64	163	166	5	1	1.1
Walnuts, English, ¼ c (60 ml)	29	470	0.9	47	103	131	1	1	0.9
LEGUMES (COOKED UNLESS STATED)									
Adzuki beans, ½ c (125 ml)	34	360	2.4	63	204	646	1	10	2.1
Black beans, ½ c (125 ml)	25	190	1.9	64	127	323	1	1	1
Black-eyed peas, ½ c (125 ml)	22	240	2.3	48	141	251	2	4	1.1
Black turtle beans, ½ c (125 ml)	54	260	2.8	48	149	423	1	3	0.7
Chickpeas, ½ c (125 ml)	42	310	2.5	42	146	252	3	6	1.3
Cranberry beans, ½ c (125 ml)	47	220	2	47	126	362	1	1	1.1
Edamame, ½ c (125 ml)	49	283	1.8	52	138	358	—	70	1.1
Falafel patties, three, 2 oz (60 g) total	32	150	2	49	115	351	1	176	0.9
Great Northern beans, ½ c (125 ml)	63	230	2	47	154	366	4	2	0.8
Kidney beans, ½ c (125 ml)	33	200	2.1	39	129	379	61	1	0.9
Lentil sprouts, raw, 1 c (250 ml)	20	290	2.6	30	141	262	0	9	1.2
Lentils, ½ c (125 ml)	20	260	3.5	38	188	386	3	2	1.3
Lima beans, baby, ½ c (125 ml)	28	210	2.3	51	122	386	5	3	1
Mung bean sprouts, raw, 1 c (250 ml)	14	180	1.0	23	59	164	1	7	0.4
Navy beans, ½ c (125 ml)	66	200	2.3	51	138	374	3	0	1
Pea sprouts, raw, 1 c (250 ml)	46	340	2.9	71	209	483	1	25	1.3
Peanut butter, 2 T (30 ml)	14	150	0.6	50	116	211	2	149	0.9
Peanuts, ¼ c (60 ml)	34	420	1.7	62	139	261	3	7	1.2
Peas, green, ½ c (125 ml)	23	150	1.3	33	99	229	2	3	1.0
Peas, split, ½ c (125 ml)	14	190	1.3	37	103	375	1	2	1.0
Pinto beans, ½ c (125 ml)	41	200	1.9	45	133	394	6	1	0.9
Soy milk, fortified, ½ c (125 ml)	158–163	110–210	0.5–1.0	19–35	55–134	138–232	3	53–85	0.3–0.6
Soybeans, ½ c (125 ml)	93	370	4.7	78	223	468	7	1	1.0
Tempeh, ½ c (125 ml)	97	490	2.4	71	233	361	0	8	1.0

FOOD	CAL-CIUM (mg)	COP-PER (mcg)	IRON* (mg)	MAG-NESIUM (mg)	PHOS-PHORUS (mg)	POTAS-SIUM (mg)	SELE-NIUM (mcg)	SO-DIUM (mg)	ZINC (mg)
Tofu, calcium-set, ½ c (125 ml)***	268–909	280–500	2.1–3.5	49–77	161–253	197–316	13–23	16–19	1.1–2.1
Veggie burger***	16	140	0.8	2	110	72	—	273	0.8
White beans, ½ c (125 ml)	85	270	3.5	60	107	531	1	6	1.3
GRAINS (COOKED UNLESS STATED)									
Amaranth, ½ c (125 ml)	58	260	2.6	80	182	188	9	7	1.1
Barley, pearl, ½ c (125 ml)	9	90	1.1	18	45	77	7	2	0.7
Bread, rye, slice, 1 oz (30 g)	22	60	0.8	12	38	50	9	181	0.3
Bread, whole wheat, slice, 1 oz (30 g)	48	—	0.7	23	64	76	11	135	0.5
Buckwheat groats, kasha, ½ c (125 ml)	6	130	0.7	45	62	78	2	4	0.5
Corn, ear, large, raw	3	80	0.7	53	127	386	1	21	0.7
Kamut, ½ c (125 ml)	9	230	1.8	51	161	184	—	5	1.6
Millet, ½ c (125 ml)	3	150	0.6	40	92	57	1	2	0.8
Oatmeal, ½ c (125 ml)	11	90	1.1	33	95	87	7	5	1.2
Pasta/spaghetti, enriched, ½ c (125 ml)	5	70	0.4	13	40	23	16	1	0.4
Pasta/spaghetti, whole wheat, ½ c (125 ml)	11	120	0.8	22	66	33	19	2	0.6
Quinoa, ½ c (125 ml)	17	190	1.4	63	149	168	3	7	1.1
Rice, brown, ½ c (125 ml)	10	100	0.4	44	86	44	10	5	0.6
Rice, white, enriched, ½ c (125 ml)	8	60	1.0	10	36	29	6	1	0.4
Spelt, ½ c (125 ml)	10	220	1.7	50	154	147	4	5	1.3
Tortilla, corn, without added calcium, 1 oz (30 g)***	24	—	0.4	22	94	56	—	14	0.4
Tortilla, wheat, without added calcium, 1 oz (30 g)***	32	—	0.7–1.0	6	57	48	—	108–208	0.2
Wheat sprouts, raw, 1 c (250 ml)	30	300	2.4	94	228	193	48	18	1.9
Wild rice, ½ c (125 ml)	3	100	0.5	28	71	88	1	3	1.2
SWEETS AND OILS									
Dark chocolate, 45–59% cacao, 2 oz (60 g)	34	—	4.8	88	124	335	—	14	1.2
Dark chocolate, 70–85% cacao, 2 oz (60 g)	44	—	7.1	137	185	429	—	12	2
Maple syrup, 1 T (15 ml)	21	0	0	4	0	42	0	2	0.3

FOOD	CAL-CIUM (mg)	COP-PER (mcg)	IRON* (mg)	MAG-NESIUM (mg)	PHOS-PHORUS (mg)	POTAS-SIUM (mg)	SELE-NIUM (mcg)	SO-DIUM (mg)	ZINC (mg)
Molasses, 1 T (15 ml)	41	97	0.9	48	6	293	3.6	7	0.1
Molasses, blackstrap, organic, Plantation or Brer Rabbit, 1 T (15 ml)***	80–200	—	0.7–3.6	32–100	—	353	—	0–10	—
Olive oil, 1 T, (15 ml)	0	0	0.1	0	0	0	0	0	0

Sources:[73, 76]

Key: Dashes indicate that no data is available.

*RDA for iron (see page 187).

**Based on recipe with kale, romaine lettuce, lemon juice, cucumber, apple, celery, and lemon (from *Becoming Raw*).

***Or see label.

For menus and delicious recipes that meet recommended intakes of all essential minerals and other nutrients, see *Cooking Vegan* by Vesanto Melina and Joseph Forest (Book Publishing Company, 2012). For raw vegan menus and recipes, see *Becoming Raw* by Brenda Davis and Vesanto Melina (Book Publishing Company, 2010).

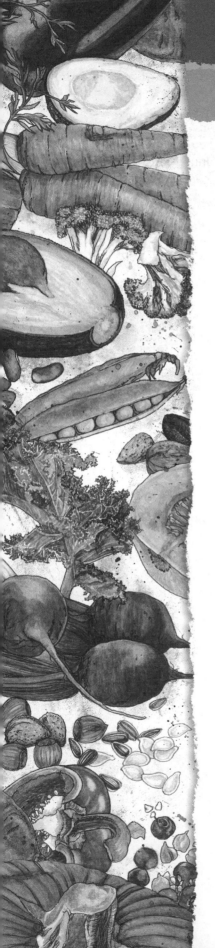

CHAPTER 7

Vitamins:
Vital for Life

On the 20th day of May, 1747, I took twelve patients in the scurvy on board the Salisbury at sea. Their cases were as similar as I could have them . . . The consequence was that the most sudden and visible good effects were perceived from the use of oranges and lemons; one of those who had taken them, being at the end of six days fit for duty.

DR. JAMES LIND, SURGEON, BRITISH ROYAL NAVY[1]

In 1900, in many urban centers in the northeastern United States, 80 percent of children had rickets; in Java during the late nineteenth century, a three-month prison sentence could lead to death from lack of thiamine. Throughout history, mankind has known that certain foods, or time spent outdoors in sunny areas, had mysterious properties that could prevent or cure illness, and that a lack thereof could threaten a person's well-being. Yet, the recognition of the existence of specific vitamins is just a century old; vitamin A was first identified in 1913.

Essential to life, vitamins can't be synthesized by the body in adequate amounts; outside sources must be obtained. Although also found in food and equally essential for health, minerals are simply single elements. Vitamins are more-complex molecules that combine carbon with other elements, such as hydrogen, oxygen, and sometimes nitrogen. The total amount of vitamins the body needs is tiny—only 0.5 gram per day—but the functions they perform are vital. Some vitamins act like hormones, with far-reaching effects in the body; vitamin A governs certain aspects of growth and vitamin D regulates mineral metabolism. Many vitamins are coenzymes that assist enzymes in vital metabolic functions. Vitamins work as teams, to protect the body from free radical damage (vitamins A, C, and E) or convert carbohydrate, fat, and protein into a form of energy the body can use (the B vitamins).

Although vegan diets deliver most vitamins in abundance, vitamins B_{12} and D invite special attention; vegans (and many nonvegans) must take care regarding issues and sources. This chapter examines the roles of vitamins in the body and explores options for meeting recommended intakes (listed for all ages on page 446).

Dodging Deficiencies

VITAMIN B_{12}*

Vitamin B_{12} in Perspective

Vitamin B_{12} has the largest molecular structure of any vitamin, with the mineral cobalt at its center. Lack of vitamin B_{12} is responsible for the lion's share of bad press that vegan diets receive. Yet a shortfall is easily averted by B_{12} supplements and/or fortified foods. Sadly, from time to time, two scenarios appear in medical literature or newspaper headlines. One features adults who don't properly supplement with B_{12}; the other documents developmental problems in infants whose mothers consumed insufficient B_{12} during pregnancy and whose intake was inadequate after birth.

Function

B_{12} is part of the vitamin team that converts carbohydrate, fat, and protein into useable energy. It's required for DNA synthesis and thus is crucial for cells that reproduce rapidly (for instance, during periods of growth) and for the red blood cells produced in bone marrow. It also maintains the protective myelin sheaths that surround nerve fibers.

As one aspect of its interaction with amino acids, vitamin B_{12} helps to rid the body of homocysteine, a potentially harmful breakdown product of protein and specifically of the amino acid methionine. Homocysteine can injure the delicate inner lining of artery walls and can trigger heart disease. Over time, such damage can occur in those who appear healthy in other respects.[2–5]

Vitamin B_{12} is produced by bacteria present in the gastrointestinal tract (for example, in the mouth and lower bowel), yet this internal production can't be relied upon to prevent deficiency. The amount made in the mouth is insufficient, and anything created in the lower bowel is too low in the digestive tract to be absorbed, so the vitamin is passed in the feces.[2, 4, 5]

Deficiency Symptoms

In cases of vitamin B_{12} deficiency (either from insufficient intake or from inadequate absorption of this vitamin), some combination of the following symptoms or conditions can appear:[2, 5, 6]

---

*Forms of vitamin B_{12} include cyanocobalamin, methylcobalamin, and adenosylcobalamin.

- **Megaloblastic anemia.** Without proper cell division, facilitated by vitamin B_{12}, abnormally large red cells appear in the blood, because the cells have failed to divide properly. This condition is called megaloblastic anemia. The blood has decreased ability to carry oxygen, which results in fatigue, weakness, decreased stamina, shortness of breath, palpitations, and skin pallor. Note that this condition can be masked in diets rich in folate (as many vegan diets are), because dietary folate is part of the process of red blood cell division.

- **Nerve damage.** The effects of vitamin B_{12} deficiency on nerve cells, the spinal cord, and the brain can cause mental changes, such as confusion, depression, irritability, mood changes, insomnia, and inability to concentrate, plus physical symptoms, such as tingling and numbness in fingers, arms, and legs, difficulty with balance, lack of sensation, and eventual paralysis.

- **Gastrointestinal disturbances.** Symptoms involving the gastrointestinal tract include a sore tongue, reduced appetite, indigestion, and diarrhea.

- **Elevated blood levels of homocysteine.** In vitamin B_{12} deficiency, homocysteine increases, atherosclerotic plaque accumulates, and arteries begin to clog, resulting in heart disease and strokes. Excess homocysteine also has a negative impact on bone health.[7]

These problems are easily avoided by ensuring a reliable source of this essential nutrient. Deficiency symptoms in adults typically can be reversed when the situation is caught and attended to early enough.[2–5, 8–10]

Deficiencies early in pregnancy may be linked to neural tube defects. Breast-fed infants whose mothers consume insufficient dietary B_{12} and other infants whose diets are low in B_{12} can develop serious and permanent damage to the nervous system. According to Dr. James Mills, a senior investigator with the US National Institute of Child Health and Human Development, any woman of childbearing age should be particularly careful to maintain adequate B_{12} levels.[11, 12]

Infants typically show a more rapid onset of symptoms than adults. A B_{12} deficiency may lead to loss of energy and appetite and failure to thrive, but there's no entirely consistent pattern of symptoms. Infants are more vulnerable to permanent damage than adults; if not promptly corrected, deficiency can progress to coma or death. Some infants make a full recovery with proper treatment, but others show delayed development.[4, 9, 13, 14]

Laboratory Tests for Vitamin B₁₂

Several lab tests are used to detect vitamin B_{12} status; the first two listed below are particularly reliable and sensitive. However, physicians and lab technicians may be unfamiliar with some of these tests. (For links to more information on such lab tests, see Resources on page 449.)[2, 4, 15–18]

- **Holo-transcobalamin (Holo-TC or Holo-TCII).** This test measures the amount of one of the binding proteins in blood, which transports B_{12} to the body's tissues. Low levels of Holo-TC may show that vitamin B_{12}

depletion is at an early stage, before stores are exhausted and clinical symptoms appear.[6, 15, 17, 18–22, 60]

- **Methylmalonic acid (MMA).** The best marker of B_{12} status when stores are depleted and deficiency has been reached is a compound called MMA. In cases of B_{12} deficiency, MMA accumulates and can be measured in blood or (taken more easily) in urine.[15, 18, 23]

- **Homocysteine.** Another compound that can build up in blood when B_{12} is in short supply is homocysteine. Though testing for homocysteine levels is more commonly used to check for increased risk of heart disease, high blood homocysteine levels can indicate vitamin B_{12} deficiency. The test lacks specificity, because high homocysteine levels can also signal a lack of folate, although most vegans get plenty of folate. (For more information on homocysteine, see page 216.)[15, 23]

- **Serum or plasma vitamin B_{12}.** A measure often used to assess B_{12} status is serum or plasma B_{12}. In the past, biological assays couldn't distinguish between the true vitamin and substances in the blood known as inactive B_{12} analogs. As a result, cases of B_{12} deficiency were missed.

  Inactive analogs are molecules that resemble B_{12} in physical structure; however, they're not identical and can't perform the vitamin's roles in the body. For example, when people who were short of vitamin B_{12} and who also consumed sources of inactive analogs (such as spirulina or seaweeds) were tested, their serum or plasma B_{12} results indicated normal B_{12} levels despite deficiency.[15, 18, 24] Modern radioisotope and immunoassay methods can more accurately measure the active form of B_{12}.

  The lower end of the reference range for serum B_{12} may have been set too low. The lower end point used by many laboratories for serum B_{12} has been 200 pg/ml (150 pmol/L); however, many experts recommend this minimum be doubled to 405 pg/ml (300 pmol/L) or more. In Japan, the low end of the serum B_{12} range considered acceptable has been as high as 550 pg/ml (400 pmol/L) for many years.[22, 25, 26] People whose lab test results are toward the lower end of the reference range yet within the range of some laboratories may still experience or develop some symptoms of vitamin B_{12} deficiency.

- **Mean corpuscular volume (MCV).** A test that can indicate possible vitamin B_{12} deficiency is MCV, an indicator of macrocytic anemia (meaning red blood cells that are larger than normal) that points to possible vitamin B_{12} deficiency. Testing MCV doesn't work for detecting B_{12} deficiency in people with high intakes of folate (from green vegetables, oranges, legumes, and other folate-rich foods), because folate helps to prevent macrocytic anemia even when a vitamin B_{12} deficiency exists. As a result, a B_{12} deficiency can remain undetected by an MCV test, while the underlying damage to nerves proceeds and homocysteine levels rise.[2, 4, 17]

For a person experiencing or wondering about symptoms of B_{12} deficiency, it can be of value to arrange to have two of the tests listed, such as serum B_{12} (a measure of the vitamin) plus MMA (a metabolic indicator). To avoid a potential deficiency, it makes even more sense to ensure that intake is adequate.[15, 17, 26, 27]

How to Obtain Adequate Vitamin B_{12}

Follow one or a combination of these approaches:

1. Every day, take a B_{12} (cyanocobalamin) supplement. Choose one that includes at least 25 micrograms (mcg) of B_{12}; most multivitamin supplements provide 25 mcg and often much more. Some experts recommend as much as 250 mcg daily for adults up to age 65, and 500 or 1,000 mcg for seniors (excess is excreted).[32–34, 37]

2. Twice a week, take 2,000 to 2,500 mcg of vitamin B_{12} in supplement form, either sublingually or swallowed. Some experts note that, taken twice a week, 1,000 mcg vitamin B_{12} supplements will suffice, with just over 1 percent absorbed. Search online for inexpensive sources.

3. Every day, consume three servings of B_{12}-fortified foods, with each serving providing at least 2 mcg of vitamin B_{12} (33 percent of the Daily Value, or DV). Typical examples are fortified nondairy milks, vegan meat substitutes, breakfast cereals, and bars (page 221). Another choice is 2 teaspoons (10 ml or 5 g) of Red Star Vegetarian Support Formula nutritional yeast, which is fortified with vitamin B_{12}.[2, 4, 16, 17, 38]

Recommended Intake

The body requires vitamin B_{12} in miniscule amounts; the official Recommended Dietary Allowance (RDA) for adults is 2.4 mcg per day, the amount needed to prevent macrocytic anemia. However, recent research suggests an intake of 4 to 7 mcg per day is necessary to prevent buildup of homocysteine and MMA.[16, 28] The RDA assumes that the total intake of B_{12} comes from two or three sources (such as fortified foods) that are eaten at different times of the day (the body's B_{12} receptors may become saturated with amounts as small as 1 to 1.5 mcg, though this varies with dose). Because the amount of vitamin B_{12} in fortified foods (page 221) can differ from one batch to another, it's wise to combine fortified foods with occasional supplement use because supplements are more tightly standardized. [29, 30]

If the whole amount of vitamin B_{12} is consumed at once (as with a supplement), the body absorbs only a fraction of the total. For example, with a 250 mcg dose, the body's B_{12} receptors only take in about 1.5 mcg and can't absorb more for four to six hours. Beyond the absorption at the B_{12} receptor sites, an entirely different mechanism—passive diffusion—allows for the uptake of about 1 percent of the B_{12} ingested.[16, 26, 31–34] As a result, the less frequently vitamin B_{12} is ingested, the higher the dose needed (see "How to Obtain Adequate Vitamin B_{12}").

Based on a lack of reports of vitamin B_{12} toxicity in the general population or during pregnancy, the Institute of Medicine (IOM) concluded there's no basis to establish a UL. Exceeding recommended intakes is considered to be safe; the excess is simply excreted in the urine.[23, 28, 35] Cobalamin itself appears to be nontoxic; at the same time, daily intake of 1,000 mcg of cyanocobalamin doses is a growing phenomenon whose long-term effects are unknown.[194]

Which form of vitamin B_{12} is best? Cyanocobalamin is most stable; it has the most proven effectiveness and research backing; a miniscule amount of cyanide is present simply to stabilize the vitamin. But there's no danger—a 2,500 mcg B_{12} (cyanocobalamin) supplement delivers 0.2 percent of the lowest daily dose of cyanide that could be toxic for a 110 lb (50 kg) person.[36] Cyanide is found in nature; 1 level tablespoon (15 ml) of flaxseeds, for example, has 30 times as much cyanide as this supplement, and toxicologists consider such tiny amounts to be insignificant. After ingestion, the body removes and detoxifies the cyanide. The cobalamin is then converted to methylcobalamin, one of the active forms of vitamin B_{12}. This conversion may be less effective in people who smoke or have kidney problems; they should use a direct source of methylcobalamin. However, less scientific research is available to determine the exact amounts needed of this less-stable coenzyme form of vitamin B_{12}; as much as 1,000 mcg daily may be needed if methylcobalamin is used.[16, 23] Note that stored vitamin B_{12} can be affected by exposure to heat and light.

These recommendations also are suitable during pregnancy or lactation; for other ages, see page 446. For updates about vitamin B_{12} and the lively field of research surrounding it, see Resources on page 449.

B_{12} Recycling and Avoiding Deficiency

As noted earlier, the effects of a vitamin B_{12} deficiency can be devastating. Fortunately, the body can be adept at recovering and reusing vitamin B_{12}. Some people are better recyclers than others; in fact, a few avoid deficiency symptoms for many years despite having no reported dietary source. However, recycling shouldn't be relied upon to maintain adequate B_{12} levels. Adult stores may last for a year or more, although deficiency symptoms can be experienced within several months.

Vegans who don't include a reliable source of vitamin B_{12} will eventually become deficient. For some, this will happen in a matter of months; for others, it could take years. The consequences of this deficiency depend on how soon the deficiency is recognized and remedied. The damage can be dramatic and—in a few unfortunate cases of long-term deficiency—irreversible.

Early symptoms, such as weakness, fatigue, and mood changes, are nonspecific and easily mistaken for stress or aging, but the longer it takes to recognize the source of the problem, the greater the risk of permanent damage. People older than 50 (on any diet) should be alert regarding signs of B_{12} deficiency, because malabsorption problems may occur with age. If a B_{12} deficiency is suspected, lab tests can be arranged by a physician (see page 215). If the tests are carried out and B_{12} deficiency is diagnosed, supplementation can begin immediately and further health consequences can be averted. However, if B_{12} isn't added to the diet at this stage, nervous-system damage will accelerate, and symptoms become more severe. A person with a B_{12} deficiency runs the risk of heart disease; in pregnant women, a deficiency could be disastrous for the infant.

Vegans whose B_{12} intake from supplements or fortified foods is at recommended levels (see "How to Obtain Adequate Vitamin B_{12}" on page 217) can expect to have serum B_{12} levels in the normal range, assuming they have normal absorption (page 221). The safest approach is to use a reliable source of vitamin B_{12} before deficiency symptoms appear. A person who hasn't had a source of B_{12} for

Liquid Gold Dressing

Makes 1½ cups (375 ml)

The name "Liquid Gold" denotes nutritional wealth that goes far beyond color; this creamy dressing is packed with riboflavin and other B vitamins. Three tablespoons (45 ml) can provide half the day's B_{12} requirement when prepared with fortified Red Star Vegetarian Support Formula nutritional yeast. (It also provides a day's supply of omega-3 fatty acids.) Use this tasty dressing on salads, rice, baked potatoes, steamed broccoli, and other vegetables. (Add 1 teaspoon turmeric for more golden color plus protective circumin, and increase its absorption with a little black pepper.)

½ cup (125 ml) flaxseed oil

½ cup (125 ml) water

⅓ cup (85 ml) lemon juice

1 tablespoon (15 ml) cider vinegar, balsamic vinegar, or raspberry vinegar

2 tablespoons (30 ml) tamari or Bragg Liquid Aminos

½ cup (125 ml) nutritional yeast

1 tablespoon (15 ml) ground flaxseeds

2 teaspoons (10 ml) Dijon mustard

1 teaspoon (5 ml) ground cumin

Put all the ingredients in a blender and process until smooth. Stored in a covered jar in the refrigerator, the dressing will keep for 2 weeks.

a time can quickly restore normal levels by seeing a physician for a B_{12} injection. Taking 2,000 mcg of oral vitamin B_{12} (cyanocobalamin) daily for several weeks also has proved effective in returning B_{12} levels to normal; one of the three regimens shown on page 217 can then be adopted.[39]

Vegan Intakes from Food and Supplements

Studies show average vegan intakes of vitamin B_{12} to be far below the RDA, with many participants having levels 25 percent or less than these recommended adult intakes.[17, 40, 41] Those who met the RDA typically included B_{12} supplements. Two of three studies assessing intakes of vegan children and teens indicated insufficient vitamin B_{12}.[17] Since these studies were conducted, responsible vegetarian societies (including raw foods groups) have recognized the need for vegans to ensure a reliable source of this essential nutrient; data from future studies should reflect improved vitamin B_{12} intakes.

Vitamin B_{12} Status of Vegans

Various studies of vegans have shown that as few as 11 percent or as many as 90 percent of those tested were deficient in vitamin B_{12} when either MMA or

Holo-TCII or both of these indicators were used. These studies were conducted in Germany, Oman, the Netherlands, the United Kingdom, and the United States. Often, the study participants had been vegan for only a few years.[16, 18, 41, 42, 61, 155] A meta-analysis found that, of seventeen studies comparing plasma homocysteine and serum vitamin B_{12} of vegans and nonvegetarians, only two studies found values to be similar between the two groups.[61] This isn't good news—and it's completely and easily avoidable.

A North American study reported results from 49 adults who had followed a vegan or near-vegan diet for two to four years without vitamin B_{12} supplementation; three-quarters of the participants had insufficient serum B_{12} or high MMA levels. Deficiencies were in the early stages, and participants didn't report having symptoms. Some participants believed they had received adequate intakes of vitamin B_{12} from raw fruits and vegetables, probiotics, fermented foods, dried greens, dulse, nori, blue-green algae, or spirulina, or from intestinal production; however, this proved not to be the case. In a follow-up study, 25 of those with vitamin B_{12} deficiency continued their diet for three weeks, but with an important adjustment. They were divided into three groups:

- One group added sublingual supplements of vitamin B_{12}.
- The second group consumed Red Star Vegetarian Support Formula nutritional yeast on a regular basis.
- The third group took probiotics.

The vitamin B_{12} supplements proved to be powerfully effective in quickly reversing deficiency. The nutritional yeast had some impact but was found to be less reliable than supplements; one person's deficiency was not completely remedied within the three-week time period. Probiotics were ineffective at reversing vitamin B_{12} deficiency.[29, 44]

Unreliable B_{12} Sources

None of the following can be relied upon as sources of vitamin B_{12}: fermented foods, sprouts, mushrooms, seaweeds, spirulina, sprouts, or raw plant foods. Little or no true vitamin B_{12} is available from these foods, and some may instead provide analog forms that are worse than useless because they fail to meet human requirements and can interfere with the action of true B_{12}. Though sea vegetables can be of value for some nutrients, they shouldn't be relied upon as B_{12} sources, because deficiency symptoms or lab results have been shown to worsen when vegans try to use nori, dulse, and spirulina as sources of this essential nutrient.[16, 17, 24, 38, 44]

Reliable B_{12} Sources

The proven vegan B_{12} sources are supplements—an excellent choice—and foods fortified with B_{12}.[44–46] B_{12} is the one vitamin that humans can't get from a varied diet of whole plant foods plus some sun exposure. B_{12} doesn't originate from animal products either; whether it exists in fortified foods, supplements, or meat, it all comes from microorganisms.

Supermarkets stock B_{12}-fortified breakfast cereals, nondairy milks, and vegan meat substitutes; check labels for the B_{12} levels in a serving. Based on a recommended intake level from the past, nutrition label listings for vitamin B_{12} use 6 mcg to mean the amount that provides 100 percent of the DV. So when a label lists vitamin B_{12} at 50 percent of the DV, a serving of the food provides 3 mcg of vitamin B_{12}.

Unproven but Possible B_{12} Sources

Research has shown *Chlorella* and *Aphanizomenon flos-aquae* (AFA) algae to have some true B_{12}, though insufficient research has been done to establish their reliability in reversing deficiency. Preliminary research suggests that *Chlorella* (a cobalt-containing algae) may be a suitable source of vitamin B_{12}. However, until *Chlorella* is tested on a significant number of B_{12}-deficient humans to determine its availability to the body and effectiveness in lowering MMA levels and reversing deficiency, it can't be considered a reliable source of vitamin B_{12}. In an initial trial, beneficial effects were seen in some, but not all, members of a small group of B_{12}-deficient vegans who used six capsules of AFA per day.[16, 17, 24, 31, 38, 47–52]

Vitamin B_{12} at the Beginning of Life

A reliable source of vitamin B_{12} is especially important for mother and child during pregnancy and lactation. When a lactating woman consumes vitamin B_{12} supplements and fortified foods, the vitamin is readily transferred to her infant via her milk. The RDA for a lactating woman is 2.8 mcg per day; amounts consumed should be greater. (See "How to Obtain Adequate Vitamin B_{12}" on page 217 for options based on several servings of fortified foods through the day, daily supplements, or biweekly supplements.)

In medical literature, the most prominent and sometimes tragic cases of B_{12} deficiency involve infants. Without vitamin B_{12}, an infant can develop irreversible brain damage in a few months. Infants who haven't built up their reserves of this nutrient must have adequate supplies. (Vitamin B_{12} drops are one option to guarantee adequate intake).[4, 11–14, 16]

Vitamin B_{12} for Older Adults

The absorption of vitamin B_{12} is a highly complex process that depends on the normal functioning of the gastrointestinal tract. However, about 2 to 3 percent of seniors (regardless of diet) fail to produce enough of a B_{12} carrier (intrinsic factor, or IF) that's essential for B_{12} absorption. IF comes from parietal cells in the stomach lining, though this production typically diminishes with age. Normally, the vitamin B_{12} from supplements and fortified foods first attaches to carriers present in saliva (called R-factors) that conduct B_{12} to the upper part of the small intestine. There, pancreatic secretions partially degrade R-factors and IF takes over, transporting the cobalamin-IF complex to the B_{12} absorption sites in the terminal ileum. For individuals whose absorption is impaired by lack of IF, monthly injections of vitamin B_{12} have been a common remedy. As it turns out, oral doses (2,000 mcg per day) are proving an easier, effective, and less invasive solution. To diagnose a lack of IF and resultant low B_{12}, people over 50 are well-advised to have their B_{12} status tested every five years.[2, 6, 15, 17, 26, 39, 53–55]

For a separate reason, the body's ability to extract and absorb the form of vitamin B_{12} present in animal products diminishes with age. In animal products, B_{12} is tightly bound to protein, and the body must use hydrochloric acid and proteases to cleave B_{12} from the protein. As bodies age, and gastritis or gastric atrophy occur, production of the gastric acid and of the enzymes lessens. (The use of protein pump inhibitors also reduces acid production.) As a result, one in three individuals age 50 or older may lose the capacity to absorb B_{12} from animal products and must rely on the B_{12} sources used by vegans, which are not protein-bound in this way. Thus, the IOM recommends that those over the age of 50 (regardless of dietary pattern) rely either on supplements or vitamin B_{12}–fortified foods to meet B_{12} needs.[2, 56] Some experts suggest that adults older than 65 increase their daily intake to 500 or 1,000 mcg of B_{12}.[16] Older vegans have an advantage if they've already developed the habit of consuming B_{12} in supplements and fortified foods. (See "How to Obtain Adequate Vitamin B_{12}" on page 217.)

Vitamin B_{12} can be effective in treating cognitive impairment and dementia in the small proportion of cases where vitamin B_{12} deficiency exists.[57, 58] Deficiency also may be related to depression in later life.[59]

VITAMIN D

Vitamin D in Perspective

From Roman times and in early China, bone deformities in children were observed and noted. The first detailed medical descriptions of rickets appeared in England around 1650, as the industrial revolution arose and families began to move from farms to smoky, smoggy cities. Many urban children worked long hours indoors, and when they got a chance to play, their play areas weren't sunlit pastures but narrow, dark alleys. It's estimated that by 1900, 80 percent of the children in Boston, New York, and other industrialized cities of the northeastern United States and northern Europe had this devastating skeletal disease.[4, 62–68]

In 1822, an observant Polish physician noted that the bowed legs and deformed skeletons of rickets were almost unheard of in rural areas, where children enjoyed plenty of exposure to sunlight for most of the year. Also, a nineteenth-century French physician noticed that a remedy used along coastal areas of northern Europe—oil from the liver of codfish—could prevent or treat this condition. As it turned out, eating fish liver directly was also protective. In Vienna, shortly after World War I, Dr. Harriette Chick and her coworkers were able to confirm two effective ways to prevent rickets in infants: ultraviolet radiation from the sun or a lamp, and a fat-soluble substance, which became known as vitamin D. In succeeding decades, researchers in the United States, England, and Germany showed that forms of vitamin D could be produced both by sun exposure on the skin and by irradiation (exposure to light) of plant sterols.[4, 62–68]

Identification of the vitamin and its effect on bone health prompted the fortification of cow's milk and then infant formula with vitamin D, creating two reliable avenues for getting this nutrient into the diets of almost all infants and children. Milk and formula were widely promoted as vitamin D sources; in regions that adopted fortification, rickets was almost eradicated. During the late 1990s, fortification was extended to nondairy beverages, such as soy milk.[4, 62–68]

In 1971, vitamin D was reclassified as a "vitamin D hormone," meaning that it can act both as a vitamin and as a hormone. In people who live near the equator and who are consistently exposed to sunlight throughout the year, "vitamin D" is a hormone that their bodies can build in sufficient amounts; for them, a dietary or supplementary source isn't necessary. So technically, the substance known as vitamin D doesn't qualify as a "vitamin" when sufficient sunlight is available. Yet for people who live far from the equator, where sunlight is limited during winter months, an alternate source becomes necessary. This is also true for people in any part of the world (regardless of location or climate) who remain indoors or completely cover their bodies with clothing. In these circumstances, foods naturally rich in vitamin D (such as liver or certain mushrooms that have been exposed to light), vitamin D–fortified foods, or supplements are essential.[4, 62–68]

The deep pigmentation of the skin of people indigenous to tropical areas absorbs shortwave ultraviolet light and acts as a natural sunscreen. As people with dark skins migrate farther from the equator, this protective melanin pigment can become a disadvantage because it also diminishes the production of vitamin D when skin is exposed to sunlight. Where sunlight is limited, paler skin can be an advantage, allowing more vitamin D production.[4, 62–68]

Function

Vitamin D enables the body to increase calcium absorption when needed, maintain critical blood levels of calcium, and limit urinary losses of this mineral. It also supports phosphorus absorption. Vitamin D's role in maintaining healthy bones has been known for decades, and the research is now flowing in on its additional functions. The body can absorb a fraction of its daily calcium requirement by passive diffusion. However, the body's calcium transport mechanism is required to meet the needs for this mineral, and that depends on vitamin D. Thus a partnership of adequate vitamin D and sufficient calcium is necessary.[69] For example, the optimal effect in reducing the risk of fractures and bone loss in people age 50 and older was seen with a combination of at least 20 mcg (800 IU) of vitamin D plus 1,200 mg of calcium supplementation daily.[70]

Many vitamin D experts suggest that significantly higher intakes of vitamin D are advantageous for overall health.[65, 69, 71, 115] Vitamin D functions throughout the body (including in the heart, brain, pancreas, thyroid, and muscles), enabling body systems to respond to everyday stresses and repairing assaults to those body systems. Vitamin D controls the growth and maturation of cells, such as those in bones and the immune system. Through its impact on the immune system, it helps to fight infectious diseases and reduce the risk of Crohn's disease, multiple sclerosis, and rheumatoid arthritis. It regulates insulin production in the pancreas and can protect against type 1 and type 2 diabetes. Due to its active role in the muscles of blood vessels, it helps to regulate blood pressure and prevent cardiovascular disease and stroke. Vitamin D is important for reproductive success and to help preserve cognitive function during aging. Evidence of its benefits continues to accumulate.[65, 69, 72, 73, 78, 79, 115, 159]

Low vitamin D intakes and low serum vitamin D levels are associated with increased risk of colon cancer and other cancers; adequate vitamin D seems to protect against breast cancer recurrence. A distinguished researcher—Edward Giovanucci of the Department of Medicine, Harvard School of Public Health—said, "I would challenge anyone to find an area or nutrient or factor that has such consistent anticancer benefits as vitamin D." He added that vitamin D may prevent thirty deaths for every death caused by skin cancer.[4, 64, 69, 74–77]

The Body's Production of Vitamin D

Either exposure to the sun on a regular basis or consumption of supplements and fortified foods—or a combination of all three—is effective in raising vitamin D levels. When skin is exposed to sunlight, ultraviolet rays stimulate the cholesterol compound called 7-dehydrocholesterol to become vitamin D_3 (cholecalciferol). Vitamin D_3 then enters the bloodstream and is carried to the liver, where it's converted to vitamin D (25-hydroxyvitamin D), the main form circulating in the blood. The latter form is inactive and is measured in lab tests. This is transported to the kidneys, where it's converted to the active form of vitamin D (1, 25 dihydroxyvitamin D). From there, vitamin D moves to the small intestine (where it stimulates calcium absorption) and to cells throughout the body.[73]

The body needs ultraviolet B (UVB), 290 to 315 nanometers in wavelength, to make vitamin D from the 7-dehydrocholesterol in skin. These light rays are plentiful all year in equatorial regions between 30 degrees north and south latitude. Yet large populations spend daytime hours indoors or reside in less-sunny locations and must resort to other options for vitamin D production. Skin production depends on geographic latitude, time of year, time of day, cloud cover, skin color, age, and body weight, as well as use of sunscreen, how much skin is exposed, and the length of exposure to UVB light.[17, 62, 66, 75, 80]

- **Latitude and time of year.** The strength of UVB radiation doesn't vary exactly with latitude; however, people who live farther from the equator than the 30th parallel generally can't get adequate vitamin D production from the sun's rays during "vitamin D winter." Serum vitamin D levels, an indicator of vitamin D status, drop significantly during vitamin D winter. As distances from the equator increase, so does the length of this winter. For example, Boston (latitude 42 degrees N) doesn't receive enough UVB light for adequate vitamin D production from November through February. In Edmonton, Alberta, (latitude 52 degrees N), the vitamin D winter extends from October through March even if skies are clear. As many as 97 percent of Canadians (on any diet) who live north of the 49th parallel show inadequate vitamin D levels at some time during the winter or spring.[81–85]

- **Time of day.** The UVB rays that stimulate vitamin D production are maximal between 10 a.m. and 3 p.m. The optimal time of day occurs when the person's shadow is shorter than the person is tall.

- **Cloud cover, fog, or smog.** A cloud cover reduces UVB radiation by approximately 50 percent. Clouds, aerosols (atmospheric particles), or thick ozone events can create vitamin D winter, even at the equator.[192]

- **Materials that block UVB rays.** UVB rays don't penetrate glass (windows), plastic, sunscreen, or clothing. People who are seldom outdoors or whose skin is covered with sunscreen will have little or no vitamin D production. Women who cover most of their bodies with clothing for cultural or religious reasons will not make sufficient vitamin D, no matter what their latitude, and can develop the adult form of rickets known as osteomalacia.

- **UVB sun lamp.** For some people, using a tanning bed with an ultraviolet vitamin D lamp once or twice a week is a suitable solution, especially in winter. The use of tanning beds is controversial; certainly, care must be taken to avoid overexposure, and many experts advise that supplements are a safer option.[65]

- **Skin color.** The minimal amount of sunlight needed is affected by skin color. As skin tone deepens, two to six times as much sun exposure is required, in terms of either length of time or area of skin exposed, with very dark skin needing two to six times as much exposure as pale skin for the same amount of vitamin D production. The skin self-regulates so the body doesn't overproduce vitamin D.[62]

- **Area of skin exposure.** The amount of skin exposed is a factor. A twenty-minute walk at lunch, with face and forearms exposed, can be equivalent to five minutes in a bikini at poolside in terms of vitamin D production.

- **Age.** Vitamin D production becomes less efficient with age. Light-skinned elderly people may need at least thirty minutes of sun exposure. However, a combination of dietary or supplement intake plus sunlight is likely to be most effective.

- **Body weight.** Being overweight or obese increases the likelihood of having a vitamin D deficiency.[86–88]

Vitamin D from Sun Exposure

Even in sunny climates, sunlight's effects can be hard to predict, with considerable variability from one individual to another. Recent studies in Hawaii, Arizona, Australia, and other sunny regions have shown inadequate vitamin D production among some residents, including a number who were regularly outdoors and without sunscreen.[86, 89–93] In a study of 93 adults (average age 24) with medium- to light-colored skin, during winter months in Honolulu (latitude 21 degrees N), 51 percent had low vitamin D status, as shown by serum vitamin D of less than 30 ng/ml, despite twenty-eighty hours of exposure per week without sunscreen. In fact, 10 percent had serum vitamin D of less than 20 ng/ml.

The risks and benefits of sun exposure are a hot topic for debate. While overexposure to the sun may increase the risk of skin cancer, inadequate vitamin D levels increase the risk of cancers of the breast, ovary, prostate, and colon. Due to the many variables, guidelines for sun exposure tend to be somewhat vague or open to interpretation. Some experts advise getting sun exposure

Guidelines for Getting Adequate Vitamin D

From Sunlight

Depending on location, on clear days in seasons with warm sunshine, a person with light skin may make sufficient vitamin D with sun exposure on the face and lower arms (without sunscreen) between 10 a.m. and 3 p.m. for an average of fifteen minutes daily. Someone with dark skin may require thirty minutes. More time or skin exposure may be needed for the elderly or the overweight. To determine effectiveness, arrange to have serum vitamin D tested. Supplementary vitamin D may be needed.

From Foods or Supplements

During "vitamin D winter" or if serum vitamin D levels are low, supplements and/or fortified foods should be relied upon. Recommended intakes of vitamin D are expressed in micrograms (mcg) of vitamin D_3. The RDA for vitamin D from foods, fortified foods, or supplements for those from 1 to 70 years old is 15 mcg (600 IU) per day, and 20 mcg (800 IU) for those over 70. For optimal health, many experts suggest 25 to 50 mcg (1,000 to 2,000 IU) or more of vitamin D_2 or D_3 per day; the Tolerable Upper Intake Level (UL) is 100 mcg (4,000 IU) without medical supervision. Recommended intakes for vitamin D are a subject of lively debate.[2, 33, 63–65, 82, 95, 96, 101, 102]

Testing

To check whether intake and/or the pattern of sun exposure is effective in meeting an individual's vitamin D requirements, serum levels of vitamin D can be checked by a physician or use of a self-testing kit.[85, 103] Currently, standards for healthy serum levels vary greatly; one expert says the serum levels of vitamin D should be at least 40 ng/ml (nanograms per milliliter in conventional units), or 100 nmol/L (nanomoles per liter in the International System of Units); however, most labs consider lower amounts "normal," and the serum range used for that classification varies.

on the face, arms, legs, or back (without sunscreen) for five to thirty minutes between 10 a.m. and 2 or 3 p.m., three times a week. Others suggest daily exposure of the face and forearms for ten to thirty minutes. (After thirty minutes, sunscreen can be applied.)[2, 17, 74, 75, 80, 89, 94, 95] A realistic approach is to spend a moderate amount of time outdoors in the sun when possible—taking care to avoid overexposure—and combine this, when needed, with a vitamin D supplement or fortified food.[2, 17, 75, 80, 95]

Vitamin D Supplements

Vitamin D is commonly taken alone as a tablet, an oral spray, in a multivitamin-mineral supplement, or in a supplement that contains vitamin D plus calcium (and perhaps magnesium).[95] Vitamin D_2 (ergocalciferol) is vegan and not of animal origin. Vitamin D_3 (cholecalciferol) has traditionally come from animal sources, such as fish, animal hides, or wool; however, vegan vitamin D_3 (from lichen) is now available. Search online for "vegan vitamin D"; specify a preference for D_2 or D_3.

Supplement amounts are expressed either in micrograms (mcg) or International Units (IU), with 1 mcg equivalent to 40 IU of vitamin D. Some research comparing vitamin D_2 and D_3 at standard daily doses (up to 100 mcg/4,000 IU per day) indicates that the two forms are equally effective at maintaining serum levels of vitamin D in adults. Other studies, particularly those using large single doses of vitamin D, found D_2 to be less potent, meaning that somewhat larger amounts may be needed.[88, 95–97] With either form, the effectiveness can vary from one person to another. A study comparing the effectiveness of supplements and of fortified juice found no significant differences between these two types of delivery.[96]

Vegan Food Sources of Vitamin D

Few foods, plant or animal, contain vitamin D. The vegan members of this select group are mushrooms exposed to UVB rays, because mushrooms contain a compound that can be converted to vitamin D_2.[98] Convincing evidence was provided by a study in which 700 mcg (28,000 IU) of vitamin D was given to two groups of people deficient in vitamin D. One group received the vitamin D in the form of irradiated button mushrooms prepared as mushroom soup (100 g of mushrooms contained 491 mcg of vitamin D.) The other group was given a supplement with the same amount of vitamin D. Both treatments were effective in raising study participants' serum vitamin D.[99]

A growing number of vitamin D–fortified vegan foods are available, including nondairy milks, juices, and breakfast cereals. The availability of fortified foods varies from one country to another, depending on legislation, advances in science, and pressures from the food industry and the public.[17, 45, 92, 95] Typical amounts of vitamin D in various fortified foods are shown in table 7.1; also check labels.[96] (Unfortified nondairy milks, margarine, and cereals provide no vitamin D). In margarines that contain vitamin D_3, the origin is typically from animals; contact the manufacturer for more specific information. Because the DV used on food labels is 10 mcg or 400 IU, a serving that provides 50 percent of the DV yields 5 mcg (200 IU) of vitamin D.

Vegan Intakes from Food and Supplements

Vegan dietary intakes of vitamin D have been far below recommended levels. Vegan intakes of vitamin D are lower than those of lactovegetarians and of

TABLE 7.1. Examples of vitamin D in fortified foods

FOOD (AMOUNT)	VITAMIN D CONTENT
Fortified breakfast cereal, 1 oz (30 g)	2.6 mcg (105 IU)
Fortified margarine, 1 tsp (5 ml)	0.5 mcg (20 IU)
Fortified soy milk, almond milk, rice milk, or fruit juice, 1 c (250 ml)	2.5–3 mcg (100–120 IU)

Sources:[44, 45]

nonvegetarians, unless vegans regularly use supplements or fortified foods. This situation of widespread deficiency isn't limited to vegans; North American, European, and Australian surveys showed half, three-quarters, or even more of adults in the general population to have low intakes and low serum levels of vitamin D, depending on the optimal ranges chosen. Most intakes ranged from 2 to 10 percent of the RDA of 15 mcg (600 IU) for adults under 70; even the highest intakes were typically a little more than half this recommended level.[17, 104–108] Food fortification policies are changing, which may help the situation.

Vegans at the greatest risk for vitamin D deficiency are breast-fed infants whose mothers are low in vitamin D, adults over 50, people of any age with dark skin, inactive people, and the obese—people with a body mass index (BMI) of more than 30 (see table 12.1 on page 363).[82, 85, 86, 91, 92, 93, 95, 109]

Laboratory Tests for Vitamin D

Debate exists concerning what constitutes optimal levels of 25-hydroxyvitamin D in the body, and the IOM has recognized the need for further research. Currently, the IOM considers serum levels of 50 nmol/L or 20 ng/ml to be adequate. Many experts and laboratories suggest that for optimal health, blood levels of vitamin D should be higher, at about 75 to 100 nmol/L (30 to 40 ng/ml).

Tests reflect vitamin D provided by diet, supplements, and the body's own synthesis.[66, 77, 85, 86, 104, 110] Tests can be arranged through a physician, or the Vitamin D Council provides a self-test kit (see Resources on page 449). Such tests can be repeated after three months to determine the effectiveness of a chosen plan in reaching desired blood levels of vitamin D.[77, 103]

Vitamin D Status of Vegans

When vegans consider vitamin D, a number of questions arise. Which standard of sufficiency for serum vitamin D should be used, that of the IOM or higher levels? Are vitamin D–fortified foods available and used? Are supplements used? What are an individual's latitude, skin color, and extent of sun exposure? Studies show that some vegans appear to be doing well when it comes to vitamin D, and some are not.

In the United Kingdom (latitude 50 to 55 degrees N), a study that included 89 light-skinned Caucasians who had followed a vegan diet for about ten years showed their average plasma vitamin D to be 55.8 nmol/L (above the IOM recommendation but below the higher optimal levels of 75 or 100 nmol/L). The study's 1,598 nonvegetarians also were somewhat low in vitamin D, though the vegan levels were lower still. The vitamin D levels of study participants dropped considerably in the winter and were insufficient. In the winter and spring, just 20 percent of the vegans had plasma vitamin D levels above 75 nmol/L. In summer and autumn, levels had risen; 45 percent of the vegans had plasma vitamin D levels above 75 nmol/L. Dietary sources available to British vegans at the time of the study included cereals, nondairy beverages, and margarines fortified with vitamin D. The vegans were slimmer (average BMI 22.3; see page 363) than the nonvegetarians (average BMI 25), and 51 percent used vitamin D supplements; those who used supplements had significantly higher plasma levels of vitamin D.[104]

A 2009 study of Seventh-day Adventist vegans and lactovegetarians living at latitudes between 30 and 50 degrees N across North America (roughly between the latitudes of New Orleans and Winnipeg) showed differences in serum vitamin D that varied with skin color. Half of the non-Hispanic whites but only one-quarter of the blacks had serum vitamin D levels in the optimal range (above 75 nmol/L or 30 ng/ml). In addition to average reported daily intakes from food and supplements of 8.8 mcg (350 IU) for those with light skin color and 9.4 mcg (375 IU) for those with dark skin color, study participants spent an average of about ninety minutes daily in the sun, with 9 percent of their skin exposed.[86] A more recent study of 100 American vegans showed none of those surveyed met recommended intakes of vitamin D through supplements.[111]

A study based in St. Louis, Mo. (latitude 38 degrees N), showed 11 men and 7 women (with an average age of 54) who had been on raw vegan diets for an average of 3.6 years to have serum vitamin D levels of 42 ng/ml despite negligible intakes of vitamin D–fortified foods or supplements. In fact, the serum vitamin D levels of these vegans were more than double those of a control group of nonvegetarians of similar age and gender. These raw foods enthusiasts made an effort to spend time in the sun on a regular basis.[105]

A study in the Netherlands (latitude between 51 and 54 degrees N) of infants in families on macrobiotic diets showed that half the infants had some signs of rickets when there was no use of vitamin D supplements or fortified foods. These babies also had low plasma levels of vitamin D, which dropped even lower in winter. Infants who regularly received a supplement and vitamin D-fortified beverages showed no signs of rickets.[17, 112]

A study in Ho Chi Minh City, Vietnam (latitude 10 degrees N), of 88 vegan Buddhist nuns older than 50 showed 27 percent of these women to have vitamin D levels below 20 ng/ml and 73 percent to have levels below 30 ng/ml. At the same time, these women experienced no more bone fractures and had slightly less bone loss than nonvegetarians.[106]

Vitamin D at the Beginning of Life

Cases of rickets have been documented where nursing mothers lived at northern latitudes and didn't ensure that infants had a source of vitamin D. To avoid this, the IOM recommends 15 mcg (600 IU) per day during pregnancy and lactation; the German-Austrian-Swiss reference values increase recommended intakes to 20 mcg (800 IU). The American Academy of Pediatrics prescribes a daily intake of 10 mcg (400 IU) of vitamin D for infants, starting from the first few days of life.[17, 85, 113] Care must be taken to avoid excess amounts; seek physician advice regarding suitable intakes.

Vitamin D for Older Adults

The body's ability to produce vitamin D diminishes with age. For example, the skin of a 70-year-old can synthesize just 25 percent as much vitamin D as that of a young person. Vitamin D deficiency is linked with muscle weakness. Research has shown supplementation with 20 mcg (800 IU) of vitamin D reduces falls in institutionalized older patients by more than 20 percent.[85] Higher intakes may be advisable.

Problems with Excess Vitamin D

Consuming excess amounts of vitamin D can cause too much calcium absorption. Taken over weeks or months, excess vitamin D can lead to unwanted calcification of the heart, kidneys, and blood vessels in adults and can harden children's bones at too early an age. Adult intakes of vitamin D above 100 mcg (4,000 IU) per day may be helpful in certain cases but aren't recommended without medical supervision. The ULs are lower for younger children.[66] Too much sun exposure doesn't produce toxic levels of vitamin D, though overexposure to UV light carries the potential risks of premature wrinkling, loss of skin elasticity, sunburn, and skin cancer.[82]

The Antioxidant Vitamins: A, C, and E

Atmospheric oxygen is necessary to survival. Yet oxygen's undesirable effects are evident when food oil becomes rancid, apple slices brown, or metal rusts. In human bodies, damaging oxidation reactions can lead to chain reactions that create rampaging molecules called free radicals. During the body's normal operating processes, moderate quantities of free radicals form and, propitiously, are inactivated by antioxidants. However, if a person smokes, consumes foods cooked at high temperatures, drinks alcohol, or is exposed to environmental pollutants, solvents, or radiation, the quantities of free radicals multiply, along with the damage they can inflict on cell membranes, genetic material (DNA), and essential proteins.

PROTECTION FROM FREE RADICAL DAMAGE

Vegan diets are outstanding sources of the diverse substances that protect against oxidative damage: antioxidants. These include certain phytochemicals (page 260); the minerals selenium, manganese, copper, and zinc (chapter 6) as part of specific enzymes; vitamins C and E; and the carotenoids that the body coverts to vitamin A (page 233). Antioxidants act synergistically. For example, vitamin C regenerates and revitalizes used vitamin E (page 237) for further action, and vitamin E protects beta-carotene from oxidation. The B vitamin riboflavin also plays a protective role against free radical damage.[4, 116–122, 137]

The body relies on a steady supply of antioxidants; if antioxidant levels are depleted, the body's cells are vulnerable to damage, disease, and aging. As people get older, an antioxidant-rich diet assumes even greater importance. A lively field of research explores the role of antioxidants in reducing the risk of cancer, cardiovascular disease, cataracts, macular degeneration, diseases of the nervous system (such as Alzheimer's and Parkinson's), and premature aging of skin due to UV light.[4, 116–122, 137]

Obtaining antioxidants from plant foods proves to be far more effective than relying on pills. In fact, high-dose vitamin A and beta-carotene supplements have been shown to increase lung cancer risk, instead of providing the protection given by the diverse, balanced antioxidant supply in plant-based diets that humans have relied upon for millennia.[116, 117, 119, 123, 124]

THE BODY'S DETOXIFICATION SYSTEM

The body eliminates some water-soluble toxins through urine or bile. Other toxins are sent to the liver, where a two-step Phase I and Phase II process renders them harmless. The enzyme activities of these two phases must be well coordinated, because intermediary compounds that form during Phase I can be even more troublesome than the original toxin. If these intermediary compounds aren't quickly processed during Phase II, cell injury or the development of cancer can ensue.

A simplified summary of detoxification in the liver is shown in figure 7.1, with the nutrients required for the different steps listed below. During Phase I, detoxification enzymes give the toxin an electrical charge that creates a type of chemical handle that can attach to another molecule during Phase II. After receiving the charge, toxins can become highly reactive and potentially dangerous molecules. However, antioxidants can prevent such changes. If all is well—as is usually the case—the reactive molecule quickly passes into Phase II and becomes attached to a large water-soluble molecule. This process creates a water-soluble complex that the body can quickly and safely dispose of via urine or bile.

FIGURE 7.1. Detoxification pathways in the liver

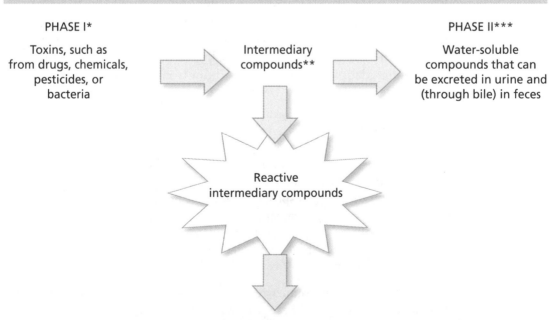

PHASE I*

Toxins, such as from drugs, chemicals, pesticides, or bacteria

Intermediary compounds**

PHASE II***

Water-soluble compounds that can be excreted in urine and (through bile) in feces

Reactive intermediary compounds

Cell damage, disease, aging

Nutrients Required for Detoxification

*The nutrients needed for Phase I include certain B vitamins (folate, niacin, pyridoxine, riboflavin, and vitamin B_{12}), iron, specific amino acids, and phytochemicals (flavonoids).

**The nutrients needed to protect against cell damage from reactive intermediary compounds and free radicals include vitamins A (beta-carotene and other provitamin A carotenoids), C, and E; the minerals copper, manganese, selenium, and zinc; and the phytochemicals found in cruciferous vegetables.

***The nutrients needed for Phase II include choline, riboflavin, selenium, sulfur, and specific amino acids (cysteine and methionine).

Sources:[119, 125–129, 137]

Diet, Lifestyle, and Detoxification

Clearly, diet and lifestyle choices can have a major protective effect against the potential damage the body's cells face from oxygen and toxins. Knowing the nutrient interactions involved will illustrate why a varied diet of plant foods goes far beyond supplements in maintaining good health. Here are some examples.

- **Phase I.** The body's first line of defense is a superfamily of enzymes—the cytochrome P-450 enzyme family—that the body builds from protein (including the sulfur-containing amino acid cysteine) and iron. These enzymes carry electrons or charges from one location to another, work in the presence of oxygen, and create a highly reactive form of oxygen that can rearrange the structure of toxic molecules. For Phase I to work properly, certain B vitamins (listed above) must be present and assisted by protective phytochemicals, such as flavonoids.[120, 125, 130]
- **Protection from highly reactive intermediary compounds.** When reactive intermediary compounds and free radicals start to accumulate, the body relies on nutrients (listed above) to block destructive chain reactions, including antioxidant vitamins, enzymes (built from protein plus the minerals copper, manganese, selenium, or zinc), and phytochemicals.
- **Phase II.** For Phase II, the body needs a supply of large water-soluble molecules that can be attached to toxins, creating a soluble complex that can be excreted. An example of such a molecule is glutathione, a chain of three amino acids that works with selenium (found in Brazil nuts). Other suitable molecules are the amino acid cysteine or the mineral sulfur. Chewing cabbage, broccoli florets, Brussels sprouts, or broccoli sprouts activates sulforaphane, a sulfur-containing molecule that protects against cancer. Several amino acids and the B vitamins choline and riboflavin also have roles in Phase II detoxification. The fiber in plant foods is another helpful component; it binds toxins, which can then be excreted in feces so they're not reabsorbed.[120, 125, 131–133]

This remarkable defense sequence protects DNA, cell membranes, and proteins. Fortunately, the supply of necessary nutrients and phytochemicals is present in fruits, vegetables, legumes, nuts, seeds, and whole grains.[119–121, 125, 126, 133–137]

The Road to Disease

The activity of certain Phase I enzymes and the resultant buildup of dangerous intermediary compounds can be increased by consumption of alcohol or polycyclic aromatic hydrocarbons, which form when foods are grilled or charred (page 271). If toxin exposure is particularly high, the assault can overwhelm the body's defenders. Then, potentially carcinogenic substances can trigger steps along the path to cancer. Protection shrinks when supersized portions of refined foods, soda pop, or alcohol crowd out antioxidant-rich plant foods. Phase I, Phase II, or both can become inefficient or overloaded. If critical nutrients needed for detoxification are depleted, the body becomes susceptible to cancer or other diseases.[119, 120, 125–128, 137–140]

VITAMIN A (BETA-CAROTENE AND CAROTENOIDS)

Vitamin A in Perspective

In developing countries where diets are severely limited and centered on breads or rice, many children and adults become blind due to insufficient vitamin A. This tragic situation occurs in one-quarter- to one-half-million children each year and could be prevented if they had access to carotenoid-rich vegetables or fruits or to vitamin A. Millions more children and adults suffer lesser forms of visual impairment due to vitamin A deficiency. Because their immune systems also are weakened, deficient children also die from measles, diarrhea, or malaria.

Two categories of vitamin A exist in the food supply: preformed vitamin A from animal products and provitamin A carotenoids from plant foods. The body can convert certain carotenoids (beta-carotene, alpha-carotene, and beta-cryptoxanthin) to the active form of vitamin A known as retinol. These carotenoids are pigments that contribute to the orange, red, and yellow colors in fresh produce. Carotenoids also are present in green vegetables, though their color is overlaid by the green of magnesium-rich chlorophyll. Other carotenoids in plant foods (lycopene, lutein, and zeaxanthin) aren't converted to vitamin A, though they have significant health benefits.[4, 116, 117, 141]

Function

Vitamin A has an important role in cell differentiation, enabling cells to become specialized and carry out specific tasks, so its effects are diverse. In the eye, vitamin A and certain carotenoids (lutein and zeaxanthin) improve night vision, prevent cataracts, and keep the cornea moist and healthy. Vitamin A is required for immune system function and to build and preserve the integrity of skin and mucous membranes so they form protective barriers against bacteria and viruses. Many carotenoids, such as the beta-carotene in carrots and the lycopene in tomatoes, are excellent antioxidants that protect against cancer and heart disease. (Preformed vitamin A has no antioxidant activity.) Vitamin A also is needed for the growth of bones and teeth, for reproduction, and for the building and regulation of hormones.[4, 116, 117, 137, 141]

Recommended Intake

The RDA is expressed in retinol (the active form of vitamin A): 700 mcg daily for women and 900 mcg for men. Because the conversion to retinol differs among the various carotenoids and forms of vitamin A, the units that measure how much active vitamin A (retinol) is derived from foods are micrograms of retinol activity equivalents (mcg RAE). In the past, the International Unit (IU) was used to measure vitamin A; 1 mcg RAE is equal to 3.3 IU.[4, 116, 117, 141]

Vegan Intakes and Status

Vegan diets, with their abundance of colorful fruits and vegetables, can easily provide more than enough vitamin A. Average intakes by vegans have been estimated at 1,500 mcg RAE for women and 1,200 mcg RAE for men.[17] However, intakes depend on the specific fruits and vegetables included. A study of plasma carotenoid levels in German vegans whose diets consisted of 95 percent raw foods (mainly fruits) showed those levels met or exceeded recommended intakes in 82 percent of the study participants. Important factors linked with good vitamin A status were the inclusion of yellow, orange, red, and green vegetables and of fat, which increases carotenoid absorption.[142, 149, 154]

The understanding of how carotenoids are converted to retinol has evolved in recent decades. Although vegan intakes of carotenoids have been reported in the past, some studies significantly overestimated the conversion of these carotenoids to mcg RAE. Any comparisons with new studies would have to factor in these discrepancies; vegan intakes over the years can't easily be compared in numerical tables.[17]

Vegan Food Sources of Vitamin A (Carotenoids)

Carotenoids are present in deep-orange vegetables and fruits (apricots, cantaloupes, carrots and carrot juice, mangoes, nectarines, papayas, peppers, persimmons, pumpkins, squash, sweet potatoes, tomatoes and tomato products, and yams), as well as broccoli, turnips, leafy greens, seaweeds, plantains, and prunes. (For other sources, see table 7.3 on page 252.) The recommended intake for the day can be derived from ½ cup (125 ml) of carrot juice, baked sweet potato, or canned pumpkin. About 470 mcg RAE is provided by ½ cup (125 ml) of cooked spinach or baked butternut squash, or half a cantaloupe.[44, 45, 137]

Special Issues

Cooking allows increased absorption of some carotenoids, such as lycopene, so there are advantages in eating some colorful vegetables cooked, along with plenty of raw vegetables and fruits. Including a little fat (from seeds, olives, avocado, or in a dressing) as part of a meal also increases absorption of carotenoids and other fat-soluble nutrients. Juicing (for example, making carrot juice) also boosts carotenoid absorption.[4, 116, 117, 143]

Although vitamin A supplements greatly benefit those who are deficient (for example, supplements can prevent blindness in impoverished children whose limited diets lack vegetables or fruits), high intakes of vitamin A from supplements are linked with a greater risk of hip fracture and other health problems and are best avoided. The best source of this vitamin is plant foods because the mix of protective compounds in plant foods works together more powerfully than any of the compounds would on their own.[144]

A perspective from Harvard Medical School concludes, "We now know that supernutritional levels of vitamins taken as supplements do not emulate the apparent benefits of diets high in foods that contain those vitamins, and we now know that taking vitamins in supernutritional doses can cause serious harm."[145–147] People should avoid high intakes of vitamin A (more than 3,000 mcg retinol) from supplements without medical supervision, especially during pregnancy, when such high intakes can lead to birth defects.[4, 116, 117, 145–148] If vitamin A supplements are used, no more than the recommended intakes should be taken. Unusually high intakes of carrot juice or other rich food sources of carotenoids aren't harmful but may temporarily turn the skin yellow.[4, 116]

VITAMIN C (ASCORBIC ACID)

Vitamin C in Perspective

During the Age of Exploration in the fifteenth and sixteenth centuries, advances in naval technology by both the Europeans and Chinese made lengthy voyages possible. Yet, during these journeys, sailors developed scurvy, a condition that caused their bodies to weaken, their joints to become painful, their teeth to loosen, and their gums to swell to the extent that eating became impossible. The sailors could barely move and, often, death followed. North American Native cultures had known about scurvy and used effective remedies, such as pine needle extracts or cranberries, to cure the disease in winter, when fresh food was scarce. Even though a few European sailors successfully adopted these remedies to facilitate recovery from scurvy, at the time, the medical profession dismissed the concept that a potent cure could have originated from "savages."

After a great deal of detective work, the exploration of numerous wrong leads, and eventual open-mindedness to new possibilities, naval commanders and physicians determined that the unhealthy factor in a sailor's life responsible for scurvy was the lack of fresh fruits and vegetables. The Chinese began to grow bean sprouts to supplement diets at sea, and the British Royal Navy adopted the practice of adding lemon or lime juice to sailors' grog. (The term "Limeys" came to refer to British seamen and, eventually, to all their countrymen.) By the time of the American Civil War, awareness had spread that citrus fruits, potatoes, or onions could prevent scurvy and save lives. A sign posted in Chicago during that period read, "Don't send your sweetheart a love-letter. Send him an onion."

The component in these fruits and vegetables responsible for preventing scurvy —vitamin C—was identified in 1912; its relationship to scurvy was established in 1932; and it was synthesized in 1935. As with other vitamins, exploration of its roles in the body continues.[4, 116, 151]

Function

Vitamin C is essential for building collagen, the protein that's a component of blood-vessel walls, scar tissue, tendons, ligaments, and bone. A lack leads to scurvy's symptoms—the breakdown of gums and other collagen-containing tissues. Vitamin C aids amino-acid metabolism and is required for the synthesis of carnitine, an amino acid that transports fat molecules to body cells (page 94). A shortage of vitamin C results in fatigue, because without it, the body is unable to use fat for energy. Vitamin C has a role in the synthesis of the neurotransmitter norepinephrine, which is essential for brain function and affects mood.

Vitamin C is a highly effective antioxidant; even small amounts can protect cells from damage. Vitamin C supports immune function, boosting the body's ability to resist infection under stressful conditions. It also helps the body to synthesize thyroid hormone and regenerate vitamin E. Vitamin C from fruits and vegetables supports heart health, protects against chronic disease, and assists greatly in the absorption of iron from plant foods.[4, 116, 137, 152]

Laboratory Tests for Vitamin C

A diagnosis of vitamin C deficiency is generally based on symptoms, not blood tests. A deficiency isn't likely in people whose diet regularly includes fruits and vegetables.

Recommended Intake

The RDA for vitamin C is 75 mg for women and 90 mg for men. Smokers are advised to get an additional 35 mg per day (or better yet, to quit smoking).[116]

Vegan Intakes and Status

Studies show that average vegan intakes of vitamin C range from 138 to 584 mg daily. Generally, these amounts reflect intakes from food rather than supplements.[17, 42]

Vegan Food Sources of Vitamin C

Good sources of vitamin C include blackberries, broccoli, Brussels sprouts, cantaloupes, citrus fruits and juices, green peas, guavas, kiwifruit, leafy greens (chard, collard greens, kale, sorrel, and spinach), mangoes, papayas, pineapples, raspberries, red peppers, strawberries, sweet potatoes, tomatoes, and vegetables in the cabbage family. Overall, five servings of fruits and vegetables per day should provide about 200 mg of vitamin C. (For additional food sources and vitamin C amounts, see table 7.3 on page 252.) Organic foods have been shown to provide significantly more vitamin C than foods treated with pesticides.[156]

Special Issues

Vitamin C is the superstar that increases the body's ability to absorb iron from natural and fortified plant foods, keeps iron in a soluble form, and overcomes factors (such as phytates) that inhibit iron absorption (page 188).[116, 157, 158]

VITAMIN E (ALPHA-TOCOPHEROL)

Vitamin E in Perspective

Vitamin E is a fat-soluble vitamin present in plant oils; it was discovered in 1922 in spinach and recognized as being essential in 1968. The term "vitamin E" actually refers to a family of related compounds; alpha-tocopherol is the form with greatest nutritional significance.

Function

This antioxidant protects fat molecules (such as those in cell membranes) from free radical damage, stabilizing cell membranes and preventing their breakage. When vitamin E neutralizes a free radical, its antioxidant function is lost; however, vitamin C can regenerate its antioxidant capacity. Vitamin E protects vitamin A (another fat-soluble vitamin) and polyunsaturated fatty acids from destruction; through these protective actions, it has a role in the prevention of many diseases. Low intakes are linked with increased risk of heart disease, possible development of cataracts, and other harmful conditions.[4, 116, 137, 160]

Recommended Intake

The adult RDA for vitamin E is 15 mg per day (equivalent to 22.5 IU).[4, 116, 160]

Vegan Intakes and Status

Before 1993, studies showed that vegan vitamin E intakes averaged 11 to 14 mg per day; since then, average intakes have increased to between 14 and 33 mg per day.[17, 42] Among the general American population, 90 percent fail to meet recommended intakes, with average intakes of 6.9 to 8.3 mg of vitamin E per day, less than is needed for optimal health.[4, 116, 162] People on low-fat diets are at increased risk for suboptimal intakes.

Vegan Food Sources of Vitamin E

Vitamin E can be found in avocados, broccoli, carrots, kiwifruit, leafy green vegetables, nuts, peanuts, seeds, whole grains, and wheat germ. (For additional sources and amounts of vitamin E, see table 7.3 on page 252). Though leafy greens don't appear to be significant sources of fat, about 10 percent of their calories come from plant oils. For those on raw or high-raw diets, big salads provide plenty of vitamin E; for example, 8 cups (2 L) of raw spinach provides a third of the RDA. When half an avocado and 3 tablespoons (45 ml) of sunflower seeds are added, the salad contains the entire recommended intake for the day. Steamed spinach cooks down to a small volume while retaining this vitamin; so 1 cup (250 ml) of cooked spinach provides close to 4 mg vitamin E. Unrefined vegetable oils—especially olive, canola, safflower, sunflower, soybean, and wheat germ oils—contain vitamin E, which protects the oils from rancidity (oxidation). However, when oils are refined, the heat in the refining process destroys vitamin E; in some oils, vitamin E is added as a preservative.[4, 44, 45, 160, 161]

Special Issues

The natural form of vitamin E in plant foods, d-alpha-tocopherol, is ideal for the body's use, offering greater protection than the forms in supplements. Some vitamin E in supplements is not well utilized by the body, so larger amounts are needed. However, high doses of these synthetic forms have adverse health consequences.[160]

What's Special about Vitamin K?

VITAMIN K (PHYLLOQUINONE AND MENAQUINONE)

Vitamin K in Perspective

A relative newcomer to the vitamin hall of fame, vitamin K's function wasn't recognized until 1974 and still is being unraveled. The "K" is derived from the German word *koagulation,* which is related to the vitamin's role in forming blood clots, an essential defense at times of injury. Symptoms of deficiency include defective blood clotting and hemorrhaging.

The first form discovered, vitamin K_1, or phylloquinone, is widely available in plant foods, especially greens. In addition, bacteria typically present in the intestine synthesize additional forms of this vitamin, known collectively as vitamin K_2, or the menaquinones. (There's also a synthetic form known as vitamin K_3, or menadione, which can be toxic.)[4, 117]

The body absorbs plenty of vitamin K_2 from the intestine. However, with the use of antibiotics, this important source may temporarily be eliminated until the bacteria population in the intestine reestablishes itself. Vitamin K_2 of bacterial origin is stored in the flesh and tissues of humans and of other animals. Because production of vitamin K in infants' intestines doesn't start for five to seven days, babies are given a vitamin K shot at birth; their intestines are soon colonized with bacteria from their mother's milk or general exposure to the environment.[4, 117, 163]

Function

Vitamin K builds the proteins that allow blood to clot and regulates blood calcium levels. It has a role in bone growth and the maintenance of bone mineral density. Data from the 1998 Nurses' Health Study showed that those who ate lettuce at least once a day had a significantly lower risk of hip fracture than those who ate lettuce once a week or less. Since then, studies have shown that 200 mcg of vitamin K—the amount present in 1½ cups (375 ml) of raw spinach, ¼ cup (60 ml) of cooked spinach, or ½ cup (125 ml) of raw kale—will reduce the risk of bone fracture.[4, 117, 163–165, 169]

Recommended Intake

Because there is inadequate scientific evidence upon which to base an RDA for vitamin K, an AI was set at 120 mcg of vitamin K per day for men and 90 mcg per day for women.[4, 117]

Is There a Need to Ingest Vitamin K₂ Directly?

A few health advocates have suggested that the body doesn't adequately convert vitamin K_1 to K_2 and that people require dietary sources of vitamin K_2. While vitamin K_1 serves blood-clotting processes and activities such as bone building, vitamin K_2 is needed for protection against heart disease, arthritis, and cancer.

Although vitamin K_2 has a wider range of biological activity, individuals with a healthy, normal supply of gut bacteria are well equipped to convert K_1 to K_2. Scientific evidence supporting a requirement for a direct source of vitamin K_2 is lacking, and the IOM doesn't suggest that any direct intake of vitamin K_2 is necessary. However, people who've had significant antibiotic therapy and are concerned about a temporary loss of ability to convert K_1 to K_2 can obtain a vegan source of vitamin K_2 by taking a supplement or consuming natto. Natto (fermented soybeans) contains 23 mcg of vitamin K_1 plus 941 to 998 mcg of vitamin K_2 per 100 grams (a little more than ½ cup).[45, 167, 168]

Vegan Intakes and Status

The average intake of the US population has been estimated at 300 to 500 mcg per day. Vegan intakes are expected to be higher still, and adequate. Although no studies have assessed the vitamin K intakes of vegans, high levels would be expected due to the generous amounts of leafy greens and other vegetables consumed by this population. One investigation reported adequate blood clotting rates among vegans, which suggests adequate vitamin K status.[17, 166]

Vegan Food Sources of Vitamin K

Leafy greens (collard greens, dandelion greens, kale, spinach, Swiss chard, and turnip greens) are the vitamin K superstars. Other excellent sources are asparagus, avocados, broccoli, Brussels sprouts, cabbage, cauliflower, grapes, green powdered tea, kiwifruit, lentils, pumpkins, peas, soybean oil, soy foods, and nori and other seaweeds. (For other sources, see table 7.3 on page 252.) Natto, a fermented bacteria-rich soy food originating from Japan, is a unique and concentrated plant source of vitamin K_2.

A day's recommended intake of vitamin K can be provided by 2 tablespoons (30 ml) of parsley or kale or 2 cups (500 ml) of romaine lettuce. Adding a little oil-containing dressing or avocado, olives, or tahini to salads increases absorption of this fat-soluble vitamin.[44, 45, 117] To minimize losses, avoid overcooking foods.

Special Issues

Anticoagulants, such as warfarin, oppose the clotting action of vitamin K. Often, people who take Coumadin and related anticoagulant medications to prevent blood clots and potential heart attacks have been advised by their doctors to avoid greens. Some physicians now take a more reasonable and healthful approach, by suggesting that patients eat moderate, consistent amounts of these nutritious vitamin K-rich foods. Patients are advised to avoid huge swings in their intakes, and their medication is monitored and adjusted if necessary.[4, 117]

Production of Energy from Food: The Roles of the B Vitamins

The body uses carbohydrates, fats, and proteins from foods to produce energy, with enzymes and the B vitamins playing roles in releasing this energy. In complex sequences that resemble a busy factory's production lines, each of the nine B vitamins assists specific enzymes. In fact, these enzymes can't function without their particular vitamin assistant or coenzyme. For energy production, the body requires dietary sources of thiamine (vitamin B_1), riboflavin (vitamin B_2), niacin (vitamin B_3), pantothenic acid (vitamin B_5), pyridoxine (vitamin B_6), and biotin (vitamin B_7). Folate (vitamin B_9) and cobalamin (vitamin B_{12}) are required to form new cells that deliver oxygen and nutrients so energy production can proceed; choline assists this duo.

When the existence of vitamins was first recognized, fat-soluble vitamin A and water-soluble vitamin B were identified. Later, scientists realized that "vitamin B" consisted of a number of distinct compounds essential to life. The B vitamins build fats needed in cell membranes, genetic material, nerve-impulse transmitters, and certain hormones. Because B vitamins are water-soluble, they can be lost when soaking or cooking water is discarded; in addition, the body excretes excess B vitamins in urine.

When individuals restrict calories (for example, during a period of weight loss), vitamin intakes can drop below recommended levels, affecting energy levels and well-being. At such times, a supplement can top up intakes from food.

THIAMIN (VITAMIN B_1)

Thiamin in Perspective

Thiamin is sometimes known as the carbohydrate burner. Symptoms of its lack were described in China as early as 2600 B.C. Thiamin deficiency came to be known as beriberi, meaning "weak, weak" or "I cannot, I cannot." Beriberi became a widespread cause of death in the poor, in prison inmates, among Asian laborers, and in the Japanese army after polished white rice became widely used in Asia during the 1870s; unfortunately the outer thiamin-containing bran layer was removed during the polishing process. Although more fortunate individuals could round out their nutrient intakes with other foods, many Asians relied on white rice—and little else—as their dietary staple.

At a time when such diseases were thought to be linked to infection or to other causes, three physicians (one of them Japanese and two Dutch), discovered the relationship between beriberi and a thiamin-deficient diet. Their insights played key roles in the discovery of vitamins in general and led to the eventual enrichment of white rice. In enriched rice, several—but not all—of the B vitamins, along with iron, are added back.[170, 171]

Function and Laboratory Tests for Thiamin

Thiamin helps with the conversion of carbohydrates to useable energy, the metabolism of amino acids, and the functioning of the nervous system. Thiamin status can be assessed by determining the activity of this vitamin in red blood cells, though this isn't a common test.[2, 4]

Recommended Intake

The thiamin RDA is 1.1 mg per day for women and 1.2 mg per day for men.[2, 4]

Vegan Intakes and Status

Studies show the average thiamin intake of vegans meets and generally exceeds recommended intakes by 50 to 100 percent.[17]

Vegan Food Sources

Thiamin is present in many plant foods in moderate amounts; it's easily destroyed by cooking, though some remains. Whole and enriched grains, products made from these grains, legumes, nuts, seeds, and nutritional yeast are excellent sources. Among the many other good sources are avocados, carrot juice, corn, dried fruit, peas, and squash (see table 7.3 on page 252).[44, 45]

RIBOFLAVIN (VITAMIN B$_2$)

Riboflavin in Perspective

Part of this vitamin's name is related to the Latin word *flavius*, meaning "blond." Evidence of this vitamin's color and water-soluble nature is often provided by the bright yellow color of an individual's urine after ingestion of a multivitamin supplement. If the body doesn't need all the riboflavin provided by the supplement, the excess is excreted in urine.

Function, Deficiency Symptoms, and Laboratory Tests for Riboflavin

Riboflavin helps to convert carbohydrates, fats, and proteins to useable energy. It interacts with and supports the action of other B vitamins (niacin, B$_6$, and folate) and iron, provides protection against free radicals and toxins, and participates in detoxification. Deficiency symptoms include sores or cracks radiating from the corners of the mouth and inflammation and redness of the tongue. Lab tests to check riboflavin levels can be done on blood and urine.[2, 4]

Recommended Intake

The RDA is 1.1 mg of riboflavin per day for women, and 1.3 mg per day for men.[2, 4]

Vegan Intakes

Studies show the average riboflavin intakes of vegans typically meet recommended levels, though intakes can be insufficient, depending on food choices.[17]

Vegan Food Sources

A day's recommended riboflavin intake is provided by ½ tablespoon of nutritional yeast.[30] Soy foods, fortified cereals, and yeast extract are excellent riboflavin sources. Moderately good sources include almonds, avocados, bananas, broccoli, buckwheat, cashews, enriched wheat flour, green beans, leafy greens, mushrooms, peas, quinoa, sea vegetables, seeds, soybeans, sweet potatoes, and whole grains. Sprouting has been shown to increase the riboflavin content of alfalfa seeds and mung beans. For other sources and riboflavin amounts, see table 7.3 (page 252).[44, 45]

The sun's UV rays or fluorescent light can destroy riboflavin. For this reason, nutritional yeast, which is high in riboflavin, should be stored in an opaque container or a dark cupboard.[30, 172–174]

NIACIN (VITAMIN B₃)

Niacin in Perspective

A deficiency of niacin causes the disease pellagra; the disease causes a worsening progression of the four "Ds": dermatitis, diarrhea, dementia, and death. Niacin deficiency was recognized among poorer people in the southern United States and southern Europe, who subsisted mainly on corn. In contrast, many Latin Americans have diets centered on corn but have long avoided this devastating disease.

The corn (maize) used for tortillas and other dishes is first treated with lime to make it more flavorful and easier to grind. Because soaking corn in an alkaline solution releases bound niacin—making this vitamin more available for absorption—this treatment has proved to be an effective defense against pellagra (and also adds calcium to the diet). In time, scientific research led to the recognition that pellagra is a dietary problem. It occurs when corn isn't treated in this manner or when corn-based diets aren't supplemented with protein-rich foods (such as peanuts and other legumes) that provide the amino acid tryptophan, which the body can convert to niacin.[2, 4, 171]

Function and Laboratory Tests for Niacin

Niacin is part of two coenzymes that are active in the production of energy. This vitamin supports the health of the skin, digestive tract, and nervous system. Deficiency can be detected by urine tests.[2, 4]

Recommended Intake

Because 60 mg of tryptophan can be converted to 1 mg of niacin, both this amino acid and the vitamin itself contribute to overall niacin intake. They're measured in milligrams of Niacin Equivalents (NE mg). The RDA is 16 NE mg

Where Is Vitamin B₄?

A substance called adenine used to hold the vitamin B₄ title, but was demoted. True vitamins can't be manufactured by the body but must be supplied by diet or supplements; however, the body can make any needed adenine, so it's not a true vitamin. This is a typical reason for gaps in the B-vitamin numbering system.

for men and 14 NE mg for women. Food tables may list only the milligrams of niacin or may list the NE mg (see table 7.3 on page 252).[2]

Vegan Intakes and Status

Studies show the average niacin intakes of vegans are at or slightly above recommended levels. Niacin intakes tend to be low among people whose diets are low in calories, as with weight-loss diets.[17, 153, 175]

Vegan Food Sources

Excellent niacin sources include good protein providers: edamame, soybeans, peanuts, peanut butter, peas, tempeh, tofu, and other legumes. Good sources are avocados, buckwheat, cherimoyas, dried fruit, durians, enriched and whole grains, fortified cereals, mushrooms, nutritional yeast, nuts, quinoa, sea vegetables, seeds, tahini, wild rice, and yeast extract spread. (For other sources and niacin amounts, see table 7.3 on page 252.)[44, 45] Seeds, nuts, legumes, and green vegetables are also high in tryptophan.

Special Issues

When intakes of riboflavin, vitamin B₆, or iron are low (as in very low-calorie diets), conversion of tryptophan to niacin can be impaired because these nutrients are involved in the conversion.[2, 4]

In supplements, the maximum tolerable upper intake level (UL) recommended is 35 mg. Pharmacological preparations of niacin are used as cholesterol-lowering agents in treating heart disease; these higher intakes may lead to uncomfortable flushing of the face, chest, and arms.

PANTOTHENIC ACID (VITAMIN B₅)

Pantothenic Acid in Perspective

The name of this vitamin hails from the Greek word *pantothen,* meaning "from everywhere." It's a component of coenzyme A, found in all living cells, so it's present in all whole plant foods and not likely to be lacking in vegan diets. However, in vegan diets that are particularly low in calories, intakes can be insufficient.[2, 4, 17, 153]

Function

Pantothenic acid plays a central role in releasing energy from dietary carbohydrate, fat, and protein. It also helps to build fats (including any cholesterol the body needs), steroid hormones, and other essential compounds. It also supports intercell communication.[2, 4]

Recommended Intake

Insufficient evidence was available to set an RDA for pantothenic acid, so an AI was set for adults at 5 mg per day.[2, 4]

Vegan Intakes

Research shows the average pantothenic acid intakes of vegans to meet or exceed recommended levels.[17, 42]

Vegan Food Sources

All whole plant foods contribute this vitamin, at least in small amounts. Avocados, nutritional yeast, sunflower seeds, and sweet potatoes are particularly high in pantothenic acid; broccoli, legumes, mushrooms, nuts, seeds, and whole grains are also good sources of this vitamin. (For other sources and pantothenic acid amounts, see table 7.3 on page 252.) The body also may absorb some pantothenic acid produced by intestinal bacteria.[4, 17, 44, 45]

PYRIDOXINE (VITAMIN B$_6$)

Pyridoxine in Perspective

Can this vitamin help individuals to dream more vividly and recall dreams more often? Does getting enough pyridoxine decrease PMS symptoms in women and reduce nausea and vomiting in early pregnancy? Do deficiencies increase vulnerability to attention deficit hyperactivity disorder (ADHD) or autism? Can a little extra B$_6$ help older adults to retain memory or can it fight depression? The reputed effects of vitamin B$_6$ are subject to rumors, some true and many with no scientific backing.

Research has shown pyridoxine does help to alleviate morning sickness. High homocysteine levels are linked with depression, and vitamin B$_6$ may help to alleviate depressive symptoms by reducing homocysteine. When B$_6$ improves these conditions, its success occurs in those who were deficient in the vitamin in the first place. A diet rich in vitamin B$_6$ might brighten dreams and improve memory as individuals age, but these effects are not certain.[59, 176–179]

Function

Pyridoxine is needed for converting amino acids to energy and for building amino acids, fatty acids, and neurotransmitters. When the body needs energy, pyridoxine retrieves glucose from stored liver glycogen. It supports the immune system and other essential processes. Pyridoxine also helps to rid the body of homocysteine, a troublesome compound created during certain metabolic processes. Pyridoxine, folate, and vitamin B_{12} convert homocysteine to two amino acids (cysteine and methionine) that the body can use in building protein. With shortages of these three B vitamins, homocysteine levels rise, arterial walls can be damaged, and blood clots form, increasing heart disease risk.[2, 4, 177]

Recommended Intake

To age 50, the adult RDA is 1.3 mg; above 50, it increases to 1.5 mg for women and 1.7 mg for men.[2, 4]

Vegan Intakes

Studies show the average vegan intakes of pyridoxine to exceed recommended levels.[17, 42]

Vegan Food Sources

Pyridoxine is well distributed among plant foods, especially fruits. For example, three bananas provide a day's supply. Vegan diets generally include plenty of foods rich in vitamin B_6; some of the richest sources are avocados, bananas, chia seeds, soybeans, and sunflower seeds. Others are bell peppers, bok choy, cabbage, carrots, cauliflower, fortified breakfast cereals, guavas, kale, mangoes, navy beans and other legumes, okra, peas, pistachios, potatoes, spinach, squash, sunflower seeds, walnuts, water chestnuts, whole grains, yams, and zucchini. (For other sources and pyridoxine amounts, see table 7.3 on page 252.)[44, 45]

Special Issues

Pyridoxine is easily destroyed by cooking and is lost in soaking water or when foods are frozen or canned. It's removed during the refining of grains and isn't added back to enriched grains.[2, 4, 17]

BIOTIN (VITAMIN B$_7$)

Biotin in Perspective

This vitamin doesn't hit the headlines because deficiencies are rare; people on plant-based diets seem to fare well. Intakes of biotin are generally sufficient unless calorie intakes are particularly low.[17, 29] Biotin also may help to strengthen fingernails.[4]

Function

In combination with other B vitamins, biotin is involved in the metabolism of amino acids, fats, and carbohydrates.[2, 4]

Is There a Vitamin B₈?

Inositol, the compound originally called vitamin B_8, went the way of vitamin B_4 when scientists discovered that the body could make it from glucose. It's no longer considered a vitamin or an essential nutrient. The most concentrated sources are plant foods, such as fruits, grains, legumes, and nuts.

Recommended Intake

Although there isn't yet an RDA for biotin, the AI for adults is 30 mcg of biotin per day.[2, 4]

Vegan Intakes

Little data is available regarding the actual biotin intakes of vegans or of any dietary group or on the biotin content of foods. One study of Seventh-day Adventists found plasma levels of biotin to be higher in vegans than in lacto-ovo vegetarians or in nonvegetarians.[17, 180]

Vegan Food Sources

Almonds, avocados, bananas, carrots, cauliflower, corn, hazelnuts, legumes, nutritional yeast, peanut butter, raspberries, oatmeal, onions, tomatoes, walnuts, and whole grains are among the many sources of biotin. (For other sources and biotin amounts, see table 7.3 on page 252.)[44, 45]

Special Issues

Biotin is manufactured by many bacteria throughout the small and large intestine and absorbed from there, adding to the dietary supply. After a course of antibiotics, intestinal synthesis may be decreased, until friendly intestinal flora flourish again.[2, 4]

FOLATE (VITAMIN B₉, FOLIC ACID)

Folate in Perspective

Both the name for this vitamin and the word *foliage* come from the same Latin root, *folium*, meaning "leaf." It's not surprising, then, to learn that leafy greens are important folate contributors. Folate is the natural form of vitamin B_9 in foods. Folic acid is the more stable form used in supplements and fortified foods; it can be converted in the liver to folate.[2-4] Folate was first isolated from spinach in 1945. Since then, numerous green vegetables have been added to the list of excellent sources, along with oranges and legumes. In recent years, grain products have been fortified with folic acid.

Function

The coenzyme form of folate transfers small segments of molecules to sites where they're needed to build DNA and amino acids. Requirements increase during pregnancy, when a great deal of cell division occurs; folate deficiencies cause neural tube defects and several other types of birth defects.

Folate works with vitamins B_{12} and B_6 to remove potentially problematic buildups of homocysteine. It's required for the synthesis of SAM (s-adenosyl-methionine), and in this role may be protective against cancer and helpful for depression and osteoarthritis. It also helps in the production of healthy sperm with less risk of chromosome damage and supports fertility in both genders.[2-4]

The synthetic form of this vitamin, folic acid, is chemically different, and scientists currently are exploring the similarities and differences in its action. While natural folate in foods is protective against cancer, the folic acid in supplements and fortified foods may actually increase the risk of breast, prostate, colorectal, and other types of cancer and of asthma, especially when total intake is greater than 1,000 mcg daily.[4, 181, 182]

Laboratory Tests for Folate

High blood levels of homocysteine may indicate either deficiencies of folate (less likely in vegans) or of vitamin B_{12} (likely in vegans who don't supplement). Lack of these two B vitamins also can cause the failure of red blood cells to mature properly. Such cells become big enough to divide, but they don't divide properly and can't transport oxygen, creating a condition known as macrocytic (big cell) anemia. As a result, sufferers become weak, tired, and short of breath.[2, 4]

Recommended Intake

The body's absorption of folate, folic acid from fortified food, or a folic acid supplement taken without food differs, with the latter showing highest absorption. These differences are reflected in the units, dietary folate equivalents (DFE), used to define recommended intakes for this vitamin.

The RDA for adults is 400 mcg (0.4 mg) of folate from food, equivalent to 400 mcg DFE per day (1 mcg DFE equals 1 mcg of food folate). A folic acid supplement of 240 mcg taken with food provides 400 mcg DFE (1 mcg DFE equals 0.6 mcg of folic acid from fortified foods or dietary supplements consumed with food). A folic acid supplement of 200 mcg taken on an empty stomach provides 400 mcg of DFE (1 mcg DFE equals 0.5 of mcg folic acid from dietary supplements taken on an empty stomach).

To protect a fetus against neural tube defects—and because more than half of pregnancies are unplanned—women who might become pregnant are advised to consume 400 mcg DFE of folic acid daily, and then 600 mcg daily throughout pregnancy.[2, 4 17, 183] See page 290 for details on getting 600 mcg of folate from orange juice, black beans, quinoa, and lettuce.

Individuals don't need higher levels than these recommended intakes.[182] In fact, it's important to be aware not only of the minimum requirement for folate but also of the UL for folic acid in fortified foods and supplements.[2, 185] The UL for adults (including pregnant women) is 1,000 mcg DFE per day from folic acid supplements or fortified foods, exclusive of food folate. No UL has been established for folate (the UL is for folic acid only), because no adverse effects have been associated with high intakes of natural folate in beans, greens, oranges, and other plant foods. An individual can easily exceed the UL by ingesting a supplement with 600 mcg of folic acid, a serving of fortified breakfast cereal that has 100 percent of the DV for folic acid (another 400 mcg), plus several slices of white bread made with folate-fortified flour (about 40 mcg each) or a cup of cooked enriched rice or spaghetti (each providing about 170 mcg DFE). Check labels for amounts to monitor intakes.[2, 4, 186]

Vegan Intakes and Status

Studies show that vegan folate intakes meet and exceed recommended intake levels.[17] A British study showed the average daily folate intake of vegans to be 420 mcg; a North American study reported average vegan intakes at 723 mcg daily.[40, 42]

Vegan Food Sources

Greens, beans, and oranges are folate champions. Other excellent sources of folate are almonds, asparagus, avocados, beets, cashews, fortified breakfast cereals, kelp, kiwifruit, legumes (beans, peas, lentils, and soy foods), mung bean sprouts, nutritional yeast, orange juice, quinoa, sunflower seeds, spinach, sprouted lentils, and yeasts. Folic acid is added to enriched flours, breads, cereals, pastas, rice, and corn meal in many countries. (For additional sources and folate amounts, see table 7.3 on page 252.)[44, 45]

Special Issues

Sprouting has been shown to more than double the folate content of seeds, such as rye.[187] To absorb folate, the body requires adequate intakes of vitamin C and iron. Folate is easily destroyed by boiling, but steaming causes little or no loss of folate from broccoli or spinach.[188]

The mandatory addition of folic acid to enriched grain products is credited with reducing the incidence of neural tube defects by 30 to 70 percent in the United States, Canada, Australia, Chile, and many African and Middle Eastern countries. However, this practice hasn't been adopted throughout the United Kingdom and Europe.[176]

The folate naturally present in plant foods is safe, beneficial, and essential; meanwhile, safety concerns exist regarding folic acid. Even though fortification has also decreased other birth defects, it has perhaps increased the risk of colon cancer in later life. Because there are limits to the body's conversion of the supplement form to folate, with high intakes from supplements, unconverted folic acid can remain in the blood, and this may increase cancer risk. High folic acid intakes also may provoke seizures in people who take anticonvulsant medications.

As previously mentioned, folic acid can mask a B_{12} deficiency, particularly when large amounts of folic acid are taken.

For these reasons, the IOM has set a UL of 1,000 mcg (1 mg) per day for folic acid. Some experts advise that intakes of 400 to 600 mcg of folic acid per day can be safe; certainly these will help to prevent birth defects that can result when a mother-to-be consumes little dietary folate. (For more information on this topic, see page 290.) An excellent choice is to get most or all of the necessary folate from foods, with the option of including some fortified grain products in the selection. This is easy to do on a vegan diet.[2, 182, 189]

CHOLINE

Choline in Perspective

Choline is present in all the cell membranes of plants and animals, including those of humans. It's present in the brain as part of a fatty compound known as lecithin. Although choline was officially recognized by the IOM as an essential nutrient in 1998, expert opinion has been divided on whether it's a true vitamin (a dietary essential) or whether the body can synthesize enough to supply its needs. People seem to need significantly different amounts from food, depending on their genetics and the composition of their diet. When intakes of folate, vitamin B_{12}, and the amino acid methionine are low, the body's choline synthesis can be limited.[2, 4]

Function

Choline helps transport fats and other nutrients through cell membranes. It's used in the construction of an important neurotransmitter, so it's crucial for the transmission of nerve impulses and it aids memory and muscle control. Choline also assists in clearing fat and cholesterol from the liver.[2, 4, 184]

Recommended Intake

An RDA hasn't been set for choline due to insufficient data; however, the AI is set at 425 mg per day for women and 550 mg per day for men. It may be beneficial for women who want to become pregnant to take a choline supplement to prevent infant neural tube defects.[2, 4] When The Vegan Plate (page 434) is used as a guide, a diet can easily meet the AIs.

Vegan Food Sources

Because it's a part of all cells, choline is widely distributed in plant foods, though data regarding exact amounts is limited. Soy foods, quinoa, and broccoli are particularly rich sources.[184] Other good sources are amaranth, artichokes, Brussels sprouts, buckwheat, corn, mushrooms, oats, wheat germ, and whole wheat products. For additional sources and choline amounts, see table 7.2 (page 250) and check online for the US Department of Agriculture (USDA) Database for the Choline Content of Common Foods.[190]

TABLE 7.2. Choline in vegan foods

FOOD (SERVING SIZE)	CHOLINE (MG)
AI for women	425
AI for men	500
LEGUMES	
Beans, cooked or canned (kidney, navy, pinto, vegetarian baked beans), ½ c (125 ml)	30–43
Edamame, ½ c (125 ml)	33
Peanut butter, 2 T (30 ml)	21
Peas, green, cooked, ½ c (125 ml)	23
Soy milk, ½ c (125 ml)	30
Tofu, firm, ½ c (125 ml)	35
SEEDS AND NUTS	
Almonds, cashews, ground flaxseeds, or pistachios, ¼ c (60 ml)	20–22
Hazelnuts/filberts, ¼ c (60 ml)	16
Pecans, ¼ c (60 ml)	10
Sunflower seeds, ¼ c (60 ml)	18
VEGETABLES (RAW UNLESS STATED)	
Asparagus, cauliflower, or spinach, cooked, ½ c (125 ml)	23–24
Avocado, medium	28
Broccoli, cooked, ½ c (125 ml)	31
Cabbage, red, ½ c (125 ml)	6
Carrot, medium	5
Corn kernels, ½ c (125 ml)	18
Pepper, bell, green or red, medium	7
Potato, baked, medium	26
Salsa, ½ c (125 ml)	16
Sweet potato, baked, medium	15
Tomato sauce, ½ c (125 ml)	12
FRUITS	
Banana, medium	12
Blueberries, ½ c (125 ml)	4
Dates, medjool, 4	10

FOOD (SERVING SIZE)	CHOLINE (MG)
Orange, medium	16
Orange juice, ½ c (125 ml)	8
Peach, medium	9
Raspberries, blackberries, ½ c (125 ml)	6–7
GRAINS	
Bread, whole wheat, slice, 1 oz (30 g)	5
Corn tortilla, small, 24 g	3
Quinoa, raw, ½ c (125 ml)	60
Rice, or oatmeal, cooked, ½ c (125 ml)	9
Spaghetti, cooked, ½ c (125 ml)	4
OTHER	
Baking chocolate, unsweetened, 1 oz (30 g)	13
Chili powder, 1 T (15 ml)	5
Mustard, prepared, 1 T (15 ml)	3
Turmeric or curry powder, 1 T (15 ml)	3–4

Sources:[45, 184, 190]

Special Issues

Lecithin (which contains choline) is a common food additive that acts as an emulsifier. Lecithin also is found in nonstick cooking sprays. Most lecithin is vegan and is derived from soy or sunflower oil; however, a certain amount can be derived from egg yolks. Check labels: the source may be included, for example, as "soy lecithin." For more information on whether ingredients are vegan, consult the online "Vegetarian Journal's Guide to Food Ingredients" by Jeanne Yacoubou (see Resources on page 449).[191]

Vitamins in Vegan Foods

T able 7.3 (page 252) lists the vitamin content of a variety of foods, using typical portions, such as 1 cup (250 ml) or one unit (for example, one apple). The USDA website lists additional nutrient data.[45]

Although tables and databases list exact numbers, nature is much more variable. For example, plants grown in plenty of sunlight contain much more vitamin C than those grown with less light.[193]

TABLE 7.3. Vitamins in vegan foods

FOOD VITAMIN (unit)	A (mcg RAE)	C (mg)	E (mg)	K (mcg)	B₁ (mg)	B₂ (mg)	B₃ (mg NE)	B₅ (mg)	B₆ (mg)	FOLATE (mcg DFE)	BIOTIN (mcg)
Recommended intake for women*	700	75	15	90	1.1	1.1	14	5	1.3–1.5 **	400	30
Recommended intake for men*	900	90	15	120	1.2	1.3	16	5	1.3–1.7 **	400	30
FRUITS (FRESH UNLESS OTHERWISE STATED)											
Apple, chopped, ½ c (125 ml)	2	3	0.1	1	0.01	0.02	0.1	0.04	0.03	2	0.7
Apple, medium	5	8	0.3	4	0.03	0.05	0.1	0.1	0.07	5	0.8
Apples, dried, ¼ c (60 ml)	0	1	0.1	3	0	0.3	0.2	0.2	0.3	0.6	2.3
Apricot, medium	34	4	0.3	1	0.01	0.01	0.3	0.1	0.02	3	—
Apricot slices, ½ c (125 ml)	84	9	0.8	3	0.03	0.03	0.7	0.2	0.05	8	—
Apricots, dried, ¼ c (60 ml)	234	1.3	5.6	4	0.01	0.01	0.3	0.1	0.2	3	—
Banana, dried, ¼ c (60 ml)	3	2	0.1	0.5	0.05	0.06	0.7	—	0.11	4	0.7
Banana, medium	4	10	0.1	1	0.04	0.09	1	0.4	0.43	24	3.1
Banana slices, ½ c (125 ml)	3	7	0.2	0	0.02	0.06	0.6	0.3	0.29	16	2.1
Blackberries, ½ c (125 ml)	8	16	0.9	15	0.02	0.02	0.5	0.2	0.02	19	0.3
Blueberries, ½ c (125 ml)	4	8	0.8	15	0.03	0.03	0.4	0.1	0.04	5	—
Cantaloupe, diced, ½ c (125 ml)	139	30	0	2	0.06	0.02	0.6	0.1	0.06	17	—
Cherimoya, ½ c (125 ml)	0	11	0.2	—	0.09	0.11	1	0.3	0.22	19	—
Crab apple slices, ½ c (125 ml)	1	5	0.3	—	0.02	0.01	0.1	—	—	—	—
Currants, black, ½ c (125 ml)	7	107	0.6	—	0.03	0.03	0.2	0.2	0.04	4	2.8
Currants, red/white, ½ c (125 ml)	1	24	7	12	0.02	0.03	0.1	0	0.04	5	2.8
Currants, Zante, dried, ¼ c (60 ml)	1	2	0	1	0.06	0.05	0.6	0	0.11	4	—
Dates, chopped, ¼ c (60 ml)	0	00	0	1	0.02	0.02	0.6	0.2	0.06	7	—
Durian, chopped, ½ c (125 ml)	3	25	—	—	0.48	0.26	1.3	0.3	0.41	46	—
Fig, fresh, medium	4	1	0.1	2	0.03	0.02	0.2	0.2	0.06	3	—
Figs, dried, ¼ c (60 ml)	0	0	0.1	6	0.03	0.03	0.2	0.2	0.06	3	—
Gooseberries, ½ c (125 ml)	11	22	0.3	—	0.03	0.02	0.2	0.2	0.06	5	0.4
Grapes, ½ c (125 ml)	2	2	0	7	0.04	0.03	0.2	0	0.05	2	—
Grapefruit, medium	143	77	0.3	0	0.11	0.08	0.5	0.6	0.13	32	2.5
Grapefruit juice, pink, ½ c (125 ml)	29	50	0.1	—	0.05	0.03	0.3	0.2	0.06	13	1.3
Grapefruit juice, white, ½ c (125 ml)	1	50	0.3	0	0.05	0.03	0.3	0.2	0.06	13	1.3
Grapefruit sections, ½ c (125 ml)	56	42	0.2	0	0.02	0.03	0.3	0.2	0.10	13	1.2

FOOD (unit)	VITAMIN A (mcg RAE)	C (mg)	E (mg)	K (mcg)	B₁ (mg)	B₂ (mg)	B₃ (mg NE)	B₅ (mg)	B₆ (mg)	FOLATE (mcg DFE)	BIOTIN (mcg)
Guava, ½ c (125 ml)	27	199	0.6	2	0.06	0.03	1.2	0.4	0.10	43	—
Honeydew melon, diced, ½ c (125 ml)	2	16	0	3	0.03	0.01	0.4	0.1	0.08	17	—
Kiwifruit, diced, ½ c (125 ml)	4	88	1.4	38	0.03	0.02	0.6	0.2	0.06	24	—
Kiwifruit, medium	3	70	1.1	71	0.02	0.02	0.4	0.3	0.05	19	—
Mango, medium	182	122	3	14	0.09	0.13	3	0.7	0.40	144	—
Mango slices, ½ c (125 ml)	47	32	0.8	4	0.02	0.03	0.8	0.2	0.10	37	—
Orange, medium	15	70	0.3	1	0.11	0.05	0.6	0.3	0.08	39	1
Orange juice, ½ c (125 ml)	13	66	0.1	0	0.12	0.04	0.6	0.2	0.05	39	0.7
Orange sections, ½ c (125 ml)	11	51	0.2	0	0.08	0.04	0.4	0.2	0.06	29	1
Papaya, cubed, ½ c (125 ml)	36	47	0.2	2	0.02	0.02	0.4	0.2	0.03	28	—
Papaya, mashed, ½ c (125 ml)	58	74	0.4	3	0.03	0.03	0.6	0.2	0.05	45	—
Peach, medium	24	10	1.1	4	0.04	0.05	1.5	0.2	0.04	6	0.3
Peach slices, ½ c (125 ml)	13	5	0.6	2	0.02	0.03	0.8	0.2	0.02	6	0.3
Pear, dried, ¼ c (60 ml)	0	3	0	9	0	0.07	0.6	0.1	0.03	0	—
Pear, medium	2	7	0.2	8	0.02	0.04	0.3	0.1	0.05	12	0.3
Pear slices, ½ c (125 ml)	1	3	0.1	3	0.01	0.02	0.1	0	0.02	5	0.2
Pineapple, diced, ½ c (125 ml)	3	42	0	1	0.07	0.03	0.5	0.2	0.10	16	0.3
Plum slices, ½ c (125 ml)	15	8	0.2	6	0.02	0.02	0.5	0.1	0.03	4	—
Prunes, dried, ¼ c (60 ml)	17	0	0.2	26	0.02	0.08	1	0.2	0.09	2	—
Raisins, seeded, packed, ¼ c (60 ml)	0	2	0.3	—	0.04	0.07	0.6	0	0.07	1	0.8
Raisins, seedless, packed, ¼ c (60 ml)	0	1	0	1	0.04	0.05	0.7	0	0.07	2	0.8
Raspberries, ½ c (125 ml)	1	17	0.5	5	0.02	0.02	0.5	0.2	0.04	14	—
Strawberries, whole, ½ c (125 ml)	0	45	0.2	2	0.02	0.02	0.4	0.1	0.04	18	0.8
Watermelon, diced, ½ c (125 ml)	22	6	0	0	0.03	0.02	0.2	0.2	0.04	2	0.8
VEGETABLES (RAW UNLESS OTHERWISE STATED)											
Arugula, chopped, 1 c (20 g)	25	3	0.1	23	0.01	0.02	0.1	0.1	0.02	20	—
Asparagus, cooked, ½ c (125 ml)	48	7	1.4	48	0.15	0.13	1.5	0.2	0.08	141	0.4
Avocado, all types, medium	15	20	4.2	42	0.13	0.26	4.3	2.8	0.52	163	7.2
Avocado, all types, puréed, ½ c (125 ml)	9	12	2.5	26	0.08	0.16	2.6	1.7	0.31	98	4.4
Avocado, all types, sliced, ½ c (125 ml)	6	8	1.6	16	0.05	0.10	1.7	1.1	0.20	62	2.8
Avocado, California, medium	10	12	2.7	29	0.10	0.19	3.2	2	0.4	121	4.9
Avocado, California, puréed, ½ c (125 ml)	9	11	2.4	26	0.09	0.17	2.8	1.8	0.35	108	4.4
Avocado, Florida, medium	21	53	8.1	—	0.06	0.16	3.5	2.8	0.24	106	—

FOOD (unit)	VITAMIN A (mcg RAE)	C (mg)	E (mg)	K (mcg)	B₁ (mg)	B₂ (mg)	B₃ (mg NE)	B₅ (mg)	B₆ (mg)	FOLATE (mcg DFE)	BIOTIN (mcg)
Avocado, Florida, puréed, ½ c (125 ml)	9	21	3.2	—	0.03	0.06	1.4	1.1	0.09	43	—
Basil, chopped, 1 c (250 ml)	118	8	0.4	185	0.02	0.03	0.7	0.1	0.07	30	—
Beans, snap, green, ½ c (125 ml)	18	6	0.2	8	0.04	0.05	0.6	0.1	0.07	17	0.5
Beans, snap, yellow, ½ c (125 ml)	3	9	—	—	0.04	0.06	0.6	0	0.04	20	—
Beet greens, 1 c (250 ml)	127	12	0.6	161	0.04	0.09	0.4	0.1	0.04	6	—
Beets, sliced, ½ c (125 ml)	1	4	0	0	0.02	0.03	0.5	0.1	0.05	78	—
Bok choy, cooked, ½ c (125 ml)	191	23	0.1	31	0.03	0.06	0.6	0.1	0.15	37	—
Broccoli, cooked, ½ c (125 ml)	64	54	1.2	116	0.05	0.10	0.9	0.5	0.16	89	0.4
Brussels sprouts, cooked, ½ c (125 ml)	32	51	0.3	116	0.09	0.07	0.9	0.2	0.15	49	—
Cabbage, green, chopped, 1 c (250 ml)	5	34	0.1	71	0.06	0.04	0.4	0.2	0.12	40	1.9
Cabbage, napa, chopped, 1 c (250 ml)	13	22	0.1	34	0.03	0.04	0.5	0.1	0.19	63	—
Cabbage, red, chopped, 1 c (250 ml)	52	54	0.1	36	0.06	0.06	0.6	0.1	0.20	17	1.9
Carrot, chopped, ½ c (125 ml)	565	4	0.4	9	0.04	0.04	0.7	0.2	0.09	13	3.4
Carrot, medium	510	4	0.4	8	0.04	0.04	0.7	0.2	0.08	12	3
Carrot juice, ½ c (125 ml)	966	11	—	19	0.11	0.07	0.7	0.3	0.27	5	—
Cauliflower, chopped, cooked, ½ c (125 ml)	1	29	0.1	9	0.03	0.03	0.5	0.3	0.11	29	0.8
Celery, diced, ½ c (125 ml)	12	2	0.1	16	0.01	0.03	0.2	0.1	0.04	19	0.1
Celery rib	14	2	0.2	19	0.01	0.04	0.3	0.2	0.05	23	0.1
Celery root, diced, ½ c (125 ml)	0	7	0.3	34	0.04	0.05	0.6	0.3	0.14	7	—
Chile peppers, hot green, ½ c (125 ml)	47	192	0.6	11	0.07	0.07	1.1	0	0.22	18	—
Chile peppers, hot red, ½ c (125 ml)	37	114	0.6	11	0.07	0.99	1.3	0.2	0.40	18	2
Cilantro, 1 c (250 ml)	1,080	4	0	50	0.01	0.03	0.2	0.3	0.02	10	—
Collard greens, chopped, 1 c (250 ml)	127	13	0.9	194	0.02	0.05	0.5	0.1	0.06	63	—
Corn, white, ½ c (125 ml)	0	6	0.1	0.2	0.16	0.05	1.7	0.6	0.04	37	—
Corn, yellow, ½ c (125 ml)	7	5	0	0.2	0.12	0.04	1.6	0.6	0.07	32	—
Cucumber with peel, sliced, ½ c (125 ml)	6	3	0	9	0.02	0.02	0.1	0.3	0.02	8	1
Dandelion greens, 1 c (250 ml)	295	20	2	452	0.11	0.15	0.5	0	0.15	16	0.2
Eggplant, cubed, ½ c (125 ml)	1	1	0.2	2	0.04	0.01	0.4	0	0.04	7	—
Garlic clove, medium	0	1	0	0	0.01	0	0.1	0	0.04	0	—
Garlic cloves, ½ c (125 ml)	0	22	0.1	1	0.14	0.08	1.3	0.4	0.89	2	—
Jerusalem artichokes, sliced, ½ c (125 ml)	1	3	0.2	0	0.2	0.05	1	0.3	0.06	10	—
Kale, 1 c (250 ml)	544	85	0.6	578	0.08	0.09	1.2	0.1	0.19	21	0.4

FOOD (unit)	VITAMIN A (mcg RAE)	C (mg)	E (mg)	K (mcg)	B₁ (mg)	B₂ (mg)	B₃ (mg NE)	B₅ (mg)	B₆ (mg)	FOLATE (mcg DFE)	BIOTIN (mcg)
Kelp, Laminaria, chopped, ½ c (125 ml)	2	1	0.4	28	0.02	0.06	0.5	0.3	0	76	—
Leeks, chopped, ½ c (125 ml)	39	6	0.4	22	0.03	0.01	0.3	0.1	0.11	30	1.3
Lettuce, butterhead, chopped, 1 c (250 ml)	96	2	0.1	59	0.03	0.04	0.3	0.1	0.05	42	1.1
Lettuce, iceberg, chopped, 1 c (250 ml)	19	2	0.1	18	0.03	0.02	0.2	0.1	0.03	22	1.4
Lettuce, leaf, chopped, 1 c (250 ml)	140	4	0.1	48	0.03	0.03	0.2	0.1	0.03	14	0.7
Lettuce, romaine, chopped, 1 c (250 ml)	216	2	0.1	51	0.04	0.03	0.2	0.1	0.04	68	0.9
Mushrooms, brown, cooked, ½ c (125 ml)	0	1	0	0	0.04	0.20	2.1	0.8	0.05	0	8.1
Mushrooms, shiitake, cooked, ½ c (125 ml)	0	0	0	0	0.03	0.13	1.2	2.8	0.12	16	—
Mustard greens, 1 c (250 ml)	311	41	1.2	294	0.05	0.07	0.8	0.1	0.1	111	—
Okra, sliced, cooked, ½ c (125 ml)	12	14	0.2	34	0.1	0.05	1	0.2	0.16	39	—
Olives, black, canned, ½ c (125 ml/70 g)	13	1	1.1	1	0	0	0	0	0.01	0	—
Onion, green	7	3	0.1	4	0.01	0.01	0.1	0	0.01	10	0.5
Onions, green, chopped, ½ c (125 ml)	26	10	0.6	109	0.06	0.08	0.9	0	0.06	68	3.7
Onions, red/yellow/white, ½ c (125 ml)	0	6	0	1	0.04	0.02	0.3	0.1	0.10	16	2.9
Parsley, 1 c (250 ml)	270	85	0.5	1,053	0.06	0.06	1.3	0.3	0.06	98	—
Parsnips, sliced, ½ c (125 ml)	0	11	0.8	1	0.07	0.04	0.6	0.5	0.08	48	0.1
Pea pods, snow, ½ c (125 ml)	28	31	0.1	13	0.08	0.04	0.5	0.4	0.08	22	—
Peas, green, ½ c (125 ml)	29	31	0.1	19	0.20	0.1	2.1	0.1	0.13	49	0.4
Pepper, bell, green, medium	22	96	0.4	9	0.07	0.03	0.8	0.1	0.27	12	—
Pepper, bell, red, medium	186	152	1.9	6	0.06	0.1	1.4	0.4	0.35	55	—
Peppers, bell, green, chopped, ½ c (125 ml)	15	63	0.3	6	0.04	0.02	0.5	0.1	0.18	8	—
Peppers, bell, red, chopped, ½ c (125 ml)	123	101	1.2	4	0.04	0.07	0.9	0.2	0.23	36	—
Potato, baked, medium	1	17	0	3	0.11	0.08	3.2	0.6	0.5	48	—
Potatoes, peeled, diced, cooked, ½ c (125 ml)	0	6	0	2	0.08	0.02	1.4	0.4	0.22	7	0.2
Radish, daikon, medium	0	74	0	1	0.07	0.07	0.8	0.5	0.16	95	—
Radish, medium	0	1	0	0.1	0	0	0	0	0	1	—
Radishes, daikon, dried, ½ c (125 ml)	0	0	0	3	0.17	0.42	2.5	1.4	0.38	181	—
Radishes, sliced, ½ c (125 ml)	0	9	0	1	0.01	0.02	0.2	0.1	0.04	15	—
Rutabaga, chopped, ½ c (125 ml)	13	17	0.4	0.3	0.07	0.04	0.8	0.1	0.09	13	0.1
Spinach, chopped, 1 c (250 ml)	149	9	0.6	153	0.02	0.06	0.4	0	0.06	62	0
Spirulina, dried, 1 T (7 g)	2	1	0.4	1.8	0.17	0.26	2	0.2	0.03	7	—

FOOD	VITAMIN (unit)	A (mcg RAE)	C (mg)	E (mg)	K (mcg)	B₁ (mg)	B₂ (mg)	B₃ (mg NE)	B₅ (mg)	B₆ (mg)	FOLATE (mcg DFE)	BIOTIN (mcg)
Squash, acorn, cubed, cooked, ½ c (125 ml)		22	12	0.2	—	0.18	0.01	1.2	0.6	0.21	21	—
Squash, butternut, cubed, cooked, ½ c (125 ml)		572	16	1.3	1	0.08	0.02	1.3	0.4	0.13	21	—
Squash, crookneck, cooked, mashed, ½ c (125 ml)		10	7	0.1	6	0.06	0.06	0.8	0.2	0.12	25	—
Squash, Hubbard, cubed, cooked, ½ c (125 ml)		363	10	0.2	2	0.08	0.05	1	0.5	0.19	17	—
Squash, winter, all varieties, cubed, cooked, ½ c (125 ml)		282	10	0.1	5	0.02	0.07	0.8	0.2	0.17	22	—
Sweet potato, dark orange, cooked, mashed, ½ c (125 ml)		1,364	22	1.6	4	0.10	0.08	1.7	1	0.29	10	7.4
Tomato, cherry		7	2	0.1	1	0.01	0	0.1	0	0.01	3	0.7
Tomato, chopped, ½ c (125 ml)		39	13	0.5	7	0.04	0.02	0.7	0.1	0.08	14	3.8
Tomato, green, chopped, ½ c (125 ml)		31	22	0.4	10	0.06	0.04	0.6	0.5	0.08	9	—
Tomato, medium		51	17	0.7	10	0.05	0.02	0.9	0.1	0.1	18	4.9
Tomato, Roma		26	8	0.3	5	0.03	0.01	0.4	0.1	0.05	9	2.5
Tomato, sun-dried, ½ c (125 ml)		12	11	0	12	0.15	0.14	3.1	0.6	0.09	19	—
Turnip, cubed, cooked, ½ c (125 ml)		0	14	0	0	0.03	0.03	0.5	0.2	0.08	11	0.1
Turnip greens, chopped, 1 c (250 ml)		337	35	1.7	146	0.04	0.06	0.6	0.2	0.15	113	—
Yam, baked, ½ c (125 ml)		4	8	0.2	2	0.07	0.02	0.4	0.5	0.16	11	—
Zucchini, cubed, 1 c (124 g)		7	12	0.1	3	0.03	0.06	0.4	0.1	0.11	16	—
NUTS AND SEEDS												
Almond butter, 2 T (30 ml)		0	2	7.9	0.	0.01	0.30	1.8	0.1	0.03	17	—
Almonds, ¼ c (60 ml)		0	0	9.5	0.	0.08	0.40	2.4	0.2	0.05	18	23
Brazil nut, large		0	0	0.3	0	0.03	0	0.1	0	0	1	—
Brazil nuts, ¼ c (60 ml)		0	0	1.9	0	0.21	0.01	0.8	0.1	0.03	7	—
Cashew butter, 2 T (30 ml)		0	0	—	—	0.10	0.06	1.9	0.4	0.08	22	—
Cashew nuts, ¼ c (60 ml)		0	0	0.3	12	0.14	0.07	1.8	0.3	0.14	8	4.5
Chia seeds, dried, ¼ c (60 ml)		—	1	0.2	—	0.26	0.07	6.4	0.4	1.11	182	—
Coconut, dried, ¼ c (60 ml)		0	0.3	0.1	0	0.01	0.02	0.4	0.2	0.06	2	—
Flaxseeds, ground, ¼ c (60 ml)		0	0	0.1	2	0.69	0.07	1.3	0.4	0.20	37	—
Hazelnuts/filberts, ¼ c (60 ml)		0	2	5.2	5	0.22	0.04	1.7	0.3	0.19	39	26
Pecans, ¼ c (60 ml)		1	0	0.4	1	0.17	0.03	0.7	0.2	0.05	6	—
Pine nuts/pignolia nuts, dried, ¼ c (60 ml)		0	0	3.2	18	0.12	0.08	2.1	0.1	0.03	12	—
Pistachio nuts, ¼ c (60 ml)		6	2	0.8	—	0.27	0.05	1.8	0.2	0.53	16	—

FOOD	VITAMIN (unit)	A (mcg RAE)	C (mg)	E (mg)	K (mcg)	B₁ (mg)	B₂ (mg)	B₃ (mg NE)	B₅ (mg)	B₆ (mg)	FOLATE (mcg DFE)	BIOTIN (mcg)
Poppy seeds, 1 c (141 g)		0	0	0.6	0	0.29	0.03	1.2	0.1	0.08	28	—
Pumpkin seeds, ¼ c (60 ml)		0	1	0.7	2	0.09	0.05	4.5	0.2	0.05	19	—
Sesame butter/tahini, 2 T (30 ml)		1	1	1.3	—	0.05	1.04	1.8	0.2	0.05	30	—
Sesame seeds, ¼ c (60 ml)		1	0	0.6	0	0.29	0.09	3.7	0.1	0.29	35	4.1
Sunflower seed butter, 2 T (30 ml)		1	1	7.4	—	0.02	0.05	3.6	0.4	0.18	77	—
Sunflower seed kernels, ¼ c (60 ml)		1	0.5	12	0	0.53	0.13	4.7	0.4	0.48	81	—
Walnuts, black, chopped, ¼ c (60 ml)		1	1	0.6	1	0.02	0.04	1.8	0.5	0.18	10	6
Walnuts, English, chopped, ¼ c (60 ml)		0	0	0.2	1	0.10	0.04	1.2	0.2	0.16	29	5.6
Water chestnuts, Chinese, sliced, ¼ c (60 ml)		0	1	0.4	0	0.04	0.06	0.3	0.2	0.10	5	—
LEGUMES (COOKED UNLESS STATED)												
Adzuki beans, ½ c (125 ml)		0	0	—	—	0.14	0.08	2.3	0.5	0.12	147	—
Black beans, ½ c (125 ml)		0	0	0	3	0.22	0.05	2.1	0.2	06	135	—
Black-eyed peas, ½ c (125 ml)		1	0	0.2	1	0.18	0.05	1.9	0.4	0.09	188	—
Cranberry beans, ½ c (125 ml)		0	0	—	—	0.2	0.06	2.2	0.2	0.08	194	—
Chickpeas, ½ c (125 ml)		1	1	0.3	3	0.1	0.05	1.7	0.2	0.12	149	—
Edamame, ½ c (125 ml)		--	5	0.5	21	0.16	0.12	0.8	0.3	0.08	241	—
Falafel patties, three, (51 g total)		0	1	—	—	0.07	0.08	0.5	—	0.06	53	—
Great Northern beans, ½ c (125 ml)		0	1	—	—	0.15	0.06	2.2	0.2	0.11	95	—
Kidney beans, ½ c (125 ml)		0	1	0	8	0.15	0.05	2.1	0.2	0.11	122	—
Lentil sprouts, raw, 1 c (250 ml)		2	13	0.1	—	0.19	0.1	0.9	0.5	0.15	81	—
Lentils, green/brown, ½ c (125 ml)		0	2	0.1	2	0.18	0.08	2.5	0.7	0.19	189	—
Lima beans, ½ c (125 ml)		0	0	0.1	2	0.15	0.05	2.2	0.4	0.08	144	—
Mung bean sprouts, raw, 1 c (250 ml)		1	15	0.1	36	0.09	0.14	1.5	0.4	0.10	67	—
Navy beans, ½ c (125 ml)		0	1	0	1	0.23	0.06	2.2	0.3	0.13	135	31
Peanut butter, 2 T (30 ml)		0	0	2.9	0	0.02	0.03	5.6	0.3	0.18	24	31
Peanuts, ¼ c (60 ml)		0	0	3.1	0	0.24	0.05	6	0.6	0.13	89	27
Pea sprouts, raw, 1 c (250 ml)		11	13	0	—	0.29	0.2	3.9	1.3	0.34	183	—
Peas, raw, 1 c (250 ml)		55	58	0.2	36	0.39	0.19	3	—	0.24	94	—
Peas, split, ½ c (125 ml)		0	0	0	5.2	0.2	0.06	2.5	0.6	0.05	67	—
Pinto beans, ½ c (125 ml)		0	1	0.8	3.2	0.17	0.06	1.9	0.2	0.21	155	—
Soy milk, fortified, ½ c (125 ml)		71	0	0.1	4	0.04	0.24	1	0.1	0.04	12	4.6
Soybeans, ½ c (125 ml)		0	3	0.6	33	0.27	0.49	0.7	0.3	0.40	93	—
Tempeh, raw, ½ c (125 ml)		0	0	—	—	0.07	0.31	5.2	0.2	0.19	21	—

FOOD (unit)	VITAMIN A (mcg RAE)	C (mg)	E (mg)	K (mcg)	B₁ (mg)	B₂ (mg)	B₃ (mg NE)	B₅ (mg)	B₆ (mg)	FOLATE (mcg DFE)	BIOTIN (mcg)
Tofu, calcium-set, firm, raw, ½ c (125 ml)	11	0	0	3	0.21	0.14	6	0.2	0.12	39	—
White beans, ½ c (125 ml)	0	0	0.9	3	0.11	0.04	1.9	0.2	0.09	77	—
GRAINS (COOKED UNLESS STATED)											
Amaranth, ½ c (125 ml)	0	—	0.2	—	0.02	0.03	0.3	—	0.14	27	—
Barley, pearl, ½ c (125 ml)	0	0	0	1	0.07	0.05	2.2	0.1	0.10	13	0.6
Bread, rye, slice, 1 oz (30 g)	0	0	0.1	0	0.13	0.10	1.6	0.1	0.02	45	0.3
Bread, white, enriched, slice, 1 oz (30 g)	0	0	0.1	0	0.13	0.06	1.2	0.1	0.02	43	0.2
Bread, whole wheat, slice, 1 oz (30 g)	0	0	0.2	2	0.10	0.06	1.8	0.2	0.06	14	1.7
Buckwheat groats, kasha, ½ c (125 ml)	0	0	0.1	2	0.04	0.03	1.6	0.2	0.07	12	—
Corn ear, yellow, raw, medium	9	7	0.1	0	0.16	0.06	1.8	0.7	0.1	43	—
Corn kernels, yellow, raw, ½ c (125 ml)	9	0	0.4	0	0.37	0.17	3	0.3	0.52	16	—
Kamut, ½ c (125 ml)	0	—	—	—	0.11	0.03	3.3	—	0.08	11	—
Millet, ½ c (125 ml)	0	0	0	0	0.10	0.08	1.8	0.2	0.1	17	—
Oatmeal, ½ c (125 ml)	0	0	0.1	0	0.09	0.02	1	0.4	0.01	7	—
Quinoa, ½ c (125 ml)	0	0	0.6	—	0.10	0.11	0.4	—	0.12	41	—
Rice, brown, ½ c (125 ml)	0	0	0	1	0.1	0.01	1.9	0.4	0.15	4	—
Rice, white, enriched, ½ c (125 ml)	0	0	0	0	0.14	0.01	1.7	0.3	0.08	81	0.8
Spaghetti, enriched, ½ c (125 ml)	0	0	0	0	0.2	0.1	2.2	0.1	0.04	88	—
Spaghetti, whole wheat, ½ c (125 ml)	0	0	0.2	1	0.08	0.03	1.4	0.3	0.06	4	—
Wheat, sprouted, raw, 1 c (250 ml)	0	3	0.1	—	0.26	0.18	5.7	1.1	0.30	43	—
Wild rice, ½ c (125 ml)	0	0	0.4	0	0.05	0.08	1.8	0.1	0.12	23	0.7
OTHERS											
Maple syrup, 1 c (322 g)	0	0	0	0	0.01	0.03	0	0	0	0	—
Oil, flaxseed, 1 c (218 g)	0	0	0	1	0	0	0	0	0	0	0
Oil, olive, 1 c (216 g)	0	0	2	8	0	0	0	0	0	0	—
Red Star Vegetarian Support Formula nutritional yeast, 1 T (15 ml)	0	0	0	0	4	4	23	8.2	3.8	80	21

Sources:[44, 45]

Key: Dashes indicate that no data is available.

*For other ages, see page 446.

**The RDA for vitamin B₆ (pyridoxine) is 1.3 mg for adults to age 50; above 50, it increases to 1.5 mg for women and 1.7 mg for men.

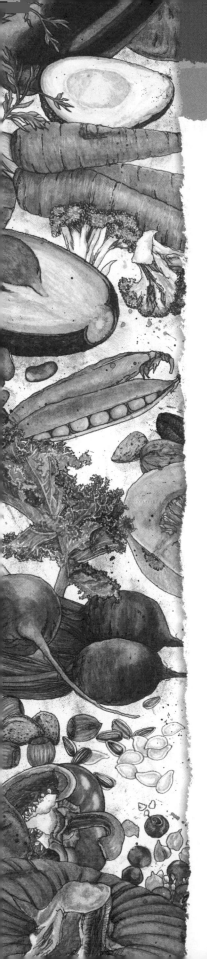

Clean, Strong Vegan Eating

A healthy body is a guest-chamber for the soul; a sick body is a prison.

FRANCIS BACON, ENGLISH PHILOSOPHER

E veryone is familiar with the saying "you are what you eat," but few recognize that the food they consume day after day is quite literally what their body is made of. Food is so much more than fuel. It provides the structural materials used to build, renew, and repair body tissues, as well as the raw resources needed to manufacture brain cells, muscles, bones, hormones, and enzymes. The only way people can ever hope to achieve and maintain optimal health is to select food as if it really matters—because it does.

Step one is to maximize the protective capacity of the diet by loading up on the foods that have the greatest potential to reduce disease risk. Step two is to minimize pathogenic factors that contribute to the onset and progression of disease. With each step, care must be taken to ensure nutritional adequacy. This is the essence of clean vegan eating.

Step One: Maximize Protective Capacity

S tep one is about making every calorie contribute to health and healing. Fortunately, plant foods are concentrated sources of the dietary components consistently linked with favorable health outcomes. Plants provide antioxidants, phytochemicals, phytosterols, fiber, enzymes, prebiotics, probiotics, essential fats, proteins, carbohydrates, vitamins, and minerals. Like a symphony, these compounds work together to turn off disease-promoting genes, reduce inflammation, boost immune function, balance hormones, enhance detoxification enzymes, maintain blood glucose levels, keep blood pressure and blood cholesterol levels in check, and support all the body's systems. Although these components are often isolated and sold as supplements, their effectiveness in supplement form is generally disappointing. Evidence suggests that their beneficial effects depend on complex synergies that exist among multiple protective compounds.

The balance and interaction among the essential nutrients—proteins, fats, carbohydrates, vitamins, and minerals—are critical in promoting and preserving health. These nutrients are aided by other protective compounds found in plant foods: phytochemicals, enzymes, phytosterols, and prebiotics. Although they're not considered essential, these compounds have a solid track record for promoting health and well-being and defending people against a vast array of chronic diseases.

PHYTOCHEMICALS

To enhance their own survival, all plants produce compounds called phytochemicals (*phyto* is the Greek name for "plant"). Some phytochemicals are responsible for plants' colors, flavors, textures, and fragrances and play a critical role in attracting pollinators and seed dispersers. Others act as an internal defense system that protects the plants from pests, pathogens, and potentially hostile environments. Because of individual plants' particular requirements, there may be as many as 100,000 different kinds of phytochemicals; often, thousands of copies of a hundred or more different phytochemicals can be found in a single plant.[1]

Fortunately, when plants are eaten, phytochemicals continue to work their magic in the human body. Whether serving as antioxidants, mimicking hormones, reducing inflammation, blocking tumor formation, eradicating carcinogens, stimulating enzymes, or destroying bacteria, phytochemicals have hundreds of mechanisms that help to prevent the onset of diseases and fight existing diseases.

Many factors can affect the quantity of phytochemicals in food, as well as their bioavailability. For example, agricultural factors, such as soil, water, climate, and the use of chemicals, influence phytochemical content. Organically grown produce must develop a more robust defense against assailants than plants protected by chemical pesticides, so its phytochemical content is correspondingly higher.[2-4] Conversely, storage methods after harvest can diminish phytochemical concentrations.

Food-refining methods dramatically reduce phytochemical content, especially when the most phytochemical-rich parts of plants (such as germ and bran from wheat grains) are removed, or when the processing involves exposure to harsh chemicals, heat, or pressure. Food preparation methods, such as cooking, sprouting, fermenting, blending, juicing, and processing, can have either positive or negative effects on phytochemical content and bioavailability.

Most phytochemicals are more efficiently absorbed from raw foods. For example, the absorption of isothiocyanates can be significantly higher from raw cruciferous vegetables than from cooked cruciferous vegetables.[5–8] In general, cooking tends to decrease phytochemical content; the greater the intensity and duration of heat exposure, the more significant the phytochemical losses. Not surprisingly, water-soluble phytochemicals are more readily lost when food is boiled, and the water discarded.

On the other hand, cooking softens or ruptures plant cell walls, making it easier for the body to extract and absorb certain types of phytochemicals, particularly carotenoids.[9, 10] For example, more lycopene is bioavailable from cooked tomatoes than raw tomatoes and more beta-carotene from cooked carrots than raw carrots.[11–17] Adding even a small amount of fat, such as avocado, tahini, or olive oil, improves carotenoid absorption from foods, raw or cooked.[18–23]

The bioavailability of phytochemicals from a raw food can be maximized by reducing the particle size of the food and increasing its surface area (by chopping, puréeing, processing, milling, mashing, or grating, or by chewing well).[21, 24, 25] Juicing is even more effective, because the process removes the plant cell walls, which contain fiber and other components known to reduce the bioavailability of nutrients and phytochemicals. Some carotenoids, such as alpha-carotene, beta-carotene, and lutein, appear to be more bioavailable from vegetable juice than from raw or cooked vegetables.[17, 26] Drinking vegetable juice can be a practical way to boost antioxidant and phytochemical intake without adding bulk to the diet.

Sprouting and fermenting significantly enhance a plant food's phytochemical content. [27–30] Scientific studies have shown that germinating a variety of plant foods yields remarkable increases in phytochemicals.[7, 29, 30–35] The rise in phytochemical content is understandable, because the life of a new plant depends on support and protection from these compounds.

Broccoli sprouts are a notable example; they contain ten to one hundred times more glucoraphanin (a glucosinolate and the precursor of sulforaphane) than mature broccoli.[7, 29] Sulforaphane (an isothiocyanate) is a potent natural inducer of the body's detoxifying Phase II enzymes, which process and eliminate carcinogens (see figure 7.1 on page 231). Sulforaphane has also been shown to be an impressive antimicrobial agent; it's highly effective against *Helicobater pylori (H. pylori),* an infective bacteria associated with gastritis, peptic ulcers, and stomach cancer.[36, 37] Recent evidence has also shown that broccoli sprouts may improve insulin resistance in patients with type 2 diabetes.[38] Finally, sulforaphane appears to reduce oxidative stress and tissue damage associated with a variety of disease states.[39]

Practical Implications: The most effective way to maximize phytochemical intake is to fill the plate with a wide variety of colorful plant foods. Including sprouts and fermented foods further boosts phytochemical content, as does choosing organic varieties.

While vegetables and fruits are commonly regarded as the primary suppliers of phytochemicals, these compounds are plentiful in all whole plant foods. Among the most celebrated phytochemical superstars are dark greens (such as kale, collard greens, and spinach), cruciferous vegetables (including broccoli, cabbage, and Brussels sprouts), sprouts (particularly broccoli sprouts), purple and blue fruits (for example, blueberries, blackberries, and grapes), allium vegetables (particularly garlic), herbs and spices (such as cinnamon, cloves, garlic, ginger, oregano, and turmeric), legumes (especially soybeans, small red beans, and other deeply colored beans), nuts and seeds (such as pecans, walnuts, and flaxseeds), cocoa beans, citrus fruits, tea, and tomatoes.

ENZYMES

The enzymes in raw plant foods promote health in two ways: they help to convert specific phytochemicals into their active forms, and they can aid digestion.

Enzymes in at least two families of plants convert phytochemicals into their highly beneficial active forms. The first is the myrosinase in cruciferous vegetables (such as broccoli, cabbage, kale, and turnips). Myrosinase converts glucosinolates into isothiocyanates, which are highly prized for their ability to induce Phase II enzymes.[40, 41] The second is the alliinase in allium vegetables (including members of the onion and garlic family). Alliinase converts alliin to allicin, its active form. Allicin fights microbes, bacteria, viruses, parasites, and fungal infections; reduces blood clots and lipid levels; curtails arthritis and cancer activity; and helps induce Phase II enzymes.[42]

Myrosinase and alliinase are released when the plant tissue is disrupted, for example, when the food is chopped, mashed, puréed, or chewed. (It's interesting to note that juicing cabbage results in high myrosinase activity in the juice; little remains in the cabbage pulp itself.)[43] Upon their release, enzymatic conversion of the phytochemicals into their active forms begins. Cooking destroys some or all of these enzymes, depending on the time and temperature used,[44] so eating some raw cruciferous and allium vegetables may provide a health advantage.

By further breaking down plant foods that were disrupted by processing or chewing, plant enzymes can make a small contribution to the digestive process. This process continues while food remains in the upper part of the stomach (it can be held there for twenty to sixty minutes after eating before being thoroughly mixed with gastric acid).[45, 46] It's unknown precisely how significant this stage of predigestion is to the entire digestive process. However, the vast majority of food digestion occurs in the small intestine, so the likely impact of food enzymes on human digestion is thought to be relatively small.[2] Once food drops to the lower part of the stomach and is exposed to gastric acid, its pH drops to about 1.3 to 2.5; at this pH level, the food enzymes are largely denatured or inactivated and don't typically survive into the small intestine.[45, 47, 48] Food enzymes with the greatest chance of surviving stomach acid and arriving intact in the small intestine are those packaged within viable microorganisms, as is the case with fermented foods.[49–51] For further information, see *Becoming Raw* by Brenda Davis and Vesanto Melina (Book Publishing Company, 2010).

Practical Implications: To maximize the amount of food enzymes present in vegetables and fruits, they should be eaten raw, with some cruciferous and allium vegetables in the mix. The addition of a variety of sprouts, as well as cultured and fermented foods, further boosts the content and functionality of food enzymes.

PHYTOSTEROLS

Plant sterols or phytosterols (including sterols and their saturated counterparts, stanols) are an essential part of cell membranes in plants, just as cholesterol is an essential part of cell membranes in animals. Phytosterols have a dual antiatherogenic effect. Because phytosterols are structurally similar to cholesterol, they compete for absorption sites with dietary cholesterol from animal products and can inhibit the absorption of cholesterol during digestion, effectively lowering total and LDL cholesterol levels. In addition, phytosterols blunt inflammatory pathways known to exacerbate atherosclerosis.[52–54]

Phytosterol intakes are directly proportional to the quantity of plant foods in a diet. Although all whole plant foods are sources of plant sterols, the most concentrated natural sources are seeds, nuts, legumes, wheat germ, avocados, sprouts, and vegetable oils. There's evidence that early human diets were rich in plant foods and provided as much as 1 gram of phytosterols per day.[55] Today, the average daily phytosterol intake in a mixed diet varies from about 150 to 450 mg.[53] Vegetarian diets are generally higher in plant sterols than mixed diets, with vegan diets supplying the most. One report noted that participants' raw vegan diets provided from 500 to more than 1,200 mg of plant sterols per day.[56]

Studies suggest that a daily intake of 2 grams of plant sterols reduces LDL cholesterol by approximately 9 to 15 percent in those with elevated blood cholesterol levels.[53] This level of intake is associated with the use of supplements or plant sterol–fortified foods.[52] The food industry now adds phytosterols to some products because of the associated cholesterol-lowering properties. Plant sterols are added to a wide variety of foods, including some margarines, mayonnaises, cereals, salad dressings, soy milks, granola bars, and fruit juices.

The US Food and Drug Administration allows manufacturers to include a health claim on the labels of these foods regarding the benefits of plant sterols. Although phytosterol-fortified products may provide some benefit for omnivores with elevated cholesterol, it makes little sense to add an unhealthy food to a diet just to boost phytosterol intake. Vegans who eat healthful diets already consume far more sterols than other dietary groups; also, they eat no cholesterol and have lower blood cholesterol levels.

For those who *do* take phytosterol supplements or use phytosterol-fortified foods, intakes exceeding 2 grams per day haven't been shown to provide added benefit; for some individuals, greater intakes are associated with adverse health effects.[53]

Practical Implications: The safest and most effective way to boost phytosterol intake is to eat a whole-foods vegan diet, including sprouts and higher-fat plant foods, such as seeds, nuts, wheat germ, and avocados. Vegans have no need for processed foods with added sterols.

PREBIOTICS AND PROBIOTICS

The intestinal tract buzzes with trillions of microorganisms. Of these, 99 percent are members of just thirty to forty species, although at least four hundred to five hundred different species are common residents. Microbial societies that reside in the gut (mainly the large intestine) are collectively called gut flora or microbiota. (These bacteria make up about 50 percent of fecal mass.)[57]

Although the body's relationship with gut flora is mutually beneficial for the most part, some guests are more welcome than others.[58] Friendly bacteria provide a number of impressive survival advantages. For example, they produce antimicrobial substances that defend against harmful bacteria. In the small intestine, good bacteria boost nutritional status by enhancing the absorption of several nutrients, recycling nitrogen, maintaining amino acid stores, and synthesizing certain vitamins (vitamin K and biotin).

Bacteria that reside in the large intestine are equipped with enzymes that can break down fiber that is resistant to human digestive enzymes. Among the by-products are short-chain fatty acids, which can provide more than 10 percent of daily caloric needs, favorably affect carbohydrate and fat metabolism,[59] and protect against colorectal cancer.[57, 60] In addition, beneficial bacteria support immune-system function, protect against food allergies, and play an important role in the development and maturation of intestinal tissues.[57] Gut bacteria and the cells lining the intestinal walls are in constant two-way communication.

If friendly gut flora aren't adequately supported, pathogenic bacteria can set up shop and multiply. These aggressive intruders can produce toxins that injure the lining of the gut (making it more permeable, or "leaky"), reduce immune function, increase chronic low-grade inflammation, generate infection, compromise metabolism, and contribute to overweight and obesity.[61–63]

Food choices influence whether the overall balance of gut flora is friendly or hostile. Foods or supplements that contain friendly microorganisms are known as probiotics; foods that support these healthy microbiota are known as prebiotics. Plant-based, high-fiber diets sustain the beneficial bacteria, while high-fat, low-fiber Western-style diets aid pathogenic bacteria. While the goal is not to eradicate harmful bacteria completely (the body needs some of them), both probiotics and prebiotics can help to shift the balance toward a more favorable mix.

Probiotics are viable microorganisms that arrive in the intestinal tract in an active form and exert beneficial health effects. Fermented or cultured foods or supplements can supply probiotics. Some of the best vegan sources of probiotics are nondairy yogurts (almond, coconut, or soy yogurt), fermented soy products (such as tempeh and miso), fermented nut or seed cheeses, fermented vegetables (sauerkraut), fermented grains (rejuvelac), and some types of tea.

Prebiotics provide indigestible, fermentable food components that stimulate the growth and activity of beneficial bacteria, usually by serving as their food supply.[64, 65] Prebiotics are particularly high in foods that contain sugars that can't be broken down by gastric enzymes (especially raw foods, such as chicory, Jerusalem artichokes, garlic, onions, leeks, bananas, asparagus, and sweet potatoes) or in foods fortified with prebiotics, such as fructooligosaccharides (inulin and oligofructose).[65, 66]

The value of both probiotics and prebiotics has been appreciated for centuries by cultures throughout the world, and is now strongly supported by research. Probiotics have been shown to prevent or diminish complaints associated with certain types of diarrhea, lactose intolerance, and irritable bowel syndrome. They reduce cancer-promoting enzymes and the toxic by-products of bad bacteria. Probiotics also appear to promote and protect the health of the gastrointestinal tract and reduce the complications associated with inflammatory bowel diseases and *H. pylori* infection. They can aid in the prevention of infectious diseases, such as respiratory tract infections (common cold or flu) and urogenital infections, as well as allergies and skin disorders in infants. There's weaker evidence that probiotics may play a favorable role in cholesterol reduction, cancer prevention, autoimmune diseases, and dental health.[64, 67, 68]

Each strain of probiotic bacteria has distinct health effects. Online research can show which strains are most effective in treating a specific condition; probiotic supplement labels include the genus, species, and strain. Experts suggest taking probiotics as soon as antibiotic therapy is initiated and for a few days after the prescribed antibiotics are finished. Generally, multispecies products are more effective than those with a single type of microorganism.[69] Most probiotics need to be refrigerated, and expiration dates are important; regardless of the particular strain, if the microorganisms are dead, they're no longer probiotics. Typical dosages vary with the product, but generally, higher dosages (from 5 to 10 billion colony-forming units [CFU] per day for children and 10 to 20 billion CFU per day for adults) are associated with better outcomes.[70]

Practical Implications: Well-planned vegan diets, which are naturally high in fiber and indigestible sugars, strongly support healthy gut flora by providing a ready source of prebiotics. Vegan diets that rely heavily on processed and refined foods fall short in this regard. Eating plenty of raw vegetables and fruits and adding some fermented or cultured foods to a diet can help to restore suboptimal gut flora, as can periodic use of a multistrain probiotic.

Step Two: Minimize Pathogenic Factors

S tep two shifts the focus to the reduction or elimination of dietary components linked with unfavorable health outcomes—not only refined carbohydrates, unhealthful fats, and excessive sodium but also allergens, chemical contaminants, and N-glycolylneuraminic acid (Neu5Gc; see page 272). Generally, these dietary constituents are more concentrated in animal products and highly processed foods. These components can threaten the goal of achieving a clean vegan diet in a variety of ways; they can turn on disease-promoting genes and can contribute to hypertension, insulin resistance, high blood cholesterol levels, inflammation, gastrointestinal disorders, and hormonal imbalances.

FOOD SENSITIVITIES

When the processes most likely to cause disease are considered, adverse reactions to food don't typically spring to mind. However, these reactions can significantly elevate disease risk.

Although the terms "food sensitivity," "food allergy," and "food intolerance" are often used interchangeably, food sensitivity is actually an umbrella term for both food allergy and food intolerance (also called nonallergic food hypersensitivity). A true food allergy is a reaction to an allergen (usually a protein) that the immune system views as a foreign invader. In most cases, this involves the release of histamine by an antibody called immunoglobulin (IgE), which leads to allergy symptoms, such as hives, eczema, runny nose, earache, shortness of breath, swelling, inflammation, and diarrhea. Eight foods account for 90 percent of food allergies: milk, eggs, peanuts, tree nuts, shellfish, fish, wheat, and soy.[71–75] Although allergies can begin at any age, most appear during early childhood and, in 90 percent of cases, are outgrown by the age of 7. The people most likely to remain allergic are those with severe life-threatening anaphylactic reactions or those with allergies to peanuts, tree nuts, or seafood.[76]

Nonallergic food hypersensitivities don't trigger an IgE-mediated immune response. Although symptoms can be similar to those listed above for a true food allergy, they're often delayed and generally less acute. While the immune system may respond, the reaction is quite distinct from the IgE-mediated immune response common to food allergies. With nonallergic food hypersensitivities, the adverse reaction is provoked by an abnormal metabolic, pharmacological, or gastrointestinal response to the food.[71, 72, 74]

Adverse metabolic reactions can occur when the body lacks the specific enzyme necessary to break down a food component. In a few cases, a serious inherited metabolic condition prevents the body from producing an enzyme. In other cases, the body may produce insufficient amounts of a particular enzyme. Symptoms arise as a result of the buildup of the unmetabolized food component or because of a resulting nutritional deficiency.

The most widespread example of such an enzyme deficiency is lactose intolerance. Beyond weaning age, about 70 percent of the global population produces insufficient lactase to completely break down the lactose in dairy products (fewer Europeans than Asians suffer from this condition).[77] When these people consume dairy products, lactose arrives undigested in the large intestine, causing gastrointestinal distress.

Pharmacological reactions result from ingesting food components that cause drug-like side effects in some individuals. For example, consumption of monosodium glutamate (MSG), a flavor enhancer commonly used in Chinese food, has been reported to cause flushing, headache, and abdominal symptoms in some people.[78] Other potentially problematic food components include sulfites in wine; tyramine in aged cheeses; theobromine in chocolate; and preservatives, colors, and flavors used in processed foods.

Gastrointestinal reactions are the category of adverse food reactions most strongly linked to chronic disease risk. Every inch of the gut provides a gateway to the body's interior in a way that no other organ does. The gut wall (lining of the gut) serves as a highly selective barrier. When it functions properly, it facilitates the absorption of essential nutrients (small molecules, such as amino acids, simple sugars, fatty acids, vitamins, minerals, antioxidants, and phytochemicals) and prevents the absorption of large, unwanted molecules (fragments of undigested protein, bacteria, and other potentially harmful compounds). This critical barrier can be breached when it's constantly in contact with food components that cause inflammation or injury.[79–82] Damage can also be induced by inflammatory diseases, such as Crohn's disease, or by stress, medications, environmental contaminants, radiation, or an excess of unfriendly gut microflora. In addition, if the epithelial cells lining the gut are injured, their ability to transport nutrients into circulation may be eroded, and malnutrition can result.

When the gut wall's integrity is compromised, a variety of unwanted molecules can leak into the bloodstream, setting off immune reactions and placing a significant burden on the body's detoxification systems. This process is often referred to as leaky-gut syndrome. Once unwanted compounds make their way into the circulatory system, hypersensitivity may manifest itself in a myriad of ways:

- anxiety or depression[83]
- asthma[84]
- autoimmune diseases[80]
- autism[85]
- cancer[79]
- cardiovascular disease[86]
- celiac disease and gluten hypersensitivity[80, 87]
- chronic fatigue[88]
- chronic low-grade inflammation[79, 81, 82]
- diabetes (type 1 and type 2)[80, 87, 89, 90]
- gastrointestinal disorders (diarrhea, bloating, irritable bowel syndrome, ulcerative colitis, Crohn's disease)[80, 91, 92]
- hormone abnormalities (leading to overweight and obesity)[90]
- insulin resistance or metabolic syndrome[82, 89, 90]
- joint and muscle issues (chronic pain, rheumatoid arthritis)[96, 97]
- liver dysfunction[93, 94]
- migraine[95]
- skin problems (itching, eczema, hives, acne, psoriasis)[98, 99]

Although any food can induce nonallergic food hypersensitivities, those most strongly associated with increased gut permeability are gluten (a protein in wheat, barley, rye, and related grains) and dairy proteins. In addition, Western diets rich in animal products and processed foods, which promote an imbalance in gut flora, are also implicated. Fortunately, when the factors responsible for increased gut permeability are removed and adequate nutrition is ensured, the intestinal lining can regenerate and heal itself. For some individuals, supplements such as L-glutamine, probiotics, zinc, and omega-3 fatty acids may be helpful.

To defend the gut, it's also important to properly identify offending foods. Traditional allergy testing (which is only moderately effective in identifying true allergies) generally isn't helpful in identifying nonallergic food hypersensitivities. Instead, an elimination diet followed by an oral food challenge is suggested.[72] This involves eliminating suspect foods for a period of time (usually two to four weeks), followed by a test dose to see if symptoms redevelop, sometimes in increasing amounts over the course of a day. When several food culprits are suspected, a few-foods elimination diet may be appropriate; a small number of low-risk foods are consumed, new foods are introduced one at a time at two-day intervals, and reactions are tracked to pinpoint the offending food. For more information on food allergies, nonallergic food hypersensitivities, gut health, and elimination diets, see *The Food Allergy Survival Guide* by Vesanto Melina, Jo Stepaniak, and Dina Aronson (Book Publishing Company, 2004) and *The Health Professional's Guide to Food Allergies* by Janice Joneja (Academy of Nutrition and Dietetics, 2013).

Practical Implications: Food sensitivities can be significant players in many disease processes. People who struggle with unsolved health issues should consider adverse food reactions as a potential contributor. In some cases, exploration using an elimination diet is warranted.

CHEMICAL CONTAMINANTS

Hazardous materials that enter the food chain unintentionally during growth, harvesting, storage, processing, packaging, or preparation can taint food. Contamination can also occur as a result of the intentional use of agrochemicals or chemicals used in food processing. Many of these substances persist in the environment, working their way up the food chain (and becoming more concentrated) as plants are eaten by animals and animals are eaten by humans. All these compounds can have adverse consequences for human health.[100] Unfortunately, the more polluted the world becomes, the greater the exposure to contaminants.

The most common sources are processed foods, animal products, and conventionally grown produce. Meat, poultry, and fish can be high in such contaminants; land animals typically consume considerable quantities in their fodder, and fish accumulate chemicals from polluted waters.

Food contaminants can adversely affect health by causing birth defects, nervous system injury, hormone disruption, damage to vital organs, and increased risk of chronic disease. Although it's impossible to eliminate food contaminants, limiting the major dietary sources of these contaminants can effectively minimize intake. Food contaminants fall into four main categories:

1. **Products of high-temperature cooking.** Heterocyclic amines, polycyclic aromatic hydrocarbons, advanced glycation end-products, and acrylamide can be formed when foods are exposed to heat.

2. **Environmental contaminants.** Heavy metals (such as arsenic, cadmium, lead, and mercury); persistent organic pollutants, or POPs (such as DDT, dioxins, and polychlorinated biphenyls, or PCBs); and chemicals in packaging materials (such as bisphenol A, or BPA, and phthalates) can move up the food chain.

3. **Agrochemicals.** Pesticides applied to plants and veterinary drugs (antibiotics and hormones) given to animals are part of the industrialized food package.

4. **Artificial food additives.** Artificial food colors, flavors, sweeteners, and preservatives (such as sodium nitrate and nitrite and sulfites) add flavor, function, and stability to processed foods.

Food Contaminants of Concern for Vegans and Nonvegans

Acrylamide

Major food sources: Processed potato products (such as chips and French fries), crackers, crispbread, pretzels, toast, cold cereal, and starchy foods processed or cooked at 248 degrees F (120 degrees C) or higher.

Associated health risks: Probable carcinogen; may damage DNA and nervous system.[101–103]

Advanced glycation end-products

Major food sources: Foods cooked or processed at temperatures of 310 degrees F (155 degrees C) or higher; fried meat (especially fried processed meat), fried chicken, processed cheese, and other fried foods, such as fried potatoes.

Associated health risks: Impaired immune-system function, accelerated aging, diabetes, cardiovascular disease, stroke, kidney disease, eye diseases, nerve diseases, and Alzheimer's disease.[104–106]

Arsenic

Major food sources: Rice (organic, conventional, brown, or white), rice products (pasta, flour, crackers, syrup, milk, cereal, bran), fish and shellfish, seaweed (especially hijiki), chicken, fruit juice, and drinking water.

Associated health risks: Hormone disruption, DNA damage, cancer, diabetes, cardiovascular disease, neuropathy, brain injury, low birth weight, stillbirth, respiratory damage, and liver diseases.[107–110]

Artificial food colors and flavors

Major food sources: Processed foods with added synthetic dyes or flavors, including beverages, snack foods, desserts, baked goods, crackers, cookies, candies, chips, spice blends, soups, sauces, salmon, beef, and oranges (which are sometimes sprayed with artificial color).

Associated health risks: Varies. In some cases, food allergy or sensitivity, learning impairment, and behavioral changes.[111–114]

Artificial sweeteners

Major food sources: "Diabetic" foods, sugar-free foods (such as gum, baked goods, frozen desserts, jam, jelly, sweets), sugar-free beverages, and sugar substitutes.

Associated health risks: Differs widely with each sweetener. Food allergy or sensitivity; some may have adverse neurological effects; may negatively affect appetite control.[115–117]

Bisphenol A (BPA)

Major food sources: Plastic food containers, plastic bags, epoxy resins used to coat food- and beverage-can interiors.

Associated health risks: Endocrine disruption (with potential adverse effects on the reproductive system, development and maintenance of the brain and nervous system, growth, and metabolism), heart problems, and possible link to some cancers; risk is highest for infants and children.[118, 119]

DDT

Major food sources: Fish, shellfish, meat, and dairy products; smaller amounts in produce.

Associated health risks: Nervous system damage, endocrine disruption, DNA damage, cancer, low birth weight, premature birth, and diabetes.[120]

Lead

Major food sources: Food or beverages cooked, served, or stored in glazed pottery (especially from Mexico or Asia), imported candies and candy wrappers, and seasonings (especially from Mexico, such as chili powder).

Associated health risks: Brain injury in children, nervous system damage, hypertension, and liver damage.[121, 122]

Pesticides (including herbicides, insecticides, fungicides, and rodenticides)

Major food sources: Conventionally grown produce (especially leafy greens and items consumed with skin, such as apples, berries, peaches, and pears). Lesser amounts in grains, legumes, nuts, seeds, and animal products.

Associated health risks: Varies. In some cases, cancer, nervous system damage, and birth defects.[123, 124]

Phthalates

Major food sources: Foods in contact with plastics and vinyls, especially high-fat foods, such as full-fat dairy products, meat, fish, and oil.

Associated health risks: Suspected endocrine disruptor, possible increased cancer risk, and developmental and reproductive abnormalities at high levels of intake.[125, 126]

Polycyclic aromatic hydrocarbons

Major food sources: Foods cooked at high temperatures (especially when blackened) grilled meats, smoked fish, processed grain products, and heated fats and oils.

Associated health risks: DNA damage; endocrine disruption; lung, skin, and genitourinary cancers.[127, 128]

Sulfites

Major food sources: Dried and glazed fruit, fruit juice, wine, cider, beer, processed foods (cheese slices, baked goods, condiments, cereal, crackers, deli meats, dressings, gravies, shellfish, snack foods, starches, sweet sauces, and shredded coconut), and dehydrated potatoes, vegetables, and herbs.

Associated health risks: Hypersensitivity, especially in asthmatics.[129, 130]

Food Contaminants Minimized or Avoided in a Vegan Diet

Antibiotics and antimicrobial agents

Major food sources: Meat, poultry, fish, shellfish, and dairy products.

Associated health risks: Antibiotic resistance in pathogenic organisms (making antibiotics less effective for humans). In some cases, allergy, alterations in intestinal flora, endocrine disruption, and DNA toxicity.[131]

Cadmium

Major food sources: Shellfish, liver, and kidneys.

Associated health risks: Kidney damage, lung damage, and stomach irritation.[132]

Dioxins

Major food sources: Fish, shellfish, meat, and dairy products.

Associated health risks: Cancer, endocrine disruption, skin problems, immune suppression, and reproductive abnormalities.[133, 134]

Heterocyclic amines

Major food sources: Muscle meat (beef, pork, poultry, and fish), especially grilled or fried; other animal products and organ meats (in much smaller amounts).

Associated health risks: DNA damage; colorectal, stomach, pancreatic, and breast cancers.[1, 135]

Hormones

Major food sources: Beef and dairy products.

Associated health risks: Endocrine disruption; some may increase risk of breast, prostate, and colon cancer.[136–138]

N-glycolylneuraminic Acid (Neu5Gc)

There's significant evidence that meat—especially red meat—increases cancer risk.[1] Scientists recently discovered one more possible contributor to this link: Neu5Gc. Neu5Gc is a sialic acid found in the flesh and milk of all mammals except humans, who lack the enzyme responsible for its formation. Scientists have observed that Neu5Gc accumulates in human tumors, particularly those of the colon, breast, and retina, and in melanocytes (dark pigments, mainly in the skin).

Although scientists aren't certain how and why Neu5Gc is associated with cancer, it appears as though antibodies to Neu5Gc trigger a chronic low-grade inflammation. This in turn promotes the secretion of growth factors that draw nutrients into the area, essentially feeding cancer cells.[146, 147]

Mercury

Major food sources: Fish (highest in large predatory fish).

Associated health risks: Nervous system damage.[139–141]

Polychlorinated biphenyls (PCBs)

Major food sources: Fish (highest in biggest, oldest fish and bottom feeders) and foods containing animal fat (milk and other dairy products, meat, eggs, and poultry).

Associated health risks: Nervous system damage, cancer, endocrine disruption, immune suppression, hearing loss, and liver, skin, and vision damage.[142, 143]

Sodium nitrite and sodium nitrate

Major food sources: Cured meat, poultry, and fish.

Associated health risks: Possible link to cancer (specifically stomach, esophageal, and colon cancers); possible link to Alzheimer's disease, type 2 diabetes, and Parkinson's disease; possible teratogen.[144, 145]

Protection against Environmental Contaminants: A Vegan Advantage

The primary reservoirs of environmental contaminants are animal products (including fish and shellfish), processed foods, conventionally grown produce, and other plant foods sprayed with pesticides. Although studies are limited, the evidence to date suggests that vegetarians and vegans have reduced exposure to chemical contaminants, compared to nonvegetarians.[148] Vegetarian women have been reported to have lower levels of environmental chemicals in their breast milk than nonvegetarian women.[149–151] One study compared the concentrations of seven contaminants in the breast milk of 12 vegans with that of the general US population. For all contaminants except PCBs, the highest vegan value was lower than the lowest value in the general population. (For PCBs, there were no significant differences between groups.) For three contaminants, the mean vegan levels were only 1 to 2 percent that of the average levels in the general population.[150]

A study from India found lower levels of organochlorine pesticides (also known as persistent organic pollutants, or POPs) in the maternal blood of vegetarians compared to nonvegetarians.[152] A second Indian study among various dietary groups examined the levels of two hormone-disrupting chemicals (PCBs and phthalate esters) associated with male infertility and deterioration of semen quality; concentrations were highest among urban fish eaters and lowest among rural vegetarians.[153]

Vegans from Hong Kong had less than one-tenth the concentrations of hair mercury than nonvegetarians.[154] A Swedish study reported that a change from a mixed to a lactovegetarian diet for just twelve months resulted in lower levels of mercury, lead, and cadmium in hair.[155] A recent Korean study reported significant reductions in urinary levels of three antibiotics, four phthalate metabolites, and one marker of oxidative stress (malondialdehyde) in 25 adults who switched to a completely vegetarian diet during a five-day stay at a Buddhist temple.[156]

One French study that calculated exposure to 421 pesticides found no advantage for vegans, vegetarians, pescovegetarians, and near-vegetarians (collectively called the veg-groups) relative to the general population.[157] In fact, participants in the veg-groups were found to have had excessive exposure to forty-one to forty-four pesticides (thirty for pescovegetarians), while the general population had excessive exposure to only twenty-nine pesticides. This difference was attributable to the higher vegetable and fruit intakes of people eating plant-based diets. On the other hand, exposure to the highly toxic organochlorine pesticides was only about half as great among veg-groups compared to the general population (these types of pesticides are concentrated in animal commodities, such as meat, eggs, and dairy products). The authors concluded that among this relatively small group of vegetarians, the intake of pesticides from plants was largely offset by the reduced intake of organochlorine pesticides from animal products. They added that even if vegetarians have increased risk of exposure to some pesticides, their diets provide better overall health advantages.

Practical Implications: Although exposure to a wide variety of chemical contaminants is reduced in vegan diets compared to omnivorous diets, additional steps can be taken to minimize risk:

- **Buy organic.** By choosing organic foods, pesticide residues are minimized. If expense is a concern, select organic for items with the highest pesticide levels and conventional for those with the lowest level. Generally, foods eaten with their skins (apples, peaches, pears, and berries) pose a greater risk of pesticide contamination than those eaten with the peel removed (pineapples, bananas, kiwifruit, and melons). (For a list of produce most likely to be high in pesticides, check Resources on page 449.)

- **Buy local.** Produce from local farmers' markets tends to have fewer pesticides, even if it's not organic.

- **Plant a garden.** Growing produce is an economical way to eat organic. Container gardens can be grown anywhere.

- **Wash or peel produce before eating.** Although pesticides can't be completely removed by washing foods (pesticides penetrate the skin), washing produce does reduce total pesticide content, as does peeling.

- **Reduce consumption of highly processed foods.** Processed foods often contain food additives, preservatives, and products of oxidation. Minimize intake of deep-fried foods and foods subjected to high heat for long periods of time.

- **Vary intake of whole grains.** Rice contains higher levels of arsenic than other grains; including a variety of whole grains helps to minimize exposure. (See page 269 for foods made from rice.)

- **Minimize use of hijiki.** Although all seaweed can be contaminated by heavy metals and other pollutants in oceans, hijiki is particularly high in arsenic. Occasional, moderate intake (for example, a small amount in a restaurant meal) is safe for most people.

- **Minimize exposure to potentially dangerous packaging materials.** Select glass containers instead of plastic for storing and reheating food. If using plastic, purchase products free of BPA. Avoid putting hot foods into plastic containers or heating foods in plastic. Avoid imported canned foods (due to potential lead seams) or foods stored in lead-glazed or leaded glassware.

- **Eat more raw foods.** Reduce exposure to the harmful by-products of cooking by eating raw foods.

- **Use methods of cooking that reduce the formation of toxic compounds.** Steaming, stewing, and braising produce fewer harmful by-products than frying, grilling, and broiling. When high heat is used, don't blacken or overcook foods.

The Power of the Plate

Regardless of age, genetic makeup, physical activity level, or state of health, people share two key dietary goals: to be adequately nourished and to avoid (or reverse) diet-induced chronic disease. What type of vegan diet best accomplishes these tasks—low-fat, macrobiotic, Mediterranean, nutrient-dense, raw, starch-based, whole foods, or fruitarian? Although different authorities offer different answers, each person's body is unique, and what works best for one may not be best for all. In addition, an individual's needs change over the course of a lifetime, and diets must be adjusted accordingly.

The optimal diet is one that's as good for the brain, bones, heart, and intestines as it is for the waistline—and it must supply all nutritional needs. Whatever pattern is selected, follow The Vegan Plate guidelines in chapter 14. Pay careful attention to vitamin B_{12} intake, and for those with insufficient sun exposure, to vitamin D needs. The ultimate goal is to design a diet that moves vegans beyond nutritional adequacy to nutritional excellence.

The following is a list of common vegan diets, their strengths and weaknesses, and how each variation works for the healthiest results.

Diet: Conventional (moderate, varied vegan diet; about 30 percent of calories from fat)

Strengths: It isn't difficult to achieve nutritional adequacy on a conventional vegan diet, which has proved protective against chronic disease. This liberal regimen is socially accommodating, and foods are relatively accessible.

Weaknesses: With poor choices, foods rich in protein, iron, and zinc (such as legumes) or calcium (such as fortified nondairy milks) may be lacking. When refined carbohydrates are used as staples, benefits are eroded.

Making it work: Eat a wide variety of raw and cooked plant foods, carefully selecting fortified foods to include in the mix. Meet the recommended intakes for each food group.

Diet: Fast Food (high use of packaged foods and restaurant fare)

Strengths: This diet is convenient for busy people. With its reliance on prepared foods that often are fortified with iron, B vitamins (including B_{12}), and vitamin D, intakes of these nutrients are boosted.

Weaknesses: Convenience foods are high in added fats, sugars, and sodium and low in protective phytochemicals, antioxidants, and fiber. These foods also may be expensive.

Making it work: Learn to read labels. Choose foods with short ingredient lists and minimal added fat, sugar, and salt. Use nutritious convenience foods, such as salads and fresh-pressed vegetable juices from the deli counter, ready-to-eat vegetable crudités, hummus with whole wheat pita bread, legume-based soups, whole-grain breakfast cereals, fortified nondairy milks and yogurts, and fruit.

Diet: Fruitarian (at least 75 percent fruit, including nonsweet fruits, such as tomatoes or avocados)

Strengths: A fruitarian diet is low in calories and fat and high in phytochemicals and antioxidants. It avoids common allergens.

Weaknesses: A fruit-based diet may not provide enough protein, essential fatty acids, or important vitamins and minerals. It's unsuitable for children. Dental erosion is common.

Making it work: Include organic greens, nuts, seeds, and sprouted or cooked legumes. Foods used in fruitarian diets aren't fortified, so a vitamin B_{12} supplement is essential; a vitamin D supplement will also be needed with insufficient access to sunshine; ensure a source of iodine.

Diet: Low-Fat (less than 15 percent fat)

Strengths: A low-fat vegan diet minimizes harmful fats and is effective for weight loss and for treating cardiovascular diseases and type 2 diabetes. It's generally rich in nutrient-dense foods, such as vegetables, fruits, and legumes.

Weaknesses: Such diets may be low in essential fatty acids and vitamin E and may not support optimal absorption of fat-soluble vitamins and phytochemicals. They may increase serum triglyceride levels if refined carbohydrates are emphasized. In addition, a low-fat diet may not provide enough calories for children or those who are underweight or very active.

Making it work: Meet the recommended servings for all food groups, including nuts and seeds that provide omega-3 fatty acids.

Diet: Macrobiotic

Strengths: A macrobiotic diet is focused on whole foods and is low in processed foods, including refined flour products.

Weaknesses: Such diets may not provide enough iron, zinc, lysine, essential fatty acids, or vitamins B_{12} and D. They may also have low nutrient density due to their heavy reliance on grains.

Making it work: Include plenty of vegetables, fruits, legumes, nuts, and seeds. Because fortified foods are typically avoided, reliable sources of iodine and vitamins B_{12} and D must be ensured.

Diet: Mediterranean

Strengths: A vegan version of the Mediterranean diet includes generous amounts of legumes, vegetables, fruits, whole grains, nuts, and seeds and limits processed foods. This diet is filling and flavorful, and its use is associated with a low risk of chronic diseases.

Weaknesses: Such diets may be too high in fat for those who are overweight or have high cholesterol. If wine is emphasized, cancer risk may be increased.

Making it work: Rely more on nuts, seeds, avocados, and olives for fat and less on oils. Select whole-grain instead of white flour products.

Diet: Nutrient-Dense

Strengths: A nutrient-dense diet emphasizes vegetables and other whole foods and provides abundant vitamins and minerals while minimizing processed foods and oils. When designed well, it's highly effective for the prevention and treatment of chronic disease.

Weaknesses: This diet doesn't necessarily take into account harmful factors, such as products of oxidation from cooking, environmental contaminants, and free radicals.

Making it work: Include the recommended servings from each food group. Use supplements when indicated. Include plenty of beans and greens.

Diet: Raw

Strengths: A raw diet minimizes the use of processed foods and avoids common allergens. It's also low in damaging dietary components and high in protective components, and avoids problems related to cooking, such as loss of nutrients and phytochemicals and formation of carcinogens. It's highly effective in the prevention and treatment of chronic disease.

Weaknesses: If not planned well, a raw diet may fall short of recommended intakes for protein, iron, zinc, calcium, iodine, and vitamins B_{12} and D. Food prep can be labor-intensive. A raw diet can be expensive if based on specialty products. Raw diets aren't recommended for infants and children.

Making it work: Ensure that all nutritional and calorie needs are met. Eat sprouted or cooked legumes to boost protein, iron, and zinc. (Raw diets may include up to 25 percent cooked foods.) Soak, sprout, juice, blend, dehydrate, and ferment foods to increase the concentration and availability of nutrients. For practical guidelines and delicious recipes with nutritional analyses, see *Becoming Raw* by Brenda Davis and Vesanto Melina (Book Publishing Company, 2010) and *The Raw Food Revolution Diet* by Cherie Soria, Brenda Davis, and Vesanto Melina (Book Publishing Company, 2008).

Diet: Starch-Based

Strengths: Starch-based diets are filling and practical; they're typically affordable and low in fat and include only moderate amounts of processed foods.

Weaknesses: Because most grains and starchy vegetables provide fewer minerals and vitamins and less protein than nonstarchy vegetables or legumes, such diets may have a low nutrient density. They may be low in essential fatty acids and lysine and can be nutritionally inadequate for people with very low caloric intakes.

Making it work: Eat nine servings of vegetables and fruits and at least 1 ounce (30 g) of nuts and seeds each day. Include legumes for more concentrated protein and select nutrient-dense starches, such as quinoa and yams. Ensure reliable sources of iodine and vitamins B_{12} and D.

Diet: Whole Foods

Strengths: When well planned, whole-foods diets are high in antioxidants, phytochemicals, fiber, vitamins, and minerals. Such diets are also affordable and low in sodium, added fat, and sugar. They're effective in the prevention and treatment of chronic disease.

Weaknesses: A diet focused on whole foods may lack iodine and vitamins B_{12} and D. Food prep can be labor intensive.

Making it work: Include some lightly processed foods (tofu, fortified nondairy milks, and nondairy yogurt) to boost nutrient intake and make preparation easier. Ensure reliable sources of iodine and vitamins B_{12} and D.

Practical Implications: To maximize the protective capacity of any vegan diet, eat more whole plant foods and fewer highly processed products. Table 8.1 (page 278) provides guidelines for making optimal food choices within each food category. For amounts and serving sizes, see The Vegan Plate on page 434.

TABLE 8.1. Clean, green food choices

FOOD CATEGORY	BEST CHOICES	CONSIDERATIONS
Vegetables	All vegetables and fresh-pressed vegetable juices, especially dark leafy greens	Choose organic when possible. Eat low-oxalate greens (bok choy, kale, napa cabbage, and watercress, as well as collard, dandelion, mustard, and turnip greens) for calcium. Eat at least half the vegetables raw. Focus on moist cooking methods and don't overcook. Include a fat source in salad dressings. Choose orange or yellow starchy vegetables (yams, squash). Add fresh vegetable juices for a boost in highly absorbable antioxidants and phytochemicals.
Fruits	All fruits, fresh, frozen, and dried	Eat mainly fresh, organic fruits; cooking depletes vitamin C. Use fresh or dried fruits as sweeteners. Fruit smoothies provide a simple, tasty way to increase fruit intake and can serve as an almost-instant meal if protein and fat sources, such as nuts, seeds, plant protein, and greens, are added.
Legumes	Beans, lentils, peas, and their sprouts, as well as soy foods and peanuts	Eat beans or lentils each day. Soak or sprout dried legumes before cooking. Enjoy sprouted mung beans, lentils, and peas. Include soy products, such as fortified soy milk, tofu, tempeh, and other traditional foods; choose organic when possible. Moderate use of meat substitutes, which often are heavily processed and high in sodium.
Whole grains	Sprouted, intact, cut, or rolled whole grains and pseudograins (amaranth, buckwheat, quinoa, wild rice)	Sprouting dramatically increases phytochemical and lysine content and reduces compounds that inhibit nutrient absorption. Pseudograins are more nutrient-dense than other grains and are gluten-free. Use intact grains when possible. Moderate the use of flour products even if whole-grain. Limit processed products, such as flaked and puffed whole-grain cereals. Minimize refined grains.
Nuts	Nuts, nut butters, and nut cheeses	Soak nuts to improve digestibility, boost phytochemical content, and decrease compounds that inhibit nutrient absorption. Walnuts provide omega-3 fatty acids. Select natural nut butters. Limit intake of roasted nuts, especially when roasted in oil and salt or coated in sugar.
Seeds	Seeds and seed butters	Sprout seeds for added nutrition. Soak to improve digestibility, increase phytochemical content, and decrease compounds that inhibit nutrient absorption. Use natural seed butters and omega-3-rich seeds (chia seeds, hempseeds, and ground flaxseeds).
Sea vegetables	All except hijiki, if from clean waters	Sea vegetables provide essential fats and iodine but may be contaminated if sourced from polluted waters. Avoid hijiki due to arsenic contamination; if used occasionally, keep servings very small.
Fats and oils	Mechanically pressed oils rich in monounsaturated fats or omega-3s	Limit use of added oils. Select organic oils to reduce toxins and store in the refrigerator. For salads, use oils rich in omega-3 fatty acids. For cooking, use small amounts of organic olive, canola, coconut, or high-oleic oils. Minimize use of processed fats, such as margarine.
Sweeteners	Dried fruit sugars, blackstrap molasses	Avoid use of refined sugars. Sugars made from whole foods, such as dates, are more nutritious options. Blackstrap molasses is the most nutrient-rich sweetener. Choose organic.

THE PALEO DIET: FACING THE FACTS

Paleolithic diets are currently the rage, attracting athletes, dieters, and health seekers of all stripes. The basic premise of the so-called "paleo" diet is simple—the diet humans ate in preagricultural, Paleolithic times is best suited for human health. Whether or not what these relatively short-lived humans ate is what's optimal for the health of today's relatively long-lived humans is a matter of considerable debate.

Preagricultural diets—which essentially consisted of wild plants, wild animals, and wild fish—varied considerably, depending on location, season, hunting and gathering skills, available tools, and so on. People didn't consume oil, sugar, or salt; anything from a box or bag; or the milk of other mammals. Today's new paleo devotees attempt to copy this diet by eating meat, poultry, fish, eggs, vegetables, fruits, nuts, and seeds and avoiding processed foods, grains, legumes, and dairy products.

Followers of the new paleo diet naturally assume that their nutrient intakes approximate that of Paleolithic humans, but their actual intakes may be wide of the mark. Nutritional anthropologists have been estimating the nutrient intakes of cavemen for several decades. As it turns out, vegan diets may actually come closer to matching the macro- and micronutrient intakes of Paleolithic diets than new paleo diets. Table 8.2 (page 280) summarizes the results of a comparison among recommended paleo menus, recommended vegan menus, and a true Paleolithic diet eaten by early humans. The data compare three days of recommended paleo menus from a popular paleo website, three days of recommended vegan menus from chapter 14 in this book, and the estimated average daily intakes of Paleolithic people.

Table 8.2 also provides dietary reference intakes (DRIs) for adult males (M) and adult females (F) who aren't pregnant or lactating. Where the DRI differs by gender, a notation is made (also see pages 446 and 447). Nutrients and other dietary factors in the new paleo or vegan diet that are more similar to the true Paleolithic diet are highlighted (dark green for the new paleo diet and light green for the vegan diet).

The comparison shows that this recommended new paleo menu supplies protein, vitamin A, and zinc in amounts closer to a true Paleolithic diet than do the vegan menus. However, its fat and saturated fat levels are about double, cholesterol almost triple, and sodium five times as much as that of a true Paleolithic diet. In addition, the new paleo menu contains about a third of the carbohydrate and fiber and half the vitamin C and calcium of true Paleolithic diets.

Even the 100 percent plant-based vegan menus deliver fiber in amounts at the lowest end of the estimated Paleolithic intake range; clearly our preagricultural ancestors ate plenty of plants (the only source of fiber). The vegan menus do provide intakes of carbohydrate, fat, saturated fat, fiber, riboflavin, thiamin, vitamin C, vitamin E, iron, calcium, sodium, and potassium that are closer to the levels supplied by a true Paleolithic diet than do the new paleo menus.

Why are new paleo diets and the true Paleolithic diet so far apart nutritionally? The answer lies in the differences between the meat and vegetables consumed today and those eaten in the Paleolithic era. The wild animals eaten back then

TABLE 8.2. New paleo, true Paleolithic, and vegan diets compared

	DRI	NEW PALEO DIET	TRUE PALEOLITHIC DIET	VEGAN DIET
Energy (cal/day)	2,200–2,900	3,000	3,000	3,000
MACRONUTRIENTS				
Protein (%)	10–35	32	25–30	14
Carbohydrate (%)	45–65	15	35–65	57
Fat (%)	15–30	53	20–35	29
Saturated fat (%)	< 10	19	6–12	6
Cholesterol (mg)		1,308	500+	0
Omega-6: omega-3 (ratio)		11:1	2:1	4:1
Fiber (g/day)	25 (F) 38 (M)	31	70–150	70
VITAMINS				
Riboflavin (mg)	1.3 (F) 1.7 (M)	2.6	6.5	2.8
Thiamin (mg)	1.1 (F) 1.2 (M)	2.7	3.9	4.6
Vitamin C (mg)	75 (F) 90 (M)	226	500	417
Vitamin A (mcg RAE)	700 (F) 900 (M)	2,436	3,797	1,513
Vitamin E (mg)	15	24	32.8	31.3
MINERALS				
Iron (mg)	8 (M) 18 (F)*	25	87.4	32.3
Zinc (mg)	8 (F) 11 (M)	33	43.4	21.3
Calcium (mg)	1,000–1,200	643	1,000–1,500	1,847
Sodium (mg)	< 2,300	4,193	768	2,005
Potassium (mg)	2,600–3,400	4,762	7,000	6,724

Sources: New paleo data: average of three days (Wednesday, Thursday, and Friday) of recommended Paleo menus, adjusted to 3,000 kcal.[158] Vegan data: average of three days from the menus on pages 439 to 442, adjusted to 3,000 calories. True Paleolithic data[159, 160]

*DRI for iron is 18 mg for women of childbearing age and 8 mg after age 50.

provided an estimated 6 to 16 percent of calories from fat compared to about 40 to 60 percent in today's domestic animals—even those that are grass-fed. They were also free of hormones, antibiotics, and environmental contaminants. All animal organs were consumed, and insects provided significant amounts of protein. In addition, virtually all fruits and vegetables available in supermarkets are more palatable, more digestible, and easier to store and transport than their wild cousins, at the expense of valuable protective dietary components. Wild or uncultivated plants provide about four times the fiber of commercial plants (13.3 grams of fiber per 100 grams versus 4.2 grams of fiber per 100 grams, respectively).[160]

Certainly, there are some benefits to switching from a standard Western diet to a paleo-type diet—highly processed foods, refined carbohydrates, fried foods, and fast foods are eliminated, and fresh fruits, vegetables, nuts, and seeds are encouraged. On the other hand, today's paleo eaters tend to include more meat than did early humans, ignoring the impressive evidence linking meat consumption to risk of chronic disease.

Grains and legumes are dispensed with, even though these foods have a long and impressive track record as valuable sources of calories and protein for the world's population. Consumption of legumes and grains is common to all Blue-Zone populations (where people live exceptionally long and healthy lives; see page 110), which validates their place in healthful diets.

Modern paleo advocates claim that these foods weren't part of Paleolithic-era diets, but new research challenges that assumption.[161] They also argue that lectins naturally present in these starchy foods are harmful to human health. Consuming too many lectins can cause significant gastrointestinal distress. However, because legumes and grains are almost always consumed in a cooked form—and lectins are destroyed during cooking—eating beans and grains doesn't result in lectin overload. Sprouting also reduces lectin levels in plants, although not as effectively as cooking. Generally, pea sprouts, lentil sprouts, and mung bean sprouts are safe to consume, as are sprouted grains, which are naturally low in lectins. Most larger legumes contain higher amounts and should be cooked.

The Bottom Line: With its emphasis on eating large quantities of meat, the new paleo diet is a poor imitation of the diets of early humans. Unfortunately, this dietary pattern also ignores the numerous health risks associated with eating meat and the ethical issues that result from an increased demand for food animals. Of the 11 billion animals killed for food every year in North America, 95 percent are raised in factory-farm conditions. While new paleo eaters encourage the use of free-range animals, these products are less affordable and less available to the average consumer than those from animals raised in confinement. Paleo proponents also ignore the looming environmental crisis that makes eating lower on the food chain an ecological imperative. People who try to imitate the diets of our ancestors are forgetting that the world is no longer home to a few million people—instead it must support several billion people. Individuals who want to move closer to a true Paleolithic diet may wish to explore plant-based diets—such diets capture the benefits of eating unprocessed foods without the immense collateral damage.

The Occasional Indulgence

Becoming vegan is like embarking on an exciting culinary adventure. Today, few foods haven't been effectively "veganized." The local natural food supermarket stocks vegan versions of peanut butter cups, chicken-style nuggets, croissants, pizza, cream cheese, marshmallows, ice cream bars, mayonnaise, spare ribs, and even calamari. Becoming vegan doesn't preclude birthday cake, ice cream sundaes, or Christmas cookies. And vegan chefs are redefining vegan cuisine with spectacular award-winning dishes. As a result, the transition to a vegan diet can be a little less daunting than it used to be.

Contrary to the impression that becoming vegan involves endless dietary sacrifices, most vegans indulge once in a while—and that's okay. However, a safe level of indulgence depends on an individual's overall state of health, as well as energy needs. Healthy and active people have more room for an occasional treat than those who are unhealthy or inactive. People fighting serious disease have far less leeway. It's best for them to ensure that every morsel that crosses their lips promotes health and healing.

When indulging in a treat, there's no comparison between the taste of manufactured foods and the flavors of fresh whole foods. For example, homemade fermented almond cream cheese is fresher and more appealing than commercial vegan cream cheese. Vegan pizza made from scratch tastes better and is less expensive than the frozen vegan pizza from the store. Banana-mango ice cream made with frozen fruit is more flavorful than commercial vegan ice cream.

Once taste buds become accustomed to the brighter flavors of fresh whole foods, commercial products begin to taste too sweet, too fatty, and too salty, and they lose their appeal over time. Preparing foods from scratch allows consumers to control intakes of desirable nutrients and monitor the levels of potentially harmful foods—the essence of clean, strong vegan eating.

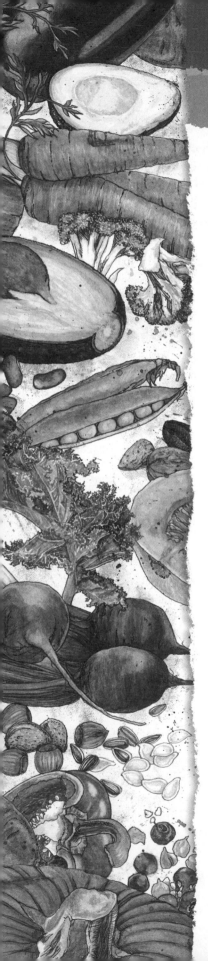

9

Expecting Vegans: Pregnancy and Lactation

Well-planned vegan, lactovegetarian, and lacto-ovo vegetarian diets are appropriate for all stages of the life cycle, including pregnancy and lactation.

POSITION PAPER ON VEGETARIAN DIETS, ACADEMY OF NUTRITION AND DIETETICS
(FORMERLY THE AMERICAN DIETETIC ASSOCIATION)[1]

During pregnancy and lactation, a well-balanced vegan diet can give a baby the best possible start and set the stage for a lifetime of good health. This is a vital stage of life for expectant parents to become savvy about nutrition. However, creating an optimal plant-based diet may be a new experience, and well-meaning friends, relatives, and even some health professionals may question or doubt the benefits of a vegan diet. Fortunately, it's a great time to be vegan because there's plenty of support available. Mothers can be well nourished during pregnancy and lactation whether they are gourmet cooks, frequent restaurants, or keep meal preparation to the barest minimum. Whatever the situation, designing a nutritionally adequate vegan diet is both possible and less challenging than one might think.

Vegan Nutrition in Pregnancy

During pregnancy, the nutrients a baby needs for growth come entirely from its mother. Because the baby will frequently draw on the mother's reserves, it's extremely important for her body to be well nourished. Women who plan to get pregnant within the next few years should start to make the necessary dietary changes now to establish eating patterns that support excellent health, so their reserves will be well stocked

283

Research on Vegan Diets and Pregnancy

The largest study to date on the health of pregnant vegans and their pregnancy outcomes was completed in 1987. Researchers examined the maternity-care records of 775 women at a vegan community known as The Farm in Summertown, Tennessee. Their diets centered on soy foods (tofu, tempeh, and vitamin B_{12}–fortified soy milk), grains, fruits, and vegetables; most foods were organic and grown on The Farm. The women took prenatal supplements with iron and calcium, had regular prenatal care, and had active lifestyles. They didn't smoke cigarettes or drink alcohol and rarely drank coffee.

Two important findings emerged from this study. First, the participants' vegan diets didn't affect infant birth weight. Second, almost no vegan women developed preeclampsia. Just one of the 775 vegan women experienced this complication of pregnancy—a rate of 0.1 percent, compared to a rate of 5 to 10 percent for this health risk in the general population. The research scientists concluded that it's possible to sustain a normal pregnancy on a vegan diet. In fact, the physician in charge of the study, James P. Carter, of the School of Public Health and Tropical Medicine of Tulane University, wrote, "Since preeclampsia in our culture is frequently associated with unrestrained consumption of 'fast foods' (foods having high levels of saturated fat) and rapid weight gain, it's possible that a vegan diet could alleviate most, if not all, of the signs and symptoms of preeclampsia."[65, 66]

In a much smaller English study, birth weights of vegan infants didn't differ from those of nonvegetarian mothers. In this small sample, there was little difference in the incidence of preeclampsia between vegans and nonvegetarians.[67]

These studies on pregnant vegans were carried out long before numerous nutritious and fortified vegan food options became widely available. While a diet centered on whole plant foods is excellent, including some carefully chosen convenience items appeals to some vegans as a way to make life a little easier.

Occasionally, less-favorable reports have appeared regarding the pregnancy outcomes of mothers who consume vegan or near-vegan diets—particularly among macrobiotic populations that were unwilling to consume supplements, such as vitamins B_{12} or D. The diets linked with poor birth outcomes were low in calories or lacked certain essential nutrients, such as vitamin B_{12}.[68–70] The conclusion is that vegan diets can support very healthy pregnancies. However, as they would on any diet, vegan mothers-to-be must take care to ensure adequate intake of calories and other nutrients.

when pregnancy ensues. Great recipes, complete with nutritional analyses, can be found in *Cooking Vegan* by Vesanto Melina and Joseph Forest (Book Publishing Company, 2012).

Calorie requirements don't change significantly during the first trimester and only increase by about 10 to 15 percent during the second and third trimesters.[2] Yet, the requirement for certain vitamins and minerals is greater from early in pregnancy, so food selections really matter. A sample menu designed to meet the nutritional needs of vegans during pregnancy is shown on page 297.

Prepregnancy Preparation Before getting pregnant, a prospective mother should reach a healthy body weight. A weight-loss diet during any stage of pregnancy is undesirable (unless done with medical supervision). To determine whether current weight is in the optimal range, check the body mass index (BMI) in table12.1 (page 363). In women who are overweight (BMI of 25 to 29.9) or obese (BMI above 29.9), weight reduction can decrease the risk of gestational diabetes, high blood pressure, and preeclampsia (a condition that includes high blood pressure, fluid retention, and protein loss in the urine). See chapter 12 for help with healthy weight loss.

In slightly underweight women, gaining a few pounds can increase the chances of becoming pregnant and decrease the risk of having a preterm birth or an underweight infant.[3] See page 362 to determine whether your current body weight is under the healthy range and page 377 for helpful tips on achieving optimal weight. For women with a large frame, the lower end of the healthy BMI range could be too low.

To protect a fetus from potential birth defects, ensure that the vegan diet is rich in folate—even before becoming pregnant. This isn't difficult; beans, greens, and oranges are excellent sources of this vitamin. Folate and the mineral zinc (present in seeds, cashews, and legumes, including soy foods) also are important for male fertility.[4, 5] For additional sources of folate and other vitamins, see chapter 7; for minerals, see chapter 6.

THE FIRST TRIMESTER:
WEIGHT, DIET, AND SUPPLEMENTS

No extra calories are required before pregnancy (unless the prospective mother is underweight) and few, if any, during the first trimester. A recommended weight gain during the first trimester is 3.5 pounds (1.6 kg). If a woman was underweight, the recommended gain is 5 pounds (2.3 kg); if overweight, 2 pounds (0.9 kg). An expectant mother's diet does require many vitamins and minerals (see table 9.1), and her food choices may need adjustment to ensure they deliver good nutrition. For example, although the recommended protein intake doesn't increase during the first trimester compared to prepregnancy requirements, foods rich in protein and iron are needed to build an increased blood supply—especially if these nutrients weren't high priorities in the past. (See chapters 3 and 6.) Legumes are a great food choice; they provide protein and iron along with fiber, which helps to prevent constipation. Legumes also can reduce the risk of gestational diabetes.[6, 7]

Eating well in the first trimester isn't always easy. In 80 percent of women, morning sickness arises between the fourth and seventh week of pregnancy; typically, it has resolved by the twentieth week. Pyridoxine (vitamin B_6) has been shown to safely and effectively alleviate nausea and vomiting for many women; fortunately, vegan diets can be rich in this nutrient (see page 245 and table 7.3 on page 252). During this period, nature gives some women a craving for bland, dry, high-carbohydrate foods.[8–10] Low-fat, high-carbohydrate foods pass rapidly through the stomach and are quickly digested, allowing less time for queasiness.

Women experiencing morning sickness may keep a few crackers by the bedside to have upon awakening. Ginger also is a time-honored remedy for nausea; consuming ginger in the form of cookies, teas, preserves, powder, capsules, and ginger ale can provide relief. Another way to limit nausea is to avoid foods that have strong odors or being around cooking; cold foods often are better tolerated, because they have less aroma.[9]

Sometimes nausea is due to hunger, so pregnant women should eat often, relying on small meals and frequent snacks. Crackers and hummus is a nutritious combination, as is toast with lentil or bean soups. If solid food can't be tolerated, expectant mothers should try to consume whatever they can; juice, fortified soy milk, or miso broth are good choices. A pregnant woman who is unable to eat or to drink adequate amounts of fluids for twenty-four hours should contact her health care provider.

Because morning sickness can interfere with proper nutrition, women who want to become pregnant or who are in the early stages of pregnancy may be advised by their health care provider to take a multivitamin-mineral supplement or a supplement specific to pregnancy. A supplement that includes the vitamins B_{12}, D, choline, and folic acid and the minerals iodine, iron, and zinc is most valuable for vegan mothers-to-be; an online search for "vegan prenatal supplement" can provide sources. For most nutrients, high doses can be harmful; avoid excessive intakes. In addition, the topic of supplementary folic acid is controversial; see page 290 for details.

The recommended intakes for minerals and vitamins change when a woman becomes pregnant and again when she's breast-feeding. Pregnant women need more copper, iodine, zinc, vitamin A/carotenoids, riboflavin, pantothenic acid, and vitamins B_6, B_{12}, and C; during lactation, even higher quantities of these nutrients are needed. The required intakes for other vitamins and minerals (magnesium, iron, thiamin, niacin, and folate) rise in pregnancy and then level off or decrease during lactation. The requirement for vitamin E also increases when a mother breast-feeds her baby. However, for a few nutrients (calcium and vitamins D and K), the recommendation stays the same. For recommended intakes for those younger than age 19 during pregnancy, see pages 446 and 447.

For many of these nutrients, just eating more of an assortment of healthy vegan foods easily takes care of such increased requirements; dietary sources are covered in chapters 6 and 7. Nutrients that need a little extra attention from pregnant women and breast-feeding mothers are addressed in this chapter. For example, omega-3 fatty acids are essential (see page 296 and chapter 4), and a daily supplement of 200 to 300 mg of DHA is often recommended during pregnancy.

In table 9.1, increased amounts of recommended vitamins and minerals are shown in bold; in addition, the periods when the greatest amounts are needed are highlighted.

By the end of the first trimester, morning sickness should be fading, at least to some extent, and expectant mothers may experience a busy bladder, notice a baby bump, and hear the baby's heartbeat through an ultrasound device.

TABLE 9.1. Recommended nutrient intakes for women from 19 to 50 (not pregnant, pregnant, or breast-feeding)

NUTRIENT	NOT PREGNANT	PREGNANT	BREAST-FEEDING
MINERALS			
Calcium	1,000 mg	1,000 mg	1,000 mg
Copper	900 mcg	1,000 mcg	1,300 mcg
Iodine	150 mcg	220 mcg	290 mcg
Iron*	18 mg	27 mg	9 mg
Magnesium**	310–320 mg	350–360 mg	310–320 mg
Potassium	4,700 mg	4,700 mg	5,100 mg
Zinc	8 mg	11 mg	12 mg
FAT-SOLUBLE VITAMINS			
Vitamin A	700 mcg RAE	770 mcg RAE	1,300 mcg RAE
Vitamin D	15 mcg (600 IU)	15 mcg (600 IU)	15 mcg (600 IU)
Vitamin E	15 mg	15 mg	19 mg
Vitamin K	90 mcg	90 mcg	90 mcg
WATER-SOLUBLE VITAMINS			
Thiamin	1.1 mg	1.4 mg	1.4 mg
Riboflavin	1.1 mg	1.4 mg	1.6 mg
Niacin	14 mg	18 mg	17 mg
Pantothenic acid	5 mg	6 mg	7 mg
Vitamin B_6	1.3 mg	1.9 mg	2 mg
Folate	400 mcg	600 mcg	500 mcg
Vitamin B_{12}	2.4 mcg	2.6 mcg	2.8 mcg
Vitamin C	75 mg	85 mg	120 mg

Sources:[6, 11–15]

*The iron RDAs are shown in table 9.1; vegans and other vegetarians may need up to 1.8 times as much; see pages 186 to 189. The Centers for Disease Control (CDC) recommends an iron supplement of 30 mg per day from the first prenatal visit.

**For magnesium, the first figure is the RDA for women from 19 to 30; the second for those 31 and older.

THE SECOND AND THIRD TRIMESTERS

Calories and Weight Gain

The need for additional calories increases during the second and third trimesters. Pregnant women should eat about 340 extra calories per day during the second trimester and about 450 calories extra per day during the third trimester; the exact amount will vary based on the mother's metabolism and activity level.[2, 6]

The recommended weight gain during the second and third trimesters is about 1 pound (0.44 kg) per week. For women who were underweight, the recommended gain is an average of 1.1 pounds (0.49 kg) per week; for overweight women, about 0.6 pound (0.3 kg) per week throughout the second and third trimesters.[2] Typical recommended weight-gain goals are shown in table 9.2; these vary based on prepregnancy weight, whether the mother is an adult or adolescent, and whether a single baby or multiple babies are expected. Women should follow the guidance of physicians and medical caregivers regarding desirable weight gain during all stages of pregnancy. (To determine prepregnancy BMI, see table 12.1 on page 363.)

Protein

During the second and third trimesters, calorie requirements increase by 15 to 20 percent over prepregnancy needs; meanwhile, protein requirements increase by 50 percent. Starting in the fourth month of pregnancy, an extra 28 grams of protein per day is required (this is 10 percent higher than the 25 grams recommended for nonvegetarians and compensates for the slightly lower digestibility of plant protein). For example, a vegan woman whose prepregnancy weight is 135 pounds (61 kg) and whose prepregnancy protein requirement is 55 grams would need to ingest a total of 83 grams of protein every day during this period of her pregnancy. A pregnant woman carrying twins would need 56 grams of added protein daily.

To meet these higher requirements, it makes sense for expectant mothers to have at least one protein-rich food at each meal and at most snacks. Table 9.3 shows foods (and serving sizes) that provide 15 grams of protein. These items typically

TABLE 9.2. Weight gain during pregnancy

FACTORS DETERMINING WEIGHT-GAIN GOALS	TOTAL WEIGHT GAIN RECOMMENDED	AVERAGE RATE OF WEIGHT GAIN PER WEEK IN 2ND AND 3RD TRIMESTERS
Normal or optimal prepregnancy weight (BMI 19–24.9)	25–35 lb (11.5–16 kg)	0.8–1 lb (0.35–0.5 kg)
Underweight before pregnancy (BMI < 19)	28–40 lb (12.5–18 kg)	1–1.3 lb (0.44–0.58 kg)
Overweight before pregnancy (BMI > 25)	15–25 lb (7–11.5 kg)	0.5–0.7 lb (0.23–0.33 kg)
Obese before pregnancy (BMI ≥ 30)	11–20 lb (5–9 kg)	0.5 lb (0.33 kg)
Adolescent	30–45 lb (14–20 kg)	(variable)
Optimal prepregnancy weight with twins	37–54 lb (17–24 kg)	(variable)

Sources:[6, 7, 16]

TABLE 9.3. Foods that provide 15 grams of protein per serving (along with iron, zinc, folate, and choline)

LEGUMES	CALORIES	IRON (mg)	ZINC (mg)	FOLATE (mcg)	CHOLINE (mg/100 g)
Black beans, cooked, 1 c (250 ml)	230	3.6	1.9	256	*
Chickpeas, cooked, 1 c (250 ml)	270	4.7	2.5	282	*
Edamame, 1 c (250 ml)	165	3.2	2	454	*
Lentils, cooked, ⅞ c (220 ml)	201	5.8	2.2	314	*
Peanuts, ½ c (125 ml)	427	1.6	2.4	106	39
Peanut butter, ¼ c (60 ml)	379	1.2	1.9	47	43
Snow peas/peas in the pod, raw, 5½ c (1.5 L)	226	11.2	1.5	226	N/A
Tempeh, ½ c (125 ml)	160	2.2	1	20	**
Tofu, firm, ⅜ cup (100 ml/100 g)	140	2.6	1.5	27	28
LEGUME (OR NUT) AND GRAIN COMBINATIONS					
Peanut butter or almond butter, 2 T (30 ml) on whole wheat bread (2 slices)	330	2	2	37–52	33
Soy milk, 1 c (250 ml) with oat cereal, 2 c (500 ml)	320	4	2.2	77	46
Veggie burger with bun (check labels)	208	1.4	1.4	100	27
Grains					
Bread, whole wheat, 4 slices	277	2.7	2	56	21–27
Rice, brown, cooked, 3 c (750 ml)	649	2.5	3.7	23	53
Pasta, white, enriched, cooked, 1¾ cups (435 ml)***	387	3.1	1.2	179	9
Pasta, whole wheat, cooked, 2 c (500 ml)	347	3	2.3	14	**
Quinoa, cooked, 2 c (500 ml)	444	5.5	4	155	85
NUTS AND SEEDS					
Almonds, ½ c (125 ml)	411	2.7	2.2	36	37
Hazelnuts/filberts, ¾ cup (185 ml)	636	4.8	2.5	114	47
Pumpkin seeds, 6 T (90 ml)	361	4.3	3.8	28	30
Sunflower seeds, ½ c (125 ml)	410	3.7	3.5	159	38

Sources:[17–19]

*Likely to be about 44 to 69 mg per 100 g of food.

**Likely to be about 31 to 35 mg per 100 g of food.

***Enriched with folic acid (check labels).

Folic Acid: Yes or No?

Based on human studies to date, it appears that the benefits of taking limited amounts of folic acid in supplement form in early pregnancy outweigh the risks. Relevant research confirms that it makes sense to take 400 mcg of folic acid during the month or so before becoming pregnant and throughout pregnancy to reduce the risk of neural tube defects in the infant—and perhaps the risks of autism, cleft lip, and cleft palate. With an additional 200 mcg of folate from her diet, a pregnant vegan easily meets the RDA.

Alternatively, a diet that includes plenty of beans, greens, and oranges, complemented by enriched or whole grains, can provide the entire RDA during pregnancy of 600 mcg of folate, as noted above. Thus, supplementary folic acid may not be necessary.

In summary, both options can work well in supplying adequate folate. (However, studies to establish effectiveness in preventing neural tube defects have been conducted only with folic acid.)

provide iron, zinc, folate, and choline too. For more extensive lists of foods with their protein contents, see table 3.5 (page 97) and table 13.3 (page 411).

SPECIFIC NUTRIENTS FOR A HEALTHY PREGNANCY

A developing baby places specific demands on a mother's body for particular nutrients. In the sections that follow, the roles and recommended intakes during pregnancy of minerals and vitamins of special interest are examined.

Folate

This vitamin is crucial for building a fetus's genetic material (DNA) and for other aspects of fetal growth, including the early evolution of the neural tube, which develops into the brain and spinal cord. The Institute of Medicine (IOM) recommends that nonpregnant women—especially those who hope to become pregnant—aim for a daily intake of 400 mcg DFE (dietary folate equivalents, which take into account the various forms of folate); a pregnant woman should receive 600 mcg DFE daily.[14, 20]

Numerous vegan foods are naturally endowed with folate; this form of the vitamin is well utilized by the body (its other name is vitamin B_9, and it is indeed "benign"). Beans, greens, and oranges provide plentiful amounts of folate.[14, 15, 21] A pregnant vegan can get her 600 mcg of folate for the day by eating a reasonable mix of citrus fruits, greens, legumes, and whole grains. For example, 1 cup (250 ml) of orange juice provides 74 mcg of folate, 3 cups (750 ml) of romaine lettuce provide 192 mcg, 1 cup (250 ml) of black beans provides 256 mcg, and 1 cup (250 ml) of cooked quinoa provides 78 mcg, adding up to a total of 600 mcg of folate.[17, 18, 22] (For more on folate, see page 246, table 9.3 on page 289, and table 7.3 on page 252.)

Although folate is required for proper cell division, it seems that an excess of folic acid may take cell division in the wrong direction and increase the risk of colon cancer and other cancers. Folic acid is a related synthetic compound used in supplements and fortified foods (such as enriched breads and baked goods, pasta, rice, flour, and cereals) because it's more stable and less expensive. Strong (and often contradictory) expert opinions exist regarding intakes of this form of vitamin B_9 in supplements, because the body processes folate and folic acid differently. Folic acid can be converted in the liver to the useable form of this vitamin by an enzyme that the body produces in limited amounts. Because of this potentially incomplete conversion, high intakes of folic acid may result in the circulation of unconverted folic acid in the bloodstream. It's wise not to exceed a total daily intake of 1,000 mcg DFE per day. Women who use folic acid supplements should choose those that provide 400 mcg—or at most 550 mcg—daily.[23, 24, 25]

Iron

The most widespread nutritional deficiency in the world is iron deficiency; it's a common concern for women on any diet, whether vegan, vegetarian, or nonvegetarian.[26] Good iron status early in pregnancy and adequate maternal intakes of this mineral during pregnancy are linked with better birth weights and less risk of preterm births.[6, 26–28]

Many otherwise healthy women fail to meet recommended iron intakes—including during pregnancy, when the body's blood supply increases by 40 to 50 percent to deliver oxygen to the fetus and surrounding tissues. Iron supports development of the brain and nervous system; deficiency can have lifelong neurological and behavioral consequences. Adequate iron also is required to build the baby's own iron stores. In fact, 80 percent of a term infant's stored iron is accrued during the third trimester; a premature infant doesn't have the advantage of this accretion and will need supplemental iron starting early in life.

The RDA for pregnant women is 27 mg of iron per day, an increase of 50 percent over the prepregnancy RDA. Because some plant foods contain substances (such as phytates) that decrease iron absorption, the IOM further advises that vegetarians consume 1.8 times as much iron as nonvegetarians—which would bring the recommended intake to 48 mg per day.[13] Some experts question whether the recommendation for vegans needs to be quite this high; plus, 48 mg is above the tolerable upper intake level (UL) of 45 mg per day, so the goal shouldn't be above 45 mg unless medically advised.

Studies in the United States have repeatedly shown that vegan diets are as high or higher in iron than lactovegetarian and nonvegetarian diets, as well as being rich in vitamin C, which greatly increases iron absorption.[31, 32] Also, during pregnancy, nature kindly steps in and greatly increases the efficiency of iron absorption from plant foods, especially during the second trimester. Iron-rich vegan foods tend to be the same foods, such as beans, peas, and lentils, that are high in protein, zinc, and the B vitamins folate and choline (see table 9.3 on page 289). (For more on iron, see pages 186 to 189 and table 6.2 on page 204.)

Building an Iron-Rich Diet

- Consume iron-rich foods, such as beans, lentils, soy foods, whole grains, fortified grain products, seeds, dried fruit, organic blackstrap molasses, and leafy greens (page 188).

- Include vitamin C–rich foods (such as bell peppers, tomatoes, and citrus fruits) in iron-rich meals to maximize absorption of the mineral (page 189).

- Avoid drinking tea or coffee with iron-rich foods; these beverages can decrease iron absorption. (For lactovegetarians and lacto-ovo vegetarians, cow's milk will have the same effect.)

- Consider taking a prenatal supplement that includes iron or a daily supplement of 30 mg of iron; the latter is necessary with iron-deficiency anemia. [6, 27, 29, 31, 34]

Supplements that provide 30 mg of iron are recommended by the Centers for Disease Control (CDC) from the first prenatal visit and are commonly prescribed for pregnant women; these are certainly needed when a woman is anemic or has low serum ferritin (iron stores). Large doses of supplementary iron can be toxic, so the amounts recommended by health care providers should not be exceeded. Some experts suggest that iron supplements are unnecessary—and, in fact, not advisable—for women who aren't anemic; however, the alternative requires the creation of an iron-rich diet.[33]

Zinc

Whether vegan or nonvegan, the diets of many North American women are low in zinc. Insufficient zinc intake during pregnancy has been linked with preterm delivery, low birth weight, prolonged labor, and other problems.[31] Zinc is involved in cell replication—the duplication of existing cells that is fundamental to growth and healthy birth weight. This mineral also is required for cell differentiation, the process during which cells change from general to more specialized forms that perform particular functions. In choosing a prenatal supplement, it's wise to choose one that provides zinc.[31]

The RDA for zinc increases from 8 mg per day before pregnancy to 11 mg during pregnancy (and to 12 mg in lactation). The expectant mother's absorption of this mineral also becomes more efficient. Good sources of zinc include seeds and seed butters, as well as nuts and nut butters and legumes.[6, 17, 18] Recent research has established that consuming nuts and peanuts during pregnancy doesn't increase the likelihood of allergies in infants; in fact, the reverse may be true.[35] Of course, a pregnant woman should avoid foods to which she is allergic. (For more on zinc, see pages 189 to 191 and table 6.2 on page 204.)

Iodine

Although iodine is an essential component of thyroid hormone, tiny amounts of this mineral are even more vital for normal development of the infant's

Ensuring Adequate Iodine Intake

Select a prenatal supplement that includes iodine; typically, it will provide 150 mcg of iodine (the amount recommended in supplement form by the American Thyroid Association during pregnancy and lactation).[40]

Plant foods in a vegan diet may well deliver sufficient iodine to top up intakes from a prenatal supplement. But because it's difficult to be sure, include another option for the remaining 70 mcg per day:

- One-quarter teaspoon (1 g) of iodized salt should add about 46 to 76 mg of iodine.[41]
- Sea vegetables (seaweeds) typically are not ideal sources, because iodine amounts can vary sixfold. However, small amounts of seaweeds, such as kombu, are an option if the label shows the iodine content; excessive intakes of iodine from kombu have led to health problems.[42]
- Iodine drops deliver a known quantity of iodine per drop.

brain and central nervous system—even a mild deficiency can affect cognitive ability. In addition, iodine deficiency during critical points in the development of a fetus and young child causes cretinism (a form of developmental disability). This form of brain damage occurs in locations throughout the world where iodine is in short supply in the soil due to losses caused by floods or, in mountainous regions, by rainfall and glaciation. Although vegetables take up iodine from the soil where they can, amounts in crops vary from one place to another.[6, 20, 31, 36, 37]

Iodine deficiency is easily prevented, and it's important to get sufficient iodine—but not too much.[13, 38] The RDA for iodine during pregnancy is 220 mcg per day. Evidence of iodine sufficiency in pregnant women is defined by iodine concentration in the urine of 150 grams per liter.[37] There also is an upper limit for daily iodine intake, which is 900 mcg for teens and 1,100 mcg for adults, pregnant or not.[11, 38]

Fortifying salt with iodine has been effective in preventing iodine deficiency in many countries. Iodization of table salt is mandatory in Canada and many other nations and optional in the United States and the United Kingdom; check labels.[38] However, a study of vegans in the Boston area found that some were at risk for iodine deficiency because the majority didn't use iodized salt or take an iodine-containing supplement. (In contrast, one of the Boston vegans had an excessive iodine intake due to high kelp intake.)[39] (For more on iodine, see pages 191 to 194.)

Calcium

Though a fetus needs calcium for building bones, a woman's RDA for this mineral is 1,000 mg whether she is or isn't pregnant, or is breast-feeding. This situation exists because calcium absorption becomes far more efficient with increased need, essentially doubling during pregnancy. Multivitamin supplements and prenatal supplements typically provide a few hundred milligrams of calcium to top up dietary intake. However, if a pregnant woman's intake is insufficient, calcium from her bones can be siphoned off to support the growth of the baby.[6, 12, 31, 43]

Many vegans have calcium intakes below the RDA, so pregnancy should instigate a habit of calcium-rich dining. Many excellent plant sources of calcium are available from each of the food groups. These include low-oxalate greens (bok choy, broccoli, napa cabbage, collard greens, kale, and okra), calcium-set tofu, almonds, blackstrap molasses, and figs, as well as fortified foods (such as calcium-fortified orange juice, soy milk, other nondairy beverages, and cereals). If necessary, a calcium supplement can top up food intakes.[18, 44] (For more on calcium, see pages 182 to 186 and table 6.2 on page 204.)

Vitamin D

This vitamin is essential for calcium absorption and bone health and for many other functions in the body. In pregnant women, insufficient vitamin D levels may increase the risk of preeclampsia and miscarriage.[20, 45, 46] The IOM recommends a vitamin D intake of 15 mcg (600 IU) whether or not a woman is pregnant.[11, 12] Some experts recommend higher intakes, advising that pregnant women should receive 50 mcg (2,000 IU) of vitamin D per day through the winter months to maintain sufficient vitamin D levels.[34, 43] (For more on vitamin D sources from sunlight, fortified foods, supplements, or a combination, see pages 225 to 228.)

Vitamin B$_{12}$

Vegans, in general, must pay special attention to ensure an adequate intake of this vitamin, and it's particularly important for pregnant vegans to consume enough vitamin B$_{12}$ to bring a healthy baby to term. The small proportion of vegans who have failed to ensure reliable sources of vitamin B$_{12}$ for themselves and their babies has created regrettable situations in which the infants weakened and had seizures, convulsions, irreversible brain damage, and nerve damage. Ultimately, some didn't survive. This is a devastating and completely avoidable tragedy.

When an infant born of a vegan mother has vitamin B$_{12}$ deficiency, the reputation of the vegan diet is tarnished. In addition, some health professionals become leery of such "restrictive regimens" and, in some cases, entire medical associations take a stand against vegan diets, discouraging their use during vulnerable periods of life, such as pregnancy and childhood. This is most unfortunate, considering the ethical, ecological, and health benefits associated with vegan diets.[11, 14, 47–49]

A pregnant woman's RDA for this vitamin is 2.6 mcg (slightly higher than before pregnancy). However, based on input from many experts, higher intakes are advised; any excess will be excreted in the urine. The vitamin B$_{12}$ consumed by the mother is passed on to the fetus (and later on, a breast-fed infant receives this vitamin through mother's milk). Without an adequate source of vitamin B$_{12}$, the baby has an increased risk of being pre-term, suffering neural tube defects, and developing other serious complications. As a result, pregnant women must ensure they have a reliable source of this essential nutrient.[47, 48, 50–52]

Ensuring Adequate Vitamin B_{12} Intake During Pregnancy

During pregnancy (and lactation), it's essential that a woman adopts one of the following practices:

- Take a daily supplement that provides at least 25 mcg of vitamin B_{12}; it's fine to take 100 or 250 mcg or more. This dose can be part of a multivitamin or pregnancy supplement.

- Two or three times a week, take 1,000 mcg of vitamin B_{12}. Taking 2,500 mcg of vitamin B_{12} twice a week also is acceptable.

- Three times a day, eat a B_{12}-fortified food (such as a breakfast cereal, a vegan meat substitute, or Red Star Vegetarian Support Formula nutritional yeast). Each choice should deliver at least 1.5 mcg per serving; a product whose label shows that a serving contains at least 25 percent of the Daily Value (DV) for vitamin B_{12} will provide that amount. It's wise to combine occasional use of a supplement with this approach.

For optimal health of both mother and baby, a healthy vitamin B_{12} status throughout pregnancy and lactation is imperative. See pages 214 to 222 to review the essential functions B_{12} performs, the effects of deficiency, and tests that determine vitamin B_{12} status. Serum vitamin B_{12} levels should be 350 pg/ml or higher. In vegans who regularly consume seaweeds, serum vitamin B_{12} may not accurately reflect true levels, depending on the test used; the vitamin B_{12} analogs present in seaweeds can result in a higher reading even though the true level of serum B_{12} is inadequate. In such situations, laboratory tests that measure holo-transcobalamin and methylmalonic acid can be conducted to verify B_{12} status.[47, 48, 50–53]

Pyridoxine (Vitamin B_6)

The recommended intake of pyridoxine during pregnancy is 1.9 mg per day. Low intakes of this vitamin may be associated with low birth weight.[54] Vegan diets contain plenty of pyridoxine-rich foods; some of the richest sources are avocados, bananas, chia seeds, soybeans, and sunflower seeds. (For more on pyridoxine, see pages 244 and 245 and table 7.3 on page 252.)

For many expectant mothers who experience morning sickness, pyridoxine—in the range of 10 mg taken three times a day for five days—has proved to be a safe and effective way to reduce symptoms.[9, 10] However, it's wise to check with a physician before beginning this regimen. Research on this remedy has proved to be a challenge, because morning sickness also seems to resolve without any treatment.

Choline

The fetus requires choline to build its cell membranes and for the transmission of nerve impulses. It accumulates in the placenta, so the baby's environment is rich in this vitamin. Because choline is a part of all cell membranes in both animals and plants, it's widely distributed in plant foods in moderate amounts. Choline wasn't classified as an essential nutrient until 1989. As a result, data regarding the choline content of many plant foods is limited, in comparison with data on other vitamins.[14, 15, 19]

Choline is available in every food group, including grains; however, it's lost during the refining process and isn't restored when grains are enriched. As long as a woman eats a diet high in unrefined foods, consuming enough choline isn't a problem. In addition, the body has some ability to manufacture choline, depending on the rest of the diet. (For more on choline, see page 249, table 7.2 on page 250, and table 9.3 on page 289.)[11, 14, 15, 19]

The recommended intake for choline increases just slightly when a woman becomes pregnant, from 425 mg to 450 mg. This amount is available in a diet centered on whole plant foods, in which few calories are wasted on sugars and oils. To prevent potential neural tube defects, it may be advisable for women who plan to become pregnant and those in the first trimester to take a choline supplement. The label of a multivitamin-mineral supplement should be checked to see if choline is listed.[11, 14, 15, 19]

Omega-3 Fatty Acids (Alpha-linolenic Acid, DHA, and EPA)

A baby requires the long-chain omega-3 fatty acids DHA and EPA for the normal development of its retinas, brain, and central nervous system. Higher levels of these essential fatty acids in pregnant women and in breast milk have been associated with improved health outcomes for babies. Although a normal body has the ability to synthesize these fatty acids (DHA and EPA) from alpha-linolenic acid (ALA), to meet the needs of the developing fetus, a pregnant woman's body develops superpowers in this regard. The baby gains most of its body fat during the last ten weeks of pregnancy and will gain fat from the essential omega-3 and omega-6 fatty acids in the mother's diet, from her body's production of DHA and EPA, and from her body's stores. It's important that expectant mothers are well nourished with these beneficial fats early in pregnancy—and even before becoming pregnant—and well equipped to pass along long-chain omega-3 fatty acids to the developing baby.[55–60]

Despite the enhanced ability of a pregnant woman's body to synthesize DHA and EPA from ALA, levels of these fatty acids are lower in pregnant vegans and in vegan breast milk, compared to the general population. The extent to which DHA and EPA can be synthesized from the ALA in foods such as flaxseeds, hempseeds, and walnuts is the subject of considerable scientific research and debate (see pages 120 to 121).

To maximize the conversion of plant-based omega-3 fatty acids to EPA and DHA, vegans should aim for a ratio of omega-6 to omega-3 fatty acids in the range of 2:1 to 4:1. Foods containing trans-fatty acids should be avoided, as should alcohol and smoking; all these factors inhibit DHA production. (Labels on margarine, crackers, cookies, pastries, and other processed foods that list partially hydrogenated vegetable oil indicate the presence of trans-fatty acids.)[55–60]

For pregnant vegans, experts commonly recommend intakes of about 300 mg of DHA (or DHA and EPA combined) per day.[57, 61–63] Vegan-friendly

DHA supplements may be used. Expectant mothers can also consume foods and oils fortified with microalgae-derived DHA, although fortification levels are generally low. According to the Academy of Nutrition and Dietetics, "Because of DHA's beneficial effects on gestational length, infant visual function, and neurodevelopment, pregnant and lactating vegans should use a microalgae-derived DHA supplement."[1] The DHA in fish is derived from marine microalgae, as is the DHA in these supplements, but the latter is uncontaminated with mercury and is a safer choice. To find suitable supplements, do an Internet search for "vegan DHA."

SAMPLE PREGNANCY MENU[17, 18, 64]

BREAKFAST

1 cup (250 ml) cereal with ½ cup (125 ml) blueberries or other fruit and 1 cup (250 ml) fortified soy milk

1 slice whole wheat toast with 2 tablespoons (30 ml) almond butter or seed butter

1 cup (250 ml) fresh-squeezed orange juice or other fruit

SNACK

½ cup (125 ml) carrot sticks with ¼ cup (60 ml) hummus

LUNCH

Sandwich with ½ cup (125 ml) seasoned tofu, 2 slices whole-grain bread, and lettuce

2 cups (500 ml) tossed salad with ½ avocado and 2 tablespoons (30 ml) Liquid Gold Dressing (page 219)

SNACK

2 figs or another choice of fruit

2 tablespoons (30 ml) almonds or other nuts, peanuts, or seeds

1 cup (250 ml) fortified soy milk

DINNER

1 cup (250 ml) beans (such as black, red, or pinto) and ½ cup (125 ml) brown rice

½ to 1 cup (125 to 250 ml) cooked kale with lemon juice

1 cup (250 ml) tomato slices

Nutritional analysis:[17, 18] calories: 2,135; protein: 97 g; fat: 85 g; carbohydrate: 271 g; dietary fiber: 60 g; calcium: 1,400 to 2,109* mg (intake depends on choice of tofu, nuts, and fruit); iron: 22 mg; magnesium: 791 mg; phosphorus: 1,817 mg; potassium: 4,938 mg; selenium: 94 mcg; sodium: 1,451 mg; zinc: 15 mg; thiamin: 3.2 mg; riboflavin: 3.4 mg; niacin: 23 mg; vitamin B_6: 2.8 mg; folate: 911 mcg; pantothenic acid: 6.1 mg; vitamin B_{12}: 5.1 mcg; choline: > 450 mg; vitamin A: 1,928 mcg RAE; vitamin C: 234 mg; vitamin D: 5.6 mcg (221 IU); vitamin E: 18 mg; vitamin K: 497 mcg; omega-6 fatty acids: 21 g; omega-3 fatty acids: 6.8 g

Percentage of calories from protein: 18 percent; fat: 34 percent; carbohydrate: 48 percent

Menu Variations

- Substitute similar items, such as other fruits, vegetables, or beans.
- For equally high-protein intakes without the use of soy, use a different nondairy milk, increase the hummus in the snack to ⅔ cup (185 ml), and replace the tofu with 1 cup (250 ml) of lentils (perhaps in a soup).
- To replace the Liquid Gold Dressing, use 2 tablespoons (30 ml) of ground flaxseeds, 2 teaspoons (10 ml) of flaxseed oil, or a handful of walnuts (thereby providing omega-3 fatty acids).

TABLE 9.4. Sample guide for pregnancy and lactation (by food groups)

FOOD GROUP	NUMBER OF SERVINGS	ITEMS IN THE MENU ON PAGE 297 (NUMBER OF SERVINGS)
Grains	6	cereal (2), bread (3), rice (1)
Legumes	4½–6	soy milk (2), hummus (½), tofu (1), beans (1)
Vegetables	6	carrot sticks (1), salad (2), avocado (1), kale (1), tomato (1)
Fruits	4	berries (1), juice (2), figs (1)
Nuts, seeds	1–2	almond butter plus nuts (1)
Calcium-rich foods (also in above food groups)	6	fortified soy milk (2), calcium-fortified juice (1), calcium-set tofu (1), figs (½), black beans (1), kale (½)

The sample pregnancy menu features protein-rich foods at every meal and snack; no calories are wasted on fats or sugars, which don't deliver valuable nutrients. Folate, potassium, and choline are provided by the assorted vegetables, fruits, and beans. The high fiber intake, aided by water and walking, helps to prevent constipation. The beans, hummus, soy foods, cereal, nuts, and seeds deliver copper, zinc, and also iron, though not quite as much iron as the high intakes recommended during pregnancy (an iron supplement may still be advisable). The ratio of omega-6 to omega-3 fatty acids is about 3.5:1.

This basic menu meets a pregnant woman's nutritional requirements, while allowing for substitutions to add variety and for additional foods to increase calories a little or to satisfy cravings. However, expectant vegans should choose treats based on whole foods, such as frozen fruit "ice cream" or nuts and dried fruit. With minor modifications (page 297), this menu also is appropriate for vegan mothers when breast-feeding. (It's a variation of The Vegan Plate (page 434), with increases in legumes from 3 to 4.5 servings, in grains from 3 to 6 servings, and in vegetables from 5 to 6 servings, with other additions as desired.)

Supplements

Prenatal or other supplements should include iron, zinc, iodine, vitamin B_{12}, and vitamin D, probably along with folate (page 294). DHA is an optional addition (page 296). Excess intakes of vitamin A in the form of supplements can be harmful; monitor intake to avoid taking too much. Also avoid herbal supplements and botanical remedies unless first discussed with a health care provider.

Fluids

Drink plenty of water and other caffeine-free fluids.

LIFESTYLE CHOICES THAT BUILD A HEALTHY BABY

• **Avoid alcohol and smoking; minimize caffeine, pesticides, and other harmful contaminants.** There's no need for a woman to become stressed over a drink consumed early in pregnancy, before the pregnancy was detected. However, once pregnancy is confirmed, alcohol should be entirely avoided throughout the pregnancy, because alcohol is toxic to developing brain cells. In addition, alcohol passes from the mother's blood through the placenta to the fetus, whose liver isn't sufficiently mature to manage this substance.

The placenta is a filter that can screen out toxins of a certain size, but it can't totally protect a fetus, so an expectant mother must do her part and shun toxic substances in the first place. Whenever possible, organic foods grown without pesticides should be chosen. Pregnant women shouldn't use powerful anti-inflammatory agents, such as chamomile tea and aspirin. Due to the risk of bacterial contamination, sprouts and unpasteurized juices shouldn't be consumed during pregnancy. Spirulina can contain unsafe contaminants from other types of algae and should be avoided.

The same goes for other habits that can potentially harm a developing fetus. Smoking tobacco or marijuana causes vasoconstriction that limits the fetal oxygen supply and should be completely avoided.[71] Although the amount of caffeine known to be safe for expectant mothers is uncertain, a limit of 200 mg daily is commonly suggested; less may be better. The amount of caffeine in 1 cup (250 ml) of coffee (100 to 200 mg) or tea (40 to 75 mg) or 1 ounce (30 g) of dark chocolate (15 mg) daily appears safe. So, expectant moms can enjoy a vegan brownie.

• **Stay active.** In Victorian times, a woman's pregnancy was called her "confinement" or "lying in." However, staying active during pregnancy has numerous advantages: feeling good, staying fit and shapely, and toning muscles for a vigorous delivery. Although expectant mothers shouldn't ski, scuba dive, roller blade, perform gymnastics, ride horses, or participate in activities where falling is a risk, many pleasant possibilities are available. Half an hour a day of swimming, water aerobics, prenatal yoga, or walking are high on the list. Mothers-to-be who jogged and cycled before pregnancy may be fine to continue. However, women who aren't accustomed to exercise—or who have a high-risk pregnancy—should check with their doctor to determine safe levels of activity.[6, 16, 31]

• **Enjoy soy.** Should soy foods be avoided during pregnancy and lactation? In general, it's important for women who are allergic to soy, or who have unresolved thyroid problems and low iodine status, to avoid soy foods. Of course, low iodine status and thyroid problems are to be resolved for a healthy pregnancy. Apart from these cautions, a maximum of three servings per day of soy foods is both safe and beneficial. In fact, their consumption may reduce the risk of breast cancer later on.[4, 72, 73] (For more on soy, see pages 105 to 106.)

For excellent books and websites on vegan nutrition during pregnancy and lactation, look through Resources on pages 449 and 451.

Vegan Nutrition While Breast-Feeding

BREAST OR BOTTLE?

One of the important decisions a new mother must make is whether her infant should be breast-fed or bottle-fed. As nature intended, breast milk is the best food for a baby. Occasionally, breast-feeding isn't possible; in such cases, parents can be confident that babies also thrive on commercial iron-fortified formulas. Such formulas have been designed to replicate breast milk as closely as possible and will support healthy development (page 307).[74-77]

Parents should never try to make their own infant formulas; because it's not so easy to duplicate nature's recipe, homemade formulas can lead to poor child development, failure to thrive, or worse. Also, plain cow's milk, goat's milk, or nondairy milks are not suitable substitutes. The only safe and nutritionally adequate primary milks for a baby's first year of life are breast milk or commercial infant formula.

Advantages of Breast-Feeding for Baby and Mom

Breast-feeding confers numerous health benefits to the baby as well as to mom. As a result, the World Health Organization (WHO) recommends exclusive breast-feeding for the first six months of life, followed by the introduction of solid foods at six months, together with continued breast-feeding (along with complementary foods) up to 2 years of age and beyond. The American Academy of Pediatrics (AAP) has similar guidelines, advising exclusive breast-feeding for the first four and preferably six months.[28, 76, 78] Even a short period of breast-feeding is beneficial.

The balance of protein, fat, and carbohydrate in human breast milk is ideal for infants. Its low protein content, digestibility, and balance of amino acids closely match infant requirements, and the proportion of sodium is ideal for the infant's kidneys. Breast milk provides ample vitamins and minerals, as well as DHA. It also contains a number of protective substances, such as antibodies, cytokines, antimicrobial agents, and oligosaccharides.

Breast milk guards against gastrointestinal illness and supports the maturation of the infant's intestines. A breast-fed baby is less likely to develop colds, ear infections, stomach upsets, allergies, and asthma. Later in life, he or she will have reduced risk of diabetes, heart disease, and childhood leukemia; will be less prone to be overweight as a child or adult; and is more likely to do well at school. Breast-feeding helps avoid excess weight gain; babies nurse until satisfied, and there's not that push on the part of parents or caregivers for the baby to finish the last half ounce in a bottle.[79, 80] In addition, breast milk composition adjusts automatically to meet an infant's changing requirements over time. Scientists continue to study this amazing fluid but have yet to duplicate it exactly.

Advantages for mom include faster postpartum weight loss—especially if breast-feeding lasts for six months or more—and reduced risk of developing diabetes, breast cancer, and ovarian cancer later in life. The slight increase in maternal food intake required to support breast-feeding is economical, compared to the cost of formulas, bottles, and equipment for safe formula preparation. Breast milk is always at the perfect temperature and is "food safe," so it isn't necessary to warm bottles and cart quite so many supplies on outings. Most importantly, breast-feeding offers superb one-on-one time with baby.

Unfortunately, potentially toxic environmental pollutants are commonly found in human milk at levels that would prevent its sale as a food for infants. Maternal intakes of meat, fish, and dairy products typically lead to higher levels of dieldrin and polychlorinated biphenyls (PCBs) in breast milk. In contrast, studies have shown that the breast milk of vegan and vegetarian mothers contains fewer toxic contaminants, compared to milk from nonvegetarian women; the breast milk of vegetarians shows lower levels of pesticides, such as DDT, chlordane, and heptachlor, and industrial by-products, such as PCBs. In an American study, the highest value for six contaminants in the breast milk of vegans was lower than the lowest value from the breast milk of women on standard American diets. Naturally, a plant-based diet composed of organic foods would be the best choice to avoid toxins.[6, 31, 81–83]

Because nursing is a new experience for both mother and baby, getting started can take a little time. Some infants begin nursing immediately, while others have some difficulty. In those cases, many mothers benefit from the help of a lactation specialist, who can help find the best position for nursing; for example, the baby's entire body can be arranged in arm and lap (now that mom has a lap again) during feeding. Many mothers find lying down to nurse a comfortable position, especially at night.

MENU FOR A BREAST-FEEDING MOM

With minor modifications, the menu that appears on page 297 can provide a general plan for a mother's diet during lactation. The Vegan Plate (page 434) also is a good guide, increasing the legumes to at least 4.5 servings for the day, upping grains to 6 or more servings, and adding carotenoid-rich vegetables and other nutritious choices listed in the sections that follow.

For the first six months, breast-feeding mothers need to consume approximately 500 calories more each day than they did before pregnancy. (To gradually lose the extra weight gained in pregnancy, a new mother may choose to get the nutrition she and baby need by consuming only about 330 extra calories a day, focusing on highly nutritious foods.) Mothers who continue to breast-feed during the baby's second six months and whose weight has returned to the desired level will need about 400 extra calories per day. The actual ideal calorie intake depends on the infant's appetite and the amount of food he or she consumes apart from breast milk.[2] With nursing twins, mothers need more of all nutrients, including calories. As in pregnancy, small frequent meals are a good way to ensure ample intakes of calories and protein.

The key dietary adjustments required during breast-feeding are increased fluid intakes; greater consumption of vitamin A (from the carotenoids in yellow, orange, red, and green foods; see page 233) and most other nutrients; and the addition of calories and small amounts of certain other nutrients. Soy foods have a negligible effect on the isoflavone content of breast milk; it's safe and reasonable to include two to three servings a day of soy foods.[6, 31, 84] (For specifics on vitamin and minerals, see table 9.1 on page 287; for food sources, see chapters 6 and 7.)

Fluids

A new mother needs plenty of fluids while breast-feeding and should keep a glass of water near the comfortable chair used during nursing. Juices, soy milk, soups, and smoothies also are suitable. (Note that avoidance of cow's milk on the part of the mother may lessen the likelihood that her breast-fed baby will experience colic.)

Protein

The word *protein* is related to the German word meaning "primary" and the Greek word meaning "first." High-protein foods (such as legumes, whole grains, greens and other vegetables, and nuts and seeds) need to be the top priority as meals and snacks because they provide plenty of iron, zinc, calcium, other minerals, and many B vitamins along with the protein. The recommended daily intake for protein is unchanged from the second and third trimesters of pregnancy—about 25 grams above the amounts the mother consumed when not pregnant. The menu on page 297 provides 97 grams of protein and can be suitable as a general meal planner for nursing mothers, who can add foods or increase portions to suit appetite and needs. (Also see table 9.3 on page 289.)

SPECIFIC NUTRIENTS FOR BREAST-FEEDING

The nutritional demands placed on a mother's body during lactation are slightly different than those of pregnancy. The following sections describe the roles and recommended intakes of minerals and vitamins during lactation.

Iron

A woman's RDA for iron is high during pregnancy, but this requirement drops dramatically during lactation. Her body is no longer building an increased blood supply, menstrual iron losses have not yet resumed (at least for a while), and breast milk contains only moderate amounts of iron. As a result, the RDA for a lactating vegan mother is 9 mg (see table 9.1 on page 287 and the section on iron on page 186).

Although the iron present in breast milk is extremely well absorbed by baby, some newborns may require iron supplements. The AAP provides the following guidelines regarding iron supplementation for infants. A preterm infant, whose iron stores are not sufficiently built up and who is breast-fed, requires supplemental iron under medical supervision; if bottle-fed, an iron-rich formula is necessary. Full-term breast-fed babies may be given iron drops starting at 4 months of age until sufficient iron-rich foods are introduced, because their iron stores start running low around 4 to 6 months of age.[28]

Zinc

A breast-feeding mother's recommended intake for zinc (12 mg) is even higher than it was during her pregnancy (11 mg). Mothers must make it a priority to include zinc-rich foods (see page 292).[11, 13, 34]

Calcium

At 1,000 mg per day, the RDA for calcium stays constant during pregnancy and lactation (see table 10.1 on page 312). Breast milk contains adequate calcium because of physiological changes in the mother's body that include doubly efficient absorption and also because she may pass some of her own stored calcium (from bones) to her baby. It's important to meet the calcium RDA, though high intakes from diet and supplementation don't seem to prevent the temporary maternal losses from bone. However, studies show that after weaning, the mother's bone mineral content is restored.[11, 12, 34]

Vitamin D

During lactation, a woman's RDA for vitamin D remains at 15 mcg (600 IU). Medical experts who advise higher intakes suggest that, through the winter months, a breast-feeding woman should receive 50 mcg (2,000 IU) of vitamin D per day to meet her own body's needs. If a mother with little or no access to sunshine were to meet both her own needs for vitamin D plus those of her infant (through her milk), it's estimated that she would need 100 mcg (4,000 IU) of vitamin D daily.[43]

Because transfer of this vitamin through breast milk can be uncertain, and breast milk is typically low in vitamin D, an infant should receive his or her own vitamin D drops directly, starting soon after birth. The AAP recommends that infants and children through adolescence have a daily intake of 10 mcg (400 IU) of vitamin D to age 1 and 15 mcg (600 IU) thereafter. (For more on vitamin D, see pages 222 to 230.)[11, 12, 55]

Vitamin A (Carotenoids)

Vitamin A has an important role in cell differentiation, allowing cells to become specialized to carry out specific tasks. Thus, the effects of this nutrient are diverse. Vitamin A is needed for the growth of bones and teeth, for reproduction, and for the building and regulation of hormones.[13]

Ensuring Adequate Vitamin B$_{12}$ Intake During Lactation

During lactation (and pregnancy), a woman should adopt one of the following practices:

- Take a daily supplement that provides at least 25 mcg of vitamin B$_{12}$; it's fine to take 100 or 250 mcg. This dose can be part of a multivitamin or pregnancy supplement.

- Two or three times a week, take 1,000 mcg of vitamin B$_{12}$. Taking 2,500 mcg of vitamin B$_{12}$ twice a week also is acceptable.

- Three times a day, eat a B$_{12}$-fortified food (such as a breakfast cereal, a vegetarian meat substitute, or Red Star Vegetarian Support Formula nutritional yeast). Each choice should deliver at least 1.5 mcg per serving; a product whose label shows that a serving contains at least 25 percent of the Daily Value (DV) for vitamin B$_{12}$ will provide that amount. It's wise to combine occasional use of a supplement with this approach.

In vegan diets, vitamin A is derived from the carotenoids in orange, yellow, and green vegetables and fruits. The menu on page 297 provides sufficient vitamin A from the carrots, lettuce, kale, and tomatoes as well as the soy milk. (For more on vitamin A, see pages 233 to 235.)

Water-Soluble Vitamins (B Vitamins and Vitamin C)

Generally, the amounts of water-soluble vitamins in breast milk reflect the mother's intake from diet and supplements. Thus, maintaining a good diet is important for the health of the child. The pattern of food groups and number of servings from each in table 9.4 on page 299 was designed to cover these vitamins.

Vitamin B$_{12}$

It is absolutely critical that lactating mothers continue to consume a reliable source of vitamin B$_{12}$ (see page 294). Babies require this nutrient for the normal development of brain, nerve, and blood cells, and their supply of B$_{12}$ comes from the mother's diet, not her body stores. The fetus stores a little vitamin B$_{12}$ obtained during pregnancy, though if the mother was deficient during pregnancy, infant stores will be negligible. At best, infant stores will last for only about three months after birth, sometimes less. Lack of vitamin B$_{12}$ can impair the infant's brain development and cause neurological problems.[85–89]

Even if a nursing mother shows no symptoms of vitamin B$_{12}$ deficiency, the situation is precarious if her vitamin B$_{12}$ intake is inadequate and her stores are low. To ensure adequate intakes, nursing mothers require supplemental vitamin B$_{12}$ or B$_{12}$-fortified foods as sources for themselves, as well as for their infants. In fact, supplements are a better choice than fortified foods, due to reliability of the delivered dosage.[47, 48, 50, 51, 85–89] The summary in the sidebar above is a duplicate of that from the pregnancy section, repeated due to its importance.

Folate

The recommended intake for folate during lactation (500 mcg) is lower than it was in pregnancy, but higher than before a woman became pregnant (see table 9.1 on page 287).[12, 14] (For more on folate, see pages 246 and 290.)

Pantothenic Acid and Vitamin E

The recommended intake for pantothenic acid increases from 6 mg in pregnancy to 7 mg during lactation.[12, 14, 18] To modify the menu on page 297 to meet this recommendation, include the remainder of the avocado, add ¾ cup (185 ml) of sweet potato or mushrooms at dinner, or make the breakfast choice 2 cups (500 ml) of oatmeal plus a big banana.

The nursing mother's RDA for vitamin E also increases to 19 mg; nuts, seeds, and avocados are great sources of both vitamin E and pantothenic acid.[12, 18] (For more information on good sources of these vitamins, see pages 237 and 243, and table 7.3 on page 252).

Choline

Breast milk is rich in choline, a nutrient that's good for baby's brain development; infant formulas, including soy-based versions, tend to provide less choline.[14] To ensure a good supply of choline, see table 9.3 (page 289) and table 7.2 (page 250).

Omega-3 Fatty Acids (Alpha-linolenic Acid, DHA, and EPA)

During lactation—as at other life stages—it's essential to consume excellent sources of alpha-linolenic acid (ALA), such as chia seeds, ground flaxseeds, flaxseed oil, hempseeds, or walnuts (see suggested quantities in The Vegan Plate on page 434). ALA can be converted to DHA, which is present in all cells and especially in the gray matter of the brain and the retina of the eye.

Certain dietary choices affect a vegan mother's ability to convert ALA to DHA, allowing her to increase the amount of DHA delivered to baby through her breast milk. The body converts ALA to DHA most efficiently when the intake of oils high in omega-6 fatty acids is somewhat limited, thereby maintaining the optimal ratio of omega-6s to omega-3s (see page 296). Avoiding trans-fatty acids, processed and deep-fried foods, alcohol, and smoking also assists the conversion process (see pages 120 to 121).

Research suggests that DHA plays an important role in the mental and visual development of infants.[57] Preterm infants need supplemental DHA because this essential fat is so important to their development during the third trimester, and a premature baby is not yet able to synthesize his or her own DHA. Formulas for premature infants have been designed to include DHA; similar formulas also are available for full-term infants.[90]

In one small UK study, the amount of DHA in the breast milk of vegans who didn't use supplemental DHA was shown to be about 38 percent that of non-vegetarians.[99] However, the balance of omega-6 to omega-3 fatty acids in these mothers' diets averaged about 18:1—far greater than what's recommended for optimal conversion. Studies from the UK have also shown reduced DHA in the breast milk of lacto-ovo vegetarians, compared to nonvegetarians, although US studies found no significant differences.[59] The amount of DHA added to formula is quite variable (check labels) and can be less than what's found in breast milk, even that of unsupplemented vegans.

Taking a microalgae-derived DHA supplement seems a reasonable option to boost the DHA levels of breast milk. (Compared to fish oil, microalgae-based supplements offer a distinct advantage for all lactating women because the plant-based supplements are free of environmental contaminants.) The amount recommended by several groups of experts is in the range of 200 to 300 mg of DHA per day.[61-63] Nursing mothers also can consume foods or oils fortified with microalgae-derived DHA, although most contain only small amounts. A combination of DHA and EPA also is suitable, because the body can covert from one to the other, to some extent.

OTHER POSTPARTUM MATTERS

Although, to a new mother, the needs of the baby come first, she shouldn't neglect her own well-being during the baby's early months.

- **Regaining a pre-baby figure.** A vegan diet is a great help in supporting a gradual return to prepregnancy weight. Women lose, on average, 1.75 pounds (0.8 kg) per month during the first six months after birth. More-rapid weight loss isn't recommended while a mother is breast-feeding, because severe cuts in calories can affect the milk supply. A better choice is to find ways to gradually include exercise in the daily routine; walking is a very good choice.

- **Diet for role models.** Whether or not a new mother chooses to breast-feed, her diet still matters—and not just for her health. An alert baby's eyes take in every move made by caregivers; mom's and dad's dietary habits can create a healthy foundation for their children's lifelong practices. Knowing the impact their habits will have, this often is the time for parents to make big improvements in food choices, if they haven't already.

- **Lack of time.** Among all the new demands that nursing mothers face, the thought of preparing elaborate meals and snacks (or any meals at all) can seem daunting. However, healthy meals don't have to be fancy, nor do they need a great deal of preparation. A nutritious meal can be as simple as a bowl of cereal and fruit with nondairy milk; crackers with peanut butter and an apple; or a baked potato and a salad with black beans or chickpeas sprinkled on top.

  To reduce preparation time, parents can use convenience foods: canned beans, frozen vegetables, mixes, chopped vegetables, and frozen veggie burgers or entrées. Stir-fries offer endless variety. Time-saving appliances, such as slow cookers and pressure cookers, can be useful when preparing big batches of favorite bean dishes or lentil or pea soups; the excess can be served as leftovers or frozen in individual portions for future meals.

A focus on easy-to-prepare foods can leave more time for other activities. For example, one smart mom whose infant is thriving chose a combination of beans, kale, and quinoa as her dietary mainstay during lactation to find time to get herself back into shape (quinoa cooks in fifteen to twenty minutes). Such a combination can be eaten for breakfast or, for variety at other meals, spiced up with salsa. Snacks add interest to such a basic menu: vegetables with hummus, tofu, or avocado dip; rice or corn cakes with nut or seed butters; or trail mix and fruit or juice.

Finally, instead of hosting a baby shower, suggest that friends or family provide the gift of time, by supplying a frozen vegan meal, a vegan restaurant or take-out coupon, an hour or two of housekeeping help or babysitting, or a massage.

HOW LONG TO BREAST-FEED

Vegetarian (including vegan) women tend to extend breast-feeding longer, compared to nonvegetarians. The WHO and the AAP support breast-feeding for two years or longer, along with the introduction of iron-rich foods and other foods starting at about 6 months of age (see page 309).[28, 76, 77] Nature seems to have intended the natural age of weaning to be between 2 and 4 years of age, when lactase, the enzyme that breaks down the milk sugar lactose, naturally declines.

In certain circumstances, mothers may need to supplement breast-feeding with the use of infant formula, either as the baby's primary source of nutrition or as an occasional option.

INFANT FORMULA

The AAP advises that the only acceptable substitute for breast milk during a baby's first year is iron-fortified infant formula. This formula choice can help prevent the development of iron-deficiency anemia. (Formula contains higher levels of iron than breast milk; however, the iron in breast milk is more readily absorbed.) Premature infants are at the highest risk of iron deficiency, because their iron stores can be very low. In full-term infants, iron stores typically last for about the first six months; solid foods—particularly those containing iron—should then be introduced.

Though infant formula lacks some of the immune-protective compounds found in breast milk, it does supply adequate amounts of vitamins D and B_{12}. The selected formula should also contain added DHA.[28, 75] (For a link regarding formula choices, see Resources on page 449.) Standard formulas are based on cow's milk or on soy milk; these are fortified carefully so they provide nutrition that's similar to breast milk, as much as possible. For parents who wish to raise vegan infants, soy formula is the best option. Both the AAP and the US National Toxicology Program have approved the use of soy formula for infants.[91-95] Soy formula is as safe as formula based on cow's milk; it ensures normal growth and has been used successfully since 1909. Soy formula isn't intended for preterm infants or for those with congenital thyroid problems.[100]

As this book goes to press, soy infant formulas currently available in North America are close to being 100 percent vegan. However, they contain vitamin D_3 derived from lanolin in sheep's wool. At least one soy formula contains oleo (beef fat), making it unsuitable for vegans, so check labels. Unfortunately, vitamin D_2, which normally is derived from irradiated yeast, can't be included in a product labeled "organic," so organic products generally contain vitamin D_3. Formula companies continually make improvements in their products, and with sufficient consumer demand, any of these companies could produce an entirely vegan formula using vitamin D_2 or using vitamin D_3 from lichen (a plant-sourced vitamin D_3).

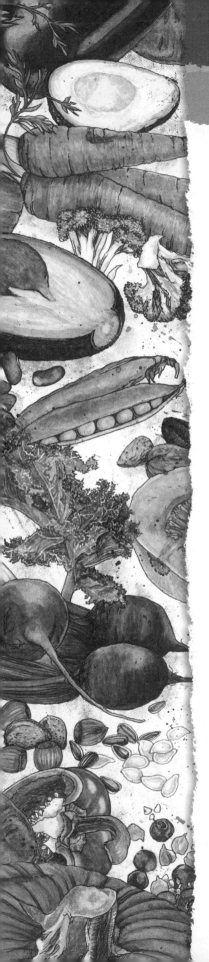

CHAPTER 10

Growing Vegans

Appropriately planned vegan, lactovegetarian, and lacto-ovo vegetarian diets satisfy nutrient needs of infants, children, and adolescents and promote normal growth.

POSITION PAPER ON VEGETARIAN DIETS, ACADEMY OF NUTRITION AND DIETETICS
(FORMERLY THE AMERICAN DIETETIC ASSOCIATION[1]

Meeting the nutrition needs of infants gives them a great start and puts in place a foundation for lifelong health. The years from birth through adolescence are characterized by growth spurts and other physical changes that result in unique physical requirements. Parents also must be prepared with strategies to navigate the challenges that arise as youngsters assume greater degrees of control over their dietary choices. This chapter provides guidelines for designing nutritionally balanced vegan diets that support each stage of the journey toward adulthood.

Baby's Big Adventure: Introducing Solid Foods

As noted in chapter 9, the World Health Organization (WHO) and major pediatric associations recommend exclusive breast-feeding during an infant's first four to six months; continued breast-feeding until the child is 2 years of age or older also is recommended.

Breast milk, iron-fortified soy formula, or both are the only foods that baby requires—when reliable sources of vitamins B_{12} and D are included—until the baby is about 6 months old. The importance of providing enough vitamin B_{12} during a baby's first six months cannot be stressed enough. Vitamin B_{12} comes through mother's milk (assuming the mother ensures an excellent B_{12} status of her own by consuming a reliable source of vitamin B_{12}). To avoid uncertainty and ensure safe levels of intake, the Institute of Medicine (IOM) suggests that vegan infants receive a B_{12} supplement from birth. A breast-fed or partially breast-fed baby should also get a vitamin D supplement of 10 mcg (400 IU) per day and may be given iron drops, starting at 4 months of age, until enough iron-rich foods are consumed, as recommended by the American Academy of Pediatrics (AAP). Soy formula provides vitamins B_{12} and D in specific quantities (check the label). [2–9] After 12 months of age (but not before), full-fat fortified soy milk is an acceptable alternative.

Breast-feeding through the next six months and up to 2 years of age or longer (with added complementary foods) confers a number of benefits. Continued breast-feeding provides protection against gastrointestinal and respiratory infection in the infant and possibly discourages overweight and obesity later in life. Longer lactation is linked with less risk of breast cancer in the mother and increased sensitivity and bonding between mother and child.

Depending on the amounts of complementary foods introduced to the baby at the same time, during the period between 6 and 8 months of age, mother's milk typically provides about 80 percent of an infant's caloric requirements; from 9 months to the first birthday, it can supply about half the calories, and one-third of the calories from age 1 to 2 years. During this stage, soy formula may be given instead of breast milk; there's abundant evidence that infants also thrive on this food. Soy formula has the approval of the AAP. It accounts for 25 percent of the formula sold in the United States; one infant in three receives soy formula during his or her first year. [3, 4, 10] (For more on formula choices, see Resources on page 449.)

The foods added midway through a baby's first year provide many important nutrients—iron in particular, which is essential for cognitive development—and also introduce a new world of sensory experiences. At the six-month point (perhaps a month or two earlier for some babies), the supply of iron stored during pregnancy is depleted. Babies indicate their readiness for solid foods when they can sit, hold up their head, clearly indicate an interest in foods that family members are eating, and the extrusion reflex disappears.

Babies younger than 4 months old should not be fed solid foods. One good reason to wait four to six months to introduce solid foods is to minimize the risk of food allergies. [6] Before then, the infant's intestinal lining has not yet perfected its filtering ability. The intestinal lining is a semipermeable membrane that blocks larger molecules and allows small molecules—the products of digestion—to pass through for the body's use. By acting as an effective barrier for undigested large molecules, the intestinal membrane prevents them from leaking into the bloodstream and triggering allergic reactions. By about 6 months of age, the baby's intestinal membrane has become an effective filter that can manage a more diverse diet. The function of a baby's intestinal lining and its connection to the development of allergies is a lively area of research. [6, 11]

Introducing solid foods at the right stage also may help to avoid weight problems in later life. For example, in children who were formula-fed, introducing solid foods before 4 months of age has been linked with six times the likelihood of obesity when the child is 3 years old. [12, 13]

The introduction of solid foods shouldn't be delayed too long after the baby reaches 6 months of age; this is a normal and optimal stage of learning for babies. If babies don't experience this period of fascination with new tastes and textures, they may develop into picky eaters and reject new foods.[14] The AAP has concluded that there is no convincing evidence that delaying the introduction of solid foods—including common allergens—beyond 6 months of age has a protective effect against the development of allergies.[12, 15]

BOOSTING BABY'S IRON STORES

The sequence and timing for introducing solid foods to babies in vegan families are similar to those in nonvegetarian households. In the past, strict sequences were suggested, but these rules have been modified as the understanding of food allergies and infant nutrition evolved; many variations work well.[4, 6, 11]

Foods rich in iron should be the first solid foods a baby consumes. Offer iron-rich foods at least twice a day. Though spinach, Swiss chard, and beet greens contain iron, little of the mineral is available for absorption (see page 181), so these aren't listed.[2, 4, 16] Instead, suitable iron-rich foods include:

- iron-fortified commercial infant cereals
- cooked and mashed lentils, beans, and tofu
- cooked and puréed or mashed kale, broccoli, and green beans (for example)
- foods listed in table 10.1 (page 312) and table 6.2 (page 214)

Parents can use a variety of iron-fortified infant cereals and grains to start baby on solid food; in fortified cereals, both ferrous fumarate and ferrous sulphate have been shown to effectively deliver iron.[17,18] Mixing iron-fortified infant formula with dry infant or family cereals will increase their iron content. Parents who prefer to start with well-cooked, puréed whole grains (mixed with breast milk or formula) can provide additional iron by giving the baby an iron supplement, in amounts advised by a physician.

Babies can thrive on home-prepared, iron-rich foods, but their digestive system may not be ready for some adult versions. For example, sprouting beans before cooking increases mineral availability; the baby (and the rest of the family) will absorb more iron, zinc, calcium, and magnesium from cooked, sprouted beans. However, the baby shouldn't be given raw sprouted beans; unwanted components (trypsin inhibitors and hemagglutinins) are present, and these are destroyed in cooking. Due to the potential for food-borne illness, other raw sprouts (alfalfa, clover, radish, and mung bean sprouts) also shouldn't be given to infants and young children.

Foods that are good iron sources also provide protein and other nutrients. Table 10.1 (page 312) shows the iron, zinc, and protein content of a number of infant foods, both commercially available and prepared at home. In commercial products, the words *enriched* and *fortified* indicate that nutrients, such as calcium, iron, or vitamins B_{12} or D, have been added to products. The label specifies which nutrients have been added.

When vitamin C–rich foods (orange, tangerine, or grapefruit sections; wedges of cantaloupe; raspberries and pieces of kiwifruit, pineapple, and strawberries) are eaten at approximately the same time as iron-fortified cereal or other iron-rich foods, these fruits can boost iron absorption. Fruit is preferable to fruit juice; if juice is given, amounts should be limited to ½ cup (125 ml) per day.[2, 4, 19] Conversely, cow's milk isn't a significant dietary source of iron, and it decreases iron absorption; the fact that its use is discouraged in infants up to 12 months old has proved to be a health benefit for babies.

The table below shows examples of foods appropriate for babies. Beans that aren't listed in table 10.1 have nutrient values in the same general range as those shown. For additional sources of protein, iron, and zinc, see table 3.5 (page 97) and table 6.2 (page 204). Check the labels of prepared foods, because their ingredients may change from time to time and vary in different countries. The infant formulas listed below were selected simply due to availability of data on the US Department of Agriculture (USDA) website; no endorsement is implied.[2, 20]

TABLE 10.1. Iron, zinc, and protein content in selected foods for infants

FOOD	AMOUNT	IRON (mg)	ZINC (mg)	PROTEIN (g)
BREAST MILK AND COMMERCIAL READY-TO-FEED FORMULAS				
Human breast milk	32 oz (976 g)	0.3	1.7	10.2
Human breast milk	6 oz (184 g)	0.06	0.3	1.9
Infant formula, Nestlé Good Start, Soy with Iron	32 oz (976 g)	12.2	5.9	15.9
Infant formula, Nestlé Good Start, Soy with Iron	6 oz (183 g)	2.3	1.1	3
Infant formula, Nestlé Good Start Supreme, Soy with Iron	32 oz (976 g)	9.7	5.2	14.2
Infant formula, Enfamil Prosobee, Soy with Iron	32 oz (976 g)	11.5	7.7	16
COMMERCIAL FORTIFIED INFANT CEREALS				
Baby food, barley cereal, dry	1 T (15 ml)	1.1	0.1	0.3
Baby food, brown rice cereal, dry, instant	1 T (15 ml)	1.8	0	0.3
Baby food, oatmeal cereal, dry	1 T (15 ml)	1.6	0.2	0.4
Baby food, rice cereal, dry	1 T (15 ml)	1.2	0.05	0.2
COMMERCIAL BABY FOODS: LEGUMES, VEGETABLES, AND FRUIT				
Baby food, peas, strained	1 jar, 3 oz (95 g)	0.9	0.4	3.1
Baby food, green beans, strained	1 jar, 4 oz (113 g)	0.8	0.2	1.4
Baby food, green beans, junior	1 jar, 6 oz (170 g)	1.8	0.3	2
Baby food, sweet potatoes, junior	1 jar, 2.5 oz (71 g)	0.3	0.2	0.8
Baby food, apricots and applesauce, strained	1 jar, 4 oz (113 g)	0.3	0.05	0.2
Baby food, prunes, strained	1 jar, 2.5 oz (71 g)	0.3	0.1	0.7

FOOD	AMOUNT	IRON (mg)	ZINC (mg)	PROTEIN (g)
GRAINS AND CEREALS PREPARED AT HOME				
Oat cereal, iron-fortified, instant, made with water; package makes ¾ c (177 g)	1 oz (28 g)	10.6	1.1	4.2
Oatmeal, unfortified, made with water	½ c (117 g)	1	1.2	3
Ready-to-eat dry fortified cereals (such as Total, puffed rice, corn flakes)	1 c (14–23 g)	4.4–13	0.14–11.2	0.9–1.4
Rice, brown, cooked	½ c (97 g)	0.4	0.6	2.5
Rice, white, enriched, cooked	½ c (79 g)	1.0	0.4	2.1
Spaghetti or macaroni, enriched, cooked	½ c (70 g)	0.9	0.5	4.1
Spaghetti or macaroni, whole wheat	½ c (70 g)	0.7	0.6	3.7
Wheat germ	2 T (15 g)	0.1	1.9	3.6
LEGUMES PREPARED AT HOME				
Black beans, cooked	½ c (85 g)	1.8	1.0	7.6
Chickpeas, cooked	½ c (70 g)	2.4	1.2	7.3
Edamame, cooked	½ c (78 g)	1.8	1.1	8.4
Green peas, cooked	½ c (80 g)	1.2	1.0	4.3
Lentils, cooked	½ c (99 g)	3.3	1.3	8.9
Lima beans, cooked	½ c (85 g)	2.1	0.7	5.8
Navy beans, cooked	½ c (91 g)	2.2	0.9	7.5
Pinto beans, cooked	½ c (86 g)	1.8	0.8	7.7
Tempeh	2 oz (60 g)	1.3	0.9	10.9
Tofu, firm	¼ c (63 g)	1.7	1.0	9.9
OTHER FOODS				
Apricots, dried	2 halves (7 g)	0.2	0.03	0.2
Applesauce, without sugar	½ c (122 g)	0.3	0.04	0.2
Avocado	¼ (50 g)	0.3	0.3	1.0
Broccoli, cooked	½ c (78 g)	0.5	0.4	1.9
Kale, cooked	½ c (65 g)	0.6	0.2	1.2
Molasses	1 tsp (7 g)	0.3	0.02	0
Peanut butter	2 T (32 g)	0.6	0.9	8
Prune juice	½ c (128 g)	1.5	0.3	0.8
Prunes, pitted	2 (19 g)	0.2	0.1	0.4
Pumpkin, canned, without salt or sugar	½ c (122 g)	1.7	0.2	1.4

Sources:[2, 20]

ADVANTAGES OF IRON FROM PLANT FOODS

Some health professionals recommend the use of red meat as a first food for infants in an effort to prevent iron-deficiency anemia in this vulnerable population. However, such a recommendation can set in place lifelong dietary habits linked with increased risk of cardiovascular disease, diabetes, certain types of cancer, dementia, and premature death.[22]

Foods that contain heme iron need not be viewed as essential iron sources. Recent research shows plant ferritin to be a significant and readily available source of dietary iron.[23] Plant ferritin is absorbed independently by the body through a separate transport system, so it doesn't compete with other dietary iron sources.[24] Iron from plant foods has the advantage of being accompanied by abundant protective phytochemicals (see page 260). This form of iron is less irritating to the intestines and doesn't promote the oxidative stress associated with heme iron. As well, the vitamin C and organic acids present in many plant foods further enhance nonheme iron absorption.

Iron Supplementation

The AAP advises that supplementation of oral iron drops before six months may be needed to support iron stores; this should be done with physician guidance.[2] Health Canada also recommends iron supplementation where necessary, for example, where intake of iron-rich foods is insufficient.[4, 25] For infants who get all their food from formula, the formula chosen should include iron; in that case, supplemental iron isn't needed.[2]

Individual recommendations for supplemental iron in preterm infants should be provided by a pediatrician.[2, 26]

Iron Deficiency

Regardless of dietary pattern, iron deficiency is the most common deficiency for infants and has been associated with developmental delays. A Norwegian study found 4 percent of infants had an iron deficiency at 6 months of age and 12 percent at 12 months of age.[27] The National Health and Nutrition Examination Survey of toddlers between 1 and 3 years old showed iron deficiency in 6 to 15 percent of these children, depending on ethnicity. The iron fortification of infant cereals, the widespread use of iron-fortified infant formula (among those using formula), and the decline in the use of cow's milk are given some credit for the reduction in iron-deficiency anemia that has occurred in the decades since 1970.[2, 25]

Introducing Baby to the World of Tastes

Babies around the world and throughout human history have proved that they can thrive on an immense variety of adult foods. Getting a baby started on solid foods requires a change in routine. For a successful beginning, it's best to offer an unfamiliar food at a time when baby is rested, awake, supported to sit up straight, and ready for a new experience. There are two ways to begin. One approach is to give puréed food from a spoon. With a purée, a baby will learn to swallow first and then chew. The other is to offer suitably sized chunks of solid, soft foods, in a method sometimes called "baby-led weaning." Often, parents use a mix of the two techniques, which are detailed below.

Bacteria can easily upset a baby's digestive system; hands and any equipment that touches the food must be absolutely clean. Use an easy-to-clean high chair on a mat; a chair that can be placed in the shower is ideal. In addition, all cooked foods must be cooled before serving.

Salt and sugar shouldn't be added to baby foods so that babies experience natural flavors. The influence of salt on the body begins early, and excess intakes during the first two years have been linked with hypertension and cardiovascular disease in later life. Immature kidneys aren't designed to cope with added salt.[28] Babies aren't born with a yen for fast food, though they quickly can develop such preferences; as a result, it's best that the introduction of added salt and sugar be delayed as long as possible.

- **Puréed food from a spoon.** A typical beginning is to offer a half-teaspoon of iron-rich food that has the consistency of cream soup one to two times per day. It may take a few weeks for a baby to grasp the concept that the food is supposed to stay inside the mouth and then be swallowed.

Though most commercial baby food is puréed, it isn't essential that all homemade baby foods be puréed, as was common a few decades ago. Foods with the consistency of mashed potato have value because they encourage the development of chewing skills. Soft fruit can be mashed with a potato masher or fork; a baby-food mill, blender, or food processor can purée peeled vegetables and fruits that have had the skin, string, and seeds removed. Puréed food may be strained, though this step isn't essential. Sources for making wholesome baby foods from scratch can be found in Resources on page 449.[29]

For convenience, larger quantities of puréed foods can be prepared and poured into the sections of a clean ice cube tray, covered with waxed paper, and frozen. For example, greens (such as kale or collard greens) can be steamed or boiled, then puréed with a little cooking water, formula, or a mixture of these. The frozen cubes can be transferred to a freezer bag or container, with a label showing the preparation date. Cubes keep for up to one month in the freezer and can be thawed and used as needed.

If not frozen immediately, prepared baby food may be covered and kept refrigerated for two days, then discarded if not used. To prevent bacteria from spoiling uneaten food, any food that the baby or the spoon has touched should be discarded.

- **Baby-led weaning.** Babies who are fed puréed food from a spoon learn the swallowing technique *before* learning how to gum soft foods into a liquid that can be swallowed. In contrast, during baby-led weaning, babies first gum and gnaw food—exploring its shape, texture, and taste. They gradually learn to move the food to the back of the mouth and then finally learn to swallow. A distinct advantage of this approach is the sensory experience provided by the new foods, such as a strawberry or slice of avocado. This feeding method is summarized in *Baby-Led Weaning* by Gill Rapley and Tracey Murkett (Vermilion Publishing, 2008). Though the book is far from vegan, the method is easily adapted to plant-based eating, and some vegan recipes are included. Vegan blogs on the subject are available online.

Babies can choke on soft pieces of food or even on puréed food; to avoid this, make sure the baby is sitting upright, not leaning back or slumping (see the "Cautionary Notes for Infant Feeding" on page 318). Fortunately, a baby's gag reflex is farther forward in his mouth than in an adult mouth; this reflex effectively moves food forward and out, protecting the baby from choking, though caregivers must be nearby and alert.

Examples of starter foods for baby-led weaning include well-cooked beans or tofu, each offered a few days apart and placed directly on the high chair tray or on a plate. Finger-shaped pieces tend to be easiest to grasp, such as toast fingers with a thin layer of peanut butter. With time, baby can manage smaller pieces and clumps of sticky rice, oatmeal, pasta (such as fusilli or rigatoni), or well-cooked peas. These can be offered between milk feedings.

When beans (such as chickpeas or lima beans) are first given to infants, they should be very well cooked, rather than having the firm consistency of canned beans, so they can be mashed between the fingers (or baby gums). (When offering processed or canned food or food from the family table, make sure it has no added salt.)

In a few months, a baby also will learn to eat from a spoon by imitating adult behavior. At some point, a blunt baby-safe fork may prove easier to use with certain foods. As increasing amounts of food end up inside the baby, he or she will automatically adjust intakes of breast milk or formula. Milk feedings (breast or iron-fortified formula) can continue as a major part of babies' diets until the age of 2 or more.

• **Finger foods.** At about 6 to 8 months of age, infants discover their amazing ability to pick up objects with their whole hand and eventually with thumb and forefinger. They often are so excited by this achievement that they'd rather explore this new skill than eat. Messy eating is normal and is a part of learning. Though parents may wonder if any food reaches their stomachs, babies often eat more when they are allowed to feed themselves.

As a precaution, solid foods should only be given to a baby seated in a high chair. The items should be soft enough to be gummed (rather than chewed) or to soften in the mouth. Examples include steamed tofu fingers; well-cooked beans or lentils; florets of boiled broccoli or cauliflower; fingers or cubes of soft-cooked vegetables or fruit; green beans (string removed); slices of raw, soft fruits, such as avocado, banana, kiwifruit, mango, melon, or papaya; chunks of pita bread or tortilla; toast fingers spread with hummus or peanut butter; teething biscuits; different shapes of cooked pasta; unsweetened ready-to-eat dry cereal; pieces of rolls or pancakes; and unsalted crackers.

The baby should be monitored after the first introduction to each individual food, to ensure the food causes no allergic reaction (see page 319). If not, the food can be mixed with other well-accepted foods. Soon the baby can share the family's tofu stir-fries, lentil curries, chilis, ratatouille, pasta dishes, stews, vegan pizza, risotto, roasted vegetables, and nut or seed "creams." (For the latter, blend nut butter with soy milk, water, or juice.) The baby's portion shouldn't have added salt, sugar, tamari, or Bragg Liquid Aminos.

Tables 10.2 and 10.3 show sample menus suitable for infants who have reached 7 months and 11 months of age, respectively. In some cases, mashing the offered food is optional. Replace breast-feeding by formula feeding where appropriate. A baby also may accept water in a cup. Before the baby reaches 6 months of age or if there's any concern about safety, the water should be boiled and then cooled.

LEARNING BABY'S SIGNALS

Healthy babies know how much to eat. Some eat a lot, some a little; variation in appetite from day to day is perfectly normal. If they're sick or teething, they may not want much food. A baby's signals, such as reaching out, turning her or his head away, or spitting food out, will indicate when to begin or stop feeding.

One way to tell whether a baby is starting to swallow any solids is to watch for intact pieces appearing in the diaper. Over time, mastication and digestion of these foods will improve. Strained apricots and prunes may cause loose stools; these can be omitted until the baby's digestive system has matured a little. For infants older than 6 months, strained apricots and prunes or a little prune juice

TABLE 10.2. Sample menu for a 7-month-old infant

TIME OF DAY	EXAMPLES OF FOODS TO OFFER
Early morning	Breast-feeding
	Breast-feeding Iron-fortified infant cereal Mashed soft strawberries or other fruit
Snack	Breast-feeding Whole-grain toast cut into small pieces or strips
Lunch	Breast-feeding Steamed tofu cubes Cooked and mashed broccoli or other vegetable
Snack	Breast-feeding Cooked unsweetened prunes or other fruit
Supper	Breast-feeding Iron-fortified infant cereal Well-cooked and mashed lentils Cooked and mashed sweet potato or other vegetable
Snack	Breast-feeding

TABLE 10.3. Sample menu for an 11-month-old infant

TIME OF DAY	EXAMPLES OF FOODS TO OFFER
Early morning	Breast-feeding
Breakfast	Breast-feeding Iron-fortified infant cereal Chopped strawberries, cantaloupe, kiwifruit, or other fruit
Snack	Breast-feeding Whole-grain bread cut into strips, muffin, or Cheerios
Lunch	Breast-feeding Steamed tofu cubes, tempeh, soy yogurt, or pea soup Cooked mashed sweet potato or squash or brown rice Cooked broccoli or other vegetable
Snack	Breast-feeding Canned peach slices or cooked unsweetened prunes
Supper	Breast-feeding Iron-fortified infant cereal Well-cooked beans or lentils Cooked and mashed carrots, yams, or other vegetable
Snack	Breast-feeding

may help in preventing constipation.[31] Beets or greens can have obvious, but harmless, color effects on the stool.

Baby's meals should be viewed as four to six small feedings, given when the child is hungry and interested, rather than scheduled as three meals a day.[31] As baby gets older, feeding times are easier when small portions of solid food are put directly on the high chair's tray; later, food can be placed on a plastic plate or in a bowl with straight sides. When the baby finishes a small portion, more can be offered; amounts can be increased gradually. Do not force solids. If solid food is rejected, due to illness, for example, focus on fluids (breast milk or formula) instead. By 11 months, though breast-feeding may be offered throughout the day (as in table 10.3), some meals or snacks may be limited to solid foods.

Cautionary Notes for Infant Feeding

- Stay nearby while the baby is eating.
- Don't let anyone other than the baby put pieces of food into her mouth, including older children who want to be helpful.
- Avoid small pieces that can cause choking, such as nuts, sunflower seeds, pumpkin seeds, peanuts, raw peas, corn kernels, popcorn, whole grapes (these can be halved or quartered), raisins, and hard candies. Avoid chunks of hard, raw fruits and vegetables (carrot can be grated) and vegan "hot dogs" or other cylindrical foods.

- Remove pits from apricots, cherries, peaches, and plums.
- Don't offer peanut butter on a spoon; spread it on a cracker or piece of toast.
- Teach children how to chew well.
- Avoid giving babies black or green tea, coffee, and foods with added salt, fat, and/or sugar.
- Check labels on baby food jars to ensure the items contain no added sugar.
- Honey should not be given to babies under 1 year of age; it can lead to botulism in the immature intestines of young infants. (Also, it's not a vegan food.)
- For ease in swallowing, thin cashew or almond butters by blending with fortified soy milk, water, or juice.
- Never give a baby unpasteurized juice or sweetened juice. Limit intake of fruit juice to ½ cup (125 ml) per day or less; more can crowd out other important foods. Juice can be mixed with an equal amount of water.
- Choose organic baby food (homemade or commercial) as often as possible.
- Don't try to persuade the baby to hurry or to eat more than she wants.
- Communicate these cautionary notes to the baby's caregivers.

DEALING WITH TEETHING

Babies as young as 3 months may begin teething, although the usual ages when teeth begin to appear can be anywhere from 6 to 12 months. During teething, babies appreciate cool items to soothe their sore gums, including:

- a clean, cold, wet washcloth
- a plastic teething ring that has been refrigerated
- spoonfuls or chunks of homemade fresh orange sherbet. (To make this, put equal parts of a peeled, chopped, and seeded orange and orange juice in a blender, process until smooth, and then freeze for about an hour until fairly firm.[29])
- commercial or homemade vegan teething biscuits (search online for products or recipes)

PREVENTING FOOD ALLERGIES

The early introduction of solid foods—especially at or before 3 months of age—has been linked with the development of food allergies; current recommendations suggest beginning the introduction of solid foods at about 6 months of age. Families with a history of allergies should seek advice from their health care provider; pediatricians and allergy specialists can help individualize the introduction of foods beyond breast milk to minimize the risks for the baby.[11, 16, 32, 33] Vegan parents should note that up to 94 percent of skin-prick allergy tests have yielded false-positive results for soybean, meaning that soy can appear to be an allergen when in fact it isn't.[11] True allergies to soy often are outgrown during childhood. Because a child is allergic to one legume (such as soy or peanuts), it doesn't follow that they'll be allergic to others in that family.[16]

Concepts regarding gluten-containing cereals and potentially allergenic foods, such as peanut and nut butters, have changed in recent years.[11, 16, 33] Introducing babies to cereals at 6 months of age and after, while they're still breast-feeding, is linked with reduced likelihood of reactions to such grains, compared to introduction either before 3 months of age or much later than 6 months. Late exposure to gluten (after 7 months of age and after breast-feeding has been discontinued) may increase risk of celiac disease. Breast-feeding seems to play a protective role in reducing reactions to gluten or to a potential allergen, perhaps by supporting the immune system and the maturation of the intestinal tract.[32–34]

For any infant, and especially those with a family history of allergies, it's wise to introduce foods one at a time and wait three or four days to see if there's any reaction before introducing another new food. (Mixed foods shouldn't be introduced unless the individual ingredients have been given without reaction.) Signs of food allergy can appear on the skin (redness or itchiness), in the respiratory tract (stuffy nose, wheezing, or runny eyes), or in the gastrointestinal tract (colic that doesn't go away, frequent spitting up, or diarrhea). Guidelines regarding the ideal time to introduce foods that tend to be allergenic have been changing in recent years; parents should follow the advice of the family physician or dietitian.[6, 11, 12]

HEALTHY CHOICES FOR BABIES

Fluids

As a baby's sole nourishment for the first six months, breast milk or formula generally supplies enough fluid. After that, sips of water may be offered from a cup, or water may be given daily in a bottle. Water intake becomes more important as solid foods replace breast milk or formula and is especially important when the weather is hot or if the baby has a fever. Because iron-fortified infant formula is so nutritious, it's preferable for babies until age 2, rather than fortified soy milk.[31]

Avoid Bedtime Bottles and Sweetened Soothers

To avert possible dental damage, a baby shouldn't be put to bed with a bottle of formula or juice or given a bottle as a daytime pacifier. Instead, a bottle of plain water or a pacifier should be used. Don't dip pacifiers in sugar, honey, or other sweet substances.[31]

OTHER ESSENTIAL NUTRIENTS FROM BIRTH TO 18 MONTHS

Vitamin B$_{12}$

When breast milk supplies most of a baby's calories, a lactating woman must ensure that she has an adequate intake of vitamin B$_{12}$ (see chapter 9) because this vital nutrient is passed to the baby through her milk. Severe B$_{12}$ deficiency can lead to irreversible brain damage in the infant, thus a reliable source is critical. To avoid uncertainty and be safe, the Institute of Medicine suggests that vegan infants receive a B_{12} supplement from birth. For entirely formula-fed infants, infant formula is fortified with sufficient vitamin B_{12}.[5]

After the baby has moved to solid foods, he or she should receive a vitamin B_{12} supplement or should have B_{12}-fortified foods or formula three times a day. Recommended vitamin B_{12} intakes are 0.5 mcg at 6 to 12 months of age and 0.9 mcg at 1 to 3 years of age; any excess is excreted in the urine. (See the appendix on pages 446 and 447 for recommended intakes of vitamins and minerals at different ages.)

Vitamin D

For breast-fed babies up to 1 year old, the recommended intake is 10 mcg (400 IU) given as a supplement; this amount is supplied by infant formula, so a supplement isn't necessary for formula-fed babies. Newborns and infants up to 6 months old shouldn't be given more than 25 mcg (1,000 IU) of supplementary vitamin D per day.[35] Current practices advise that infants younger than 1 year of age avoid direct sunlight, due to the risk of skin cancer.

For children from 1 to 3 years of age, the recommended vitamin D intake is 15 mcg (600 IU).[35] In addition to its requirement for bone mineralization, vitamin D is believed to be important for prevention of development of type 1 diabetes as well as other chronic diseases later in life.[36]

Omega-3 Fatty Acids

Although there's no Recommended Dietary Allowance for essential fatty acids, Adequate Intakes (AI) (see page 182) have been set at 0.5 grams of alpha-linolenic acid (ALA) for babies from 6 to 12 months old and 0.7 grams for children from 1 to 3 years old; higher amounts may be advisable for vegan children.

Sufficient omega-3 fatty acids can be obtained from breast milk or DHA-fortified infant formula. Additional steps can be taken to maximize long-chain omega-3 fatty acid DHA, which may be preferable.

- If a breast-feeding mother consumes a supplemental source of DHA, her intake should be at least 200 to 300 mg of DHA per day.
- If infant formula is used, one with added DHA should be selected.
- If no direct DHA sources are provided double the AI for ALA. ALA sources include ground flaxseeds, chia seeds, hempseeds, and walnuts (walnuts could be ground and added to cereals, spreads, cookies, or other foods). Quality oils that provide a 1:1 or 2:1 ratio of omega-6 to omega-3 fatty acids are available; some provide DHA in addition to ALA. Read the label to determine appropriate serving sizes. The source of ALA can be an oil blend that provides a mixture of omega-3, -6, and -9 fatty acids.
- If breast-feeding stops between 1 and 3 years of age and the child gets full-fat fortified soy milk rather than formula, then he or she should either obtain 0.7 grams of ALA from the foods listed above plus 70 mg of supplemental DHA

or receive double the ALA, meaning 1.4 grams per day.[37–39] (For more on omega-3 fatty acids, see table 4.5 on page 129 and other sections in chapter 4.)

Toddlers and Preschoolers

When young children leave breast or bottle behind (at least some of the time), their nutrient needs change again. They move from a reliance on breast milk or formula to family foods, and expand their exploration of textures, tastes, and their ability to feed themselves. They can be nutritionally vulnerable during this time of change, of growth spurts, and of discovering the power of saying "No!" The key to a successful transition to healthy vegan foods is to be flexible, adjusting for the child's individual preferences, while following a balanced diet plan. This can be averaged over time.

FORTIFIED FOODS OR SUPPLEMENTS

Vitamin B$_{12}$

The recommended intake is 0.9 mcg per day. From a larger dose, a smaller fraction is absorbed. Children should receive B$_{12}$ from one of the three sources below:

- a daily supplement that provides 10 to 40 mcg of vitamin B$_{12}$
- a twice-a-week supplement of 375 mcg of vitamin B$_{12}$
- a food fortified with at least 0.3 mcg of vitamin B$_{12}$ (or 5 percent of the DV) three times a day. (This could include some combination of infant formula, fortified soy milk, fortified cereals, and nutritional yeast; check labels. Because the amounts of vitamins in fortified foods can vary, some experts suggest also giving a daily or weekly supplement that provides B$_{12}$.)

Vitamin D

The recommended intake is 15 mcg (600 IU) per day. Parents should select one of the following options daily to provide adequate vitamin D:

- a daily supplement that provides 15 mcg (600 IU) of vitamin D
- foods fortified with 1.7 mcg (70 IU) of vitamin D three times a day (such as 6 ounces or 180 ml of infant formula or fortified soy milk) plus a daily supplement that provides 10 mcg (400 IU) of vitamin D
- sun exposure on face and forearms between 10 a.m. and 3 p.m.; ten to fifteen minutes for light-skinned children and twenty minutes for those with darker skin

A combination of sun exposure, fortified foods, and supplements can work well. Because adequate sun exposure isn't an option in winter months at latitudes above 37 degrees N (see page 224), children living in these locations should receive vitamin D using supplements and/or fortified foods. Excess sun exposure and vitamin D intakes above 63 mcg (2,520 IU) per day should be avoided (see pages 222 to 230).[35, 40]

FIGURE 10.1. Typical daily vegan food guide for 1- to 3-year-old children

Include a wide variety of foods. Offer water from a cup between meals.

Milks and formula: Total 20 to 24 oz (600 to 700 ml)

Five servings of breast milk, commercial infant formula, full-fat fortified soy milk, or a combination of these.

Breads and cereals: 4 or more toddler-sized servings

1 toddler-sized serving =

¼ c (60 ml) cooked cereal, grain, or pasta

½ c (125 ml) ready-to-eat cereal

½ slice bread or a similar-sized piece of tortilla, pita bread, or roll

Vegetables: 2 or more toddler-sized servings

1 toddler-sized serving =

¼ c (60 ml) cooked vegetables

⅓ c (85 ml) vegetable juice

½ c (125 ml) salad or other raw vegetable pieces

Fruits: 2 or more toddler-sized servings

1 toddler-sized serving =

½ to 1 fresh fruit

¼ cup (60 ml) cooked fruit

¼ cup (60 ml) fruit juice (limit to ½ cup total per day)

Beans and alternatives: 2 or more toddler-sized servings

1 toddler-sized serving =

¼ cup (60 ml) cooked beans, peas, or lentils

2 oz (60 g) tofu or tempeh

½ to 1 oz (15 to 30 g) meat substitute

2 oz (30 ml) soy yogurt

1 to 2 T (15 to 30 ml) peanut butter

Nuts and seeds: 1 or more toddler-sized servings

1 toddler-sized serving =

1 to 2 T (15 to 30 ml) nut or seed butter

2 T (30 ml) nuts or seeds

Omega-3 Fatty Acids

The AI for essential fatty acids has been set at 0.7 grams of ALA. Many experts suggest that this should be doubled to 1.4 grams of ALA for vegan toddlers to support conversion of ALA to DHA, or that additional DHA may be beneficial. Options for getting these essential fats are:

- breast milk (see page 305 for a mother's DHA sources)
- infant formula that includes DHA
- nuts, seeds, or oils in quantities that provide 0.7 grams of ALA (see table 4.5 on page 129) plus a supplement that provides 70 mg of DHA (vegan DHA sources are available online)
- nuts, seeds, or oils in quantities that provide 1.4 grams of ALA, such as ½ teaspoon (2 ml) of flaxseed oil, 1 teaspoon (5 ml) of an oil that contains a blend of omega-3, -6, and -9 fatty acids, 2 teaspoons (10 ml) of chia seeds, 2 tablespoons (30 ml) of hempseeds, or 3 tablespoons (45 ml) of walnuts (see table 4.5 on page 129).

Oils rich in omega-3 fatty acids are unstable and have a low smoke point, so they shouldn't be used for cooking. Meanwhile, chia seeds can be added to cooked cereal; hempseeds; to smoothies and cereals; and walnuts to cereals, loaves, patties, and other foods, such as vegan pesto and other spreads.

Iodine

The recommended intake is 90 mcg, which can be obtained from ⅓ teaspoon (2 g) of iodized table salt. However, this amount of iodized table salt also delivers 388 mg of sodium—or more than one-third of a child's recommended intake for the day (800 mg sodium).

Another reliable way to provide the recommended amount of iodine is in supplement form or by a using a combination of supplement (which may provide only 50 mcg of iodine) plus a little iodized salt. Kelp is an option only if the amounts of iodine are listed on the label; otherwise, the kelp's iodine content may vary greatly and be insufficient or excessive.

Multivitamin-Mineral Supplements

Toddlers can be given a vegan multivitamin-mineral supplement that includes vitamins B_{12} and D and iodine, as well as calcium, iron, and zinc, to top up their intakes of these nutrients from foods, especially during a stage when meals seem unbalanced or insufficient.[41-43] Vegan supplements can be found in local natural foods stores or sourced online. All supplements should be safely stored away from children.

MEAL AND SNACK PLANNING

At weaning, little ones are nutritionally vulnerable. It's hard to beat human milk and infant formula, which are so well suited to the first years of life. Toddlers are switching from these easily digested fluids—which are tailored to infant needs and in which approximately half the calories come from high-quality fat—to an assortment of foods that can be more challenging to eat.

Children have small stomachs and may need meals or nutritious snacks every two to three hours. Youngsters thrive on healthier high-fat plant foods, such as tofu, nut and seed butters, avocado, soy yogurt, soy formula, and fortified full-fat soy milk. In contrast, bulky foods (such as salads) can fill a child's small stomach while providing few calories. For good nutrition, foods from three to five of the food groups listed in figure 10.1 on page 323 should be included at each meal; at least two food groups should be represented at snack time. Any of the foods can be served any time of day. For example, in some parts of the world, lentils are regularly served at breakfast. Though whole grains are excellent choices, vegan parents may be surprised to learn that refined breads, cereals, crackers, and pastas, which are lower in fiber and bulk, also can be healthful parts of a toddler's diet. Iron-rich foods, such as iron-fortified dry cereals and other items listed in tables 10.1 (page 312) and 6.2 (page 204), should be provided often.[44]

It's best to offer meals at regular times. Children shouldn't eat while running or playing; avoid or keep to a minimum other distractions (such as television or tablets). To prevent choking, seat children at the table with an adult nearby. It's natural for children to take time to finish their meals, and adults may want to match their children's pace at the table instead of hurrying them along. Leisurely mealtimes are viewed as one of the health benefits of the Mediterranean diet.

Healthy snack ideas include muffins (made with nutritious ingredients and kept handy in the freezer), soy yogurt, a tray of cut-up veggies with an avocado or bean dip, or a smoothie with hempseeds.

Avoiding Power Struggles

If a child isn't hungry, he or she shouldn't be forced to eat. Although regular meals are important for children, it's acceptable if they miss a meal occasionally. By deciding when and how much to eat, a child learns self-confidence and independent thinking.

Meal and snack times provide an arena in which children and parents work out issues of independence (feeding oneself) and dependence (being fed). A creative approach can have better results than efforts to force feeding. For example, when one small girl stubbornly refused to be fed with a spoon, her parent gave her the spoon and let her feed the adult instead. As food dribbled down the adult's chin, the pair dissolved in laughter, harmony was restored, and the meal proceeded.

Children shouldn't be punished for not eating; such actions can override their natural cues regarding hunger and fullness. Parents who try to force a child to eat will likely fail—and possibly steer the child toward eating problems. Instead, parents and caregivers can decide which foods to serve and allow the child to choose whether and how much to eat. Offering a selection within a food group (such as bananas, blueberries, or papaya; or bread, tortillas, or noodles) provides choice, as well as motivation to eat something. A child may reject a food on one or many occasions yet accept and enjoy it in the future.

On the other hand, parents needn't cater to every wish. Nor should dessert be used as a bribe; this raises the status of sweets so they seem more desirable. Instead, it's best to remove uneaten food without comment. This portion or another nutritious choice can be offered again at snack time.

By 12 months of age, children can become independent eaters and feed themselves. Parents encourage autonomy and avoid conflict by providing nutritious finger foods and allowing children to accept or refuse what they wish. Though the "Vegan Food Guide for 1- to 3-Year-Old Children" (see figure 10.1 on page 323) is helpful, a child's diet won't always follow the guide's recommendations. Adults can model good eating habits and be confident that their example will be followed.

Picky Eaters

It may seem that five foods favored by children can't possibly sustain a child's life. Yet over the course of a day, if a child that weighs 25 to 33 pounds (11 to 15 kg) consumes 3 cups (750 ml) of fortified soy milk, two peanut butter sandwiches, two sliced bananas, and ½ cup (125 ml) of peas, he or she receives enough calories and triple the recommended intake for protein. These foods provide more than enough B vitamins, vitamins A, C, E, and K, calcium, iron, magnesium, phosphorus, selenium, and zinc, plus 85 percent of the potassium and more than half the recommended intake for vitamin D. Even though this "picky eater" firmly rejects every other food in the house, these simple choices are packed with nutrition.

Though children may appear to be fussy eaters, examining their food intake, energy, and growth often proves they're managing well and even thriving. They may reject much on their plate at meals, while between-meal snacks disappear easily. That makes snack choices important.

Parents can employ other strategies to pique a child's appetite, such as inviting them to participate in simple food preparation. One vegan father overcame concerns about his daughter's lack of interest in food by inventing a concoction he called Sneaky Dad's Pudding. He helped his daughter to climb up on a stool by his side to add nutritious ingredients to a blender. These included strawberries, a banana, cocoa or carob powder, hempseeds, nut butter, a wedge of avocado, a little orange juice, and fortified soy milk to thin the mixture to the desired consistency. He then allowed her to push the button to start the blender. As cocreator of this tasty combination, she enjoyed sharing it with her dad, while the father could rest assured that she wasn't developing a deficiency.

Creativity can ensure that children consume vegetables, even if they've put a ban on them; children do outgrow such temporary distastes. Meanwhile, muffins can be prepared with grated carrots, cooked squash, or pumpkin as an ingredient. Children often will add avocado, tomato, or sprouts to a veggie burger or taco, at the same time that they might shun cooked spinach. Parents can set out platters of cut vegetables for snacking.

To encourage picky eaters, one of the best tools is perseverance. Mealtimes can be made pleasant and include at least one favorite food. The child can be encouraged to try something different, and his or her success in trying new foods celebrated. Table 10.4 suggests solutions to a few of the common challenges.

Food, Nutrition, and Health:
From Toddlers to Teenagers

Although most parents didn't learn how to prepare wholesome and delicious vegan food as children, this may be the ideal time to develop this skill.[45] If they're good role models, parents and caregivers can inspire their children to develop healthy diets. Research associated with 1,254 people from 61 to 90 years old whose diets and health had been tracked since childhood

TABLE 10.4. Food challenges and solutions

NORMAL PHASES OF GROWING UP	AS THE CHILD MAY SEE IT	AS THE PARENT MAY SEE IT	WHAT TO DO ABOUT IT
Refusal to eat	I'm not hungry, I'm asserting my independence, or I want attention.	The child must somehow be made to eat; growing children need food.	Respect the wisdom of the child's own body (and spirit). A skipped meal won't hurt a healthy child; remove the food without a fuss after a reasonable length of time. If the child's weight gain is inadequate, see the doctor or visit the health clinic.
Food jag; getting hooked on one food	What a great new food this is!	Children need balanced diets.	Food jags aren't unusual in children; they occur in adults, too. If no issue is made of them, eating patterns tend to balance out after a few days.
Dislike of new foods	I don't like the taste, or I don't feel up to trying something new today.	Children should learn to like everything and adjust to family eating patterns.	Children have a right to a few dislikes. If the dislike is treated casually, the same food may be accepted at a later date. The youngster may eat that food without question when offered at play school or at the home of a friend. Parents can provide a substitute from the same food group, if readily available.
Dislike of cooked vegetables	Those aren't appealing, or they taste funny.	Vegetables are packed with good nutrition. Furthermore, children are supposed to be given variety.	It's not essential to eat cooked vegetables every day. Vitamins, minerals, and protective nutrients come in all sorts of foods. Children may prefer raw or lightly steamed vegetables. If a child rejects everything except, for example, raw peas from a pod, carrot sticks, or bananas, or papaya, or mango, note that each of these is highly nutritious. A child will notice a parent's enjoyment of nutritious foods.
Dawdling or playing with foods	The color, taste, texture, and squishiness of these foods is fascinating! Also, I may not be hungry.	Food isn't a toy. Besides, eating shouldn't take all day.	Exploring foods is different than playing with food. Touching foods with fingers is a natural way to explore a food before putting it in the mouth. Allow exploring in this way. Parents who eat too quickly could use this as an opportunity to slow down a little themselves. When the child is clearly done eating, simply remove the food.

showed that good habits, such as vegetable consumption, were set in place early in life.[46]

Adults who spend time with youngsters in shared food preparation can reap a rich harvest in good nutrition habits. Meal planning and preparation can become a time for quality instruction and interaction—even if little helpers who are fascinated by the process cause these jobs to take longer. Meals needn't be exotic or complicated. In fact, most youngsters reject fancy foods and prefer easily identified finger foods: raw vegetables, fruit, simply prepared chunks of tofu, and toast or crackers with a spread. By encouraging consumption of these foods and guiding youngsters' developing palates, vegan parents can ensure their children will continue to build on the healthy start they've provided.

OPTIMAL GROWTH

There's no "ideal" rate of growth for children, despite the prevalence of growth charts and percentile rankings. At certain stages, children seem to shoot up a few inches overnight or change from a roly-poly toddler to a lean older child. During other periods, increases in height or weight are tiny and development occurs mainly in other realms, such as language or motor skills. If one or both parents are small or tall, their genetic influence probably will appear in the next generation.

Bigger isn't always better, and slightly slower development can be healthier overall. For example, the fastest rates of growth and early puberty in girls may be linked to a higher risk of breast cancer later in life. However, if there's a marked, significant change in a growth pattern, there may be other possible causes.

The standard growth charts used in medical clinics have been developed by the Centers for Disease Control and Prevention (CDC) and the World Health Organization (WHO) and are available online. They include WHO Growth Charts (birth to 24 months) that reflect growth among children who were predominantly breast-fed for at least four months and who were still breast-feeding at their first birthday. The CDC Body Mass Index (BMI) Percentile Calculator for Child and Teens also is available. See Resources on page 449).[47, 48, 69]

Growth of Vegan Children

Several decades ago, the CDC studied the growth of 288 vegan children ranging in age from 4 months to 10 years old. These children lived in a community called The Farm in Summertown, Tennessee. Researchers viewed their parents as "relatively well informed regarding issues related to vegetarianism." The resulting data showed that the average weights and heights of the children in the study group were within normal ranges and were between the 25th and 75th percentile.

Infants born at The Farm had normal birth weights, and their growth was typical of predominantly breast-fed children. The importance of weaning vegan children on to nutritious foods that provide plenty of calories was emphasized.[49] The children received full-fat soy milk fortified with vitamins B_{12}, D, and A, plus other nutritious vegan foods. Peanut butter sandwiches were a favorite food at lunchtimes. Many children consumed Red Star Vegetarian Support Formula nutritional yeast in a variety of dishes (a product made popular in the marketplace by this predominantly vegan community).

NUTRITION-PACKED FOODS

For healthy growth throughout childhood and adolescence, children need foods and beverages that are concentrated sources of calories, minerals, and vitamins,[1] including:

- avocados, nut butters, seed butters, hemp hearts, and bean-based spreads, such as hummus
- fortified full-fat soy milk, tofu, or soy yogurt
- whole-grain breads, cereals, and baked goods, such as healthful muffins, energy bars, and cookies
- refined, enriched grain products (such as pasta); used occasionally, these can increase caloric intake
- thick soups or stews (a cup of pea soup provides 136 calories and 9 grams of protein, whereas a cup of snow pea pods provides 26 calories and 2 grams of protein)
- puddings, frozen desserts, and shakes made with healthful ingredients

Consuming soy foods during childhood and/or the teen years may reduce cancer risk in later life by as much as 60 percent. In girls, soy isoflavones impact breast cells during breast development in ways that confer some protection against breast cancer. Most girls in Asia grow up eating soy foods, which may help to explain the lower rates of breast cancer in those countries.[50, 51]

Eating Away from Home

By setting vegan children apart, a vegan diet may cause difficulties at school, but many parents find this isn't a big hurdle to overcome. Many nonvegan parents have children with food allergies; others wish to have healthier foods at special events. When parents collaborate to help school staff plan food-related events that support children's health, would be accepted by the children, and don't involve extra work for the staff, improved dietary choices can be integrated smoothly.

For those who wish to make more-permanent positive changes in local school meals, allies may include vegetarian-friendly teachers, school food-service personnel, or other parents. Naturally, the school food-service staff will appreciate supportive ideas, input, encouragement, and praise for their efforts. It may interest school personnel to know that there's a widespread movement to improve the healthfulness of school meals and to include entirely vegetarian options for those who want them. The Vegetarian Resource Group offers numerous practical and helpful resources,[52] as does the Physicians Committee for Responsible Medicine (see Resources on page 449).

To make lunch box challenges a little less daunting, invest in BPA-free containers of various sizes and with spill-proof lids, of the type available at outdoor equipment stores. These will safely transport a serving of fortified soy milk, a protein-rich vegan soup or stew, hummus, a veggie burger, or marinated tofu to school and special events. Hot foods, such as soups, stews, chilis, beans, and veggie wieners, can be packed in a thermos bottle and will keep safely for several hours (preheating the thermos bottle with boiling water helps it to retain heat). Perishable cold foods can be placed in an insulated lunchbox or bag with frozen gel packs.

When children dine away from home, it often helps to supply them with a high-protein item to help hosts who are unfamiliar with vegan foods. Typically, the rest of the meal presents no problems.

What about Raw Food and Fruitarian Diets for Children?

The safety of more restrictive diets, such as fruitarian and 100 percent raw diets, has not been established for infants and children, although there have been a few unfortunate case reports in the medical literature. These diets can be very low in energy, protein, some vitamins, and some minerals and cannot be recommended for this vulnerable population.[1]

If parents are consuming a well-balanced raw diet—as described in *Becoming Raw* by Brenda Davis and Vesanto Melina (Book Publishing Company, 2010)—their diet can be adapted and extended for children with the addition of more energy-dense food, including cooked legumes, grains, and starchy vegetables, such as steamed yams. It's essential that reliable sources of vitamin B_{12}, vitamin D, and iodine are provided.

Restaurant Dining

When children are involved, dining out can be a pleasure or a nightmare. Some children are natural explorers; others want familiar foods. For the latter, it can make a big difference to bring favorite crackers, individual packs of chocolate soy milk, mini portions of peanut butter, a well-liked sandwich, or a favorite trail mix. With one or two items brought from home for the child, the rest of the meal can come together easily.

When possible, advance planning helps, including online searches for vegan-friendly restaurants (see Resources on page 450). A good alternative may be an ethnic restaurant, including Chinese, East Indian, Mexican, Middle Eastern, Japanese, or Thai.

Breakfast can include oatmeal, cereals, fruit, toast, jam, peanut butter, and juices, which are all widely available. Cereal can be eaten dry, with juice, or with fortified nondairy milk brought separately. For lunch or dinner, most food outlets typically serve rice, baked potatoes, pasta, vegetables, or salad; salad bars often include peas, chickpeas, beans, and tofu.

For car travel, a big bottle of water is helpful to wash berries, cherry tomatoes, or peas in the pod purchased en route; a knife to cut fresh fruit or vegetables is useful, too.

Appropriate Treats

Based on observations of what their friends may be eating, children are likely to ask for treats. Sometimes, when the treats requested are unhealthy, a gentle, firm "no" is essential.

However, is it essential that a treat be a sugary or fatty food that undermines health? In establishing lifelong eating patterns, the definition of a healthy treat—and the appropriate time to enjoy it—is worth considering. Though children ask, adults don't have to buy unhealthful foods and beverages. Instead, the meaning of "treat" can be redefined to include nutritious choices, organic foods, fresh berries, or fruit juice. A healthy alternative to soda pop can be made with sparkling water plus a fresh-squeezed orange or a small amount of fruit juice. Frozen popsicles can be prepared with blended fresh mango and orange juice or with fruit and nondairy yogurt. This doesn't mean that the occasional serving of chips, chocolate, or candy is forbidden—they're just not regular fare.

Some adults try to numb their feelings with unhealthful foods or beverages. If youngsters know where these "treats" are and whether or not they're prized, a message is relayed to impressionable minds that "treats" are the best solution to life's problems. However, if a child is upset, but not hungry, the use of food shouldn't be a remedy. Attention and affection might be the appropriate reward instead.

Healthy Weight for Life

Grocery shopping can be a challenge when children push for nonnutritious products. Before giving in, a parent or caregiver should reflect on typical North American diets and their troubling effects. Among children between 6 and 19 years of age, one in six is overweight or obese. During the last two decades, the proportion of American children who are overweight has doubled; the proportion of overweight teens has tripled.[53, 54]

Trends that have accompanied this startling weight gain among youngsters include increased soft drink consumption, low fruit and vegetable consumption, and inactivity. Although seeing an infant drinking cola from a baby bottle is shocking, this situation is more common than most parents would care to imagine. By adolescence, 32 percent of girls and 52 percent of boys drink three or more 8-ounce (240 ml) "servings" of soda per day. Meanwhile, just 21 percent of children eat as many as five servings a day of fruits and vegetables, whereas at least six to nine servings are recommended for school-age children.[55] When an American child eats a vegetable, 46 percent of the time, they consume fried potatoes. When children are awake, one hour out of four is spent watching television; those who watch the most TV are most likely to be obese. Worse, high-calorie snacks tend to accompany the TV viewing.[54, 56]

These habits are largely responsible for the 300 percent escalation in health care costs directly attributable to childhood obesity. Compared to children with an optimal BMI, those who are overweight are more likely to become obese adults, with a correspondingly greater likelihood of developing coronary heart disease, hypertension, diabetes, gallbladder disease, respiratory ailments, orthopedic problems, and some cancers. In addition, children who carry excess weight often experience psychological stress, poor body image, and low self-esteem.[54]

Besides shifting to a healthier diet, other strategies can redirect societal trends toward physical fitness and optimal weight. For example, activity levels have been shown to increase when bike lanes are installed on streets, when walkways are well lit, and when space is created for indoor and outdoor recreation. Even a little more exercise is beneficial.[54] Parents should take the lead by providing healthier meals and snacks and initiating appropriate physical activity to instill good habits at an early age.

CHILDREN TO AGE 12

The nutritional needs of rapidly growing children are quite different from those of adults. Youngsters are involved in a remarkable bodybuilding project, which eases off slightly through the preteen years and then revives with new force in early adolescence.

At around 2 years of age, a toddler may weigh 27 pounds (12 kg) and be 34 inches (86 cm) tall. Three years later, that child may weigh 50 percent more and be 9 inches (23 cm) taller. To support this growth, the child's diet must be rich in protein, minerals, essential fats, and the other nutrients required to form new cells. Vegan food choices throughout the day can meet these demands.

Breakfast

Starting the day with a healthy meal helps children pay attention, concentrate, remember, and do better in English, science, and overall test scores.[57] Appealing and nutritious breakfasts can include scrambled tofu or a smoothie with hempseeds, pumpkin seed protein, sunflower seeds, or another type of smoothie booster (see page 387). A breakfast bar (similar to a salad bar) consisting of muesli, granola, or flaked unsweetened cereal, along with jars of seeds, nuts, and shredded coconut, can be left in place near the breakfast table (this arrangement also provides convenient snacks). These choices can be supplemented by cooked cereal, fresh fruit, and fortified nondairy beverages in the morning. When there's time for a leisurely breakfast, prepare pancakes together, and top them with fruit or fruit sauce. (For an instant version, warm vegan frozen waffles in the toaster.)[58] Such activity gives children skills and confidence about cooking.

Advance planning can help to ensure that children do have breakfast. For those who are too sleepy to eat before heading to school or day care, prepared items (such as a nutritious home-made muffin or a nut butter sandwich) can be eaten in the car or during a morning break with a cup of fortified soy milk.

Bagged Lunches

If lunches are packed at home, they should include protein-rich foods and whole grains to supply energy through the afternoon. Some children prefer the security of the same sandwich every weekday. Others prefer a rotation of favorite foods. Nutritionally, an important feature of any lunch is that it gets eaten, so children should participate in choosing the lunch menu; packing lunch bags or boxes can then be a pleasant evening (or morning) task.

Choices that can be packed in insulated lunch bags include soy yogurt and bean, potato, pasta, or grain salads. Leftover pizza, pasta, and rice dishes, including gluten-free options, are also nutritious. If a child prefers sandwiches, table 10.5 provides a selection that meet a child's nutritional needs when combined; start with a grain product from the column on the left, then add a spread or two and a protein filling. Where appropriate, garnish with a few vegetables or provide them on the side.

TABLE 10.5. Grain products, spreads, protein fillings, and vegetables for vegan sandwiches

GRAIN PRODUCTS	SPREADS	PROTEIN FILLINGS	VEGETABLES
Baguette	Dijon mustard	Cashew cheese (homemade)	Avocado slices
Corn cakes	Guacamole	Commercial vegan cheese	Cucumber slices
Crusty roll	Ketchup	Curried tofu spread	Green onions
Multigrain or whole wheat bread	Olive tapenade	Falafel patties	Green, red, or yellow bell pepper slices
Pita bread	Pickle relish	Flavored tofu slices	Lettuce
Rice cakes	Vegan margarine	Hummus (homemade or commercial in a variety of flavors)	Olive slices
Rice paper wrap	Vegan mayonnaise	Marinated tofu strips	Pickles
Rye bread or roll	Yellow mustard	Nut butters	Red onion slices
Sourdough roll		Peanut butter	Sauerkraut
Tortilla (plain, tomato, or spinach)		Refried beans	Shredded carrots
		Sesame tahini	Sprouts (alfalfa, sunflower)
Whole wheat roll or sub		Sunflower or pumpkin seed butter	Tomato slices
		Tempeh bacon or burgers	
		Tofu salad	
		Vegan burger (hot or cold)	
		Vegan meat substitutes (deli slices, ham, pepperoni, salami, or turkey)	
		Vegan pâté or spreads	

Lunches and Suppers

It's well-known that most people return repeatedly to six to ten favorite meals. Time-tested meals that children love include vegan pizza, chili (with or without veggie meat), pasta sauce (with cooked red lentils) and spaghetti, veggie burgers, falafels, and tacos or burritos. With the right ingredients, these meals are very nourishing.

Children also should be introduced to a wider variety of healthful foods. They can be encouraged to try ethnic or international meals, perhaps with an occasional theme day that includes music, a movie, or a dinner guest from the region where the food originated. If children aren't fond of homemade soups, cooked vegetables, or stir-fries, involving them in preparation can help them to become more "vegetable friendly"; they can harvest lettuce from the garden, wash carrots, and (when capable of handling a knife safely) chop avocado, celery, or zucchini.

Desserts aren't a necessary part of daily meals. If dessert is served, it should be a nutritious choice, such as frozen fruit "ice cream," fresh fruit salad, or fruit crumble.

Snacking

As alternatives to peanut butter and jelly sandwiches or expensive junk-food snacks, leftovers from lunch and supper (or the breakfast bar) make nutritious snacks when hunger strikes after school, or at any time. Although many children don't mind eating cold grains or pasta, these may be warmed with a little tomato sauce or peanut sauce. Provide fresh fruit in a bowl on the countertop and jars of dried dates, apricots, or figs to satisfy a sweet tooth. (Children should brush their teeth after eating these sweet treats.)

The "Perfect" Food Day

There's no need (and it's virtually impossible) for children to achieve perfect nutrition every day—a more realistic approach averages healthy intakes over time. Good nutrition is a worthy goal, and menus that meet recommended intakes for all nutrients leave little room for junk foods.

Table 10.6 shows sample menus that more than meet the nutrient needs of children at three stages of growth. Each menu provides more protein than required (the protein content of each food is shown). Vitamin and mineral amounts can be compared with the recommended intakes for different ages shown in the appendix (pages 446 to 447). Although a complete nutritional analysis for each menu is provided, the exact amount of protein, minerals, and vitamins can vary, depending on which soy milk, veggie burger, or other product is chosen (check labels for specific amounts). Analysis is based on metric measures.

Menu 1 relies on fortified foods, such as iron-fortified cereals, with dry cereal on some days and cooked cereal on other days. This menu can suit a child with a soy allergy; soy milk and tofu are not included. When relying on nondairy beverages, check the labels for calcium and vitamin B_{12}, D, and A. Be aware that soy milk is far higher in protein and several other nutrients than most other nondairy beverages. One cup (250 ml) of soy milk provides 6 to 8 grams of protein per cup, compared to only 1 to 2 grams for most other nondairy milk choices. So, if using the lower-protein milks, be sure to provide plenty of other protein-rich options as part of the standard daily fare. Menu 2 includes whole, natural foods, along with fortified soy milk and soy yogurt. Menu 3 features meals that are quick to prepare (though all three menus are simple). Active children are likely to burn more calories than the amounts supplied by these menus; for these youngsters, parents can increase portions or add foods.

Supplementing Healthy Menus

Ensuring reliable sources of vitamins B_{12} and D is essential for children. The menus in table 10.6 include fortified foods that contain these nutrients. However, the amounts of vitamins and minerals provided in supplements are more tightly controlled than those in fortified foods.[44, 60] Children should obtain vitamins B_{12} and D in supplement form every few days or during periods when their intake may be less than adequate.

- **Vitamin B_{12}.** In the menus in table 10.6, fortified nondairy beverages and a veggie burger provide vitamin B_{12}; some fortified breakfast cereals also are sources of B_{12} and of many other nutrients.

TABLE 10.6. Sample menus for children at three weights

MENU 1, FOR CHILD WEIGHING 44 POUNDS (20 kg) APPROXIMATE RECOMMENDED PROTEIN INTAKE: 21 grams	PROTEIN (g)	MENU 2, FOR CHILD WEIGHING 62 POUNDS (28 kg) APPROXIMATE RECOMMENDED PROTEIN INTAKE: 28 grams	PROTEIN (g)	MENU 3, FOR CHILD WEIGHING 80 POUNDS (36 kg) APPROXIMATE RECOMMENDED PROTEIN INTAKE: 34 grams	PROTEIN (g)
Breakfast	8 g total		16 g total		16 g total
1 serving iron-fortified cereal	1 g	1 c (250 ml) oatmeal	6 g	1 English muffin	4 g
2 T (30 ml) hemp hearts	5 g	1 T (15 ml) ground flaxseed	2 g	1 T (15 ml) almond butter	3 g
1 c (250 ml) fortified nondairy milk	1 g	1 c (250 ml) fortified soy milk	7 g	Smoothie, made with ½ c (125 ml) blueberries, 1 banana, 1 c (250 ml) fortified soy milk	9 g
½ c (125 ml) calcium-fortified juice	1 g	1 banana	1 g		
Lunch	9 g total		16 g total		17 g total
¾ cup (185 ml) black bean soup	5 g	1 c (250 ml) minestrone soup	6 g	Sandwich with 2 slices whole-grain bread, 2 T (30 ml) peanut butter, and 1½ T (22 ml) jam	15 g
3 whole wheat crackers	1 g	4 rye crackers	1 g		
½ c (125 ml) guacamole	2 g	1 orange or other fruit	1 g	1 carrot	1 g
½ c (125 ml) raw vegetable strips	1 g	1 c (250 ml) fortified soy milk	7 g	6 oz (180 ml) orange or grape juice	1 g
		2 fig bars	1 g		
Supper	14 g total		22–24 g total		25–34 g total
¾ c (185 ml) pasta	6 g	1 tortilla	1–3 g	1 veggie burger	9–18 g
½ c (125 ml) tomato sauce with 2 T (30 ml) cooked lentils	2 g / 2 g	¾ cup (185 ml) refried pinto beans	12 g	1 whole wheat hamburger bun	4 g
¼ c (60 ml) green peas	2 g	⅓ avocado	1 g	¼ c (60 ml) lettuce, 2 slices each red onion and tomato, 2 T (30 ml) ketchup or relish	1 g
1 c (250 ml) fortified nondairy milk	1 g	¼ c (60 ml) chopped tomato, ¼ c (60 ml) chopped lettuce, and 1 T (15 ml) salsa	1 g		
1 c (250 ml) raspberries	1 g	1 c (250 ml) fortified chocolate soy milk or strawberry soy yogurt	7 g	½ c (125 ml) baked yam or yam or potato fries	4 g
				1 c (250 ml) fortified soy milk	7 g
Snacks	3 g total		7 g total		14 g total
1 c (250 ml) fortified nondairy milk	1 g	¼ c raisins or currants	1 g	¼ c (60 ml) walnuts	4 g
1 banana	1 g	1 T (15 ml) sesame tahini and 1 tsp (5 ml) blackstrap molasses on 1 slice toast	6 g	1 c (250 ml) fortified soy milk	7 g
¼ c (60 ml) dried apricots	1 g	½ cup (125 ml) papaya	0 g	2 slices watermelon	3 g
Water		Water		Water	

Nutritional analysis: calories: 1,403; protein: 34 g; fat: 38 g; carbohydrate: 245 g; calcium: 1,369 mg; iron: 14 mg; magnesium: 422 mg; phosphorus: 1,148 mg; potassium: 3,338 mg; zinc: 7.7 mg; thiamin: 1.3 mg; riboflavin: 6.4 mg; niacin: 14 mg; vitamin B$_6$: 1.9 mg; folate: 404 mcg; pantothenic acid: 5 mg; vitamin B$_{12}$: 4.8 mcg; vitamin A: 963 mcg RAE; vitamin C: 132 mg; vitamin E: 13 mg; omega-6 fatty acids: 8 g; omega-3 fatty acids: 5 g

Nutritional analysis: calories: 1,754; protein: 61 g; fat: 44 g; carbohydrate: 295 g; calcium: 1,336 mg; iron: 17 mg; magnesium: 458 mg; phosphorus: 1,453 mg; potassium: 4,144 mg; zinc: 10 mg; thiamin: 1.6 mg; riboflavin: 1.7 mg; niacin: 12 mg; vitamin B$_6$: 1.8 mg; folate: 602 mcg; pantothenic acid: 4 mg; vitamin B$_{12}$: 7.6 mcg; vitamin A: 600 mcg RAE; vitamin C: 146 mg; vitamin E: 11 mg; omega-6 fatty acids: 16 g; omega-3 fatty acids: 3 g

Nutritional analysis: calories: 2,009; protein: 72 g; fat: 61 g; carbohydrate: 320 g; calcium: 1,402 mg; iron: 14 mg; magnesium: 536 mg; phosphorus: 1,284 mg; potassium: 4,843 mg; zinc: 9 mg; thiamin: 1.5 mg; riboflavin: 2.5 mg; niacin: 21 mg; vitamin B$_6$: 2.3 mg; folate: 391 mcg; pantothenic acid: 6 mg; vitamin B$_{12}$: 6.6 mcg; vitamin A: 2,975 mcg RAE; vitamin C: 203 mg; vitamin E: 11 mg; omega-6 fatty acids: 24 g; omega-3 fatty acids: 4 g

Sources:[20, 59]

- **Vitamin D.** Fortified nondairy beverages provide about 2.5 mcg (100 IU) of vitamin D per cup (cow's milk is fortified with the same amount), and usual menus typically fall short of the RDA, which is 15 mcg (600 IU) from age 1 to adulthood. Thus, vitamin D must be topped up with a supplement, exposure to sunlight, or both. For children who live at latitudes above 37 degrees N, sunlight is insufficient for vitamin D production during the winter, so supplements are especially important from October or November through March or April (see pages 224 to 226). Children should be out in the sunshine for ten to fifteen minutes without sunscreen. Then, for longer exposure, add a protective layer of sunscreen.

- **Iodine.** Iodine could come from ¼ teaspoon (1.5 g) of iodized salt used in cooking, at the table, or as part of a supplement.

- **Potassium.** Plenty of fruit is needed to meet recommended potassium levels; vegetables also provide potassium (see table 6.2 on page 204). If more foods are added to the menus to satisfy a need for additional calories, fruit is a wise choice to increase intake of this mineral.

TEEN NUTRITION: GETTING IT RIGHT

A major task for adolescents is to achieve a sense of their unique identity and individuality; as a result, the teen years can be a period of challenge. Issues related to nutrition can become an arena for conflict—or shared learning for all concerned—if parents and caregivers can relax and allow teens to gradually increase their independence (along with more responsibility). In some homes, vegan families find that their teen has decided to experiment with being a meat eater. On the other hand, some teens become vegans, independent of their family's way of eating. Nonvegan parents do well to support such a position if the youngster is willing to eat a nutritionally adequate vegan diet.

It helps if a teen has an honest commitment to a healthy vegan diet, perhaps preparing his own veggie burger or other foods to complement the plant foods the rest of the family eats. Typically, when a teen adopts a vegan lifestyle, he needs to add protein-rich beans, peas, lentils, and veggie meat substitutes. Fortunately, vegetarian teens aren't doing too badly, compared to their nonvegetarian counterparts.

Studies comparing teens at Adventist schools (whose diets are predominantly vegetarian, including vegan) with children in public schools found that BMIs were lower among vegetarians, especially girls. Vegetarian teens were found to have better dietary intakes than their nonvegetarian counterparts and were less likely to be overweight and obese. (Although some teens who suffer from eating disorders follow a vegetarian diet [see pages 390 to 402], the diet is typically adopted after the onset of the disorder as a means of limiting caloric intake.)[61, 80]

Studies also have found that vegetarian girls, and girls with higher intakes of soy foods, began menstruating an average of seven months later than their nonvegetarian counterparts. Later onset of menstruation is linked with two health benefits: longer life and less risk of breast cancer as adults.[62]

An Australian study compared teens who were predominantly vegetarian with those who were nonvegetarian. Findings showed that, on average, the vegetarian and near-vegetarian adolescents had a lower BMI, smaller waist circumference, lower LDL levels, and a better ratio of total cholesterol to HDL. Heights, hemoglobin levels, and activity levels were similar in the two groups; the one disadvantage of the predominantly vegetarian group was lower levels of vitamin B_{12}.[63, 64]

Teen Topics

Adults and teens share a common desire: for teens to gain skills in decision-making. Learning from mistakes can provide important and long-lasting lessons. A key is helping teens to avoid irreversible mistakes while adults and teens establish new patterns and boundaries. Food-related concerns that can affect long-term health include:

- use of supplements
- the need for increased nutrients during a major growth spurt
- rebellion against family food traditions
- lack of interest or being uninvolved in food preparation
- not prioritizing good nutrition
- lack of interest about skin problems or premenstrual syndrome (PMS)
- anxiety about body weight (see chapter 12) and shape (see chapters 12 and 13)
- development of eating disorders (see pages 390 to 402);
- eating to improve athletic performance or participation in sports (see chapter 13)

Do Vegan Teens Need Vitamin-Mineral Supplements?

The short answer is yes. As at any age, adequate intake of vitamin B_{12} is essential; because a consistent level is provided in a supplement, getting this vitamin in supplement form is ideal. Vitamin D supplements are important for teens (on any diet) who spend little time outdoors or who live farther from the equator than 37 degrees latitude; supplements are especially needed during winter, when sunlight is limited. Research is accumulating on the numerous advantages of adequate vitamin D status. In this age group, higher vitamin D intakes (as from fortified beverages and supplements) are associated with fewer stress fractures in girls from 9 to 15 years old who participate in high-impact sports.[65] (For more information on these vitamins, see chapter 7; also see the appendix on page 446.)

Iron, zinc, and calcium (see chapter 6) also are important during teen years.[66] Though these and all other essential nutrients are available in a balanced vegan diet, a multivitamin-mineral supplement can top up any potential nutrient shortfalls. For example, iron deficiency is common among teens on any diet (including vegan patterns), especially among menstruating girls. Also, although a teen's recommended intake of calcium (1,300 mg) can be obtained from several servings of fortified nondairy milk plus some combination of calcium-set tofu and other calcium-rich plant foods (see "Calcium, Vitamin D, and Bone Building," below), those who consistently fall short of the RDA are well-advised to make up the difference by using a daily supplement.

Growth Spurts in Boys

Before puberty, a boy may weigh 100 pounds (45 kg) and be 5 foot 2 inches (157 cm) tall. Four years later, he may have gained 50 pounds (23 kg) and 7 inches (18 cm). To accomplish this, he needs plenty of proteins, vitamins, minerals, carbohydrates, and essential fats—and this is reflected in a markedly increased appetite. Teenage boys have been known to consume a dish intended for the whole family, mistaking it for a single portion. They may devour double servings of dinner at home and then have another meal elsewhere. Such a voracious appetite is the body's normal response to the demand for additional building materials during this stage.

Growth Spurts in Girls

Girls aged 11 to 14 begin their growth spurt at about the same average weight (100 pounds or 45 kg) and height (5 foot 2 inches or 157 cm) as boys of the same age—in fact, girls might be an inch or so (2 to 3 cm) taller than the boys. During the growth spurt that lasts about four years, their growth is typically less than that of boys. They may gain about 20 pounds (9 kg) and 2 inches (5 cm). This 20 percent increase in weight still requires plenty of nutritious food. In addition, with the onset of menstruation, their iron requirements are greater.

Calcium, Vitamin D, and Bone Building

Obtaining enough calcium during adolescence is crucial for heightened bone mineralization; this process lasts through several decades, lessening the risk of osteoporosis in later years. Youngsters from age 9 to 19 years have particularly high requirements (1,300 mg of calcium per day). Vegan diets can be short of calcium unless care is taken to ensure adequate intakes.[1, 67]

Good calcium sources include fortified nondairy milks and juices, low-oxalate greens (kale, collards, napa cabbage, bok choy, broccoli, and okra), beans (soy, white, navy, great Northern, and black turtle), blackstrap molasses, and figs. Some corn tortillas are fortified with calcium, too; check labels. The Vegan Plate (page 434) gives additional guidance regarding calcium-rich foods and serving sizes. Following the recommendations in this food guide also delivers many other nutrients involved in bone building.

Bone health relies on more than proper nutrition. Participating in outdoor activities is advantageous in two ways. First, the effect of sunlight on skin encourages the body's vitamin D production, supporting calcium absorption, utilization, and retention. Second, weight-bearing exercise encourages the body to respond by maintaining stronger bones.

Nourishing Healthy Skin

Along with other matters of appearance, skin health is a major interest to adolescents. A surge in the level of sex hormones (androgens) can enlarge and stimulate oil glands in the skin, particularly around the nose and on the neck, chest, and back. Despite similar levels of hormones, some bodies produce more oil than others, and some people's skin is less efficient at exfoliation (clearing away discarded cells). The result can be acne and pimples.

To deal with such blemishes, it's important to clean the skin gently and regularly with water and mild soap, to avoid oil-based cosmetics, and to keep the skin dry. Some teens find that certain foods (such as sweets, processed foods, artificially flavored beverages, and fried foods) can cause skin reactions. Vegan teens have an advantage, because they avoid whey, cow's milk, and fish, all of which are known to cause skin problems in some people.

In contrast, many vegan foods are beneficial to skin health. Soy foods, such as tofu, tempeh, and soy milk, not only are sources of protein, iron, and zinc, but also contain isoflavones that may protect skin health. Foods that provide essential fatty acids support healthy skin (see pages 117 and 436). Fruits and vegetables help keep skin clear, partly because they contribute nourishing vitamins and phytochemicals. Carotenoid-rich yellow, orange, red, and green vegetables and fruits also give skin a warm, healthy glow, which scientists have found increases attractiveness to others; this fact can increase the appeal of such foods.[68]

Consumption of fruits and vegetables also helps to meet the body's demand for water; fruits and vegetables consist of 80 to 95 percent water by weight. Water is an important cleanser inside the body; it carries away the toxins flushed out through the kidneys. The effectiveness of drinking 6 to 8 cups (1.5 to 2 L) of water daily in promoting skin health shouldn't be underestimated.

Premenstrual Syndrome (PMS)

Although menstruation is a natural body function, some girls experience excruciating cramps at its onset each month. Attention to some diet-related factors may help to ease or eliminate such discomfort.

- **A low-fat, high-fiber vegan diet.** A study conducted at Georgetown University in Washington, DC, found a plant-based diet to be beneficial in relation to PMS. When girls and women who experienced mild to moderate PMS pain switched from meals that included animal products and fatty foods to a pattern of whole grains, beans, vegetables, and fruit plus a vitamin B_{12} supplement, their PMS symptoms were reduced. These included the intensity and duration of pain, water retention, and weight gain. An added advantage of the dietary switch was more energy. Researchers suggest that these benefits may be related to the impact of diet on hormone levels.[70] To lessen the effects of PMS, follow the recommendations of The Vegan Plate (page 434), avoid fried foods, and limit added fats and oils.

- **Plant foods rich in thiamin and riboflavin.** Research has shown food sources of the B vitamins thiamin and riboflavin to be effective in reducing pain and improving mood. These vitamins are found in whole grains, fortified cereal products, nutritional yeast, legumes, soy foods, seeds, and nuts (see pages 240 and 241).[71]

- **Beneficial oils.** Though a PMS-prevention diet should be moderately low in fat, it's important to include recommended levels of omega-3 fatty acids. For example, 2 tablespoons (15 ml) of ground flaxseeds or ¼ cup (60 ml) of hempseeds or walnuts are excellent additions to daily menus.[72] On the other hand, several well-designed studies have shown oils that contain gamma-linolenic acid, such as borage oil and evening primrose oil, are ineffective in alleviating the symptoms of PMS.[73]

- **Vitamin D.** A pilot study of college-age women showed that those with higher intakes of vitamin D had lower rates of PMS. This may be related to improved calcium absorption and retention, or the vitamin's impact on hormones or neurotransmitters.[74]

- **Avoidance of alcohol.** Researchers have found links between greater alcohol intakes and higher incidence of PMS among female students.[75–78]

Keeping an Eye on Teen Nutrition

Because adolescents may crave privacy and independence, it can be a challenge for parents to ensure that teens are eating a well-balanced diet. Parents can respect the need for personal space while balancing this with a required half hour together at dinner, not only to share family time but also to monitor their dietary intakes. Teens that have regular breakfast, lunch, and supper meals fare best in terms of fruit and vegetable intake.[30]

A variety of eating styles can effectively deliver the nutrients teens need. Samples are described below; all are supplemented with vitamin B_{12}.

- **The "convenience" lifestyle.** Parents can cope with teens who are determined to survive on fast foods by stocking the freezer with vegan burger patties, "hot dogs," and individual portions of favorite entrées that can be warmed at a moment's notice. The freezer also can hold muffins plus fruit crumbles, based on seasonal fruit.

Families with little time for food preparation can enlist teens in chopping quantities of raw vegetables once or twice a week; the vegetables should be kept in a container near the front of the refrigerator for easy snacking, along with several flavors of hummus or guacamole from the supermarket. Fortified non-dairy milks, prepared bean soups, pea soups, vegan chilis, trail mixes, and other ready-to-eat choices can be obtained from grocery stores; deli departments offer delicious seasoned tofu, wraps, salads, and main dishes. On days when there's time to cook, if each family member has learned how to make his or her own special dish, such as a stir-fry, pasta dish, Thai curry, or burgers and salad, the unique combinations will result in diverse, healthy, and tasty meals.

Take-out pizza is the ultimate convenience food, and it can be a delightful family treat. Check with local pizzerias, because many now offer vegan pizza using meltable vegan cheese and meatless pepperoni; request that they start to supply vegan pizza if it's not yet being offered. Of course, cheeseless pizza can be ordered and toppings added at home—just heat for a few more minutes and serve.[79]

- **The athletic lifestyle.** Teens often participate in numerous sports and add workouts to improve their performance. A vegan teen athlete who is working to develop a powerful, healthy body is likely to have high caloric demands. Although a high-protein diet helps to increase muscle mass, carbohydrates are the body's preferred fuel.

A young athlete's goals may include a protein intake of at least 1.5 grams per kilogram of body weight per day. Preparing vegan chili in quantity and freezing portions, or learning a few quick ways to prepare tofu can provide a series of high-protein meals. Dishes from ethnic restaurants, such as samosas, chickpea dishes, and dahl, can supplement homemade foods, while prepared items, such as marinated or seasoned tofu from the deli or supermarket, can deliver a quick source of protein. Adding soy protein or vegan smoothie enhancers to shakes and smoothies can help to meet that goal.

Baked potatoes, rice, pasta, cereals, and breads are ideal for the constant stream of energy needed by active athletes. Trail mix that consists of dried fruits, nuts, and seeds provides extra calories, while serving as a nutritious snack.

To deal with team travel, vegan athletes can bring containers with leak-proof lids (available from an outdoor-equipment store) to carry items from home or from local supermarkets. To discover options for vegan-friendly restaurants in various locations, an app for helpful websites can be added to a cell phone, or a search can be done online (see Resources on page 450).

- **The weight-conscious lifestyle.** Teens concerned about their weight and appearance may consider a vegan diet to be a valuable tool that prevents weight gain.[80, 81] Designing a diet that limits calories while meeting requirements for vitamins and minerals can be a valuable learning experience for teens.[80] Deficiencies can cause unwanted health concerns. For example, insufficient dietary iron results in brittle nails and goes on to cold hands and feet, dizziness, headaches, frequent infections, and extreme fatigue.[66] Shortages of several nutrients can lead to depression.

Weight-conscious teens need information about healthy eating as well as easy access to nourishing foods, such as whole-grain or fortified ready-to-eat cereals (for iron). They need confirmation that vitamin C–rich fruits and vegetables help to absorb iron as well as provide a foundation for clear, glowing skin; a bowl of fresh fruit on the kitchen counter is a good reminder. Avoid keeping high-calorie, low-nutrient snack foods, such as chips, cookies, or vegan ice cream in the house; these tempt teens and undermine their efforts.

Parents can help their weight-conscious teens by noting that beans, peas, and lentils are very low in fat and high in iron and zinc. A practical approach is to work with teens to cook batches of bean or lentil soup, freezing extra portions for quick meals in the future. Chopped salads with a variety of healthy vegetables can keep for several days when refrigerated (in a container with a tight lid) and provide a series of nutritious instant meals. Parents can ensure that teens get enough calcium by keeping on hand fortified soy milk, calcium-set tofu, beans, leafy greens, and tahini dressing for salads.

For family recipes accompanied by a complete nutritional analysis, see *Cooking Vegan* by Vesanto Melina and Joseph Forest (Book Publishing Company, 2012).

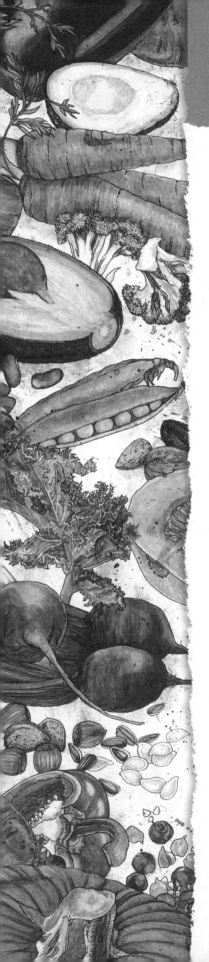

CHAPTER 11

Prime of Life: Nutrition for Seniors

I don't understand why asking people to eat a well-balanced vegetarian diet is considered drastic, while it is medically conservative to cut people open and put them on cholesterol-lowering drugs for the rest of their lives.

DEAN ORNISH, MD

T hanks to the baby boomers, the ranks of "senior citizens" are growing rapidly (but don't call this group old—60 is the new 40). Today, one in eight Americans is over 60, and that proportion is expected to skew older; by 2030, one in five people will be above the age of 65.[1]

At 65, people have an average life expectancy of 18.8 more years. Men who live to 85 can expect to live 5.7 additional years, and 85-year-old women 6.8 additional years. In fact, in 2001, 48,000 people in the United States were 100 or older; eight years later, their number had risen to more than 64,000.[2] Due to a variety of lifestyle factors, vegans may expect to live a few more years than the general population.[3] Compared with nonvegetarians, vegetarians have been shown to have somewhat longer telomeres, an indicator of biological aging, showing a slight slowing of the aging process.[4]

Of every one hundred Americans over age 65, one is vegan; three consume no meat, poultry, or fish; and forty-six eat one or more vegetarian meals per week.[5] Many are aware that a plant-based diet is linked with longevity. Some make this dietary choice to reduce their risk of cardiovascular disease, diabetes, hypertension, obesity, and certain types of cancer; others choose it to prevent a recurrence of one of these conditions. Some studies have shown avoiding meat reduces one's risk of dementia, making a plant-based diet more attractive.

For a few seniors, environmental concerns were the primary inspiration to make a lighter footprint on the planet. For others, ethics, religion, or a wish to avoid harm to animals provided the motivation. Whatever led to their dietary shift—early in life or more recently—a nutritious diet of plant foods has proved to be a wise choice. Studies of older vegetarians, including vegans, indicate that their intakes of many minerals and vitamins are similar to or better than those of nonvegetarians, their body weight is more likely to be in the optimal range, and they're likely to live longer in good health. (See chapters 1 and 2.)[6–8, 82]

Age-Related Changes in Nutrient Needs

Relative to the needs of young adults, seniors require fewer calories but more calcium, vitamins D and B_6, and possibly additional protein. Meanwhile, the recommended intakes for other nutrients remain the same as those of a younger person, with the exception of iron for postmenopausal women, which is reduced. (For more on recommended intakes of vitamins and minerals, see the appendix on pages 446 and 447). Overall, the diets of seniors must have greater nutrient density.

DECREASED CALORIC REQUIREMENTS

There are two primary reasons behind seniors' lower calorie requirements: reduced muscle mass and decreased physical activity.

Muscle tissue burns calories; fat tissue doesn't. Lean body mass (the amount of muscle tissue) tends to shrink with age, while the percentage of body fat typically increases. As a result, at 60, women have an average of 3.5 pounds (1.6 kg) less muscle tissue than they did at 20. Men lose even more, with 7 pounds (3.2 kg) less muscle at age 60. This shift from muscle tissue to fat occurs for a variety of reasons: hormonal changes, a change in basal metabolic rate, and less exercise. Loss of muscle mass and strength (sarcopenia) can set in motion a cascade of consequences, including worsening of diseases, increased disability, malnutrition, and death.[2, 8–10]

The body's basal metabolic rate decreases by about 1 to 2 percent per decade from age 20 to 40 if body weight is constant, then starts to decline more rapidly. Each following decade, a man expends 100 fewer calories per day and a woman expends 70 fewer calories daily; in many cases, and the decline in total energy expenditure is greater. However, instead of adjusting menus accordingly, many adults gradually gain weight. Women often gain an extra 10 pounds (0.45 kg) around the time of menopause and may lose more muscle mass at this time.[9, 10] Among American adults over 65, one in three is obese.[2]

Although some factors can't be completely controlled, the reduction in activity, conversion from muscle to fat, and accumulation of excess weight in seniors is strongly influenced by lifestyle choices. According to the Academy of Nutrition and Dietetics' Position Paper on Food and Nutrition for Older Adults, "Older adults who follow a dietary pattern of high-fat dairy products and sweets and desserts have a higher risk of mortality than those that follow a healthy dietary pattern."[2] Using evidence from the National Health and Nutrition Examination

Survey (NHANES), vegan diets are suggested by registered dietitians as one way to avoid overweight and obesity and to achieve a body mass index (BMI) within the optimal range (see table 12.1 on page 363).[12] Lifestyle choices that support a healthy old age include choosing a protein-rich and nutritious vegan diet, eating a little less each decade, and participating in regular exercise.

Dr. Ruth Heidrich (born 1935), author of *Senior Fitness* and *Lifelong Running*, says, "I'm convinced that our lifestyle choices make the difference between thriving and dying." After a devastating diagnosis of advanced breast cancer (with metastasis to the bones, liver, and one lung) in 1982, she looked at the research and immediately adopted a low-fat vegan diet. Signs of her cancer's spread reversed and her energy soared. She had been a runner but added Ironman Triathlons; over the next thirty years, she won nine hundred medals and was named "One of the Ten Fittest Women in North America." She remains cancer-free and continues daily running, biking, swimming—and her plant-based diet.[13, 14]

EXERCISE AND FITNESS

Regrettably, less than 5 percent of adults participate in thirty minutes of daily physical activity, and this small proportion declines with age. Yet maintaining fitness is as much a key to wellness as avoiding excess calories, and even moderate amounts of exercise are helpful. A Texas study of adults with an average age of 70 showed that participants experienced improved blood flow and muscle-building effects after forty-five minutes on a treadmill.[15, 16]

Regular exercise promotes physical and psychological well-being and better sleep quality. It reduces the risk of disability and vulnerability to a variety of conditions among older adults, including coronary heart disease; type 2 diabetes; metabolic syndrome; stroke; hypertension; colon, breast, endometrial, and lung cancers; overweight; loss of cognitive function; and depression.[2, 17, 18] Regular physical activity can keep the muscles and bones strong, metabolic rate up, and weight in check, and it can also help to prevent falls.

For good health, adults should aim for an hour of physical activity each day. The variety of recommended activities for seniors include weight-bearing exercise that helps maintain bone mass (walking, jogging, dancing, tennis, and hiking); aerobic or endurance activities that keep the heart strong (any of the weight-bearing exercises, plus swimming, aquatics, cycling, and kayaking); strengthening activities to retain muscle tissue (weight lifting, carrying groceries, stair climbing, and gardening); and activities that support flexibility and balance (yoga, tai chi, stretching, and Pilates). Seniors also should work on their balance (such as standing on one foot), which helps to prevent falls and retain cognitive function.[16, 17, 19] (For specific guidelines for seniors adapted from the *Physical Activity Guidelines for Americans*, see page 429.)[16]

Some people acquire a new interest in fitness at this stage of life. British vegetarian and centenarian Fauja Singh rediscovered his passion for running at the age of 81 and thereafter took part in marathons every two to three years, running in London, New York, and Toronto. He gained a spot in history by completing the Toronto Waterfront Marathon in 2011 at the age of 100, becoming the oldest person ever to complete the twenty-six-mile run; he completed the course in just over eight hours, less than his nine-hour goal. He also carried the 2012 Olympic torch on part of its route.

Although some expense may be associated with keeping fit, it can be a thrifty choice. A California study reported on 424 older adults who were at risk for mobility disabilities (losing the ability to walk safely and independently). The study participants followed a program that involved 30 minutes of activity on most or all days and included 150 to 210 minutes per week at a gym, as well as at home. The study estimated that the physical activity program (with center-based educational and exercise sessions that lasted 34 to 52 weeks) cost $1,309—but avoided disability-related annual costs of $28,206.[20]

PROTEIN FOR MUSCLE MAINTENANCE

Research has established that plant protein intake is suitable for building and retaining muscle. A study of 60- to 70-year-old men who engaged in resistance training reported that a soy-rich diet is as effective as a beef-rich diet in improving muscle strength and power. The men were overweight (average BMI just over 28), nonvegetarians, and weighed an average of 197 pounds (89.3 kg). For the study's purposes, either soy or beef was added to a vegetarian diet; in both cases, the men's daily protein intake averaged 1.1 grams per kilogram of body weight over twelve weeks. Their program included resistance training, done at a gym three days per week.[21, 22]

Muscle mass increased equally and significantly in both the beef and soy groups. Researchers found no added benefit from components, such as creatine, that are present in meat but not in soy. It was concluded that either soy or beef protein plus exercise interventions can delay muscle loss and increase muscle quantity, tone, and strength.[21, 22]

A study of pre- and postmenopausal Boston women found vegan diets provided essential amino acids and maintained muscle mass as well as lacto-ovo vegetarian (LOV) or nonvegetarian (NV) diets. Average protein intakes on the vegan and LOV diets were 1 gram per kilogram of body weight daily (g/kg/day) compared with 1.3 g/kg/day on the NV diet; nonetheless, muscle mass and intakes of the indispensible amino acids (IAAs) were similar for participants. Researchers concluded that vegan intakes of protein and IAAs were sufficient to maintain muscle mass.[24] (For more on vegan protein sources, see chapter 3.)

Although a senior's recommended dietary allowance (RDA) for protein doesn't differ from a younger adult's, many experts suggest a daily protein intake of at least 1 g/kg/day for seniors; some experts suggest 1.1 g/kg/day. This is slightly more than the recommendation for vegan adults of 0.9 g/kg/day (see page 85).[2, 24–26] Because this recommendation is based on a healthy weight, an overweight person of any age should use his or her healthy body weight to calculate the desired protein intakes (see table 12.1 on page 363).

The Adventist Health Study-2 (AHS-2) included 5,694 vegans; 60 percent were 55 or older, and 63 percent were women. Their average BMI was 24.1, and protein intake was about 72 grams in a diet of about 1,800 calories daily, with protein providing 14 percent of calories.[27]

Muscle Maintenance

To support muscle maintenance, a daily intake of at least 1 gram of protein per kilogram of healthy body weight may be optimal in seniors. For those who want to build muscle, short-term intakes that are somewhat higher can help. [24–26]

The menus in chapter 14 (pages 439 to 442) easily provide enough protein for most seniors, along with enough iron, zinc, and other nutrients. The 1,600-calorie menu provides 80 grams of protein; for a person whose healthy body weight is 176 pounds (80 kg), this menu provides 1 gram of protein per kilogram of body weight; for a person whose healthy body weight is 160 pounds (72 kg), it provides 1.1 grams of protein per kilogram of body weight. The 2,000- and 2,500-calorie menus provide 76 grams and 97 grams of protein, respectively.

For seniors, vegan diets may offer a special advantage over diets high in meat, poultry, and fish by providing sufficient, but not excessive, protein; consuming too much protein can accelerate the decline in kidney function that some seniors experience. [6–8]

IRON AND ZINC

For senior men, the RDA for iron is 8 mg per day (unchanged from earlier in life). Postmenopausal women, who no longer have monthly menstrual iron losses, have the same RDA for iron as men. [28] Iron from plant sources can be less well absorbed than that from meat; however, the high vitamin C intakes that are typical of many vegan diets substantially increase iron absorption. [8, 12]

Due to lower absorption of the nonheme iron present in plant foods, the Institute of Medicine (IOM) suggests that for vegetarians, the RDA should be multiplied by a factor of 1.8, making the recommended intake for iron for vegan seniors 14.4 mg per day. This recommendation remains controversial (see page 187). [8, 28–31] However, numerous studies show vegetarians (including vegans) have iron intakes that exceed this level. For example, in AHS-2, the vegans' median iron intake was 20 mg per day. [27]

In the general population, iron deficiency (as shown by low hemoglobin levels) occurs mainly in the elderly who are hospitalized, institutionalized, or chronically ill; it can be linked with chronic bleeding in the gastrointestinal tract, dental problems, diminished sense of taste and smell, poor appetite, challenges in obtaining food or making meals, or poverty. [32] Anemia can result from chronic inflammation, chronic kidney disease, or insufficient dietary iron. Thus, it may be expected that some elderly vegans will similarly be anemic. Complications of anemia in the elderly include greater risk of mortality, cardiovascular disease, cognitive dysfunction, falls, fractures, longer hospitalizations, and reduced bone density. [33–35] Anemia is associated with "restless leg syndrome"; this condition can be corrected with iron supplements (and with foods listed below). [32]

The RDA for zinc is unchanged from earlier in life for seniors of both genders, at 8 mg per day for women and 11 mg per day for men. In the AHS-2 study, the average vegan intake met or exceeded these levels. In the elderly, insufficient zinc can cause poor wound healing, reduced immune function, and dermatitis; it also affects the ability to taste and thus can have a deleterious effect on appetite. Zinc deficiency can result from poor absorption or from use of certain medications. With increased intake of zinc-rich foods, an elderly person may find that the ability to taste returns, dermatitis heals, and other deficiency symptoms improve. Zinc supplements also can help someone who is deficient; however, these supplements can interfere with the absorption of other minerals, so zinc-rich foods should be the first option.[32]

The same foods that are good protein sources tend to be rich in iron and zinc: oats, whole-grain products, fortified breakfast cereals, legumes (beans, peas, or lentils), fortified vegan meat substitutes, soy foods, seeds (especially pumpkin seeds), and seed butters. Other iron sources include dried apricots and raisins, dark chocolate, and blackstrap molasses. Additional sources of zinc include cashews, pecans, pine nuts, wheat germ, and fresh and sun-dried tomatoes. Cashews can be blended with water and added to soups and sauces; when heated, they thicken, giving a creamy texture. (For more on iron, zinc, and vegan sources of these minerals, see chapter 6.)

CALCIUM, VITAMIN D, AND BONE HEALTH

Broken bones are a top health hazard for the elderly and often spell an end to independent living. Maintaining strong bones depends on a broad spectrum of nutrients: calcium, vitamin D, and protein are key components. (Weight-bearing exercise also helps the body to retain the calcium in bones.) Adequate calcium is linked with prevention or reduced risk of osteoporosis, colon cancer, hypertension, and other conditions.[8, 32, 36, 67] In women, bone loss is particularly high during the perimenopausal stage, although these losses can be lessened with adequate intakes of key nutrients.

For people older than 50, the recommended intake for calcium increases from 1,000 to 1,200 mg per day.[37] Some experts suggest it should be further increased to 1,500 mg per day after age 65, because the body's ability to absorb this mineral declines over the years.[32]

It can be a challenge for people to meet recommended calcium intakes—let alone the levels advised for seniors—with food alone. Thus, increased use of fortified foods or a supplement can help.[68] Numerous studies show calcium supplementation at levels between 500 and 1,200 mg per day is associated with reduced bone loss and less risk of fracture.[36]

Vegans in the AHS-2 met the RDAs for calcium and vitamin D, on average.[27] The German Vegan Study, which examined the diets of 154 vegans aged 21 to 75, reported that their intake of nutrients related to bone health met recommended intakes, except for calcium (which averaged 840 mg) and vitamin D (which averaged 0.65 mcg per day).[38] In many studies that were conducted over six decades in the United States, Canada, Finland, France, Great Britain, and New Zealand, reported daily vegan intakes are well below the RDAs, often averaging about 500 mcg of calcium and substantially less than 2 mcg of vitamin D.[8] Nonvegetarians also tend to be low in these two nutrients.[8] At northern latitudes, these low intakes of vitamin D matter (as does the calcium).

The 1,600-calorie menu on page 439 provides approximately 1,964 mg of calcium (depending on one's choice of calcium-set tofu) and the 2,000-calorie menu on page 440 provides 1,294 mg of calcium.

To absorb calcium, the body needs vitamin D. In addition to regulating bone mass, this vitamin plays an essential role in immune function and is protective in many other ways. For people age 70 and older, the RDA for vitamin D increases from 15 mcg (600 IU) to 20 mcg (800 IU); however, many experts recommend significantly higher intakes (see page 223.) Various studies have shown that seniors reduce the risk of fractures and falling or increase bone mineral density with daily supplemental intakes in the range of 500 to 1,200 mg of calcium along with 800 to 900 IU (20 to 22.5 mcg) of vitamin D.[36, 39, 40] Serum vitamin D concentrations of at least 75 to 99 nmol/L are suggested for optimal bone health.[41]

The benefits of adequate vitamin D intake go beyond bone health. For example, daily supplementation with 1,000 IU (25 mcg) of vitamin D along with about 1,000 mg of calcium has been shown to reduce periodontitis and is linked with shallower dental pockets. (Of course, consistent dental care helps too.)[42] An Austrian study of 961 female nursing-home residents (whose average age was 83) found 49 percent greater mortality among those with low serum vitamin D levels.[43] Low vitamin D levels also may predispose a person to gain excess weight.[44]

Poor vitamin D status among older people has numerous causes, related to the vitamin's primary sources: sunlight, supplements, and fortified foods. With age, the skin's production of vitamin D from sunlight drops, and vitamin D production by the liver and kidney is less efficient.[32, 36, 45] Thus, at age 70, the body has only about 25 percent of the capacity to make vitamin D that it had at age 20.[45] Another factor that impacts vitamin D production can be avoidance of sun exposure due to fear of skin cancer.[67]

Walking and other forms of outdoor exercise have multiple benefits that include bone health and vitamin D production. Despite spending time outdoors, however, people of any age who live at latitudes above 37 degrees north have little or no vitamin D production in winter months. Adequate vitamin D status can result from some combination of thirty minutes of exposure to warm sunshine between 10 a.m. and 3 p.m., vitamin D-fortified nondairy beverages and cereals, and supplements. It may be of value to have vitamin D levels checked at an upcoming physical examination.[36, 39, 45, 67]

Vitamin K, found in leafy green vegetables, helps to maintain the complex protein-mineral structure of bones.[36, 46] Adding just 2 tablespoons (30 ml) of kale to a smoothie or having ½ cup (125 ml) of broccoli, 1 cup (250 ml) of romaine lettuce, or 2 cups (500 ml) of chopped cabbage at lunch or supper is beneficial.[36, 47, 48]

VITAMIN B$_{12}$

The RDA for vitamin B$_{12}$ is 2.4 mcg. However, due to updated research and to seniors' limited absorption, larger amounts are advised; see pages 217 or 434 for adult options. Some experts suggest that for optimal status, those aged 65 and older should take at least 500 mcg of vitamin B_{12} per day and that some do best with 1,000 mcg daily.[29, 49, 50, 52, 83]

The body requires vitamin B_{12} to keep the myelin sheaths around nerves in good repair. Because B_{12} is needed for a healthy nervous system, symptoms such as confusion, disorientation, and memory loss may be related to a shortage of this vitamin. In cases when a B_{12} deficiency caused these symptoms, such symptoms reversed when vitamin B_{12} status was restored, sometimes through B_{12} injections. Other signs of deficiency are fatigue, depression, irritability, mood swings, restlessness, apathy, insomnia, and perhaps poor hearing.

B_{12} also is involved in ridding the body of homocysteine, a troublesome by-product of metabolism that increases the likelihood of a heart attack or stroke, depression, and perhaps dementia. Lack of vitamin B_{12} is linked with megaloblastic anemia and with damaged DNA strands that increase susceptibility to cancer.[52-55] In vegetarians whose vitamin B_{12} levels are below normal, vitamin B_{12} supplementation has been shown to improve arterial function and reduce risk of atherosclerosis.[55, 56]

One might imagine that vegan seniors are at greater risk for vitamin B_{12} deficiency than nonvegetarians. However, vegans may have the advantage when habitual use of supplements or fortified foods provides their B_{12} source. Non-vegetarians may assume that they're getting all their required vitamin B_{12} from meat and other animal products, while in fact many seniors no longer can absorb that form of the vitamin. These people can become B_{12}-deficient, while vegans who are supplementing get plenty of absorbable vitamin B_{12}. Among 80-year-olds in the general population, one in five has been reported to have low B_{12} status.[52-58]

In fact, all people over 50 are advised to consume B_{12} supplements or B_{12}-fortified foods. Because as many as 30 percent of people in this age group may be unable to absorb vitamin B_{12} from animal products, the IOM states, "it is advisable for those older than 50 years to meet their RDA mainly by consuming foods fortified with vitamin B_{12} or a vitamin B_{12}-containing supplement."[49]

Absorption of this vitamin requires the normal function of the stomach, pancreas, and small intestine. In animal products, vitamin B_{12} is bound to protein. Hydrochloric acid and the digestive enzyme pepsin (both produced in the lining of a well-functioning stomach) are required to split the complex for later absorption in the intestine. The vitamin then becomes attached to R proteins that carry it to the small intestine, where pancreatic enzymes free the B_{12} from the R protein, allowing it to bind to intrinsic factor (a glycoprotein) in a form that can attach to receptors in the intestine and be absorbed. With age and possible inflammation (gastritis), secretion of acid and pepsin by cells in the stomach lining may be decreased, and the bound form of vitamin B_{12} from meats, eggs, dairy, and other animal products isn't absorbed.[52, 59] A decrease in gastric acid production can lead to gradual depletion.

The vitamin B_{12} in supplements and fortified foods isn't bound to a protein in this way; it can be absorbed in the intestine in the normal manner, with the help of intrinsic factor. Because people typically know little about the state of their stomach lining, those older than 50 should use supplements or fortified foods to obtain vitamin B_{12}, regardless of diet.[49]

Boosts for the Brain

Vegan diets have been shown to reduce the risk of dementia—as long as good vitamin B_{12} status is maintained (see pages 72 and 436). Lifestyle choices that help to avoid cognitive decline include:

● choosing foods rich in antioxidants and vitamin B_6—plenty of fruits and vegetables

● taking a vitamin B_{12} supplement

● ensuring optimal omega-3 fatty acid status, perhaps with 200 to 300 mg DHA daily or at least twice a week

● continuing to exercise both body and mind

For someone whose vitamin B_{12} status is marginal, circumstances that can further deplete B_{12} include intestinal surgery; use of nitrous oxide during surgery; use of laxatives, antacid medications, and alcohol; diminished thyroid function; and deficiencies of iron, calcium, and vitamin B_6. Measuring vitamin B_{12} status is complicated by the lack of a gold-standard assay; ideally tests should be done in combination. Laboratory diagnosis may show low serum vitamin B_{12} levels or elevated serum methylmalonic acid or homocysteine levels (see page 215).[50, 55, 59]

Approximately 2 percent of people over 60 develop an entirely different B_{12} absorption problem known as pernicious anemia. This is an autoimmune disease characterized by destruction of the gastric mucosa and failure to produce intrinsic factor, the transport glycoprotein that takes vitamin B_{12} to intestinal receptor sites where the vitamin is absorbed. Pernicious anemia can occur regardless of dietary choice or supplement use; it seems to run in families and to have a genetic component. With time, B_{12} deficiency symptoms appear and the condition can be fatal.[52, 55, 59]

The most common and effective remedy for pernicious anemia is intramuscular injections of the vitamin at regular intervals (such as once a month) for life, bypassing any need for intestinal absorption. Alternatively, a high-dose oral vitamin B_{12} supplement of 1,000 to 2,000 mcg per day can be taken. These large doses appear sufficient for a lower-efficiency absorption system in the intestine that doesn't require the presence of intrinsic factor. Vitamin B_{12} status should then be monitored by a physician.[55, 60] (For more on vitamin B_{12} functions and sources, see pages 214 to 222.)

VITAMIN B_6

For people older than 50, the RDA for vitamin B_6 (pyridoxine) increases from 1.3 mg to 1.7 mg for men and to 1.5 mg for women. Vitamin B_6 is involved in the metabolism of amino acids, carbohydrates, and fats and in building hemoglobin.[52] The body's need for this vitamin can be met by including four servings of fruit per day (recommended in The Vegan Plate on page 434); fruit also provides potassium and fiber.

The many vegan sources of vitamin B_6 include avocado, chickpeas and other legumes, fortified breakfast cereals, fruits (other than citrus), nutritional yeast, nuts, potatoes, seeds, spinach, and whole grains. (Also see pages 244 to 245 and table 7.3 on page 252.)

ANTIOXIDANTS

Older adults who consume generous amounts of antioxidant-rich plant foods are likely to enjoy better overall health and greater protection against disease than those with lower antioxidant intakes. Antioxidants are linked to a reduced risk of heart disease, various forms of cancer, cataracts, macular degeneration, and even wrinkles.[2, 61] The antioxidant vitamins A, C, and E and the mineral selenium are powerful protectors against the free radical damage that contributes to these conditions. RDAs for these antioxidants are the same for seniors as for younger adults. The concentration of antioxidants in vegan diets—due largely to increased intake of vegetables, fruits, seeds, and nuts—can provide vegans with a considerable advantage.

For example, by consuming an abundance of carotenoid-rich yellow, orange, red, and green plant foods, vegetarians have a significantly reduced risk of developing cataracts, and vegans have even less.[62] It's advisable to get vitamin A in the form of beta-carotene from colorful plant foods; in contrast, intakes of preformed vitamin A (which has no antioxidant potential) from supplements have been linked with bone and liver problems.[32] (For more on antioxidants, see pages 230 to 238.)

Studies show vegan diets to contain abundant antioxidants. Nonvegetarians who changed to a low-fat vegan diet for fourteen or twenty-two weeks significantly improved their intakes of vitamins A and C (and of folate, magnesium, potassium, and fiber).[12] Vitamin E intakes also improved but were still a little low; this can be expected if a diet is low in fat, because vitamin E is a fat-soluble vitamin. Including some higher-fat plant foods, such as avocado, seeds, nuts, olives, or fresh-pressed oils, quickly brings vitamin E to recommended levels.

Other than some allergies, I've gotten rid of every one of a half-a-dozen or so chronic conditions, including obesity, fatty liver, high uric acid (gout), heartburn/ulcers/stomach acid, nervous tension, sleeping problems, and rising cholesterol.

JOI ITO, VEGAN VENTURE CAPITALIST, MULTIMILLIONAIRE, AND GLOBAL LEADER FOR TOMORROW (WORLD ECONOMIC FORUM), COMMENTING ON HEALTH CHANGES SINCE HE BECAME VEGAN

For good sources of selenium, see page 200. (For additional sources of these nutrients, see table 6.2 on page 204 and table 7.3 on page 252.)

Unfortunately, if dental problems develop in the elderly, they may start to shy away from fresh vegetables and fruits. However, soft fruits, cooked vegetables and fruits, and fresh-squeezed or bottled juices can take the place of foods that are more difficult to chew (see page 356). Baked sweet potatoes and winter squash are rich in protective carotenoids (vitamin A), as are fresh or frozen mangoes and papayas. The day's RDA for vitamin C is available from 1 cup (250 ml) of

Potential Advantages of Vegan and Vegetarian Diets in the Senior Years

"Populations of vegetarians living in affluent countries appear to enjoy unusually good health, characterized by low rates of cancer, cardiovascular disease, and total mortality. These important observations have fueled much research and have raised three general questions about vegetarians in relation to nonvegetarians:

1) Are these observations the result of better nondietary lifestyle factors, such as a lower prevalence of smoking and higher levels of physical activity?

2) Are they the result of lower intakes of harmful dietary components, in particular, meat?

3) Are they the result of higher intakes of beneficial dietary components that tend to replace meat in the diet?

Current evidence suggests that the answer to all three questions is 'yes.'"

Walter C. Willett, Department of Nutrition, Harvard School of Public Health, Boston

cooked potato plus ½ cup (125 ml) of cooked broccoli. Antioxidants are well absorbed from blended vegetable soups, either raw or cooked. (For delicious and nutrient-rich soups, sauces, and pâtés based on puréed vegetables, seeds, and nuts, see *Becoming Raw* by Brenda Davis and Vesanto Melina (Book Publishing Company, 2010) or *The Raw Food Revolution Diet* by Cherie Soria, Brenda Davis, and Vesanto Melina (Book Publishing Company, 2008).

FIBER, FLUIDS, AND INTESTINAL HEALTH

Because constipation is linked with too little fiber, water, and/or exercise, some older adults find themselves battling irregularity. Plant foods provide dietary fiber; as a result, vegan diets help to maintain regularity. The fiber in legumes, whole grains, vegetables, and fruits keeps waste and toxins moving through the intestine and out. (Although whole grains are most beneficial, some intake of refined grains can help to increase caloric intake for the frail elderly or those with poor appetites.[2])

The high fiber intakes of plant-based diets are linked with a reduced risk of diverticular disease[63] and colorectal cancer.[84, 85] A vegan diet has been shown to alter the balance of the bacteria in the gut. Unwanted microorganisms, such as *E. coli*, are reduced, and microorganisms that reduce inflammation are increased. Such a change has been shown to reduce the risk of type 2 diabetes, hypertension, and rheumatoid arthritis.[64–66]

Fiber also helps to maintain blood glucose levels and thus sustains energy between meals.[2] However, vegans are generally advised to avoid adding wheat bran to foods; the additional fiber is unnecessary and can significantly compromise mineral absorption.

Thirst and dehydration can be a problem for older people, especially those older than 85 or who are institutionalized; also, medications can affect hydration. With age, the sensation of thirst may become less acute. The kidneys become less adept at concentrating urine, trips to the bathroom may become more frequent, and fear of incontinence can lead to decreased fluid intake. Fortunately, many fruits and vegetables contain more than 90 percent water. Seniors also should regularly drink water, fortified nondairy beverages, and herbal teas, with a focus on beverages that are calorie-free or low in added sugars.[2]

Meals and Menus

In planning meals and menus for the later years of life, The Vegan Plate (pages 434 to 435) is a useful guide. For many people, minimum servings from each group provide a suitable caloric intake.

For example, seniors often find that three servings from the grains group are sufficient; also, this approach tends to be ideal for those who want to lose weight. There are significant differences in the speeds at which carbohydrates from different foods are absorbed, digested, and enter the bloodstream. Compared with grains, the carbohydrates in legumes are released in a slow and gradual manner, maintaining more even blood glucose levels between meals and making beans, peas, lentils, and soy foods a priority in meal planning.

It's especially important for older consumers to emphasize legumes and vegetables, because these are so rich in protein and a wide variety of vitamins and minerals. An international study of people aged 70 and older found consumption of legumes to be "the most important dietary predictor of survival in older people of different ethnicities."[69]

Various plant foods have other benefits. The isoflavones in soy foods may help keep skin healthy and lessen wrinkles,[70] as do antioxidant-rich vegetables and fruits. Fruit is important for its contribution of potassium, vitamin B_6, and other nutrients. Nuts, seeds, and their butters provide important minerals, and their fat helps with absorption of protective phytochemicals, minerals, and fat-soluble vitamins. The sample menus in chapter 14 provide adequate intakes of these nutrients at various caloric levels.

CHANGES THAT AFFECT NUTRIENT INTAKE

Although a highly nutritious diet is needed in the later years, certain factors can work against achieving this goal. In older people, chewing, swallowing, digesting food, and absorbing nutrients may be impaired. Poor oral health, loss of teeth, ill-fitting dentures, and dental problems can make chewing difficult; a dental referral may be advisable. Changes in the stomach and intestinal lining can affect digestion and nutrient absorption.[32]

At the age of 70, people have just 30 percent of the taste buds that they did as young adults. Sensitivity to taste also can decline due to use of certain medications or due to zinc deficiency (for vegan zinc sources, see pages 191 and table 6.2 on page 204). Unfortunately, the loss of taste may encourage seniors to use excessive amounts of salt to flavor foods; excess sodium can increase the risk of hypertension, and thereby contribute to heart disease, stroke, and kidney disease.[2, 8] Instead, foods should be flavored with herbs, spices, lemon juice, and other low-sodium seasonings, and seniors should monitor the sodium content in canned, frozen, and ready-to-eat items by checking the labels.

Besides such sensory loss, a reduction in appetite can be related to poor health, diminished cognitive status, or isolation. Some seniors may have enjoyed food preparation when it involved shopping and cooking for a family or partner, but have lost interest in these activities when dining alone. Physical disabilities, loss of mobility, or lack of transportation may make it a challenge to assemble a meal. Poor eyesight can render direction-reading difficult; limited hand strength and coordination makes opening packages difficult.

Other aspects of declining health influence nutritional well-being. Besides affecting taste buds, medications can directly affect nutrient status. For example, proton pump inhibitors prescribed for peptic ulcer disease and gastroesophageal reflux disease (GERD) are linked with infectious complications and deficiencies of calcium and other nutrients.[71]

A vegan diet is an ally in combatting certain problems. Some elderly people are motivated to switch from meat to tofu because the latter is far easier to chew and swallow. When seasoned or marinated, tofu becomes a welcome part of lunch and dinner menus. Soft or firm tofu is easily incorporated into smoothies for breakfast and snacks, providing a tasty and easily consumed source of protein, iron, zinc, calcium, and numerous other nutrients. If the combination includes mango, orange juice, and strawberries, the smoothie also becomes an excellent source of vitamins A and C.

Quinoa and oatmeal are whole grains that are easy to prepare and swallow. In addition, refined products, such as soft enriched white bread or rolls, couscous, and white rice, may be easier to chew and thus better accepted than some of the coarser whole grains. The use of some refined grains can provide a suitable balance for elderly consumers, because vegan diets provide so much fiber from vegetables, fruits, legumes, and nut and seed butters.

Digestive difficulties, swallowing problems, hypertension, and other disease conditions can require dietary modifications that are beyond the scope of this book; a few resources that can address these difficulties include:

- For those with type 2 diabetes or metabolic syndrome, *The Kick Diabetes Cookbook* by Brenda Davis, RD, and Vesanto Melina, MS, RD (Book Publishing Company, 2018), and *Kick Diabetes Essentials* by Brenda Davis, RD (Book Publishing Company, 2019) kickdiabetescookbook.com

- For those with fibromyalgia or rheumatoid arthritis, raw (and gluten-free) vegan diets have proved helpful to some; *Becoming Raw* by Brenda Davis and Vesanto Melina (Book Publishing Company, 2010)

- For vegan recipes that are SOS-free (free of sugar, oil, and salt) and used effectively for those with type 2 diabetes, hypertension, and rheumatoid arthritis, *Bravo: Health-Promoting Meals from the TrueNorth Kitchen* (Book Publishing Company, 2012) and *Bravo Express* (Book Publishing Company, 2019) by Chef Ramses Bravo of TrueNorth Health Clinic in California

- For healthful, delicious, and easy recipes, each with a nutritional analysis, *Cooking Vegan* by Vesanto Melina and Joseph Forest (Book Publishing Company, 2012)
- For how to veganize recipes and more recipe ideas and health tips, *Never Too Late to Go Vegan* by Carol Adams, Patti Breitman, and Virginia Messina (The Experiment, 2014)[61]

In addition, the list that follows includes meal ideas that deliver good nutrition and are affordable, appealing, simple to prepare, and easy to chew.

EASY-TO-PREPARE VEGAN MEAL ITEMS

Breakfast or Snacks

- Bagel, toast, or soft bread with nut butter (or with sesame tahini plus blackstrap molasses), accompanied by fresh fruit
- Fortified ready-to-eat dry cereal with fortified nondairy milk and fruit or juice
- Fruit smoothie made with tofu, hempseeds, or protein powder
- Hot cereal with fresh, canned, or dried fruit, and fortified nondairy milk
- Nondairy yogurt parfait: yogurt with berries, fresh fruit, and nuts, seeds, or granola sprinkled on top
- Scrambled tofu with sautéed onions, garlic, spinach, mushrooms, bell peppers, or other vegetables, seasoned with nutritional yeast and turmeric, and served with rye bread toast and fruit or juice

Lunch and Dinner

- Avocado and tomato sandwich on whole-grain or white bread, served with bean soup
- Baked potato with steamed broccoli and chickpeas, drizzled with Liquid Gold Dressing (page 219) and sprinkled with toasted sunflower or pumpkin seeds (optional)
- Baked yam with black beans and steamed kale
- Baked tofu with barbecue sauce, green salad, and steamed yam
- Canned low-sodium soup with beans, peas, or lentils, with added chopped greens
- Canned low-sodium baked beans or chili served atop a baked sweet potato, accompanied by spinach salad
- Veggie burger with green beans and baked potato wedges or yam fries
- Vegan pizza and green salad
- Tacos or burritos made with soft tortillas, refried beans, avocado, lettuce, salsa, and vegan cheese (optional)
- Hummus, crackers, and raw vegetables
- Flavored rice mix with added vegetables, peas, beans, or edamame

- Soup with a side of raw vegetables and dip
- Marinated three-bean salad, green salad, and soup
- Pasta with prepared sauce and lentils
- Pasta with prepared sauce, greens, and chickpeas
- Peanut butter or nut butter and banana sandwich
- Quinoa with chopped vegetables and lima beans
- Vegetable stir-fry with seasoned or baked tofu over brown rice
- Sandwich of avocado, tomato, and vegan meat substitute on a roll

Preparation Tips

- For a creamy texture, add cashews to vegetable soups and blend. (Blended cashews thicken when heated.)
- Add cubes of tofu to soups to enhance nutrition; for a creamy texture, blend the tofu into the soup.
- Mix crumbled tofu with vegan mayonnaise and seasonings for a sandwich filling.
- To prevent spoilage, keep bread in the freezer. Remove a slice or two at a time for toast or a sandwich.
- When preparing foods, make enough to provide a foundation for tasty meals for the next few days. For example, bake a variety and larger quantity of root vegetables (potatoes, yams, beets); bake slices of tofu with barbecue sauce, peanut sauce, or another sauce at the same time; or make large batches of hearty soups or stews. Freeze in serving-sized portions.
- Dried beans are economical; soaking them for a few hours and then discarding the soaking water before cooking will reduce flatulence (double soaking will do the job even better). Cook beans in quantity and freeze in serving-sized portions. If using canned beans, buy a low-sodium variety or rinse well to remove some of the sodium.
- Red lentils, a great source of iron, protein, and zinc, take just fifteen to twenty minutes to cook and can be added to tomato sauce, other sauces, and soups.
- Mild curry paste adds a superb blend of flavors to cooked lentils and beans.
- Substitute quinoa for rice or other whole grains in a variety of dishes. It's higher in protein and minerals than other grains and cooks in only fifteen minutes; rinse the quinoa before cooking.
- Buy ripe soft fruits, such as papayas, peaches, nectarines, mangoes, pears, bananas, melons, kiwifruit, and berries; for convenience, freeze in serving-sized portions.
- Grate harder fruits (such as apples) for salads; also stew or bake such fruits.
- Well-cooked vegetables usually are easier to eat, including soft-cooked squash, yams, sweet potatoes, zucchini, eggplant, and potatoes.
- After removing stems, slice kale into thin strips or chop it in a food processor, then add it to salads.

- Keep canned and frozen fruits and vegetables on hand for snacks, as side dishes, or for use in recipes. Because potential spoilage is reduced, these tend to be an economical choice.

- When ordering Chinese food, such as vegetables, tofu, and rice, purchase enough for leftovers for another meal or two.

- Invest in a good juicer; fresh juices provide easily absorbed nutrients.

- Adapt the 1,600-, 2,000-, and 2,500-calorie menus in chapter 14 (pages 439, 440, and 441) to individual preferences.

VEGAN RESTAURANT FARE ABROAD OR NEAR HOME

Seniors who have the freedom to travel and dine out may foresee challenges in locating vegan options. Yet, thanks to technology, travelers can quickly find excellent vegan fare in Paris, Prague, Portland, Perth, and points beyond. The websites listed in Resources on page 450 can be accessed via the Internet or downloaded apps for mobile phones. They provide articles and reviews, as well as vegetarian or vegan restaurant choices.[72]

Community Support for Seniors

Apart from those who live in care facilities, about one older adult in three lives alone. While these seniors have mobility and independence, they have viable choices about preparing food at home and dining at restaurants. However, as mobility declines, the possibilities of gradual isolation and poor nutrition may arise.

In some cases, a lack of funds may be the problem. Fortunately, in the United States, through state and tribal agencies, the Senior Farmers' Market Nutrition Program provides low-income seniors (over age 60) with coupons that can be exchanged for eligible fruits, vegetables, and fresh herbs at farmers' markets, roadside stands, and community-supported agriculture programs.[73]

For an elderly person who has difficulty getting to a store or market, other options exist. Many supermarkets and some natural foods stores offer grocery delivery services, which can include prepared vegan items from the deli. Food-delivery programs, such as Meals on Wheels, tend to have vegetarian but not vegan meal choices; however, menus are based on local demand. If encouraged, local meal providers may be interested in implementing a four-week menu cycle developed by the Vegetarian Resource Group specifically for Meals on Wheels (see Resources on page 449).[74]

The Older Americans Act directed the US Department of Health and Human Services Administration on Aging to provide funding for nutrition education, as well as home-delivered meals for low-income seniors. The US Department of Agriculture's Supplemental Nutrition Assistance Program, as well as other programs, also provides options for seniors with limited incomes, and these may include vegan items.[2, 75, 76]

Most people prefer to continue living in their own home as long as possible, yet some wish to also enjoy a greater sense of community. In some areas, community meal programs allow older people to meet in a central location to enjoy a meal in the company of others; often, transportation is provided. In other areas, cohousing communities successfully address the problem of isolation while retaining the best aspects of independent living.

Cohousing is a type of collaborative housing in which residents live in their own homes but actively participate in the design and operation of their own neighborhoods. Cohousing communities typically serve optional group meals in a "common house" at least two or three times a week, with small groups of residents taking turns to prepare meals; efforts usually are made to accommodate vegetarians and vegans. One book on this topic is *Senior Cohousing: A Community Approach to Independent Living* by Chuck Durrett (New Society Publishers, 2009). For more on cohousing, see reference.[77]

Vegetarian Food in Care Facilities

There may come a time when living at home is no longer safe or healthy for an elderly person. For those in search of a suitable care home for a vegan, it's worth exploring those run by the Seventh-day Adventists, perhaps through a local Seventh-day Adventist church.[78] Mainstream facilities are beginning to recognize the need for vegetarian and vegan options. For example, the Goodman Group, a company with senior living, health care, and residential communities throughout the United States, has made the incorporation of plant-based options in all facilities a top priority. The company's goal is to enable residents to achieve optimal health and well-being, and to fully support residents who elect to use diet and lifestyle choices as therapeutic tools. Also, the Living Well Bistro in Portland, Oregon, offers a model of an entirely vegan hospital restaurant.[79]

Nursing homes and assisted-living facilities often are willing and able to accommodate a vegan or vegetarian senior, especially if the kitchen staff is provided with practical solutions to the challenge of providing vegan entrées along with their main menu. Examples of protein-rich foods that can be heated for one or a few individuals include marinated tofu; veggie burgers or other vegan meat substitutes (such as veggie chicken, frozen falafel patties, and vegan entrées); or hearty bean, pea, or lentil soups made in quantity and then frozen in individual portions. Staff could also use veggie ground round in pasta sauce, tofu cubes in stir-fries, or chickpeas in curry to replace meat. A resource on quantity cooking for staff at care facilities is *Vegan in Volume: Vegan Quantity Recipes for Every Occasion* by Nancy Berkoff (Vegetarian Resource Group, 2000).[80]

Vegan and Vegetarian Diet Specialists

For the elderly who suffer from various diseases or chronic conditions, working with a registered dietitian can be helpful. Dietetic associations in the United States, Canada, the United Kingdom, Europe, and Australia list consultant dietitians who are vegetarian and vegan specialists, provide counsel regarding therapeutic nutrition, are knowledgeable about food-related assistance, and can be contacted through the individual association's website.[81] For example, the Academy of Nutrition and Dietetics (AND) has a strong vegetarian dietary practice group with numerous online resources. AND and Dietitians of Canada have websites with links to "Find an RD" (Registered Dietitian); see reference.[81]

Vegetarian Associations for Support and Connection

Though this book focuses on nutrition, other lifestyle factors also are keys to achieving and maintaining good health throughout life: the habit of regular exercise, the maintenance of loving relationships (whether of long-term family or of new-found friends), a positive attitude, and a good sense of humor. Belonging to a community that encourages a quality lifestyle can help people achieve and maintain health goals. "Community" no longer means solely one's immediate surroundings; thanks to the Internet, a quick e-mail can connect people whose lifestyles and ethical values are in line.

Still, face-to-face contact helps to establish stronger relationships. Fortunately, many communities have lively vegetarian associations whose members span the spectrum from newborns to those dancing through the doors in their nineties; those in wheelchairs are most welcome too. Vegetarian associations often are open to new ideas, such as the creation of a seniors' support or social group. The associations typically host regular potluck dinners, meetings, restaurant ouings/ get-togethers, and annual festivals or food fairs. Such events provide opportunities to meet like-minded people, begin new friendships, and offer support as a volunteer. These associations can easily be found via an Internet search, using the name of the town, city, or country, plus the words *vegetarian* or *vegan;* local librarians can help seniors with such a search.

For those interested in widening their horizons, larger gatherings are held at national levels and international levels; these events typically feature great food, excellent speakers, and fascinating people. One is Vegetarian Summerfest held in Pennsylvania each July; travelers also can explore the International Vegetarian Union website for vegfests held in different parts of the world (for links to these events, see Resources on page 450).

For people who are more comfortable in small groups, Meetups provide an opportunity to get together with others based on shared interests, such as vegan food or animal rights. Internet dating also can be a way to get to know potential partners or friends. A search using the words *vegan online dating* will quickly turn up numerous vegan-friendly websites, as well as regular websites that include vegans. Dating can be an exciting and heartwarming adventure for the old and wise, ensuring that all the years added by a healthy diet also are happy ones.

I truly believe that if we were to adopt a whole-foods, plant-based diet, we could cut hospital costs by 70 to 80 percent.

COLIN CAMPBELL, PROFESSOR EMERITUS OF NUTRITIONAL BIOCHEMISTRY, CORNELL UNIVERSITY, AND AUTHOR OF *THE CHINA STUDY*

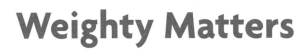
Weighty Matters

The way you treat yourself sets the standard for others.

SONYA FRIEDMAN, AUTHOR, PSYCHOLOGIST

Although vegans are generally leaner than their nonvegan counterparts, becoming vegan doesn't guarantee thinness—vegans come in all shapes and sizes. As a result, for an overweight individual, it can be frustrating to adopt a vegan diet and not lose an ounce. For people who struggle with being too thin, it can be even more challenging to gain weight on a vegan diet. However, well-planned vegan diets are powerfully effective in helping to support and promote healthy body weights, regardless of a person's starting point.

Americans certainly need help in the weight-control realm; they're among the fattest people in the world. Nearly 70 percent of American adults who are 20 or older are overweight or obese. More than one-third of American adults are obese, and less than one-third are at a normal weight.[1, 2] In contrast, approximately 1.6 percent of the US population is underweight,[3] a steady decline from about 4 percent in the early 1960s.

Eating disorders also are a growing concern. An estimated 0.5 to 1 percent of American women suffer from anorexia nervosa,[4] and roughly 3 percent will suffer from bulimia during their lifetime. Rates of eating disorders are higher among young women; about 6 percent of teen girls and 5 percent of college-age women are affected.[5] Many people believe that being vegan can trigger eating disorders. However, anorexia nervosa, bulimia, and other compulsive eating behaviors are the result of a state of mind rather than of a particular diet.

The following discussion addresses the causes and consequences of weight problems, provides a guide for helpful and healthful eating behaviors, and offers practical advice for overcoming specific weight issues.

Healthy Body Weight Defined

There's no one "ideal" weight for individuals who are the same height, because healthy weight depends on a combination of factors besides height: bone structure, muscle mass, body fat, and body build. However, general guidelines—along with additional indicators, such as body mass index (BMI) and percentage of body fat—can be helpful in determining if a person is overweight, obese, or underweight:

- **Overweight.** At least 10 percent above healthy body weight (for most people, about 10 to 30 pounds above healthy body weight).

- **Obese.** At least 20 percent above healthy body weight (for most people, 30 pounds or more above healthy body weight).

- **Underweight.** At least 15 to 20 percent below healthy body weight (for most people, 20 to 30 pounds under healthy body weight).

The percentage of body weight composed of fat can indicate whether a person's weight is within a healthy range. Body fat of more than 17 percent in men and 27 percent in women indicates overweight; body fat of greater than 25 percent in men and 31 percent in women indicates obesity. Low body fat doesn't necessarily predict underweight in men, because male athletes can achieve body fat under 8 percent and still be healthy. However, low body fat can induce amenorrhea (cessation of menstruation) in women at levels below 13 to 17 percent (the exact percentage varies among individuals).

Getting accurate body fat measurements can be difficult and costly. Instead, BMI is commonly used as a simple, noninvasive way to estimate total body fatness. This is generally done using a chart or BMI calculator (both widely available online). BMI is determined by dividing a person's mass (weight in kilograms) by the square of their height in meters (kg/m^2).

A BMI of 18.5 to 24.9 is in the healthy weight range. A BMI of 25 to 29.9 is considered overweight. Obesity is defined as a BMI of greater than or equal to 30, with further designations made according to degree of obesity (class 1 obesity: BMI 30 to 34.9; class 2/severe obesity: BMI 35 to 39.9; class 3/extreme obesity: BMI $\geq$ 40). A BMI below 18.5 is deemed underweight; mild underweight ranges from 17 to 18.49, moderate underweight from 16 to 16.99, and severe underweight is any BMI under 16. (Table 12.1 charts the BMI for a range of heights and weights.)

While useful for most people, BMI has several significant limitations. Foremost, it doesn't take into account differences in body composition due to age, gender, race, or ethnicity.[6] BMI may be most accurate for Caucasian women and small-boned men. For men with more muscle mass or larger bone structure, it's less reliable. For example, a man might register a BMI of 25 or more (considered

TABLE 12.1. Body mass index (BMI)

Weight (lb)	Height (in)																
	60	61	62	63	64	65	66	67	68	69	70	71	72	73	74	75	76
100	20	19	18	18	17	17	16	16	15	15	14	14	14	13	13	12	12
105	21	20	19	19	18	17	17	16	16	16	15	15	14	14	13	13	13
110	21	21	20	19	19	18	18	17	17	16	16	15	15	15	14	14	13
115	22	22	21	20	20	19	19	18	17	17	17	16	16	15	15	14	14
120	23	23	22	21	21	20	19	19	18	18	17	17	16	16	15	15	15
125	24	24	23	22	21	21	20	20	19	18	18	17	17	16	16	16	15
130	25	25	24	23	22	22	21	20	20	19	19	18	18	17	17	16	16
135	26	26	25	24	23	22	22	21	21	20	19	19	18	18	17	17	16
140	27	26	26	25	24	23	23	22	21	21	20	20	19	18	18	17	17
145	28	27	27	26	25	24	23	23	22	21	21	20	20	19	19	18	18
150	29	28	27	27	26	25	24	23	23	22	22	21	20	20	19	19	18
155	30	29	28	27	27	26	25	24	24	23	22	22	21	20	20	19	19
160	31	30	29	28	27	27	26	25	24	24	23	22	22	21	21	20	19
165	32	31	30	29	28	27	27	26	25	24	24	23	22	22	21	21	20
170	33	32	31	30	29	28	27	27	26	25	24	24	23	22	22	21	21
175	34	33	32	31	30	29	28	27	27	26	25	24	24	23	22	22	21
180	35	34	33	32	31	30	29	28	27	27	26	25	24	24	23	22	22
185	36	35	34	33	32	31	30	29	28	27	27	26	25	24	24	23	23
190	37	36	35	34	33	32	31	30	29	28	27	26	26	25	24	24	23
195	38	37	36	35	34	33	32	31	30	29	28	28	27	26	25	24	24
200	39	38	37	35	34	33	32	31	31	30	29	28	27	26	26	25	24
205	40	39	37	36	35	34	33	32	31	30	29	29	28	27	26	26	25
210	41	40	38	37	36	35	34	33	32	31	30	29	28	28	27	26	26
215	42	41	39	38	37	36	35	34	33	32	31	30	29	28	28	27	26
220	43	42	40	39	38	37	36	35	34	33	32	31	30	29	28	27	27
225	44	43	41	40	39	37	36	35	34	33	32	31	31	30	29	28	27
230	45	43	42	41	39	38	37	36	35	34	33	32	31	30	30	29	28
235	46	44	43	42	40	39	38	37	36	35	34	33	32	31	31	29	29
240	47	45	44	43	41	40	39	38	36	35	34	33	33	31	31	30	29
245	48	46	45	43	42	41	40	39	37	36	35	34	33	32	32	30	30
250	49	47	46	44	43	42	40	39	38	37	36	35	34	33	32	31	30

UNDERSTANDING BMI	
BMI < 16: indicates severe underweight	BMI 25–29.9: indicates overweight
BMI 16–16.9: indicates moderate underweight	BMI 30–34.9: indicates class 1 obesity
BMI 17–18.49: indicates mild underweight	BMI 35–39.9: indicates class 2 or severe obesity
BMI 18.5–24.9: indicates healthy weight for most people	BMI ≥ 40: indicates class 3 or extreme obesity

overweight), but if he has a large frame and muscular build, he could actually be very lean. For many men and some large-boned muscular women, BMI might be more accurate if the cutoffs for overweight were shifted up by about 2 points to 27. BMI is also less accurate for some black people, who have denser, more muscular builds, and for whom a high BMI also wouldn't indicate overweight. However, genetic diversity is even more pronounced in blacks than Caucasians, so this assumption wouldn't apply to all black people.

Likewise, individuals with smaller bone structure and lower muscle mass may not be underweight, even if their BMI dips below 18.5. For such individuals, the cutoffs for overweight also may need to be dropped a couple of points. This is especially true for Asians, who commonly experience the adverse consequences of overweight—such as high blood pressure and insulin resistance—when their BMI is only 23.[7] In both Japan and Singapore, BMI tables show cutoffs for overweight at 22.9 instead of 24.9.[8, 9]

In addition, BMI is only considered valid for those between 20 and 65 years old, is less precise for very short people (less than 5 feet/1.5 meters), and is of little value to body builders or other individuals with extremely large muscles. Pregnant women shouldn't use BMI tables but should follow their physician's advice on healthy weight during pregnancy.

THE EFFECT OF BODY SHAPE ON WEIGHT

Factoring in body shape can help to eliminate some of the inconsistencies associated with BMI. The most common descriptors of body shape are "apple" and "pear." People who carry the bulk of their weight above the hips (mainly in the abdomen) have an apple shape. This body shape is more prevalent in men. Apple-shaped people sometimes have a larger waist than hip measurement and tend to gain weight in the abdomen first. People with apple-shaped bodies are more likely to accumulate visceral fat, a dangerous type of fat that accumulates in and around body organs. Conversely, people who carry excess weight below the waist (on hips, thighs, and buttocks) have a pear shape. This body shape is more common in women. Pear-shaped people generally have larger hips than waists and tend to have more subcutaneous fat. While not without health risk, subcutaneous fat isn't as harmful as visceral fat.

Measuring and calculating the waist-to-hip ratio confirms an apple or pear shape. To arrive at the ratio, divide the waist measurement by the hip measurement. A ratio of 0.8 or less for women and 0.9 or less for men is considered a pear shape. Higher ratios indicate an apple shape.

Having an apple or pear shape isn't a concern unless a person is carrying excess weight. In the overweight or obese, having an apple shape results in a much higher risk for heart disease, type 2 diabetes, hypertension, and several types of cancer. For those who naturally become apple shaped with weight gain, it's particularly important to maintain a healthy body weight.

Using the waist measurement alone can determine whether a person is carrying excess baggage. Waist measurements of more than 32 inches in women and 37 inches in men are commonly used as upper limits, over which further weight gain is ill advised. A measurement of 35 inches for women and 40 inches for men indicates a likelihood of overweight, and that health improvements could be expected with weight loss. Once again, these numbers would need to be adjusted for those with very large or very small frames.

Lifelong Solutions for Weighty Matters

Today, a majority of Americans are actively attempting to change their body weight. Most are consumed with losing weight, while a handful want to gain a few pounds. For most people, "diets" are a lesson in frustration because they eventually end, and the same weight problem seems to return.

There are more-effective, permanent solutions. Whether a person is overweight, underweight, or struggling with an eating disorder, three simple steps can set the course to a healthy body weight for life:

1. **Make great health the #1 goal.** To permanently overcome an unhealthy body weight, the first and most critical step is to redirect focus from weight to health. When health and wellness become the top priority in food selection, overall body weight responds predictably in a positive direction. Foods shouldn't be chosen on the basis of calories or their perceived effectiveness as weight-change aids. Instead, nourishing foods should be selected to help and protect the body, and offer enjoyment and satisfaction while maintaining a healthy weight.

2. **Build healthy habits.** Habits are simply behaviors repeated so often that little conscious thought is required. Habits that erode health can be replaced with those that restore health. To create a habit, choose a new routine and follow it diligently for at least a month. After a behavior is repeated for a month, it's well on the way to becoming a good habit.

3. **Think positive.** In the journey toward a healthy weight, there are no interviews, no exams, and no reprisals. Slips should be met with a review of, and appreciation for, all the constructive changes already made, and a renewed commitment to press on. Positive affirmations can push out negative thoughts. Consider every constructive step taken as cause for celebration.

PREPARING FOR THE JOURNEY

Before significant diet and lifestyle changes are undertaken, make the appropriate mental and physical preparations:

- **Have a physical examination.** Check blood cholesterol, triglyceride, blood glucose, and CRP (measure of inflammation) levels. Get vitamin B_{12}, vitamin D, and iron levels tested. Check blood pressure and body weight. Review any prescription medications with health care providers; medications may need to be adjusted or eliminated once a healthy diet supports the body, so close monitoring may be necessary.

- **Record diet and lifestyle for three days.** Track food and beverage intakes for three full days (including one weekend day); be specific about preparation methods and amounts. Note the time of day a food was eaten, where it was eaten, and hunger level at the time.

Record all activities, from gardening and grocery shopping to exercise and answering e-mails, and document sleeping patterns. Also note other positive activities, including massages, pedicures, prayer time, meditation, and enjoyable social activities. Finally, record all addictive substances used (cigarettes, alcohol, and recreational drugs). Such a record provides a powerful reality check, as well as a valuable baseline.

- **Set realistic health goals.** Set short- and long-term goals that are specific, measureable, and attainable. Goals can include weight loss or gain, but this shouldn't be the primary focus. Instead, select goals that encourage health gains, such as improving fitness; increasing fiber intake; eating more leafy greens and beans; improving blood cholesterol, triglyceride, or blood glucose levels; more effectively managing stress; improving energy and mental alertness; curtailing mood swings; stopping smoking or reducing alcohol consumption; getting better at time management; sleeping at least seven hours a night; or being more patient and kind. Tackle goals one at a time, so the tasks don't become too overwhelming. Even small changes can produce big health rewards.

- **Restock the pantry.** Get rid of foods and other items that don't promote health; ultraprocessed fat-, sugar-, and salt-laden foods are analogous to addictive drugs. Instead, shop for healthy and tasty items. Select health-promoting recipes that sound appealing and gather the ingredients required. Consider investing in high-quality food preparation equipment, if possible.

Dietary guidelines specific to individual weight challenges have been provided in the following sections on overweight, underweight, and eating disorders. However, lifestyle factors beyond food can undermine dietary efforts if neglected. Although there are additional considerations for those with eating disorders, the following issues pertain to everyone who struggles with body weight.

Overweight

One of the great attractions of a vegan diet is the promise of slimness. This is an established part of the vegan stereotype. However, being vegan doesn't preclude overweight or obesity, and becoming vegan doesn't guarantee weight loss or even weight maintenance.

For many overweight vegans, the stereotype only adds stress to an already demanding lifestyle, because some may feel embarrassed not to be living up to expectations. However, the only prerequisite for being vegan is a compassionate heart.

Still, do vegans really have an advantage in regard to ideal body weight? Do plant-based diets offer a solid solution to the current weight crisis? In general, the answer is "yes."

THE PREVALENCE OF OVERWEIGHT IN VEGANS

Being vegan provides remarkable protection against overweight and obesity. In a Swedish study of more than 55,000 women, self-identified vegans had about one-third the risk of overweight or obesity compared to omnivores, while vegetarians and semivegetarians had close to half the risk.[10] More than twenty studies have reported that vegans are leaner than other dietary groups, have lower BMIs, and have lower percentages of body fat.[11] Two large studies—EPIC-Oxford in the United Kingdom and the Adventist Health Study-2 (AHS-2) in the United States—compared the BMIs and obesity rates of vegans with other dietary groups, including health-conscious meat eaters, fish eaters, and lacto-ovo vegetarians. In these studies, vegans had the lowest BMIs (page 39). Vegan BMIs ranged from 21.98 to 23.6, compared to 23.49 to 28.8 for health-conscious meat eaters.[12, 13] In the EPIC-Oxford study, vegan obesity rates were under 2 percent compared to more than 5 percent in health-conscious meat eaters.[12]

What gives vegans the advantage? Vegans tend to eat more fiber; more vegetables, fruits, and legumes; and more whole foods in general. They also tend to eat fewer highly processed and fast foods, and they eat no meat or dairy products, factors that have been associated with better weight management.[14, 15] While the science is reassuring, it may offer little consolation to vegans who are overweight or obese. So, why aren't kale-munching vegans entirely protected?

CAUSES OF OVERWEIGHT IN VEGANS

Everyone knows that overeating and underactivity are at the root of the global overweight and obesity epidemic. The solution is clearly a matter of energy balance. Although it's true that overweight and obesity are the result of energy imbalances, these imbalances are the product of a complex interplay of physical, environmental, and emotional factors.

Although the statement "if you eat more than you need, you gain weight; if you eat less than you need, you lose weight" sounds simple, a number of things can throw a monkey wrench into this "energy in, energy out" theory. For example, cutting 500 calories per day can cause a weight loss of 1 pound per week for a few weeks, but the body quickly adjusts to the new normal, and weight loss slows or stops. As it turns out, adults with greater fat reserves can expect to lose more weight by reducing calorie consumption than people with fewer fat reserves. However, small changes in energy intake can still result in significant weight loss over time.

The standard view that "a calorie is a calorie" has also come under fire. Accumulating evidence suggests that not all calories behave the same way in the body.[16] For example, some foods and food combinations promote calorie-burning more effectively than others. In addition, sleep, stress, and exposure to environmental toxins can disturb hormones that influence fat storage, fat breakdown, calorie-burning, and body weight. These factors can weigh as heavily on vegans as on nonvegans.

Physiological Factors

Some people are metabolically efficient. The good news for such individuals is this: if they were dropped on a desert island with no food, their metabolism would slow, preserving every ounce of fat and releasing stored energy gradually to prolong survival. The bad news is that they're more likely to live in places with endless supplies of tempting, energy-dense food. Those who are best able to survive famine are the least able to survive excess. For metabolically efficient people, moderate food intake and vigorous physical activity are necessary.

Not surprisingly, risk for weight gain can be affected by genes, age, and gender. Men tend to burn more calories than women and, for most people, metabolism gradually declines after age 40. Very low-calorie diets and yo-yo dieting only make matters worse, because they signal the body to put on the metabolic brakes and conserve precious energy stores.

Less commonly, overweight and obesity are triggered by hypothyroidism. This condition reduces metabolic rate, triggers weight gain, and often makes its sufferers feel cold, tired, weak, and depressed. Hypothyroidism can be triggered or worsened by chronic iodine deficiency, which is rare in North American omnivores due to the addition of iodine to table salt. However, risk may be increased among vegans who avoid iodized salt (perhaps choosing sea salt, tamari, or Bragg Liquid Aminos instead) and who fail to ensure a reliable source of iodine in the diet (for more information on iodine, see pages 191 to 194).

Medications, such as corticosteroids, antidepressants, and seizure medicines can also slow metabolism, increase appetite, or cause water retention, all of which can lead to weight gain.

Environmental Factors

Humans are hardwired to like the taste of fat, sugar, and salt. Highly dilute in nature, these flavors once assured people that a food was safe and nourishing to consume, and that it would sustain them through lean times, give them energy, or replenish losses. However, when the sources of these flavors are concentrated and used as the principal ingredients in processed foods, the body's innate ability to control appetite becomes unhinged. Vegan versions of such foods can be just as problematic. This is no mere coincidence. These foods are all physically addictive. Foods that contain hyperconcentrations of sugar, fat, and salt (all of which are vegan ingredients) stimulate the same pleasure centers in the brain as heroin, nicotine, and alcohol. Essentially, they provide such pleasure that they trigger cravings.[17-19]

To further challenge self-control, portion sizes keep expanding. According to the Centers for Disease Control and Prevention (CDC), the average restaurant meal today is four times larger than it was in the 1950s. Not surprisingly, evidence confirms that as portion sizes increase, people eat more.[20] Also, it doesn't seem to matter if the dietary choices are vegan. Vegan versions of almost every convenience food, snack food, and fast food are now available, and the word *vegan* is used to provide products with a "health halo" regardless of portion size.

On the other hand, physical demands have dwindled dramatically since the 1950s. Every possible convenience has been developed to help reduce the need for physical activity. Even if people wanted to increase activity, many neighborhoods lack sidewalks and safe places for exercise. In these environments, staying slim is an ever-greater challenge.

Another less well-recognized potential trigger for weight gain is lack of sleep.[21] Although less sleep would seem to imply greater caloric expenditure, evidence suggests that lack of sleep promotes weight gain. Sleep-deprived people seem to crave more energy-dense foods. In addition, there's some evidence that lack of sleep reduces insulin sensitivity, increases levels of ghrelin (a hormone that promotes hunger), and reduces levels of leptin (a hormone that curbs hunger).

Emotional Factors

For many people, weight gain has as much to do with self-preservation and social pressure as it does with overeating and underactivity. Difficult interactions, disappointment, embarrassment, stress, overwork, or hardship all seem to be eased by food, even in the complete absence of physical hunger. Of course, social events and festive experiences are often celebrated with favorite foods and beverages too. Eating in response to feelings rather than physical hunger is known as "emotional eating," and it's a well-recognized factor in overweight and obesity. In its most severe form, emotional eating can lead to eating disorders, such as compulsive overeating or binge eating disorder (see page 392 for more information).

THE HEALTH CONSEQUENCES OF OVERWEIGHT

The economic and health burdens associated with overweight and obesity are immense. In 2008, medical costs associated with obesity in the United States were estimated at $147 billion.[22] Contrary to popular opinion, "healthy obesity" is not a benign condition. Compared to healthy normal-weight individuals, obese people are at increased risk for long-term adverse health outcomes, even when they appear metabolically healthy.[23] Excess body fat causes unwanted changes to the body's basic physiology, adversely affecting blood pressure, cholesterol, triglycerides, respiration, fertility, skin and joint health, hormones, and insulin action. Gaining excess fat significantly increases risks for many debilitating and often fatal conditions:[24–26]

- **Type 2 diabetes.** The risk of type 2 diabetes is directly linked to degree of body fat, particularly for people with an apple shape. As body fat increases, insulin sensitivity declines, and insulin resistance increases.
- **Coronary artery disease, congestive heart failure, and stroke.** Being overweight contributes to high blood pressure, high cholesterol, high triglycerides, and angina (chest pain), and can markedly increase the chances of sudden heart attack, stroke, or congestive heart failure.
- **Cancer.** Overweight women suffer more breast, uterine, cervical, ovarian, gallbladder, and colon cancers, while overweight men are at elevated risk for cancers of the colon, rectum, and prostate.
- **Osteoarthritis.** Excess body weight increases the risk of osteoarthritis, probably by placing extra pressure on joints and eroding the cartilage tissue that cushions and protects the joints.
- **Sleep apnea.** Sleep apnea triggers pauses in breathing during sleep and is often marked by heavy snoring and snorting breaths that follow sometimes

fairly prolonged lapses in breathing. Risk for sleep apnea is significantly higher in overweight individuals.

- **Gout.** The product of high levels of uric acid in the blood, gout causes painful swelling in the joints, usually affecting one joint at a time. The most common site affected is the big toe, but it's also seen in the ankle, knee, elbow, wrist, and finger joints. The risk for gout increases progressively with excess body weight.

- **Gallbladder disease.** Being overweight significantly increases the risk of both gallbladder disease and gallstones. However, rapid, significant weight loss can also increase the chance of developing gallstones.

- **Polycystic ovarian syndrome.** This painful disorder is marked by small cysts on the ovaries, menstrual irregularities, facial hair, acne, patches of dark skin on the neck, and weight gain in women of reproductive age. It's associated with insulin resistance and abdominal obesity and strongly increases the risk of type 2 diabetes, heart disease, and stroke.

Although published research doesn't exist to answer whether being vegan protects against the adverse consequences of overweight and obesity, evidence suggests that healthy lifestyle habits are associated with a significant reduction in mortality in normal-weight, overweight, and obese individuals, with the greatest benefits being observed in obese individuals.[27] Because vegan diets are generally associated with reduced risk of chronic disease, one may expect that overweight and obese vegans would enjoy some advantages over overweight and obese omnivores. However, vegans who consume unhealthful diets could certainly fare worse than health-conscious omnivores.

Nutritional Health Goals

It's common knowledge that dietary modifications are an essential component of weight management, but the extent of the modifications necessary for long-term success are often underestimated. While caloric restriction is generally necessary, many other dietary factors must interact to produce the desired results. Some dietary choices essentially set up a chain reaction of metabolic dysfunction that compromises all body systems. Consuming a rich variety of healthful foods builds a powerful defense against this type of assault. Six health goals are fundamental to achieving and maintaining healthy body weight for life:

1. **Overcome food addictions and cravings.** Where food addiction is concerned, ultraprocessed and fat-, sugar-, and salt-laden foods are essentially equivalent to drugs. To break the cycle, the addictive foods must be eliminated. When these foods are replaced with foods of real value to health, the body restores its balance and frees itself from the addiction. At this point, the body can better handle the occasional "addictive food" and is less likely to crave it.

For success in overcoming a food addiction, blood sugar levels must be stable. Eating meals with a good balance of protein, carbohydrate, and fat helps. For example, breakfast cereal should be topped with nuts, seeds, and unsweetened nondairy milk. Beans at breakfast yield staying power through the morning. Eat legumes, tofu, or tempeh at lunch and dinner. Avoid caloric beverages, sugar, and artificial sweeteners. Eliminate deep-fried foods.

One less well-recognized cause of cravings is allergies or sensitivities; for a number of people, gluten is an issue. Ironically, people often crave the very foods to which they're sensitive. Consider eliminating suspect foods for two to four weeks, then gradually adding them back, one at a time, at two- to four-day intervals.

2. Control inflammation. Inflammation is one of the key driving forces behind overweight and obesity, as well as many other chronic diseases. Dietary factors, including overeating itself, can generate inflammation in many ways. When fat cells become bloated, production of proinflammatory hormones increases and production of anti-inflammatory hormones decreases. This imbalance promotes insulin resistance.[28]

Other common contributors to inflammation are foods to which individuals are sensitive or allergic. Environmental contaminants, chronic stress, and deficiencies of certain nutrients, such as vitamin D and omega-3 fatty acids, can also promote inflammation. Fortunately, the vegetables, fruits, legumes, whole grains, nuts, seeds, herbs, and spices in a whole-foods plant-based diet provide an array of anti-inflammatory compounds that help to keep inflammation at bay.

3. Improve digestion. An inflamed gut—which can result from allergies or sensitivities, intestinal diseases, parasites, chronic or acute diarrhea, and other factors—may contribute to obesity and disease. "Leaky gut," a popular term that describes increased intestinal permeability, allows fragments of food proteins to penetrate the intestinal lining and enter the bloodstream. When proteins circulate in the bloodstream, they can accumulate almost anywhere in the body, potentially leading to insulin resistance or other adverse conditions. The foods most commonly associated with leaky gut are ultraprocessed packaged convenience items, including products with refined sugar or flour, and those linked to hypersensitivities, such as gluten-containing grains and dairy products. [29–34]

Unhealthy intestinal flora also adversely affect digestion, metabolism, and immune function. Evidence suggests that these bacteria produce toxins with the potential to injure the gut lining and contribute to leaky gut.[35–37] Conversely, beneficial bacteria may help to promote leanness by manufacturing short-chain fatty acids that reduce fat accumulation in cells, boost metabolism, and promote the production of satiety hormones.[38] Low-fat, high-fiber, vegetable-rich diets encourage good bacteria to flourish. In addition, high-quality probiotics will support the reestablishment of healthy gut flora.

4. Reinforce detoxification systems. Scientists are just beginning to recognize a connection between body fat accumulation and environmental contaminants, such as bisphenol A (BPA), heavy metals, persistent organic pollutants, and pesticides. Consumers can't completely eliminate exposure to these compounds, but they may take steps to minimize it. In addition, body systems that help to excrete these compounds can be reinforced.

Fortunately, vegans may be at an advantage on both counts. First, because they're high on the food chain, animal products (including fish) are significant sources of environmental toxins. Not surprisingly, preliminary evidence suggests

that exposure to such toxins may be reduced in vegetarian and vegan populations.[39, 40] Second, cruciferous vegetables, which tend to be heavily consumed
by vegans, are rich in phytochemicals that support the body's detoxification
processes. Numerous vitamins, minerals, amino acids, phytochemicals, and
antioxidants play a role in this process, so good nutritional status is important.
Finally, eating organic foods, when possible, reduces exposure to pesticides.

5. Balance hormones, boost metabolism. Optimal health and metabolism depend on the proper functioning of the body's many systems that produce and
release hormones, including thyroid, stress, and sex hormones. Thyroid hormones control metabolism and can have a significant impact on body weight.
Vegans—especially those who avoid iodized salt and sea vegetables—may be
low in iodine, which is needed in the production of thyroid hormones. Insufficient selenium and vitamin D can also adversely affect thyroid function.[41, 42]

The stress hormone cortisol helps to deliver the appropriate type and quantity of carbohydrate, fat, or protein to body tissues. Under conditions of chronic
stress or calorie deprivation, cortisol levels rise. Elevated cortisol levels are associated with increased appetite and cravings for foods rich in fat and sugar.[43–45]
In addition, fat is shuttled into visceral fat deposits in the abdomen, which promotes cardiovascular disease and insulin resistance.

Insulin resistance impacts sex hormones. In women, insulin resistance can
trigger polycystic ovarian syndrome, causing masculinizing symptoms, such as
unwanted hair growth and infertility. In men, elevated insulin levels can depress
testosterone levels and sex drive.[46, 47]

A whole-foods, low glycemic-load, nutrient-dense, plant-based diet (with
appropriate supplements) plays a critical role in balancing hormones and boosting metabolism. Stress management and physical activity also are vital.

6. Enhance nutritional status. Much of the developed world is overfed and
undernourished. People consume too many calories and environmental contaminants; too much fat, salt, and sugar; and not enough of the elements necessary
for optimal health. Vegans tend to have higher intakes of vegetables and fruits,
fiber, and a number of nutrients, phytochemicals, and antioxidants. But, even so,
nutrient shortfalls aren't uncommon among vegans.

When curtailing calories for weight control, foods with high energy density
(many calories per gram) should be deemphasized. More important are foods
with high nutrient density (many nutrients per calorie). Fueling the body with
high-quality organic whole plant foods shifts gene expression, reducing the risks
for overweight, obesity, and chronic disease. The best choices are vegetables (especially leafy greens), legumes, fruits, nuts, seeds, and intact whole grains (rather
than grains ground into flour).

Food Choices for Health

1. Eat at least five servings of nonstarchy vegetables per day. In their natural
state, vegetables are the most nutrient-dense foods on the planet. One serving
equals 1 cup (250 ml) raw or ½ cup (125 ml) cooked. Aim for color and variety:
at least one serving each of green (including dark leafy greens), red, orange-yellow,

Allies and Enemies in the Battle for Health

TOP TEN HEALTHY-WEIGHT ALLIES	TOP TEN HEALTHY-WEIGHT ENEMIES
Leafy greens	Overeating
Nonstarchy vegetables; sea vegetables	Sugary beverages
Sprouts	Sugar-laden treats (e.g., frozen desserts, candy, pastries)
Legumes of all kinds	Refined starches (e.g., white-flour breads, bagels, crackers, cookies)
Fresh fruits	Ultraprocessed convenience foods
Nuts and seeds	Fast and/or fried foods
Herbs and spices	Salty snack foods
Unrefined starchy foods—intact whole grains, starchy vegetables	Concentrated fats and oils
Herbal teas (e.g., green tea)	Environmental contaminants
Water	Alcohol

purple-blue, and white-beige vegetables; include raw vegetables daily. Cooked vegetables are most nutritious when lightly steamed. Limit the serving sizes of starchy vegetables, such as sweet potatoes and corn, to no more than ½ cup (125 ml) once or twice a day. Include sprouts, which are highly nutritious and inexpensive to grow.

2. **Learn to love legumes.** Eat at least three ½ cup (125 ml) servings of legumes per day. (New consumers should begin with smaller servings to allow the gut bacteria to adjust to the increased fiber intake.) Beans, lentils, and peas are among the richest fiber sources, providing satiety and staying power between meals. Lentils and split peas or fresh peas (in or out of the pod) are extremely low in fat but high in nutrients. Lentils, mung beans, and whole peas are excellent candidates for sprouting. Other nutrient-rich legume-based products include tofu and tempeh, unsweetened soy milk, protein powders, and vegan meat substitutes (check the labels, though). Add beans to stews, soups, and salads or use them to make patties, loaves, or spreads. If using canned beans, opt for those in BPA-free cans.

3. **Go easy on grains.** As calorie needs decrease (e.g., with age, menopause, reduced physical activity, and so forth), intake of all grains should be reduced as well. Especially avoid refined grains, such as white rice and products made from white flour and white rice, as well as processed cereals with added sugar and salt. Minimize the use of ground grains (e.g., flour) of all types, even whole-grain flours. (This includes whole-grain breads, crackers, cookies, pretzels, and other flour-based baked goods.)

Choose intact whole grains, such as quinoa, wild rice, buckwheat, oat groats, and barley, and, for most people, limit portion sizes to ½ cup (125 ml). One of the most healthful ways to use grains is to sprout them. Add the sprouts to salads or enjoy as a breakfast cereal (add fruit, nuts, seeds, and nondairy yogurt or milk). Although less desirable than intact whole grains, cut grains (e.g., bulgur) and rolled grains (e.g., rolled oats) also can be part of the diet.

4. Satisfy a sweet tooth with fresh fruit. Although the thought of an apple for dessert may seem boring, there are many ways to turn fruit into a tantalizing after-dinner treat. Simply slicing fruit and creatively arranging the pieces on a plate makes it seem special. Topped with a little cinnamon and plain nondairy yogurt or nut cream, chopped fruit or berries turn into a delightful parfait. Fruits can be poached, baked, or grilled for fabulous flavor. And, who wouldn't appreciate the taste of ice cream—minus the fat and sugar? Freeze peeled bananas, berries, pineapple, mango, and other fruit; process these through a juicer to make a soft-serve ice cream for instant consumption. Alternatively, blend together frozen fruit with just enough nondairy milk or yogurt to make a smooth ice cream.

Because fruit skins and seeds are especially rich sources of fiber and phytochemicals, edible varieties should be consumed. Limit use of dried fruits to ¼ cup (60 ml) or less per day; these foods are more concentrated in naturally occurring sugars, and are higher in calories. People with elevated blood glucose levels are well-advised to limit fruit to not more than four servings a day (see page 335 for recommended serving sizes).

5. Select nuts, seeds, and avocados as primary fat sources. Although high-fat plant foods are calorie packed, in both population studies and clinical trials, they're inversely associated with weight gain.[48] Loaded with protective compounds, including essential fatty acids, these higher-fat plant foods are vital health allies. Eat about 1 to 2 ounces (30 to 60 g) of nuts and seeds a day. Select a mix of nuts and seeds that provides a good balance of essential fatty acids, such as chia seeds, flaxseeds, hempseeds, and walnuts. Include a Brazil nut for selenium.

One of the best ways to eat nuts is straight from the shell, because the effort required to retrieve the nut discourages overconsumption. In addition, soaking nuts and seeds reduces antinutrients and increases their nutritional value. Soaked nuts can then be dehydrated to add crunchiness without adding the harmful products of oxidation formed during roasting.

Minimize the use of fats and oils. They provide about 120 calories per tablespoon (15 ml) but very few nutrients, because minerals, phytochemicals, fiber, and most fat-soluble vitamins are left behind during processing. Partially hydrogenated oils contain harmful trans-fatty acids—read labels, and avoid them completely.

6. Make the most of herbs and spices. Herbs and spices are the most recently hailed health heroes. They enhance food flavor without increasing sodium or fat intake. Several herbs and spices also may boost metabolism, calm inflammation, or balance blood glucose levels. Among the spicy superstars are black pepper, cardamom, cayenne, cinnamon, cumin, cloves, ginger, ginseng, mustard seeds, oregano, rosemary, and turmeric. Freshly grown herbs can be frozen or dehydrated for later use.

7. Keep a lid on ultraprocessed and convenience foods. Such foods are generally the result of many stages of processing, such as grinding, refining, and/or partial hydrogenation. To enhance the final products, food manufacturers also may add sugar, salt, additives, colors, or preservatives. Because of the body's natural affinity for these flavors, individuals overconsume calorie-dense foods. Good examples include chips and other salty snacks, sugar-laden breakfast cereals, and salt- and fat-rich frozen dinners.

Not all processed foods are harmful. To meet consumer demands for healthful options, food manufacturers have responded with better choices. For example, some foods may be partially prepared to help reduce cooking time, but their processing is kept to a minimum and few ingredients are added. Good examples include frozen herbs, beans canned with little salt in BPA-free cans, shelled frozen edamame, some sprouted breads, organic sugar-free fruit-and-nut bars, and some jarred tomato sauces. To find such minimally processed foods, read the ingredient list.

8. Minimize the use of sugar and avoid artificial sweeteners. Whether sugar comes from high-fructose corn syrup or organic dehydrated cane juice, the type of sugar matters less than the amount ingested. Besides being a source of empty calories, sugar offers few or no nutrients. Be aware of added sugars in foods; read the labels on packaged foods to find and avoid them. In most cases, if a commercial vegan product contains no fruit (fresh or dried), it's likely that any sugar listed on the label is added sugar.

Avoid artificial sweeteners; they provide no real assistance in a quest for health and may negatively affect metabolism and appetite control, undermining efforts to achieve a healthy body weight.

9. Choose the right beverages. Water is the best thirst quencher—and it's calorie-free. If possible, dispense the water through a filter that eliminates chlorine, lead, nitrates, microorganisms, and other environmental contaminants without removing minerals, such as calcium and magnesium.

Herbal teas can be healthful beverage choices. Green tea has been shown to boost metabolism and may aid in weight loss.[49] For added nutrition with minimal calories, vegetable juice (especially green juices or tomato juice) or wheatgrass juice are good options. Nutritious but higher-calorie beverages (fresh fruit juices and fortified soy, rice, or other nondairy milks) provide 100 to 150 calories per cup. Homemade smoothies made from some combination of fruit, greens, and seeds can make healthful meal replacements providing 400 to 500 calories per 24-ounce (750 ml) serving. They should be looked upon as meal replacements and limited to not more than one per day. Commercial smoothies often are loaded with concentrated juices and can contain up to 800 calories in a 24-ounce (750 ml) serving and 75 grams (18 teaspoons) of sugar—unless you can control the ingredients, avoid them.

Although some beverages add nutritional value to the diet, in general, whole foods provide greater satiety value for weight management. Fluids don't fill the

Vegan Victory: The Game Plan

- Eat at least five servings of nonstarchy vegetables a day.
- Eat at least three servings of legumes daily.
- Limit grains to not more than three servings a day—eat only intact whole grains.
- Eat four servings of fresh fruit per day.
- Eat 1 to 2 ounces of nuts and seeds per day. Include at least one serving of omega-3 rich walnuts, flaxseeds, chia seeds, or hempseeds. Limit added fats and oils.
- Spice it up—use herbs and spices liberally.
- Steer clear of ultraprocessed foods.
- Skip added sugars.
- Drink water. Minimize consumption of caloric beverages.
- Take supplements, as needed.

stomach the way solid food does, so it's easy to underestimate a beverage's contribution to calorie intakes. A 12-ounce serving of lemonade, fruit punch, or soda pop contains 120 to 150 calories but provides little, if any, nutritional value. Alcoholic beverages can also send calorie intakes soaring.

Artificially sweetened calorie-free beverages aren't the answer, nor are the sweeteners themselves. Stevia is a reasonable option to sweeten coffee or tea, if necessary. (For more information, see page 167.)

Adequate hydration is vital to healthy body functioning and peak performance. Dehydration can be mistaken for hunger and can trigger overeating. Water is generally the best beverage choice, so having a water bottle handy is a good habit to develop.

10. Consider nutritional supplements. Whole-foods vegan diets can be low in vitamin B_{12}, iodine, and vitamin D (depending on exposure to sunshine). Unless reliable sources of these nutrients are obtained from fortified foods, it's wise to take supplements. Targets for these nutrients are about 1,000 mcg of vitamin B_{12} two or three times per week (see pages 214 to 222 for more options), 150 mcg of iodine per day, and 1,000 mcg of vitamin D per day (see pages 222 to 230 for more options). A multivitamin-mineral supplement is also an option, although unnecessary if reliable sources of iodine and vitamins B_{12} and D are ensured.

Changing Food Behaviors

Even when consumers are acutely aware of which foods are nutritious, today's obesogenic environment can lead to less-healthful choices. Strengthening the resolve against this constant temptation requires a heightened awareness of the body's needs, and consciousness of the enticing environment that can weaken judgment. Consider these proven strategies:

- **Listen to body signals.** Learn the body's natural hunger signals to reclaim the lost skill of intuitive eating. Avoid these twin temptations: eating when not hungry or fasting when famished. Sometimes thirst is mistaken for hunger. When hunger strikes, first drink a glass of water and wait fifteen minutes. If hunger is still present, then eat. Plan for regular mealtimes, but be flexible. In the absence of hunger, skip a meal or eat very lightly. Eat slowly and stop when comfortable, but not full.

Recognize when nonphysical "hunger" is triggered by emotions or environment. Fill that "hunger" with an appropriate nonfood option. For example, if you recognize a temptation to indulge in emotional eating, go for a walk, call a friend, or take a bubble bath instead. If a strong emotion, such as anger, triggers hunger, take it out on a punching bag or stomp around the block.

- **Eat mindfully.** Build healthful habits that make mindless eating less harmful (such as mindlessly eating greens instead of candy). Create a relaxing atmosphere to make meal times special. Eat slowly and chew food well to aid digestion, enhance appreciation of the foods' flavors, and reduce total food intake. Be conscious of everyone involved in getting food to the table and consume the meal with a grateful heart. Buy from local farmers and local producers and avoid foods that support practices inconsistent with your values.

- **Build healthful habits.** Keep mealtimes regular; skipping meals can lead to overeating at the next meal. Avoid eating within two to three hours of bedtime; eating drives up insulin levels, triggering fat storage. The body doesn't need much fuel to sleep, so satisfy true hunger with vegetables or a piece of fruit.

Portion control can be a challenge. Placing serving bowls or platters of food on the table at mealtimes often results in larger servings than those portioned onto plates or into bowls. Begin by using smaller cups, plates, and bowls. Always serve recommended portions on a plate or in a bowl, and sit down to eat. Put the salad and vegetables on the table and leave other foods on the counter or stove after preparing plates or bowls. Because it's easy to overeat while standing, especially during food preparation, suck on a cinnamon stick or chew some mint to avoid excessive "tasting."

Be careful not to fall into the "health halo" trap by eating larger servings of foods labeled low-calorie, low-fat, natural, or organic. While such replacements may contain 10 or 15 percent fewer calories, eating larger quantities easily eliminates that advantage.

Finally, keep food out of sight, unless it's superhealthy and increased intake is desired. Ditto for eating while watching TV. To keep hands occupied, do a craft, catch up on ironing, or do some stretching exercises during viewing.

Underweight

While being underweight affects people of both genders, it's less often recognized as a serious problem for women, in whom thinness is prized. Men feel a different sort of pressure when it comes to body shape. For them, low body fat is desirable, but being skinny isn't. Their goal is usually a buff body, so their quest involves accumulating sufficient muscle mass.

Fortunately, a well-planned vegan diet can support weight-gain goals for both men and women. While modern culture tends to promote the consumption of meat for increasing muscle mass, similar rewards can be reaped by consuming protein-rich plants foods.

PREVALENCE OF UNDERWEIGHT IN VEGANS

Vegans typically have lower BMIs and less body fat than lacto-ovo vegetarians or the general population; most vegans fall within the healthy weight range.[12, 13, 50–53] However, vegans do seem to experience higher rates of underweight compared to the general population, although data is currently very limited.

A German study reported that among 572 individuals eating raw food vegan diets, 25 percent of the women and 14.7 percent of the men were underweight (BMI <18.5).[54] Chronic energy deficiency (CED) grade II or III affected 5.7 percent of women and 2.6 percent of men. Generally, those eating a higher percentage of raw foods (90 to 100 percent of calories from raw food) were at greater risk for underweight compared to those eating more moderate raw food diets (70 to 89 percent of calories from raw foods). A study on followers of a mostly raw vegan diet promoted by the Hallelujah Acres Foundation reported average BMIs of 21.5 for women and 22.9 for men. Sixteen individuals (9.1 percent) were underweight (BMI<18.5).[55] EPIC Oxford reported higher rates of low BMI (<20) in vegans compared to other dietary categories. Approximately 2.4 percent of meat eaters had BMIs of less than 20, compared to 9.5 percent of fish eaters, 5.4 percent of lacto-ovo vegetarians and 16.8 percent of vegans. Rates of underweight (BMI <18.5) were not reported.[56]

DETERMINATIONS OF UNDERWEIGHT IN VEGANS

While the BMI chart on page 363 provides useful guidelines, its cutoffs aren't accurate for everyone. Careful consideration of the following factors will help determine whether or not low body weight poses a health risk and warrants treatment:

- **State of health.** After ruling out an underlying disease (such as cancer) in someone who lacks energy or is weak, often sick, and requires long recovery periods, chances are good that body weight is too low. On the other hand, an individual who is generally in good health, is energetic and seldom sick, and quickly recovers from illness may be at a healthy body weight even if BMI is low.

- **Body frame.** In people with small frames, BMI sometimes suggests underweight, even when the person is at a healthy weight for his or her size. For example, a healthy, small-boned Asian woman who is 5 feet 4 inches (1.63 m) and weighs 107 pounds (52 kg) has a BMI of 18.4, which is technically underweight. However, considering her bone structure and health status, this woman is likely at a healthy weight. On the other hand, a 5 foot 4 inch (1.63 m) woman with a large bone structure may be underweight at 116 pounds (56.4 kg), despite a BMI well within the healthy range at nearly 20.

Underweight versus Calorie Restriction

If underweight is associated with increased mortality, why do studies on calorie restriction (CR) suggest increased longevity? While it's not certain, one explanation is that the adverse health outcomes associated with underweight populations are actually a consequence of poverty, malnutrition, poor lifestyle habits, and illness. In contrast, participants in CR studies are generally healthy and reasonably well nourished. Not surprisingly, these associated benefits are lost if the study subjects become malnourished.[70]

CR is a long-term dietary intervention in which energy intake is reduced by 10 to 30 percent but adequate nutrients are provided. Most epidemiological studies of calorie-deprived human populations are associated with malnutrition and aren't useful for CR research. The most notable exception is in Okinawa, Japan, where traditionalist Okinawans purposefully restrict their caloric intake by eating until they're only 80 percent full. Yet, they maintain good nutritional health. In fact, they're known to live extraordinarily healthy lives and boast one of the largest populations of vigorous centenarians in the world. The Okinawan experience suggests considerable potential for CR diets in maintaining human health.

In clinical studies of animals and organisms, CR has been shown to delay the onset of aging and to increase longevity. CR effectively reduces age-related changes in subject's energy metabolism, inflammation, and subjects' many other mediators of health. Two research groups are currently conducting investigations in humans: the National Institute on Aging (NIA) and the Calorie Restriction Society (CR Society). The NIA is performing short-term CR studies in humans. Preliminary evidence suggests that during periods of CR, people exhibit similar adaptive responses as other calorie-restricted species. The CR Society is carrying out long-term studies of adherents who maintain a strict CR-lifestyle regimen. These individuals have been reported to have had favorable changes in metabolic markers for disease.[71, 72]

Although the data on disease-risk indicators have proven favorable, experts are not yet recommending CR as a long-term therapeutic diet for humans. Concerns remain about variability among individuals and safety at their various life-cycle stages (e.g., children, adolescents, pregnant and lactating women, and seniors who are at greater risk for malnutrition). While common sense would suggest avoiding CR during stages of growth and development (e.g., infancy, childhood, adolescence, pregnancy, and lactation) and for those at increased risk for malnutrition, it's possible that moderate CR will prove useful for some individuals. It's not easy to meet the needs for all nutrients on low-calorie diets, thus caution is warranted.

- **Gender.** Men tend to have larger bones and muscles than women, so at any given height, lean men generally weigh more than lean women, even when their body fat percentage is lower. Although the BMI cutoffs are the same for men and women, it's relatively common for men to be underweight when their BMI is at the lower end of the normal range (i.e., between 18.5 and 20).
- **Lifestyle.** Underweight is more of a concern in those whose low body weight is due to unhealthy lifestyle practices, such as substance abuse or a poor diet. However, underweight people who eat nutritious plant-based diets, avoid addictive substances, and engage in regular physical activity have low risks for illness.

CAUSES OF UNDERWEIGHT IN VEGANS

Underweight is relatively rare in populations with abundant food supplies. Still, hunger due to food scarcity, the most common cause of underweight worldwide, is more prevalent in affluent countries than many realize.

Technically, underweight is the result of insufficient energy intake relative to energy output. However, the causes of weight imbalances are far more complex than textbook calculations might suggest. Physical factors, such as genetics, illness, and chemical dependency, can all play a role. In addition, some individuals are born with lean genes.[56] If their metabolic rate is naturally high, these people require more calories than others of similar height and weight to avoid underweight. Psychological factors—depression, eating disorders, stress, abuse, and cultural pressure—also can undermine healthy eating patterns, reduce energy intake, and result in significant, sustained weight loss. Other environmental factors, such as overactivity, social isolation, and poor eating habits (such as restrictive eating or skipping meals), can also lead to underweight.

A vegan diet makes weight maintenance even more challenging because plant foods, which are high in fiber and generally low in fat, cause feelings of fullness with fewer calories. Fortunately, simple steps can ensure healthy weight maintenance after animal products are removed from the menu (see pages 381 to 390).

THE HEALTH CONSEQUENCES OF UNDERWEIGHT

While most people would rather be underweight than overweight, being underweight is associated with increased mortality. Underweight individuals are generally at greater risk than people who are normal weight or overweight, although they're at lower risk than the obese.[57] In the Oxford Vegetarian Study, the death rate of participants with BMIs below 18 was more than double the death rate of those with BMIs between 20 and 22.[58] Research suggests that the association between underweight and mortality is most pronounced in people with poor lifestyle habits, such as smoking, inactivity, and poor vegetable and fruit intake.[59] Deaths from respiratory diseases and illnesses (apart from cancer and circulatory diseases) are increased in the underweight compared to people in other weight categories. In contrast, mortality from cardiovascular diseases, diabetes, kidney diseases, and some cancers is increased in those who are obese.[60]

Underweight can also negatively affect immune response and resistance to infection. Poor intakes of protein and calories can compromise the production of antibodies, cytokines, and other compounds necessary for optimal immune function. Even mild single-nutrient deficiencies can threaten immune response. A lack of zinc, selenium, iron, copper, essential fatty acids, and vitamins A, C, D, E, B_6, and folic acid can have significant negative impact on the immune system.[61-64]

Being underweight can also compromise hormone production and action in both males and females. In females, low body fat can prevent ovulation, induce amenorrhea, and reduce fertility.[65, 66] If conception does occur and weight gain during pregnancy is insufficient, the baby's development is put at risk, and it's

Where Can I Find Great Recipes?

For nutritious menus and delicious high-protein recipes, all with nutritional analysis, see *Cooking Vegan* by Vesanto Melina and Joseph Forest (Book Publishing Company, 2012).

more likely to be small for its gestational age. In underweight men, sperm count and semen quality can be significantly reduced.[67]

Underweight is often associated with multiple nutritional deficiencies. For example, underweight individuals—particularly women of child-bearing age—are at increased risk for iron deficiency, resulting in weakness, fatigue, irritability, and paleness. In some individuals, iron deficiency leads to hair loss and intolerance to cold.

When the body doesn't receive sufficient calories, it mobilizes energy from glycogen stores (carbohydrates); when these are exhausted, fat is used. Then, the body relies upon stored protein for amino acids and energy, resulting in decreased muscle mass, leading to weakness and fatigue. Underweight can also trigger bone breakdown and decreases in bone density, elevating the risk for osteoporosis.[68, 69]

Great Gains for Vegans

Deciding to actively pursue weight gain depends on personal body perception. For the most part, men are more inclined to correct an underweight problem than are women because of cultural preferences for muscular men and thin women. The most effective approach to weight gain isn't so different than it is for weight loss: permanent lifestyle changes that promote and sustain health and wellness.

Underweight vegans also should consider the ultimate goals of a vegan lifestyle. A positive personal example is a powerful tool to motivate others toward adopting a more compassionate and sustainable lifestyle. However, underweight and generally unhealthy vegans fail to provide the kind of inspiration for dietary change that is often hoped for.

Eating to Gain

1. **Increase food intake.** In theory, adding 500 calories per day results in a gain of 1 pound per week, but in reality, caloric needs for weight gain can vary considerably from person to person. Most underweight adults require between 2,500 and 4,000 calories per day to gain weight, and competitive athletes need more. To reach this goal, select energy-dense vegan foods and increase serving sizes. Begin by following The Vegan Plate (see pages 434 to 435); include extra servings from each group, as needed. This will not only increase calorie intakes to recommended levels but also will ensure that nutrient needs are being met. A 2,500- to 2,800-calorie menu is provided on page 441, and a 4,000-calorie menu is provided on page 442. Table 12.2 (page 382) presents general guidelines on

TABLE 12.2. Suggested servings for weight gain

FOOD GROUP	AVERAGE CALORIE CONTENT (kcal) PER SERVING*	NUMBER OF SERVINGS* FOR 2,500-CALORIE DIET	NUMBER OF SERVINGS* FOR 4,000-CALORIE DIET
Legumes	120	5	9
Grains	75	8	13
Nuts and seeds	160	4	6
Vegetables	40	5	7
Fruits	75	4	6
Calcium-rich foods	Varies	6	8
Fats and oils**	40	4	7

Source:[73]
*Serving sizes provided in The Vegan Plate (pages 434 to 435)
**1 serving = 1 tsp.

the daily number of servings from each food group needed to achieve 2,500- and 4,000-calorie diets. Ideally, these foods should be consumed throughout the day, including a bedtime snack (with other snacks as desired).

2. Eat more often. Snacking between meals and before bedtime plays an important role in weight gain. It's difficult to consume sufficient calories when eating only one or two meals a day. Aim for three meals a day, plus two or three hearty snacks. Avoid skipping meals or going to bed on an empty stomach. A timer can be used to remind those who are likely to forget to eat. If mornings are rushed, a lunch and snacks can be made the night before.

Add at least 500 calories more per day to the current diet. These snack options provide approximately 500 calories each:

- ¾ cup (185 ml) of trail mix (nuts, seeds, and dried fruits)
- ⅓ cup (165 ml) of nuts
- a smoothie (see recipe on page 387)
- 1 almond butter and banana sandwich plus 1 cup (250 ml) of fortified soy milk (or hot chocolate made with soy milk)
- ¾ cup (185 ml) of granola, 1 banana, and 1½ cups (375 ml) of fortified soy milk
- 20 crackers, 2 ounces (60 g) of vegan cheese, 4 veggie meat slices, and 10 olives
- 1 vegan muffin or energy bar, 1 cup (250 ml) of coconut yogurt, and an apple
- 2 ounces (60 g) of baked pita chips and ½ cup (125 ml) each of salsa, refried beans, and guacamole

3. Sneak in extra calories. Whole plant foods, especially fruits and vegetables, can be high in fiber, low in fat, and relatively low in calories. When such foods predominate in the diet, they can be filling without providing sufficient calories for weight gain. When more high-calorie foods are consumed, not only does energy intake improve, but favorite dishes also become more appealing. The following suggestions will add calories, nutrients, and flavor:

- Garnish a salad with beans, nuts, seeds, tofu, and avocado. Prepare a dressing using nut or seed butters, avocado, or high-quality oils.
- Add a creamy sauce to steamed vegetables.
- Include tofu, nuts, or seeds in stir-fries, casseroles, and pasta dishes.
- Top diced fruits with soy yogurt, granola, and cinnamon.
- Cook breakfast cereal (e.g., whole grains or oats) in nondairy milk. Add chopped nuts, seeds, and dried fruits.
- Spread nut butter on muffins or toast.
- Use full-fat nondairy milk (such as soy milk) instead of lighter varieties.
- Top vegan ice cream with nuts, dark chocolate pieces, and berries.
- Dip cut-up fruit in a vegan avocado/chocolate mousse.
- Add cashew cream (purée ½ cup/125 ml cashews with 1 cup/250 ml water) or coconut milk to soups and sauces.

4. Use beverages to boost calories. Including nutritious calorie-rich fluids increases total energy intake with little effort. One cup (250 ml) of fruit juice (fresh-squeezed is best) provides 120 to 180 calories, 1 cup (250 ml) of soy milk about 100 to 120 calories, and a soy/fruit shake about 400 to 500 calories. Limit the amount of other liquids taken with meals, because low-calorie soups or calorie-free coffee and tea take up space in the stomach and can reduce consumption of higher-calorie solid foods. Those who have difficulty eating larger portions at mealtime can try reserving fluids for between meals.

TABLE 12.3. Energy content of selected high-fat foods

FOOD	SERVING SIZE	ENERGY (CALORIES)
Nuts, mixed (without peanuts)	½ cup (125 ml)	443
Peanuts, raw	½ cup (125 ml)	414
Soy nuts	½ cup (125 ml)	405
Tofu (firm)	½ cup (125 ml)	183
Soy milk	1 cup (250 ml)	104
Avocado	7 oz (201 g)	322
Dark chocolate (70–85% cocoa solids)	2 oz (60 g)	340
Chocolate SaviSeed Protein Bar (Vega)*	1 bar	240
Oatmeal raisin cookies (Alternative Baking Company)*	1 package 4.5 oz (120 g)	480
Vegetable oil	1 T (15 ml)	120

Source:[73]

*Calorie count for commercial products from package labels.

5. Eat higher-fat whole vegan foods. Because vegan diets are generally higher in fiber and lower in fat than nonvegan diets, the easiest way to add energy without adding too much extra food volume is to increase fat intake. Aim for 20 to 35 percent of calories from fat. Among the most energy-dense plant foods are nuts, seeds, soy nuts, tofu, coconut, nondairy products (milks, creams, cheeses, and yogurts), avocados, oils, energy bars, nutritious baked goods, and dark chocolate. Table 12.3 (page 383) provides the approximate calorie content of a variety of high-calorie vegan foods. Specific suggestions on how to add energy-dense foods to meals and snacks are listed below:

Nuts, seeds, and their butters. Nuts and seeds are convenient snacks. Eat ½ to 1 cup (125 to 250 ml) daily.

- Keep a bag of nuts and/or seeds wherever you spend most of your time (work, school, and so forth).
- Use nuts and seeds to make vegan cheeses or sauces.
- Add nuts and seeds to vegetable-based roasts, patties, and stir-fries.
- Sprinkle roasted nuts and seeds on salads.
- Add nuts and seeds to baked goods, pancakes, and waffles.
- Eat nut- and/or seed-based power bars.
- Use nut butters on toast and bread and in dressings.
- Give soy nuts a try.
- Spread nut butter or tahini on apple slices or celery sticks.

Tofu. Tofu is a wonderfully versatile, low-fiber, relatively high-fat vegan food.
- Add soft tofu to shakes and smoothies.
- Enjoy scrambled tofu for breakfast.
- Use flavored tofu or tofu-based eggless salad in sandwiches.
- Sauté chopped or grated tofu with a little oil, tamari, nutritional yeast, and herbs to make a salad topping.
- Add tofu to stir-fries, stews, curries, Asian soups, and lasagne.
- Use tofu to make vegetable-based roasts and patties.
- Enjoy marinated baked or barbecued tofu.
- Make tofu puddings and cheesecake; use tofu in cakes, muffins, and cookies.

Nondairy products. Nondairy foods can significantly increase energy intakes. Vegan replacements for most dairy products—including milk, cream, sour cream, ice cream, hard cheese, cream cheese, yogurt, and butter—are widely available. Some are soy-based, while others are made from almonds, rice, coconut, hempseeds, grains, or root vegetables. These products continue to evolve and are often both tasty and nutritious. Avoid dairy substitutes based on partially hydrogenated oils, sugar, and preservatives; always read the ingredient list before buying. Instead, for example, choose full-fat commercial soy milk made from whole organic soybeans.

It's not difficult to prepare nondairy foods for complete control over ingredients. Make almond or hempseed milk, fermented cashew cheese, fruit-based ice cream, or soy yogurt.

Work more of these products into a daily menu:

- Choose fortified nondairy milk and/or yogurt for smoothies instead of water.
- Use nondairy milk and yogurt in cereals, puddings, soups, pancakes, and baked goods.
- Enjoy nondairy yogurt as a base for desserts; add berries and granola or nuts.
- Add vegan mayonnaise to sandwiches and salads, and use vegan sour cream as a base for dips or a topping for soups (make versions that use cashews or tofu).
- Experiment with nut-based cheeses; both hard cheeses and cream cheese can be prepared from scratch.

Avocados. Avocados pack a lot of calories into a small package and provide exceptional flavor and incredible versatility:

- Dress up a salad with wedges of avocado.
- Mash with lemon or lime juice for dips, sandwich spreads, and toppings.
- Add avocado chunks to salsa.
- Use avocado pieces in vegetable pita sandwiches.
- Add diced avocado to pasta or quinoa salads.
- Use blended avocado to add richness to chocolate pudding.
- Add to mashed potatoes.

Sweet treats. With the right ingredients, sweet treats can make a valuable contribution to a daily calorie count:

- Raw versions of cheesecakes, pies, cookies, and brownies are based on nuts, coconut, and dried and fresh fruits, so they generally provide nutrient-dense calories. See recipes in *Becoming Raw* by Brenda Davis and Vesanto Melina (Book Publishing Company, 2010.)
- Include nuts, seeds, coconut, and their butters as some or all of the fat in baked goods.
- Use ground flaxseeds as an egg replacer.
- Select recipes that use dates and other dried fruits for a sweetener instead of sugar.
- Use high-quality oils instead of hydrogenated fats in baking.

6. **Be generous with carbohydrates.** Aim for about 55 to 65 percent of calories from carbohydrates. The most concentrated sources are grains and starchy vegetables. Excellent choices are high-protein pseudograins (such as amaranth, buckwheat, and quinoa) and nutrient-dense, colorful, starchy vegetables (such as corn, squash, yams, and purple potatoes).

- Soak and sprout grains to use in cereals and salads, breads, and raw or baked treats.
- Cook intact grains and use in salads, stews, pilafs, and cereals.
- Top baked yams or sweet potatoes with spicy black-bean peanut sauce.
- Add cooked yams or sweet potatoes to salads.
- Enjoy breads with hummus or other legume-based spreads.
- Add potatoes to curries, stews, and scrambled tofu.
- Use whole-grain flours with added wheat germ to make breads, muffins, pancakes, and waffles.
- Add corn to marinated salads, soups, and stews.

7. **Push plant protein.** For the underweight who have lost muscle, an intake of approximately 1.2 to 1.7 grams of protein per kilogram of body weight per day is recommended to regain muscle mass. For a person who isn't aiming for big muscle gains, an intake of 1.2 g/kg/day is usually sufficient.

TABLE 12.4. Protein-rich food replacements

INSTEAD OF	PROTEIN CONTENT (g)	CHOOSE	PROTEIN CONTENT (g)
Brown rice, 1 c (250 ml)	5	Quinoa, 1 c (250 ml)	8
Corn nuts, 2 oz (60 g)	5	Soy nuts, 2 oz (60 g)	24
Cornflakes, 1 c (250 ml)	2	Oatmeal, 1 c (250 ml)	6
Garden salad with Italian dressing, 4 c (1 L) salad and 2 T (30 ml) dressing	4	Kale salad with tahini dressing, 4 c (1 L) kale and dressing made with 1 T (30 ml) tahini	12
Margarine, 2 T (30 ml)	0	Peanut butter, 2 T (30 ml)	8
Orange juice, 1 c (250 ml)	2	Protein Power Smoothie, page 387	40
Pretzels, 1 oz (30 g)	3	Pumpkin seeds, 1 oz (30 g)	9
Vegetable soup, 1 c (250 ml)	2	Lentil soup, 1 c (250 ml)	9
Rice milk, 1 c (250 ml)	1	Soy milk, 1 c (250 ml)	8
Tomato sandwich on whole-grain bread	6	Tomato sandwich on whole-grain bread with 2 oz (30 g) deli slices	21
Tomato sauce, 1 c (250 ml)	3	Tomato sauce, 1 c (250 ml) with 2 oz (60 g) veggie ground round	15
Vegan mayonnaise-based dip, ¼ cup (60 ml)	0	Hummus, ¼ cup (60 ml)	5
Vegetable stir-fry, 3 c (750 ml)	6	Vegetable-tofu stir-fry, 3 c (750 ml) with ½ c (125 ml) firm tofu	26

Source:[73]

Protein Power Smoothie

MAKES 1 SERVING

Smoothies are an exceptional vehicle for adding protein, calories, and nutrients to a vegan diet. Blending foods breaks down plant cell walls, making the nutrients highly available for absorption. For ice-cold smoothies, use frozen fruit (peel bananas before freezing) or add a few ice cubes before blending.

    1 scoop protein powder

    1 banana

    1 cup (250 ml) berries, peaches, or other fruit

    1½ cups (375 ml) fortified soy milk or other nondairy fortified milk

Put all the ingredients in a blender and process until smooth. Drink immediately.

Provides approximately 400 to 500 calories and about 30 to 40 grams of protein, depending on milk selected.

Superb Smoothie Boosters

Smoothie boosters and variations can add significant fat and calories (e.g., seeds, nuts, seed or nut butters, avocado, tofu, or oils); some add phytochemicals and antioxidants (e.g., kale, cocoa or carob powder, herbs, spices, or goji berries); others add beneficial bacteria (e.g., probiotic powder or nondairy yogurt). Add any one or more of the following items to the basic recipe above:

- 2 cups (500 ml) chopped kale for a green smoothie
- ½ small avocado (best in a green smoothie)
- Fresh herbs, such as mint, oregano, and basil (in green smoothies)
- ½ cup (125 ml) soy yogurt or other nondairy yogurt; reduce soy milk in the basic recipe to 1 cup (250 ml), if desired
- ¼ to ½ cup (60 to 125 ml) soft tofu
- 2 tablespoons (30 ml) goji berries (soak dried berries at least 4 hours or overnight)
- Cinnamon, nutmeg, ginger, and/or cloves (in fruit smoothies)
- 2 tablespoons (30 ml) hempseeds, flaxseeds, or chia seeds
- 1 to 1½ tablespoons (15 to 22 ml) cocoa or carob powder
- 1 tablespoon (15 ml) cold-pressed EFA oil (try one with added DHA)
- 1 tablespoon (15 ml) almond or other nut butter
- ¼ teaspoon powdered probiotics

Calculate protein needs based on ideal body weight, not actual body weight. For example, a person who weighs 120 pounds (55 kg), whose healthy weight is 145 pounds (66 kg), should aim to eat at least 80 grams of protein per day (66 kg x 1.2 g/kg = 79.2 g). This intake level isn't difficult to achieve on a weight-gain diet. If 2,500 calories and 80 grams of protein are consumed daily, approximately 13 percent of calories are provided by the protein (80 grams of protein x 4 calories per gram = 320 calories; 320/2,500 = 12.8 percent). This target puts protein intake in the recommended range of 10 to 15 percent of calories from protein, which is sufficient for good health. (See protein contents of menus on pages 439 to 442.)

Vegan diets can fall short on protein, particularly when legume-based foods, nuts, and seeds are avoided. With a diet of cold cereal and rice milk for breakfast; a tomato sandwich and fries for lunch, and pasta with pesto for dinner, protein intake will be insufficient. Ensure a good source of protein with every meal. Table 12.4 (page 386) provides suggestions for replacing low-protein foods with higher-protein options. For a comprehensive list of the protein content of plant foods, see table 3.5 on pages 97 to 103.

For people who have difficulty meeting protein needs, vegan protein powder is an option. A wide variety of products are available (protein derived from hempseeds, peas, rice, soy, and other plant foods). Adding protein powder to a smoothie is easy and delicious (see recipe on page 387).

8. Make healthy eating a priority. For those who often find their cupboards bare, and who eat mainly out of boxes and bags, significant lifestyle adjustments may be necessary to achieve weight-gain goals. To succeed, begin with a plan:

- Make a weekly menu, prepare a shopping list, and select a weekly shopping day.
- Order in bulk, if possible. Look into co-ops, buying clubs, and organic delivery services.
- Learn to cook. Take lessons; go with a friend to make it fun.
- Make eating a social event. Eat with friends and family more often. Host a potluck, invite someone to dinner, or enjoy a meal at a vegetarian or vegan restaurant. (See links to vegan-friendly restaurants in Resources on page 450.)
- Invest in simple vegan cookbooks and try new recipes periodically to increase variety.
- Buy a slow cooker. Put ingredients in the slow cooker in the morning (following the manufacturer's recommendations) and come home to a hot meal. Use slow cookers to prepare dishes with grains, beans, vegetables, and/or tofu; try a variety of slow-cooker recipes to make best use of this appliance.
- Cook ahead on weekends to prepare meals that can be easily reheated later. Make one or two main dishes, a soup, and some healthy baked goods and prepare enough to last several days. Freeze the extras for days when there's no time to cook.
- Keep the pantry, refrigerator, and freezer well stocked with healthy snacks: trail mix, power bars, muffins, healthy cookies, frozen bananas covered in chocolate and rolled in nuts, raw cheesecake, and similar foods. Keep a few goodies in the car, in a purse or backpack, at work, or anywhere you spend a lot of time.
- Keep the blender handy; use it daily to prepare smoothies, sauces, and homemade nut or seed milks and creams.

The Vegan Game Plan for Conquering Underweight

- Increase food intake.
- Eat more often.
- Sneak in extra calories.
- Use beverages to boost calories.
- Eat higher-fat whole vegan foods.
- Be generous with carbohydrates.

- Push plant protein.
- Make healthy eating a priority.
- Feed hunger; fuel appetite.
- Carefully consider the pros and cons of supplements and weight-gain aids.

9. Feed hunger; fuel appetite. Some people rarely feel hungry; they may have a small appetite or a small stomach. However, hunger and appetite can be affected by moods, stress levels, and physical activity. Try these strategies to improve appetite:

- Increase food intake gradually, allowing the stomach to expand slowly over time.
- Focus on energy-dense foods that take up less space in the stomach per calorie. Good examples are nuts, seeds, dried fruits, beans, avocado, and tofu. Mashing and puréeing foods can also help reduce their volume.
- Stimulate hunger with tempting aromas. Make bread or buy frozen dough and bake it. Put a few cinnamon sticks and cloves in water and simmer on the stove. Inhale enticing aromas at fresh food stands, bakeries, and restaurants.
- Peruse magazines and cookbooks with beautiful photographs of food and try the recipes.
- Choose larger bowls, plates, cups, and cutlery. Using bigger dishes, forks, and spoons has been shown to increase total food intake.
- Eat several courses; instead of one big plate of food, have four courses at the main meal. A variety of different aromas and tastes is more appetizing.
- Honor hunger. At the first signs of hunger, eat as soon as possible. If hunger doesn't strike by mealtime and a full meal is unappealing, consider having a nutritious beverage (such as a smoothie) or a substantial snack instead.
- Notice if certain foods cause gastrointestinal distress (gas, bloating, or stomach upset), which can reduce appetite and food intake. Some people discover that their body can handle these foods when it's functioning at its best (for some, that's in the morning, for others, it's at night). Some foods, such as beans, are naturally gas-forming, and it can take the body time to adjust to increased consumption. If this is an issue, eat small servings and gradually increase portion sizes. See pages 157 to 160 for tips on reducing gas production from beans.

10. Carefully consider the pros and cons of supplements and weight-gain aids. Dozens of weight-gain aids are available, though most are designed for body builders who aren't underweight. Investigate the risks and benefits before trying a new supplement. Although some may prove helpful, others are a waste of money or are potentially harmful. The US Food and Drug Administration provides information online regarding bodybuilding products that contain hidden ingredients considered unsafe. Supplements intended for bodybuilding athletes are reviewed on pages 422 to 425.

Health care providers may suggest appetite stimulants to support weight-gain efforts. Although these can be effective, some have undesirable side effects. It's best to use other strategies to increase food intake.

A multivitamin-mineral supplement may be helpful, especially for individuals struggling to improve the quality and consistency of their diet. Select a supplement that provides zinc, magnesium, chromium, selenium, and possibly iron (have iron levels tested to see if additional iron would be beneficial). Vegans require supplements of vitamin B_{12} (if insufficient fortified foods are selected), vitamin D (if sunshine exposure is limited), and iodine (if iodized salt isn't used).

Eating Disorders

When constant thoughts of food and eating, and unnatural concerns about weight and body shape, negatively affect a person's physical or emotional health and day-to-day functioning, the possibility of an eating disorder must be considered.

The image that most often springs to mind when people think of eating disorders is that of a young, emaciated woman with anorexia nervosa. Unfortunately, it's been rumored that being vegan is a trigger for eating disorders. However, whether an individual has an eating disorder isn't determined by body weight, gender, or dietary pattern, but rather by state of mind. Eating disorders are characterized by extreme emotions, attitudes, and behaviors toward food, eating, and body weight and shape. They're serious psychological conditions, and their presence can result in life-threatening physical consequences. In fact, eating disorders have the highest death rates of all mental illnesses.[73]

The good news: eating disorders are highly treatable and completely curable. For someone at risk, this section provides the information, support, and reassurance needed to start down the road to recovery.

TYPES OF EATING DISORDERS

The American Psychiatric Association recognizes eight distinct eating and feeding disorders—the three most widely recognized are anorexia nervosa, bulimia nervosa, and binge-eating disorder (BED).[75]

Anorexia Nervosa

Anorexia nervosa is characterized by self-starvation that results in extreme thinness. There are two distinct subtypes of anorexia nervosa: the restricting type (weight loss is achieved by restricting food intake) and the bingeing/purging type (weight loss is achieved through bingeing and purging or a combination of restricting and bingeing/purging). Of those suffering from anorexia nervosa, 90 to 95 percent are female. The disorder generally appears in adolescence, with 40 percent of newly identified cases being 15- to 19-year-old girls.[76] Death rates are as high as 5 to 20 percent, although one recent report estimated the death rate at 4 percent.[77]

Affected individuals go to great lengths to achieve weight loss, often building elaborate rituals around food, eating, and exercise. Food is generally viewed as the enemy, and the ultimate goal is to achieve complete control over eating, calories, and body weight. Cessation of menstruation is a common feature in females but was removed as a diagnosis criteria in 2013, because it can't be applied to males or to females who are premenarchal, postmenopausal, or taking oral contraceptives. Three primary criteria are used for diagnosis:[75]

1. **Weight loss.** Persistent restriction of energy intake leading to significantly low body weight (in the context of what's minimally expected for age, sex, developmental trajectory, and physical health).

2. **Fear of weight gain.** Either an intense fear of gaining weight or of becoming fat, or persistent behavior that interferes with weight gain (even though significantly low weight).

3. **Distorted body image.** Disturbance in the way one's body weight or shape is experienced, undue influence of body shape and weight on self-evaluation, or persistent lack of recognition of the seriousness of the current low body weight.

Bulimia Nervosa

Bulimia nervosa or bulimia is typified by recurrent cycles of binge eating and behaviors that attempt to compensate for calories consumed. There are two primary methods of compensation: purging (which includes vomiting or taking laxatives, diuretics, or enemas) and nonpurging (which generally involves fasting or exercise). The primary feature that distinguishes bulimia nervosa from anorexia nervosa is body weight. Although people with bulimia experience considerable weight fluctuations, their weight is generally within a normal weight range and they aren't underweight. While bulimia affects a disproportionate number of females, as many as 20 percent of sufferers are male.[78] Some evidence suggests that those with a history of addictions, compulsive disorders, or affective conditions may be at increased risk. Diagnosis of bulimia nervosa is dependent on five criteria:[75]

1. **Binge eating.** Recurrent episodes of binge eating (eating an unusually large amount of food; a lack of control over eating during the episode).

2. **Compensatory behaviors.** Recurrent, inappropriate compensatory behavior to prevent weight gain (e.g., self-induced vomiting; excessive exercise; fasting; and misuse of laxative, diuretics, enemas, or medications).

3. **Frequent binge/purge episodes.** Episodes occur at least once a week for three months.

4. **Self-evaluation is unduly influenced by body shape and weight.**

5. **Absence of anorexia nervosa.**

Binge-Eating Disorder

Binge-eating disorder (BED) is characterized by periods of obsessive, uncontrolled consumption of large amounts of food. Eating often takes place quickly and in isolation and is frequently followed by feelings of guilt, disgust, and/or shame. While people with BED don't purge, many do attempt to periodically restrict food intake through dieting or fasting. BED is much more severe than overeating and is associated with distress regarding the eating behavior and co-occurring psychological issues. It's more common in men than other eating disorders, with about 35 percent of those affected being male.[79] Approximately two-thirds of sufferers are obese, although some are just overweight or even normal weight.[80] While BED is even more common than anorexia nervosa or bulimia nervosa, it was only in 2013 that it was acknowledged as a diagnosis in its own right (it had previously been considered an eating disorder not otherwise specified (EDNOS). Diagnosis of BED is dependent on five criteria:[75]

1. **Binge eating.** Recurrent episodes of binge eating (eating an unusually large amount of food; a lack of control over eating during the episode).
2. **Unusual eating behaviors and feelings associated with behaviors.** Binge-eating episodes are associated with at least three of the following:
   - eating much more rapidly than normal
   - eating until feeling uncomfortably full
   - eating large amounts of food when not feeling physically hungry
   - eating alone because of feeling embarrassed by how much one is eating
   - feeling disgusted with oneself, depressed, or very guilty afterward
3. **Marked distress regarding eating is present.**
4. **Frequent binge episodes.** Binge eating occurs, on average, at least once a week for three months.
5. **Lack of compensatory behaviors.** Not associated with compensatory behaviors, as in bulimia nervosa or anorexia nervosa.

Other Eating Disorders

Eating disorders that don't meet the diagnostic criteria for anorexia nervosa, bulimia nervosa, or BED generally fall into "other" categories, such as Other Specified Feeding or Eating Disorder (OSFED) or Avoidant/Restrictive Food Intake Disorder (ARFID). The body weights of people suffering from these less well-recognized eating disorders can range from seriously underweight to morbidly obese. It's important to note that just because these eating disorders categories are less well-known, it doesn't mean that they're less severe. A recent study reported death rates of 5.2 percent among those suffering from these "other" eating disorders, compared to about 4 percent for those with anorexia nervosa or bulimia.[77]

An eating aberration that doesn't fit into any of the recognized eating-disorder categories is called Unspecified Feeding or Eating Disorder (UFED). Examples may include orthorexia and diabulimia. Orthorexia describes an extreme obsession with eating a perfect diet, often leading to instability and social isolation.

The obsession is with health and purity rather than body weight. Only foods viewed as clean or health supportive are consumed. Food preparation techniques are selective and often exclude the use of frying and barbecuing. While these are wise choices, the person with orthorexia takes the pursuit of a healthful diet to a pathological level, harming emotional—and possibly physical—well-being. Diabulimia refers to a condition in which people with type 1 diabetes minimize insulin doses in an effort to reduce fat storage (insulin encourages fat storage). This action can cause chronically elevated blood sugars, increasing the risk of ketoacidosis and other complications of diabetes.

CAUSES OF EATING DISORDERS

Eating disorders are the product of a complex interplay of biological, psychological, family, social, and cultural factors, as well as a manifestation of unresolved emotional challenges. The complexity is compounded by the fact that eating disorders involve an obsession with or an addiction to food—a substance absolutely essential to life.

Biological and genetic factors at least partly determine character and psychological makeup. If a close family member, such as a mother or sister, suffered from an eating disorder, risk is consistently elevated.[81]

Certain psychological traits also increase risk. People with a natural tendency toward obsessive-compulsive behavior or perfectionism are more susceptible. Affected individuals are often overly concerned about how others perceive them and have difficulty dealing with criticism. In spite of intelligence, work ethic, and notable achievements, they see themselves as inadequate. Many lack self-esteem, personal identity, and independence, and the eating disorder serves as a source of personal control. Often, sufferers see the world as black and white. For example, if being thin is good, being thinner must be better, and being the thinnest is clearly best.

Some families contribute to eating disorders by being overprotective, controlling, rigid, and enmeshed. These tendencies reinforce problems with self-esteem and personal identity. Other families contribute by being emotionally cool or absent, while at the same time having high expectations surrounding physical appearance, achievement, and success. This can leave the affected individual feeling judged, misunderstood, and alone. Difficulty with conflict resolution and failure to share doubts, fears, and anxieties are also commonly reported. Finally, some evidence suggests that parents who set very restrictive rules around food and eating may inadvertently increase risk.[82]

Socially vulnerable individuals can be pressured into an obsession with weight and food by friends, lovers, or colleagues. Peer pressure can extend into the classroom, the gym, a college dorm, or a dance company. People who feel like outsiders, outcasts, or recluses may lack the kinds of deep social connections needed to allay doubts, fears, and insecurities.

Culture has a profound and powerful influence on the risk of developing an eating disorder. The Western world so highly prizes thinness in women that body weight has a tangible impact on success, employment, power, popularity, and romance. Many women become conditioned to link their self-worth with a number on weight scales. The pressure is further strengthened by the media;

You are not in control of your life when you have an eating disorder; the eating disorder is completely in control of you.

The disorder masquerades as an ally that helps a person reach an ultimate goal. But in reality, it serves only to make sufferers feel like failures, by convincing them that thinness is the only ticket to being beautiful and valued as a human being. The truth is so much sweeter.

"The beauty in your heart is permanent and pure. The exterior is temporary and fleeting. Beauty shines from a light in your heart."

HEATHER WAXMAN,
NUTRITIONIST, RECOVERED ANOREXIC

the ideal woman is portrayed as young and thin, while the ideal man, regardless of age, is portrayed as strong and fit.

These gender differences help to explain why the vast majority of eating disorders occur in women. Although girls and women attempt to emulate popular celebrities, few recognize that about a third of these women are technically underweight. This compares to less than 5 percent of the adult female population.[83] Fashion models are even more underweight, with a dangerously low average BMI of about 16.8. The discrepancy between the body weight of models and the general population has widened over the years; models have become thinner and the public has become fatter. The average American woman was at the upper limit of normal weight in the early 1960s with a BMI of 24.9; she's now overweight with a BMI of 28.4.

The pressure to achieve and maintain a lean physique is magnified in athletes (e.g., dancers, gymnasts, skaters, distance runners, swimmers, and divers). The term "female athlete triad" is commonly used to describe female athletes who exhibit eating disorders, amenorrhea, and eventual osteoporosis. Overzealous coaches and teachers, who encourage dieting and weight loss, often only compound the problem.

A full-blown eating disorder can be initiated by something as trivial as a derogatory comment, as traumatic as a rape, or anything in between. One of the most common triggers is dieting. If weight is lost, the fear of regaining the lost weight can spark an obsession. Often, the disorder begins during a period of increased challenges or responsibilities that the affected individual feels ill-equipped to handle. This may involve a significant life change or loss. Examples include the death of a family member or friend, a move, a change of school, graduation, a divorce, relationship problems, or the onset of puberty. In a fruitless effort, the person attempts to gain control by restricting food intake, bingeing, purging, and exercising or otherwise manipulating food and eating.

RED FLAGS FOR EATING DISORDERS

How can "normal" concerns about weight and shape be distinguished from those that cross the dangerous line of an eating disorder? In the early stages, it can be challenging for family and friends to know for sure, but the sooner a diagnosis is made, the better the person's chances of a full recovery.

Many red flags suggest the presence of an eating disorder. Some relate to eating and purging behaviors, others to exercise, attitudes, and social behaviors. For example, an individual might create multiple rituals and rules around food and eating, be obsessive about label reading, or lie about food intake. A sufferer may have a nervous response if "caught" eating or may run water in the bathroom to cover the sounds of vomiting. The person may never be satisfied that her body is thin enough and may compulsively exercise beyond what is necessary or healthy. A vegan with an eating disorder might refuse to consume healthy high-calorie vegan food. When taken together, many such warning signs can point to a serious problem (see Resources on page 450).

Eating disorders can lead to serious physiological changes that signal the need for medical intervention. The physical signs and symptoms of eating disorders can be broadly divided into three categories. Those stemming from starvation (as seen with anorexia nervosa) include swelling of the abdomen, cold hands and feet, and extreme thinness. Purging (as seen with bulimia nervosa and binge/purge anorexics) can result in erosion of the teeth, disorders of the esophagus, and swelling of the hands and face. Binge eating or overconsumption (as seen with BED) can lead to many of the same health concerns as being overweight. For all these disorders, there's increased risk of heart disease, digestive problems, and liver and kidney damage.

RISK OF EATING DISORDERS
AMONG VEGANS AND OTHER VEGETARIANS

Many experts believe that vegan diets (and other types of vegetarian diets) can increase the risk of eating disorders. Some treatment centers consider the reintroduction of meat a necessary part of recovery.

These beliefs are based on data released between 1997 and 2009 that reported significantly higher rates of disturbed-eating attitudes and behaviors, restrained eating, and disordered eating among vegetarians compared to nonvegetarians.[84–88] Currently, approximately 50 percent of adolescents and young women with anorexia nervosa eat some form of vegetarian diet; whereas only 6 to 34 percent of their nonanorexic peers in the general population eat a vegetarian diet.[89]

Although one might logically conclude that vegetarian diets cause eating disorders, evidence indicates that vegetarian diets are typically adopted after onset and simply mask eating disorders. In other words, vegetarian diets are used as a means to facilitate calorie restriction and legitimize the removal of high-fat, high-calorie animal products, and processed or fast foods made with these products.[89, 90] One research team quite appropriately labeled this phenomenon "pseudovegetarianism."[91]

This isn't to say that vegetarians can't develop eating disorders or that individuals with eating disorders won't decide to become bona fide vegetarians while they're ill. Both possibilities exist. However, true vegetarians can typically be distinguished by their motivation. A 2012 study of 160 women (93 with eating disorders and 67 controls) examined the motivation for becoming vegetarian in those who were vegetarian or who had ever been vegetarian. Almost half the participants with a history of eating disorders cited weight concerns as a primary motivation for becoming vegetarian; in the control group, none of the participants became vegetarian as a result of concerns about body weight.[89]

In 2012, two research papers provided valuable insights into the supposed link between vegetarianism and eating disorders. The first paper reported that vegetarians and pescovegetarians weren't more restrained in their eating patterns than omnivores; however, semivegetarians (no red meat consumption) and flexitarians (occasional red meat consumption) were significantly more restrained than omnivores or vegetarians.[92] In addition, the fewer animal products the vegetarians ate (in other words, the more vegan they became), the less likely they were to exhibit signs of disordered eating. The authors noted that while the semivegetarians and flexitarians were motivated by weight concerns, vegetarians and pescovegetarians were motivated by ethical concerns.

The second paper (which included two separate studies) carefully separated true vegetarians and vegans from semivegetarians and omnivores.[93] The findings added to the evidence suggesting that semivegetarians are at greater risk for disordered eating than omnivores or vegetarians. The investigators found that vegans had the healthiest scores of all dietary groups and speculated that vegan diets may actually be protective against developing eating disorders.[93] Although these are preliminary findings, they do effectively challenge conventional thinking. Furthermore, the conclusion makes sense, given the other-directedness of vegans (their concern for animals and the environment) as opposed to the inner-directed nature of eating disorders.

To provide effective treatment for vegetarians with eating disorders, the first determination must be whether the patient is a true vegetarian or a pseudovegetarian. If the individual is a pseudovegetarian, the reintroduction of animal products can reasonably be considered a valid step in the normalization of eating. On the other hand, the reintroduction of animal products is unnecessary and potentially damaging for true vegetarians or vegans. Individuals who are ethically committed to a vegetarian or vegan lifestyle will resist any attempts to force them to forgo their values. They'll feel disrespected and disconnected, making it difficult for them to trust their health care providers and work honestly at recovery. For true vegetarians, the addition of higher-fat, higher-calorie vegetarian foods is recommended. For vegans, this includes nuts, seeds, nut butters, avocados, tofu, legumes, starchy vegetables, and whole grains.

Vegans and vegetarians who have eating disorders should ask themselves this question: Was the decision to become vegetarian influenced by a desire to achieve a lower body weight—and is this still true? Some who initially select a vegetarian or vegan diet as a means of eliminating fattening food end up becoming convinced by the ethical, ecological, or health arguments in favor of this eating pattern. Although returning to an omnivorous diet is a part of recovery for some individuals, it's not necessary for everyone; recovery doesn't require eating animal foods again. Vegans and vegetarians can achieve complete recovery without forsaking the beliefs and values of this empathetic lifestyle.

OVERCOMING EATING DISORDERS

The first step to reclaiming a healthy lifestyle is acknowledging the eating disorder. Sufferers may resist taking this first step because they're terrified that getting help means getting fat or losing what seems like the only part of life under their control.

Recovery requires the acceptance of a simple truth: An eating disorder can result from a quest for perfection in everyday life. However, affected individuals must realize that an eating disorder is not a means of control. If fact, being controlled by an eating disorder results in forgoing opportunities to realize other hopes and dreams. When a quest to be the thinnest of the thin succeeds, the only "reward" may be death. No one will celebrate this as an achievement. Instead, they'll mourn the tragic loss of a kind, intelligent, and beloved daughter, sister, mother, friend, and colleague.

To overcome an eating disorder, vegans must learn to treat themselves with the sort of compassion that they strive for in their interactions with people and with animals. They need to celebrate each step toward health, even if it's a single step; to be positive, patient, and gentle with themselves; and to redirect their focus from food to other essential components of a truly meaningful life.

Unfortunately, BED sufferers may have an even harder struggle, because health authorities are just beginning to recognize this condition as a bona fide eating disorder. Health care providers may assume that overweight is the result of overeating and laziness, and instruct sufferers to simply eat less and exercise more.

The various eating disorders are separated by a very fine line. However, the first step in overcoming any eating disorder is to admit there's a problem and to seek help.

The Road to Recovery

Eating disorders begin as psychological disorders that can produce serious physiological consequences, becoming a disease of both mind and body. Treating only the mind can be a grave error, because malnutrition itself can create alterations in the mind. However, treating only the body is an even more serious error; such treatment neglects the roots of the problem and may mask the symptoms but aggravate the condition.

A complete recovery is possible; however, the healing process may take months or even years. An effective treatment program requires a holistic approach that addresses both causes and consequences. This is best accomplished by a multidisciplinary team that offers consistent, ongoing support.

A trusted family doctor can provide a reference to the appropriate treatment center, where the physiological and psychological consequences of the particular disorder will be medically assessed. For many affected individuals, initiation of appropriate treatment and monitoring by an experienced eating-disorders team is necessary. For those suffering anorexia nervosa, hospitalization is often required for initial treatment, while those with bulimia less often need crisis intervention. For those with BED or an EDNOS that's less well recognized by health professionals, it's essential to collect information on these eating disorders to present to the doctor.

Soon after a medical assessment is completed, individual counseling with an experienced therapist should begin. This part of treatment addresses the underlying issues of control, ineffectiveness, and autonomy and explores any traumatic events or abuse that may have contributed to the disorder. Such treatment assists in building self-confidence and independence and in regaining control over daily life. Some individuals also benefit from group therapy, which can help build relationships and break down feelings of isolation and alienation.

Family therapy, while not essential for everyone, is extremely important for younger patients, for whom the family is still a strong influence. Family therapy addresses many of the destructive patterns of interaction that feed the disease, in turn helping to create new and healthier family dynamics.

Nutrition counseling is an integral part of recovery; the primary goal is the normalization of eating. This part of treatment directly addresses food and eating behaviors. Normal eating helps to restore a healthy nutritional status, emotional state, and overall well-being. This means eating a wide variety of foods in amounts that support appropriate body weight and reintroducing foods that have been eliminated due to their caloric and/or fat content. Vegans with eating disorders will need to incorporate higher-fat, higher-calorie plant foods in their diet.

During treatment, ethically committed vegans may experience some pressure to add meat, eggs, and dairy products to their diets. However, such additions aren't essential; a person can uphold his or her vegan values and consume a diet that's balanced and nutritionally adequate. Gather resources for support; this section and the articles referenced in it would be a good starting point. Conversely, for pseudovegetarians, the reintroduction of animal products is generally considered an important step in recovery.

GUIDELINES TO NORMAL EATING

Although the next section is meant as a guide, it isn't a replacement for proper treatment by a team of experts on eating disorders. Vegans who want to bolster any formal treatment can follow the suggested steps to return to normal eating, and refer to The Vegan Plate on page 434 for further information. In addition, the "Lifelong Solutions for Weighty Matters" section on page 365 offers helpful advice.

OVERCOME RESTRICTIVE EATING

1. **Eat at least three meals a day, plus one to three snacks.** Smaller meals are easier to eat and are less likely to lead to a bloated feeling. Ideally, include breakfast, a small mid-morning snack, lunch, a mid-afternoon snack, dinner, and a small evening snack.

2. **Practice mechanical eating until the body heals itself.** Normal hunger and satiety signals may be performing poorly. Until normal function of these signals returns, eat set amounts of food at predetermined times. (A registered dietitian can set up an acceptable program that meets nutritional needs.) A sample mechanical program follows:

- Breakfast (7 a.m.): 1 cup (250 ml) of whole-grain cereal, 2 tablespoons (30 ml) of walnuts, 1 cup (250 ml) of fortified soy milk, ½ cup (125 ml) of berries.
- Morning snack (10 a.m.): 1 fresh apple with 1 tablespoon (15 ml) of almond butter
- Lunch (12:30 p.m.): 1 vegetable and hummus wrap or sandwich with tahini dressing
- Afternoon snack (3 p.m.): 6 ounces (180 g) of nondairy yogurt with 2 tablespoons (30 ml) of pumpkin seeds and 1 small sliced banana

- Dinner (5:30 p.m.): 2 to 3 cups (500 to 750 ml) of stir-fry with vegetables and tofu, and ¾ cup (185 ml) of brown rice or quinoa.
- Evening snack (9 p.m.): 12-ounce (375 ml) Protein Power Smoothie (page 387).

3. **Reintroduce "unsafe" foods slowly.** Foods that were avoided due to their high fat or energy content might be considered "unsafe" by many vegans with eating disorders. This food group includes nuts, seeds, avocados, olives, oils, soy foods and other legumes, and many grain products. Reintroduce these foods slowly and in small portions: slice avocado onto a salad, toss toasted almonds into stir-fries, or add black beans to a soup.

4. **Stop counting calories.** To end food obsessions, avoid counting calories. During recovery, rely on body signals to guide hunger and satiety. Eat meals and snacks in locations that have no distractions. Enjoy the pleasures of food once more and get reacquainted with foods that provide the greatest satisfaction.

5. **Avoid "diet" foods.** Buy tasty foods that nourish the body; avoid buying foods solely based on fat or calorie content.

6. **Let food be the body's medicine.** Food is the body's ally, not its enemy. Let it be the fuel that provides nourishment, boundless energy, radiance, and health.

Eliminate Binge Eating

1. **Don't skip meals or otherwise become famished.** Hunger is the most powerful binge trigger of all. Skipping breakfast and/or lunch sets the stage for a binge. Eating more frequently will help ensure that hunger doesn't lead to bingeing. Try eating four to six small meals each day.

2. **Practice mechanical eating until comfortable with normal eating.** For binge eaters, it's easy to forget what normal portions look like. A dietitian or nutritionist can develop an eating plan that lists specific foods and quantities for meals and snacks. (It will probably look much like the meal plan described on page 398.) To locate a local vegan-friendly dietitian, see Resources on page 449.

3. **Avoid temptation.** Don't keep "trigger" foods in the house. If consumed, such foods should be limited to meals shared with others, for example, at a restaurant. This can help to eliminate feelings of deprivation. Eating reasonable portions can help develop confidence that such foods can still be safe and enjoyable parts of the diet.

4. **To subdue overwhelming urges to binge, develop a strategy to avert the unwanted behavior.** The most effective plan may require a change of location to escape the trigger food. Take the dog for a walk, go shopping, visit a friend, or make a trip to the library. If a change of location isn't possible, call a chatty friend, meditate, or read a book. Start a craft project or learn a skill to keep hands busy when the urge to eat strikes. Keep some mints or chewing gum handy to get through difficult moments.

5. **Have a plan B: a reasonable, nonbinge snack.** Be prepared for real hunger, when the risk for a binge is high. Make a list of five or six reasonable snacks

for those occasions and stick to the list. Select foods that take a little effort to consume. Good choices include:

- a handful of nuts in the shell
- a bowl of popcorn
- frozen grapes, apple slices, or a pomegranate
- a slice of toasted pumpernickel bread with almond butter and banana
- sliced strawberries topped with nondairy yogurt and walnuts
- a green smoothie or green juice (drink slowly)
- protein pudding (one scoop of plant-based protein powder stirred into unsweetened almond milk)

6. **Break the cycle of eating in secret.** Eating alone is an invitation to binge. As much as possible, eat with other people. Bring lunch to the park, plan regular potlucks with friends, and go out to lunch or dinner at a restaurant.

Replace Destructive Behaviors with Healthy Ones

- **Get rid of scales.** Scales don't weigh human value; they may reinforce an eating disorder.

- **Get involved in nonfood-related activities.** Replace eating with pleasurable activities. Rekindle lost enthusiasms and enjoy every accomplishment.

- **Monitor exercise activities.** For those prone to exercising excessively, routines should be appropriately adjusted, especially if underweight. For example, cut back on disproportionate aerobic activity; don't exceed thirty to sixty minutes a day. Alternate aerobics with strength-building and stretching activities; weight gain is healthier if it springs from increased lean muscle mass, which results in a fit, healthy look. For overweight individuals who don't exercise regularly, adding enjoyable activities can reduce bingeing and help to control appetite. Join a hiking club, take up tennis, or find a walking partner. Exercise at least three or four times a week.

- **Adopt lifestyle changes that enhance success.** Read through the suggestions in the section on "Lifelong Solutions for Weighty Matters" on page 365.

SUPPORTING THE EATING-DISORDERED VEGAN

The family and friends of a person with an eating disorder can do a number of things to support recovery and to avoid making things worse, including becoming educated about the disorder. Supporters need to be patient and encourage good habits and personal responsibility, without being judgmental. The required medical assistance should be given to a sufferer younger than 18. Those who are 18 or older can't be forced to get help, but they can be encouraged, provided with educational information, and offered ongoing support.

Information on eating disorders, organizations, websites, support groups, and recovery centers abound at the local library as well as on the Internet; search on the term "eating disorders."

Lifestyle Choices Beyond Food

T o reach exceptional health, everyone—regardless of body size or weight challenges—needs to carefully consider making additional changes beyond dietary alterations.

1. Make exercise a part of daily life. Exercise thirty to sixty minutes daily or at least five to six days a week. Best activity choices depend on age, current fitness level, state of health, and personal preferences. Include a wide variety of exercises—walking, jogging, biking, swimming, hiking, yoga, racket sports, and aerobic classes. To stick with exercise in the long term, choose enjoyable activities.

For people who have been sedentary a long time, walking or another comfortable activity is appropriate. Start with ten or fifteen minutes of walking two or three times a day, increasing the duration of workouts gradually. Include a balance of cardio, strength, and flexibility exercises, as well.

For overall health, moderate aerobic activity (such as brisk walking) combined with moderate resistance training (such as light weight training) is ideal. To get the most from aerobic activity, consider interval training; alternate bursts of intense activity with a less-intense activity. For example, alternate walking with bursts of jogging or running; or alternate slower walking with speed walking.

Include strength training at least two times a week on nonconsecutive days. When choosing training weights, pick up enough weight to challenge muscles; at the end of each set of repetitions, the muscle group should be fatigued. Gradually increase the weights to maintain muscle development. For flexibility, stretch well after workouts and consider adding deeper stretching routines, such as yoga or Pilates.

Beyond exercise, every physical movement the body makes increases its energy expenditure. Such nonexercise activity thermogenesis (NEAT) includes energy burned during physical movements, such as gardening, walking at work or while shopping, cleaning house, and even foot-tapping when seated. NEAT can make an even bigger difference in energy expenditure than planned exercise. People with high NEAT burn as many as 2,000 calories more per day than people with low NEAT. Research shows that lean sedentary controls stand and move their bodies for 2½ hours longer per day than obese individuals.[93]

For overweight individuals, it's helpful to be active after eating. Muscles at rest have limited use for sugars that circulate in the bloodstream, but working muscles quickly use them without requiring a huge insulin surge. Being physically active after a meal prevents excess sugar from being stored as fat and keeps sugar from damaging body tissues. Even very light activity can lower blood glucose as effectively as an oral hypoglycemic drug.[94, 95]

Some underweight people may need to cut aerobic activity to thirty to sixty minutes just two or three times a week (at least temporarily). Aerobic activity boosts metabolism and burns calories, which can offset efforts to gain weight, but it shouldn't be completely avoided because it enhances cardiovascular and respiratory function and keeps body fat low. On the other hand, building and maintaining lean body tissue is critical to successful weight gain. Moderate resistance training is the best way to promote muscle growth and ensure that any weight gained includes a healthy balance of muscle and fat. Resistance training is often performed with free weights or weight machines, but it can also be done using body weight alone (e.g., push-ups or pull-ups) or resistance bands.

To optimize the effectiveness of any weight-training program:

- work with a professional trainer who can tailor a program to meet personal goals and abilities, and track progress
- train two to three times a week on nonconsecutive days to allow muscles sufficient time to recover and grow between workouts
- aim for thirty- to sixty-minute workouts, because short, intense workouts are more effective than long, leisurely sessions
- begin with light weights, gradually increasing them as form is perfected and muscles need new challenges
- change exercise routines every six to eight weeks to prevent plateaus
- warm up for five to ten minutes before strength training and cool down for five to ten minutes afterward
- keep well hydrated by drinking plenty of water

2. Get adequate sleep. Insufficient sleep can compromise physical and mental performance, contribute to death and disease, and undermine efforts to achieve a healthy body weight. For most adults, seven to nine hours a night is reasonable. Choose a regular bedtime and observe it as often as possible. Make the bedroom peaceful and inviting, and plan bedtime activities that calm and soothe, such as taking a warm bath or reading a good book. Waking up spontaneously and feeling refreshed and alert for the whole day indicates a good night's sleep.

3. Manage stress. Physical and emotional stress can affect metabolism, appetite, and hormones and wreak havoc with the body's immune system. In some people, stress triggers mindless eating; in others, it leads to missed meals. Incorporating stress management into a daily routine prepares a person to handle challenges as they arise. Of course, a healthy vegan diet, exercise, fresh air, sunshine, and sleep are all important, but attitude trumps these factors when it comes to dealing with stress. Healthy relationships and an appreciation of kind and thoughtful acts by others can help. For many people, a spiritual practice—prayer, meditation, yoga, or tai chi—forms the cornerstone of daily stress management. Learning from mistakes, forgiving mistakes in oneself and others, and moving on can subdue the stresses of daily life.

4. Avoid addictive substances. Addictions to alcohol, cigarettes, or other drugs aren't only damaging to health, they also alter metabolism and appetite. Alcohol, which provides about 7 calories per gram, or almost twice that of carbohydrate or protein, contributes to excess energy intakes for some, while displacing nutritious foods for others. Although cigarette smoking increases the body's metabolic rate slightly, it also acts as a developmental obesogen in humans, significantly increasing risk of overweight and obesity in infants of mothers who smoked during pregnancy.[96] A struggle with any addiction may contribute to an individual's challenges. To overcome such addictions, consider all available support systems.

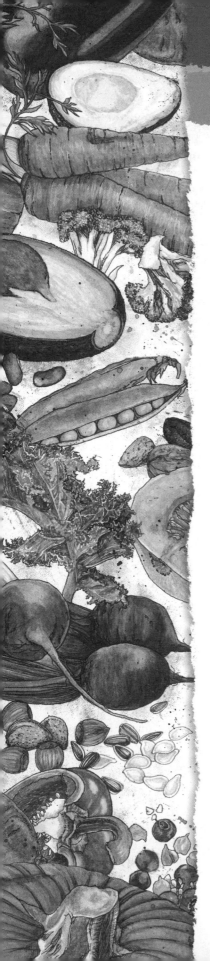

CHAPTER 13

The Vegan Athlete

Almost two years after becoming vegan, I am stronger than ever before, and I am improving day by day . . . Go vegan and feel the power!

PATRIK BABOUMIAN, STRONGMAN

Vegan athletes are among the most persuasive ambassadors of plant-based diets. Without uttering a single word, they effectively silence naysayers by proving there's no need to eat chickens, pigs, or cows to be fast, strong, and fit.

Some athletes believe that vegan diets provide a competitive edge, particularly for endurance sports; others argue that vegan diets put athletes at a disadvantage, especially in strength-based sports. Although the evidence is limited, plant-based diets haven't been shown to be particularly better or worse than any other diet for athletic performance.[1–3]

As a result, aspiring athletes who want to join the ranks of world-class competitors, as well as recreational athletes aiming to begin entering competitions, can rest assured that a varied and well-planned vegan diet will provide all the nutrients needed to meet performance goals. In fact, a meat-free diet can fuel elite athletes, boost performance, and provide sufficient protein to sustain big gains in muscle mass. Consider just a small sampling of world-class vegan athletes (search the Internet to discover elite vegan athletes in many other sports):

- **Cam Awesome.** Amateur superheavyweight boxer; captain of the American team; winner US men's national competition and national Golden Gloves; winner of more medals than any other American amateur boxer in history.
- **Patrik Baboumian.** Strongman; European champion in powerlifting, having set three world records in the 125 to 140 kg (275 to 310 lb)

category; winner of the German loglift championships; record holder for fronthold and keg lift.

- **Brendan Brazier.** Professional Ironman triathlete and author; two-time winner of the Canadian 50 km ultramarathon.

- **Robert Cheeke.** Vegan body builder and author; winner of the 2005 International Natural Bodybuilding Association Northwestern USA, Overall Novice Bodybuilding Championship.

- **Mac Danzig.** American mixed martial artist; national amateur mixed martial arts (MMA) champion, Gladiator Challenge lightweight champion, International Fighter Championship lightweight champion, five-time King of the Cage world lightweight champion, The Ultimate Fighter season-six winner.

- **Steph Davis.** Rock climber; the only woman to have free-soloed at the 5.11+ grade; featured in an extreme-sport film, climbing the Mineral Canyon in Utah; and appeared on the March 2013 cover of *Climbing* magazine.

- **Ruth Heidrich.** Triathlete champion; winner of more than nine hundred gold medals for running, marathons, ultramarathons, and triathlons; holder of three world fitness records in her age group; listed as one of the "Top Ten Fittest Women in North America" in 1999 at the age of 64 (all others named were in their 20s and 30s).

- **Scott Jurek.** American ultramarathon champion; winner of multiple elite ultrarunning titles, including US all-surface twenty-four-hour run title holder (165.7 miles—6.5 marathons in one day), the 153-mile Spartathlon, the Hardrock 100, the Badwater 135-mile Ultramarathon, the Miwok 100K, and the Western States 100-Mile Endurance Run, which he won seven straight times. *The Washington Times* named him one of the top runners of the decade, *Runner's World* awarded him a Hero of Running, and *Ultrarunning Magazine* named him Ultrarunner of the Year three times.

- **Fiona Oakes.** Marathon runner; world record holder for fastest woman to run aggregate marathons on seven continents plus the polar ice cap; winner of the 2013 Antarctic Ice Marathon (broke the course record by six minutes); winner of the North Pole Marathon (broke the course record by forty-four minutes); Guinness world record holder for the fastest woman to run the Seven Continents Marathon (combined times for each continent), breaking the world record by almost two hours and thirty minutes; sanctuary owner; firefighter.

- **John Salley.** Retired professional basketball player, actor, and talk-show host; first player in NBA history to play on three different championship-winning franchises.

Fueling Peak Performance

Four main factors drive athletic performance: genetics, training, diet, and drive. While there isn't much an individual can do about genetics, the other factors are largely a matter of choice. Each variable can be developed to provide a competitive edge.

A vegan diet alone won't guarantee athletic success, but enriching the fuel mix that sustains physical activity improves efficiency. A key to achieving peak performance is consuming a healthful balance of all the necessary nutrients while meeting energy needs.

ENERGY TO BURN

Two main sources of energy feed muscles: carbohydrates (glucose and glycogen) and fats (fatty acids). These fuels are readily available in the bloodstream and are provided both by foods consumed and from body stores. Glucose is stored as glycogen in skeletal muscle and in the liver; these stores provide approximately 5 percent of the body's energy reserves. Protein accounts for only about 2 percent of the fuel burned in activities lasting less than an hour. In exercise lasting three to five hours, the contribution of protein can increase to as much as 5 to 15 percent as stores of glucose and fatty acids become depleted.[4-6] The lion's share of fuel is stored as fat.[7] Although fat stores vary dramatically from one individual to the next, they're generally sufficient to last for many hours or even days of exercise.

During the first few minutes of exercise, the body relies almost exclusively on carbohydrates for energy. As exercise continues, more fats are used. Within twenty to thirty minutes of activity, the fuel supply is about half carbohydrates and half fats. With high-intensity exercise, the balance shifts in favor of carbohydrates, and with low- or moderate-intensity exercise, fatty acids soon become the more dominant fuel sources. A benefit of aerobic training is that it increases the proportion of energy derived from fat, preserving precious glycogen stores.[8-11]

Carbohydrates continue to provide much of the fuel for higher-intensity activities because people can't metabolize fat at a high enough rate to provide all the energy needed for more-demanding activities. However, the ability to use fat as a fuel during more-intense activities improves with physical training.[11, 12] Glycogen stores are typically depleted within two to three hours of continuous moderately intense exercise, and in as little as fifteen to thirty minutes of highly intense exercise.[11] When glycogen stores are depleted, consuming carbohydrate-containing foods or beverages promotes rapid repletion of the stores. Athletes who train regularly and eat sufficient carbohydrates generally have higher resting glycogen stores than sedentary individuals.[13]

The fuel the body uses depends on the type, intensity, and duration of the activity performed, as well as fitness level. The body has two distinct pathways that unlock energy: aerobic and anaerobic.

The Aerobic Pathway (Endurance Activities)

Aerobic means "with oxygen." For the body to enter the aerobic pathway to generate energy during exercise, sufficient oxygen must be delivered to the muscles. When exercise lasts for more than two or three minutes, the aerobic mode predominates.[12] The primary fuels used during aerobic activities are fatty acids from the blood, muscles, and fat tissue and glycogen from the liver and muscle tissue.

Measuring Physical Fitness

Physical fitness is a function of strength, flexibility, and aerobic capacity. VO_2 max is the most widely used test of aerobic capacity. It's simply a test of the body's ability to use oxygen; it measures the maximum volume of oxygen an individual can use per minute of extreme exertion. It's reported as milliliters of oxygen used in one minute per kilogram of body weight (ml/kg/min). The more oxygen consumed per minute, the fitter the individual. Elite endurance athletes generally have the highest VO_2 max, with results averaging about 70 ml/kg/min, compared to inactive individuals, who average about 35 ml/kg/min.

Regular aerobic exercise can boost a person's VO_2 max by increasing the capacity of the heart and lungs to deliver oxygen to the muscles and organs. Other factors, such as genetics, age, gender, and altitude, also influence VO_2 max. Although accurate VO_2 max measures are done under strict conditions in a sports lab, they can also be estimated using treadmill, timed-run, cycling, or step-fitness tests. VO_2 max can help to assess a person's potential to perform, but it's only one of several factors that determine success. Exercise intensity is often expressed as a percentage of VO_2 max:

Low-intensity exercise: < 30% VO_2 max (example: walking)

Moderate-intensity exercise: 31–69% VO_2 max (example: jogging)

High-intensity exercise: > 70% VO_2 max (example: running)

Any exercise that uses large muscle groups over an extended period of time is an aerobic or cardio activity. Good examples include distance running, swimming, biking, cross-country skiing, rowing, hiking, and canoeing. Aerobic activities train the heart, lungs, and cardiovascular system to process and deliver oxygen more quickly and efficiently to every part of the body. As a result, a fit individual can work longer and more vigorously, and achieve a quicker recovery at the end of the aerobic exercise session.

The Anaerobic Pathway (Speed and Power Activities)

When the heart and lungs can't provide muscles with sufficient oxygen for aerobic metabolism, the muscles rely on anaerobic ("without oxygen") metabolism to generate energy. Anaerobic metabolism uses only muscle glycogen and glucose as fuels. However, this fuel-consumption process doesn't completely metabolize glucose, and fragments of lactic acid can build up, causing burning pain and muscle fatigue. When sufficient oxygen becomes available, that lactic acid can be completely broken down or converted back to glucose.

During the first two or three minutes of exercise or when the activity is so intense that energy demands outstrip the oxygen supply, the body operates in anaerobic mode. For example, during a 30-second sprint, approximately 25 to 35 percent of muscle glycogen stores are used up.[12] The anaerobic pathway predominates in speed sports, such as sprinting and other quick track events, short-distance swim races, basketball, hockey, volleyball, football, baseball, lacrosse, and speed skating, and in power sports involving sudden intense movements, such as weightlifting, powerlifting, bodybuilding, field events, and wrestling.

Meeting Energy Needs of Active Vegans

E nergy needs vary with age, gender, and metabolism and body size, weight, and composition, as well as the amount and type of physical activity performed. Most athletes require 2,000 to 6,000 calories per day.[3] For elite endurance athletes, such as ultramarathoner Scott Jurek, energy needs may reach 5,000 to 8,000 calories per day.[14] High-fiber plant-based diets may reduce energy availability, so additional calories may be needed to compensate for losses,[12] especially in athletes with a high metabolism. Although one study reported an 11 percent higher resting metabolic rate (RMR) in young male vegetarians,[15] two studies found no difference in RMR when comparing similar vegetarians and nonvegetarians.[16, 17] A fourth study assessing RMR in vegans and nonvegetarians reported a lower RMR among vegans.[74]

An athlete's ability for optimal performance can be compromised if the body's energy needs aren't met. When the proper fuel is unavailable, lean tissue can serve as an energy source, reducing muscle mass and endurance.[12] Athletes who lack energy or can't improve their performance despite consistent training efforts may need to increase their caloric intake.

The best indicators of adequate caloric intake are body weight and composition. Unfortunately, some athletes purposely restrict calories in an effort to reduce body fat and improve their body's aesthetics or to make a specific weight class. This practice can seriously impair performance by lowering metabolic rate; reducing energy available for exercise; and compromising the body's nutritional, immune, and endocrine status. In young athletes, insufficient energy intake can also hinder growth and development.

A constant state of negative energy balance in female athletes is of particular concern, because it's a warning sign for a combination of conditions known as the "female athlete triad" (page 421). For example, when a female's body fat dips below a critical level, menstruation ceases. Generally, the minimal level of body fat compatible with health is 12 percent for female athletes and 5 percent for male athletes.[12] An athlete's optimal percentage of body fat can be determined by the level at which overall health and performance are most effectively supported.

The Institute of Medicine has developed equations that help provide a reasonable estimate of energy requirements. Although the equations are rather cumbersome, several websites provide a handy calculator that does the math to suggest a healthy level of calories (see Resources on page 449 for links.)

Vegan foods can meet the high energy needs of athletes, including those who engage in extreme sports. However, many plant foods are bulky, so it's important that athletes with high caloric requirement include plenty of energy-dense vegan options. In addition, during heavy training, athletes may need to take advantage of every eating opportunity, including large snacks before bed. Great choices include smoothies, sandwiches (see table 10.5 on page 333), whole-grain cereal, marinated salads, stir-fries, healthy baked goods, bean soups and stews, seasoned tofu, sushi, avocados, trail mix, toast with nut butter, power bars, yogurt with fruit and granola, and pasta dishes. Some athletes may find it easier to meet energy needs by eating more frequent meals and snacks.

For those who have difficulty consuming sufficient calories, incorporating more liquid calories (e.g., smoothies) and some refined low-glycemic foods (such as pasta) may prove helpful. Athletes who have recently shifted to a vegan diet may need to introduce higher-fiber foods (such as legumes) gradually to minimize gastrointestinal discomfort.[3, 12] (See pages 381 to 390 for ideas on how to increase energy intake and pages 441 to 442 for 2,500- to 2,800- and 4,000-calorie menus.)

On the other hand, athletes who eat more than necessary can increase body fat, potentially compromising performance. Injured athletes or those who reduce the intensity of their training need to reduce their intakes to avoid an undesirable weight gain.

Managing Macronutrients

The ideal distribution of carbohydrate, protein, and fat in the diets of athletes isn't necessarily different from that of the general population. Although aiming for the Dietary Reference Intakes' Acceptable Macronutrient Distribution Range (45 to 65 percent carbohydrate, 10 to 35 percent protein, and 20 to 35 percent fat) is considered appropriate for most athletes, some experts suggest a lower limit of 50 percent of energy from carbohydrates.[12, 18, 19] Athletes are currently cautioned against using a specific intake target, such as 60:10:30 (carbohydrate: protein: fat), because the most appropriate balance varies with an individual's energy and training needs.

CARBOHYDRATE

Carbohydrates provide the primary fuel for athletes because they help to sustain blood glucose levels during exercise, improve exercise capacity, and maintain glycogen stores. Evidence suggests that carbohydrate restriction is detrimental to performance. An athlete should eat sufficient carbohydrates to provide ample energy for training and to replenish glycogen stores after exercise and between competitions.

It's best for athletes to rely on whole plant foods as their primary source of carbohydrates. Vegans have an advantage where carbohydrate intakes are concerned, because both the quantity and quality of carbohydrates tend to be high in plant-based diets. Whole grains, vegetables, fruits, legumes, nuts, and seeds not only provide carbs but also a healthful complement of protein, fat, vitamins, minerals, and phytochemicals—all of which contribute to peak performance. Although some refined carbohydrates can be useful for training purposes, these foods are best used judiciously, especially by athletes with lower energy requirements.

TABLE 13.1. Vegan foods that provide 50 grams carbohydrate per serving

FOOD	SERVING SIZE
Almond yogurt with apples, cinnamon, and granola	1 c (250 ml) yogurt, 1 apple, ¼ c (60 ml) granola
Bowl of cereal, blueberries, and soy milk	1 oz (30 g) cold cereal, ¾ c (185 ml) blueberries, 1 c (250 ml) fortified soy milk
Brown rice with tofu and vegetables	¾ c (185 ml) rice with 2 c (500 ml) vegetables and 2 oz (60 g) tofu
Fruit smoothie	1 banana, 1 c (250 ml) fortified soy milk, 1 scoop protein powder, 1 c (250 ml) strawberries
Muffin with almond butter and fresh orange juice	1 healthy muffin, 1 T (15 ml) almond butter, ½ c (125 ml) fresh orange juice
Pea, lentil, or bean soup and rye bread	1¼ c (310 ml) pea, lentil, or bean soup, 1 large slice rye or other bread
Peanut butter and banana sandwich	2 slices bread, 2 T (30 ml) peanut butter, 1 small banana (or ½ large)
Pita bread and hummus	1 pita bread, ½ c (125 ml) hummus
Power bar	1 bar

(For more on carbohydrates, see chapter 5; for the proportion of carbohydrates, protein, and fat in foods, see table 3.5 on page 97.)

Recommended carbohydrate intakes for athletes range from 5 to 12 grams per kilogram of body weight per day, depending on the day's activity level. On low-intensity workout days (sixty to ninety minutes of moderate exercise), most athletes will need about 5 to 7 g/kg/day. On days of moderate to heavy endurance training (one to three hours per day), needs increase to about 7 to 12 g/kg/day. On days of extreme endurance training (four to six hours per day), requirements can reach 10 to 12 g/kg/day.[20] Table 13.1 lists a variety of foods or combinations that provide 50 grams of carbohydrate. The refined options may be more suitable as part of a pre-event meal.

PROTEIN

A commonly held notion among athletes, coaches, and trainers is that protein is the most vital of all nutrients—and the more the better. Some athletes hesitate to make the switch to a vegan diet due to concerns about whether plant protein is adequate for best performance. While athletes often need more protein, these requirements are easily met by a well-designed vegan diet.

Although protein plays a very small role as a fuel source for exercise, adequate protein is critical to maintain lean body tissue and exercise performance. The current recommended dietary allowance (RDA) for protein (0.8 g/kg/day) is thought to be adequate for fit and active individuals. However, in a position statement on nutrition and athletic performance, the American Dietetic Association (ADA), Dietitians of Canada (DC), and the American College of Sports Medicine (ACSM) recommend that protein intakes be increased by 10 percent for vegetarian (including vegan) athletes. Most vegetarian athletes meet or exceed recommendations for total protein intake; this increase is suggested to compensate for the reduced digestibility of protein from plant foods, relative to animal products.[12] Thus, for active vegans, protein intakes of at least 0.9 g/kg/day are recommended. Endurance athletes require more—especially during training and recovery—as do strength athletes, particularly during the early stages of training and while building muscle. Vegan endurance athletes are advised to consume 1.3 to 1.5 g/kg/day, and vegan strength athletes are advised to consume 1.3 to 1.9 g/kg/day (these figures have been adjusted by 10 percent above those of nonvegan athletes).

For example, an endurance or strength athlete who weighs 150 pounds (68 kg) would need a minimum of 88.4 grams of protein per day (68 kg x 1.3 g/kg/day). Vegans who consume less than 12 percent of calories from protein could fall short. For example, if that 150-pound athlete ate 3,000 calories per day, with 10 percent of calories from protein, total protein intake would be only 75 grams (3,000 calories x 0.1 = 300 calories; 300 calories ÷ 4 calories/gram = 75 grams). So, while vegan diets can provide plenty of protein for athletes, this nutrient deserves attention. The 2,500-, 2,800-, and 4-000-calorie menus on pages 439 to 442 provide 97 and 128 grams of protein, respectively. Table 13.2 provides a summary of recommended protein intakes for vegans.

Insufficient protein intake can compromise the maintenance, repair, and synthesis of skeletal muscle after training.[12] Vegan athletes at greatest risk for low protein intakes are those who restrict calories or who eat few legumes, tofu, tempeh, and other meat alternatives. While it's not necessary to eat specific combinations of plant proteins at each meal, it's important that vegan athletes do consume good sources of protein at each meal.[5] Vegans who have difficulty eating enough protein may find it helpful to add a vegan protein powder—such as hemp, rice, pea, or soy protein—to a smoothie to boost protein intake. Table 13.3 provides a list of foods that provide approximately 10 grams of protein per serving. Table 13.4 provides some suggestions for improving the protein content of common meals. (Also see table 9.3 on page 289 for foods that provide 15 grams of protein, and table 12.4 on page 386 for further ideas on boosting protein.)

TABLE 13.2. Recommended protein intakes for vegans (whole-foods diet)

ACTIVITY CLASS	PROTEIN (GRAMS PER KILOGRAM OF BODY WEIGHT PER DAY)
Active vegan	0.9 g/kg/day
Endurance athlete	1.3–1.5 g/kg/day
Strength athlete	1.3–1.9 g/kg/day

Source:[12]

TABLE 13.3. Vegan foods that provide 10 grams of protein per serving

FOOD	SERVING SIZE
Almonds	⅓ c (80 ml)
Black bean soup	⅔ c (160 ml)
Deli slices*	3 slices
Firm tofu	4 oz (120 g)
Hempseeds	3 T (45 ml)
Hummus	½ cup (125 ml)
Peanuts	⅓ c (80 ml)
Peas, raw	1¼ c (310 ml)
Power bar	1
Pumpkin seeds	¼ c (60 ml)
Veggie patty*	½–1

Sources:[21, 22]
*Check label.

TABLE 13.4. Increasing protein content of meals

INSTEAD OF	CHOOSE	PROTEIN INCREASE (APPROXIMATE)
BREAKFAST		
1½ c (375 ml) cornflakes, 1 c (250 ml) rice milk	1 c (250 ml) natural granola, 1 c (250 ml) fortified soy milk	19 g
3 pancakes, 2 T (30 ml) maple syrup	3 pancakes, 3 vegan sausages, ½ c (125 ml) cooked blueberries	14 g
LUNCH		
1½ c (375 ml) vegetable soup, 2 slices whole wheat toast with 2 tsp (10 ml) margarine	1½ c (375 ml) lentil soup with 2 slices whole wheat toast and 2 T (30 ml) peanut butter	23 g
3 c (750 ml) green salad, 2 T (30 ml) Italian dressing and 2 slices garlic bread	3 c green salad with 4 oz (120 g) grilled tofu and 2 T (30 ml) tahini dressing, 2 slices multigrain Italian bread	13 g
DINNER		
2 c (500 ml) pasta with 1 c (250 ml) marinara sauce	2 c (500 ml) pasta with 1 c (250 ml) marinara sauce and 6 meatless balls	16 g
3 c (750 ml) vegetable curry with 1 c (250 ml) brown rice	3 c (750 ml) chickpea/vegetable curry with 1 c (250 ml) quinoa	15 g
SNACK		
2 c (500 ml) green smoothie with banana, blueberries, kale, and water	2 c (500 ml) green smoothie with banana, blueberries, kale, hemp protein, and water	20 g
2 oz (60 g) pretzels or popcorn	Vegan power bar	6–14 g*

Sources:[21, 22]
*Check label.

FAT

After carbohydrate and protein needs are met, the remainder of energy will come from healthy fat sources. According to the joint position of the ACSM, ADA, and DC, athletes should consume 20 to 35 percent of calories from fat. An important energy source, fat also is the body's sole source of essential fatty acids and carries protective phytochemicals and the fat-soluble vitamins A, D, E, and K.

Reducing fat intake below 20 percent of calories hasn't been found to benefit performance and isn't generally recommended for athletes.[12] In fact, there's some evidence that low-fat diets (less than 15 percent fat) contribute to exercise-induced amenorrhea and reduce the supply of energy from fat stored within muscle cells (necessary for optimal performance in prolonged moderate- to high-intensity training).[5] However, athletes are advised not to exceed the upper limit of 35 percent of calories from fat; high fat intakes could compromise carbohydrate and protein intakes, especially in lower-calorie diets.[12] Optimal fat intakes vary with energy needs; in general, those with lower energy needs are advised to meet recommended intakes for protein and carbohydrate first.

Vegan athletes should rely primarily on whole plant foods for fat, because these foods also provide protein, carbohydrate, and valuable vitamins, minerals, and phytochemicals. Excellent choices include nuts; seeds; nut and seed butters, milks, and creams; avocados; olives; and soy foods. Judicious use of fats and oils can help athletes to meet their energy needs without adding bulk to the diet. Processed foods that contain trans-fatty acids are best avoided, as are deep-fried foods.

Micronutrients: Vitamins and Minerals for Vegan Athletes

Not surprisingly, an athlete's need for vitamins and minerals is higher than the amount inactive individuals require. These micronutrients play key roles in the body's use of macronutrients. Vitamins and minerals are also needed to synthesize, maintain, and repair muscle and bone tissue, as well as for immune function, the production of hemoglobin, and minimizing oxidative damage to cells.[12]

When energy needs are met, athletes generally meet or exceed requirements for vitamins and minerals without the need for supplements. This is true for all athletes, including vegans, with the possible exception of vitamins B_{12} and D. Vitamin B_{12} and vitamin D supplements are recommended for vegan athletes, unless sufficient amounts of these nutrients are provided by fortified foods (or in the case of vitamin D, through sunshine). Although multivitamin-mineral supplements provide some assurance that micronutrient needs will be met, they aren't essential. Supplements may prove advantageous for vegan athletes who restrict energy intake (or are dieting), have disordered eating, consume poorly planned diets, are pregnant or lactating, or are recovering from injury. In some situations, single-nutrient supplements can address specific medical or nutritional challenges, such as iron deficiency.

Vegan diets are naturally higher in certain vitamins and minerals and lower in others when compared to omnivorous diets. For vegan athletes, some nutrients deserve special attention.

VITAMINS

B Vitamins

B vitamins serve two primary functions for athletes. First, thiamin, riboflavin, niacin, pyridoxine, pantothenic acid, and biotin are necessary to metabolize energy-giving nutrients. Second, vitamin B_{12} and folate are needed to synthesize protein, for tissue repair, and to produce red blood cells.[12]

Of all the B vitamins, insufficient intakes of two in particular are of special interest to vegan athletes: B_{12} and riboflavin. Because whole plant foods lack vitamin B_{12}, all vegans—including athletes—must rely on fortified foods and/ or supplements to ensure an adequate, reliable supply (for more information, see pages 214 to 222). Some athletes take B_{12} shots to boost oxygen delivery to tissues and enhance performance. However, although B_{12} shots can be highly effective for vegan athletes who are B_{12}-deficient, no evidence shows that athletes with good B_{12} status benefit from this practice.[5]

The need for riboflavin increases with training, due to its role in energy production. While most vegan diets provide ample riboflavin, some studies have reported suboptimal intakes. So, it's important for vegans, particularly very active individuals, to include reliable sources of this nutrient. Excellent sources of riboflavin are listed on page 242.[5, 18]

Vitamin D

In addition to its critical role in calcium absorption and bone health, vitamin D is directly involved in forming and maintaining skeletal muscle and the nervous system. Vegan athletes who consume few fortified foods, who train indoors, or who have limited sun exposure are at increased risk for vitamin D deficiency.[12] While the RDA for vitamin D is 600 IU (15 mcg) for adults from 19 to 49, a growing number of experts suggest intakes of at least 25 to 50 mcg (1,000 to 2,000 IU) per day. (For more on vitamin D, see pages 222 to 230.)

Antioxidant Vitamins (Provitamin A Carotenoids, C, and E)

Athletes consume oxygen in volumes ten to fifteen times greater than nonathletes. This may trigger exercise-induced oxidative stress, which can be controlled, at least to some extent, by antioxidant nutrients. While oxidative stress can be harmful to health over time, some may actually be beneficial. Recent evidence suggests that continuous training (as opposed to sporadic training) stimulates antioxidant defense systems, thereby providing long-term protection against oxidative stress and disease.[12, 23]

Generally, vegans have superior vitamin antioxidant intake and status compared to nonvegetarians.[2, 24, 25] Athletes at greatest risk for poor antioxidant vitamin status are those who consume too few fruits, vegetables, legumes, nuts, seeds, and whole grains. Calorie restriction also may compromise vitamin intake, while low-fat diets can inhibit antioxidant absorption.[12] (See page 379 for further information.)

If dietary intakes are adequate, little evidence suggests that antioxidant supplements improve performance, and they're not generally advised.[12] However, insufficient dietary intakes have been shown to compromise athletic performance. Prolonged, strenuous exercise increases the need for vitamin C, so the joint position of the ACSM, ADA, and DC suggests that athletes who participate in habitual prolonged, strenuous exercise consume 100 to 1,000 mg of vitamin C per day.[12] The menus on pages 439 to 442 provide between 283 and 425 mg of vitamin C; see the nutritional analysis below the menus for this and other nutrients. Excellent sources of vitamin C are listed on page 236 and in table 7.3 (page 252).

Limited evidence suggests that vitamin E may help to reduce exercise-induced DNA damage and improve recovery. Vitamin E is present in avocados, nuts, seeds, and fresh pressed oils (page 237). Currently, athletes are advised not to exceed the upper intake levels (UL) for antioxidants, due to the potential for adverse effects from higher doses.[13]

MINERALS

An athlete's mineral status can have profound effects on overall performance. Although a vegan diet can adequately meet mineral needs, some minerals warrant special attention from vegan athletes.

Iron

Iron deficiency is the most common mineral deficiency among athletes, especially female endurance athletes. The body requires iron to handle and transport oxygen and for the enzymes involved in energy production. Poor iron status reduces the oxygen-carrying capacity of blood, in turn increasing muscle fatigue; decreasing work capacity, endurance, and overall performance; and adversely affecting nervous, behavioral, and immune system function.

When athletes embark on an aerobic training program, serum ferritin and hemoglobin levels often drop. This condition, commonly referred to as "sports anemia," is caused by an increase in blood volume and the resulting dilution of red blood cells. Sports anemia is a beneficial adaptation to aerobic training and shouldn't be confused with true iron deficiency, because it's usually transient and doesn't negatively affect performance.[12] In athletes who have iron-deficiency anemia, iron supplementation is advised because it not only improves lab measures but also increases oxygen uptake, reduces heart rate, and boosts performance. There's some evidence that iron-deficient athletes who don't have anemia also may benefit from iron supplementation.[12, 26]

At similar levels of iron intakes, vegetarian athletes have reduced iron stores compared to nonvegetarian athletes, because iron is less well absorbed from plant foods.[27, 28] However, although there are currently no reports on the iron status of vegan athletes, iron intakes are higher in vegans than in lacto-ovo vegetarians or omnivores, though vegan iron stores are commonly lower than those of omnivores.[5, 18]

Iron requirements in endurance athletes, particularly distance runners, are increased by an estimated 70 percent.[12] High-impact exercise, particularly the footstrike in distance running, can induce iron losses through hemolysis (the rupturing of red blood cells in the bloodstream).[29] Iron also is lost during intense endurance activity through perspiration or gastrointestinal bleeding (often associated with analgesics).[30, 31]

The joint position of the ACSM, ADA, and DC suggests that "athletes who are vegetarian or regular blood donors should aim for an iron intake greater than their respective RDA (i.e., > 18 mg and > 8 mg, for men and women respectively)."[12] It's unclear whether the authors considered the increased recommendations for vegetarians; however, distance runners might be prudent to aim for these higher levels (i.e., 32 mg for women and 14 for men). In addition, all female endurance athletes are well-advised to monitor their iron status. The menus on pages 439 to 442 provide from 22 to 37 mg of iron.

Vegan athletes (especially menstruating females and endurance athletes) can ensure sufficient iron intake and absorption by eating plenty of iron-rich plant foods and iron-fortified foods, and consuming these with a rich source of vitamin C. Iron-deficient athletes can take supplements to restore iron status and significantly enhance performance.[12] However, some individuals absorb iron very efficiently, resulting in high iron levels. Excess iron can act as a prooxidant, negatively impacting health, so iron status should be checked before beginning iron supplementation. (For more on iron, see pages 186 to 189.)

Zinc

Zinc is involved in energy production, immune function, and the healing of injuries through muscle repair. Intense exercise induces zinc losses in urine and sweat, increasing zinc requirements.[3] Suboptimal zinc status can reduce muscle strength, cardiorespiratory function, endurance, metabolic rate, and protein use, adversely affecting athletic performance.[12] Zinc deficiency in athletes can also lead to loss of appetite, weight loss, decreased endurance, and increased risk of osteoporosis.[32]

Female athletes and endurance athletes who adopt high-carbohydrate, low-protein, low-fat diets are considered at risk for zinc deficiency.[12, 32] Vegetarian and vegan diets are associated with lower zinc intakes and reduced zinc absorption, so the risk may be even greater among vegetarian and vegan athletes.[3, 18]

To maintain adequate zinc status, vegan athletes may need to exceed recommended intakes. The best plant sources of zinc include legumes, tofu, nuts, seeds, whole grains, and wheat germ. The menus on pages 439 to 442 provide from 12 to 24 mg of zinc. (For more on zinc, see pages 189 to 191.) Single-nutrient zinc supplements aren't generally advisable because they often exceed the UL of 40 mg. Excess zinc may result in nutritional imbalances and a drop in HDL cholesterol.[12] If supplemental zinc is needed to meet the RDA, the best choice is a multivitamin-mineral supplement with zinc.

Calcium

Calcium is critical to bone health, muscle contractions, nerve conduction, and numerous other body reactions, so athletes should strive to meet the current RDA for calcium (1,000 to 1,300 mg per day, depending on age). For many vegans, this means incorporating some fortified foods, such as nondairy beverages and fruit juice, into the diet, in addition to eating plenty of calcium-rich plant foods.

Poor calcium status is linked to stress fractures and reduced bone density.[12] At increased risk of calcium deficiency are female athletes who limit calories, have eating disorders, or are postmenopausal or amenorrheic. The joint position of the ACSM, ADA, and DC suggests increasing calcium intakes to 1,500 mg per day for female athletes at high risk for early osteoporosis.[12] A calcium supplement is suggested for those who can't meet recommended intakes through diet alone. (For more on calcium, see pages 182 to 186.)

Magnesium

Magnesium has a profound effect on muscle function. Evidence suggests that even marginal magnesium deficiency diminishes performance and exacerbates the adverse effects of strenuous exercise. For example, magnesium depletion may result in muscle cramps.[31] Athletes who restrict energy intake, including those in weight-class and body-conscious sports, are at increased risk for deficiency.[12, 34]

Intense endurance activities can increase magnesium requirements by 10 to 20 percent, due to losses in urine and sweat.[34] Although vegans generally consume adequate magnesium, it's important that sufficient magnesium-rich plant foods, such as nuts, legumes, greens, and whole grains, are included in the diet. Supplements are an option (either alone or in combination with other nutrients) for those who don't meet recommended intakes. (For more on magnesium, see pages 196 to 197.)

Electrolytes

Requirements for electrolyte minerals, including potassium, sodium, and chloride, are highly variable among athletes, depending on fluid losses. Although potassium is plentiful in vegan diets—as long as ample amounts of fruit, legumes, and vegetables are included—sodium and chloride quickly become depleted during intense endurance sports, and insufficient repletion of these nutrients can seriously impair performance. Endurance athletes commonly require significantly more sodium and chloride than the UL (more than 2,300 mg of sodium and more than 3,600 mg of chloride). For endurance events that last more than two hours, sports drinks containing sodium and potassium are recommended.[12]

Eating to Win

T he foods and fluids athletes consume before, during, and after events or training sessions can make or break their performance. Compared to the general population, athletes require more energy to fuel physical activity and more fluids to compensate for perspiration losses.

Depending on an athlete's individual needs, meals, snacks, and beverages are best selected and times based on the intensity and duration of the workout or event. Hydration is extremely important; a loss of more than 2 percent of body mass through perspiration and dehydration can adversely affect performance, especially in warm climates and high altitudes. Dehydration is also associated with heat exhaustion and heat stroke.[12]

PRE-EVENT FOOD AND FLUID

Ideally, a pre-event meal will provide sufficient fuel to sustain an athlete throughout the event. Timing is everything: the trick is to eat just enough to maximize performance but avoid having undigested food in the stomach. To help hasten digestion, the chosen meal or snack should be relatively low in fat and fiber; to boost fuel availability, it should be high in carbohydrate.[35] The closer the meal is to an event, the smaller the meal ought to be. Liquid meals may be more convenient and digestible within an hour of an event.

Consuming 200 to 300 grams of carbohydrate three to four hours before an event has been shown to enhance performance (see table 13.1 on page 409 for examples of foods and food combinations that provide 50 grams of carbohydrate).[12] In general, four hours before an event, the rate of carbohydrate consumption should be about 4.5 grams per kilogram of body weight; one hour before an event, it should be about 1 g/kg of body weight.

Pre-exercise or pre-event foods are best chosen based on individual tolerance. Athletes who experience nausea, cramps, or vomiting may need to avoid solid foods within three to four hours of an event. Those prone to reflux are advised to steer clear of foods that exacerbate their symptoms prior to competition (e.g., caffeine, chocolate, fatty or fried foods, or carbonated beverages). Individuals who frequently experience diarrhea may wish to reduce fiber intake twenty-four to thirty-six hours before an event.[36]

Generally, an athlete's muscle glycogen stores are sufficient for events that last sixty to ninety minutes. During events longer than ninety minutes (marathons, triathlons, long-distance swims, and similar demanding activities), athletes can experience extreme fatigue (often referred to as "hitting the wall") when glycogen stores become completely depleted. Not surprisingly, athletes often attempt to boost glycogen stores before longer competitions.

For many years, athletes used a strategy known as carbohydrate (or carb-) loading, which involved a period of relatively low carbohydrate intakes and intense exercise to deplete muscle glycogen. This was followed by a period of tapered exercise and high carbohydrate intakes to supercompensate for the reduced stores. More-recent studies suggest that athletes don't need the depletion

Are Sports Drinks Useful?

Although the value of sports drinks is hotly debated within scientific and athletic communities, most experts agree that for the average active consumer, hydrating with water is preferable. For inactive consumers, sports drinks can serve as one more source of empty calories.[38] However, such drinks can play a useful role in refueling and rehydrating endurance athletes or people who participate in intense activities that last for more than an hour.

Sports drinks contain water, sugar and other sweeteners, electrolytes (e.g., sodium, chloride, and potassium), colors, flavors, preservatives, and sometimes vitamins and minerals. They're often categorized as isotonic, hypotonic, or hypertonic, based on the amount of carbohydrate they contain. Isotonic drinks are 6 to 8 percent carbohydrate; they can help athletes quickly replace fluids lost by sweating and provide a boost of energy. They're the beverage of choice for endurance athletes (e.g., distance runners, triathletes, soccer players) who engage in activities that last an hour or more. Hypotonic beverages contain only 3 to 4 percent carbohydrate, and are useful for athletes who need fluid and electrolytes, but not extra calories (e.g., gymnasts and wrestlers). Hypertonic beverages contain the greatest amount of carbohydrate (often 10 percent or more). They're generally reserved to boost glycogen stores after exercise, although some ultra-endurance athletes use isotonic beverages to replace fluids and hypertonic beverages to meet high needs for energy.

For athletes who prefer to avoid sports beverages, coconut water, vegetable juices, homemade sports drinks, or a combination of solid foods and water provide reasonable options. Coconut water's sodium and carbohydrate content is lower than that generally recommended for endurance events, but athletes can combine coconut water with vegetable juices for an excellent balance. Coconut water and fruit juice combinations are also available and are significantly higher in carbohydrates than plain coconut water. Homemade sports drink recipes (generally containing fruit juice, water, sugar, and salt) are also accessible online.

Recent research suggests that due to its nitrate content, beet juice may enhance performance by reducing the amount of oxygen needed during exercise.[39–41] Beets aren't the only nitrate-rich vegetable—arugula, spinach, Swiss chard, collard greens, bok choy, radishes, carrots, rhubarb, and celery also provide hefty doses. Table 13.5 provides a nutritional comparison of various beverages.

phase to boost glycogen stores. Simply tapering exercise and eating a high-carbohydrate diet (about 10 g/kg/day) for thirty-six to forty-eight hours before a competition is sufficient. Of course, carbohydrates consumed just before and during the event provide additional fuel.[36]

Athletes need to drink water or a sports beverage in the amount of 5 to 7 milliliters per kilogram of body weight at least four hours before competition or training (although excess fluid intake is discouraged before an event, because this increases the need to void during competition).[12] For example, a 160-pound (73 kg) athlete should drink 1½ to 2 cups (375 to 500 ml) of liquid. Athletes who compete in intense, long-duration events (more than an hour) with minimal opportunity to hydrate may require fluids fifteen minutes before the start of the event.[36]

TABLE 13.5. Nutritional comparison of selected sports drinks

BEVERAGE (1 c/250 ml)	CALORIES	CARBO-HYDRATES (g)	PROTEIN (g)	SODIUM (mg)	POTASSIUM (mg)	COMMENTS
Vegetable juice*	54	12	2	137	467	Including beets, carrots, and apples increases the carbohydrate content
Carrot juice	48	11	1	119	310	Fresh
Beet juice	83	19	3	472	571	Fresh
Coconut water (average of 3 brands**)	41	9	0	42	410	Also available with juice or fruit flavors; check labels for nutritional content
Fresh coconut water	46	9	2	252	600	Liquid from fresh coconut
Gatorade	50	14	0	110	30	Original contains a variety of sugars, salt, flavors, and colors
Powerade lemon-lime flavor	78	19	0	54	44	Contains high-fructose corn syrup and artificial sweeteners
HydraFuel	66	16	0	25	50	Powder form contains a variety of sugars
Soft drink (cola)	103	27	0	6	0	Too high in sugar to be useful as a sports drink

Sources: Product labels[21, 42]

*Nutritional analysis is based on a green vegetable juice containing kale, romaine lettuce, apples, carrots, beets, celery, cucumber, and lemon.

**Coconut waters analyzed: O.N.E. Plain, vita coco 100% pure coconut water, ZICO Natural Coconut Water

EVENT FOOD AND FLUID

Although sports drinks and other sources of calories are generally unnecessary for activities lasting less than an hour, they may provide benefits during intense endurance events. The additional carbohydrates can help to maintain blood glucose levels and can be particularly useful if the event or activity takes place in the early morning on an empty stomach. Beverages that supply no more than 6 to 8 percent of carbohydrate are recommended; fluids that provide more than 8 percent of carbohydrate content (such as soda) can reduce gastric emptying.[12]

To extend endurance during events or activities that last more than an hour, carbohydrates in the approximate amount of 0.7 grams per kilogram of body weight per hour are advised. For most people, this means consuming 30 to 60 grams of carbohydrate per hour during the event.[12] Some experts recommend intakes as high as 90 grams per hour for events or activities that last three hours or longer.[37] In that case, it's more effective to consume the carbohydrates every fifteen to twenty minutes, rather than having larger amounts at one time.

Including carbohydrates during exercise is especially important for athletes who haven't carb-loaded before the event, who haven't eaten three to four hours before the event, or who have limited caloric intake for weight loss. The carbohydrates consumed should yield primarily glucose (as opposed to primarily fructose, because fructose is a less-effective fuel and may cause diarrhea in some athletes). Whole foods and products made from whole foods, including fruits, are acceptable; beverages sweetened with fructose aren't recommended. Because the body can use only about 60 grams of any single carbohydrate source per hour (e.g., glucose), foods and beverages that provide a mixture of different types of carbohydrates may be preferable. The carbohydrate can be consumed as a beverage, snack, or gel. However, if a snack or gel is selected, adequate water must also be provided.

Athletes also need to maintain adequate hydration, which means getting sufficient fluids and electrolytes (especially sodium). Perspiration rates can vary from 0.3 to 2.3 liters per hour, depending on climate, body weight, genetics, and metabolic efficiency, making it impossible to formulate one fluid- and electrolyte-replacement schedule for all athletes. However, serious athletes can establish sweat rates for specific activities and conditions.

Sometimes athletes become dehydrated because their sweat rate exceeds their ability to absorb fluids from the stomach. Many experts suggest drinking sufficient fluids during an event to limit dehydration to less than 2 percent of body weight,[12] although some athletes can withstand greater losses.[38] It may be helpful to replenish sodium during endurance events that last more than an hour, because an average of 1 gram of sodium is lost per liter of perspiration. Athletes also lose modest amounts of potassium, magnesium, chloride, and other minerals in sweat.

Common signs of dehydration include muscle cramps, muscle fatigue, low blood pressure, dizziness, and headaches. While most cases of dehydration result when fluid loss exceeds fluid intake, some athletes may begin a competition in a dehydrated state, because they have too little time between events to rehydrate or they're limiting foods and fluids to make a weight class for the competition.[12, 36]

Athletes must maintain hydration without drinking to excess. Overhydration can lead to hyponatremia (low sodium levels), a serious and sometimes fatal condition. Although it can occur in any athlete who consumes too much fluid, hyponatremia is more common in slow, less well-trained athletes who sweat less and drink excess fluids before, during, and after an event.[12, 36]

Competitors can replenish carbohydrates, fuel, and electrolytes during endurance events by consuming water and solid foods (such as energy bars), although this approach isn't always convenient. A more practical option for many athletes is to consume beverages that provide fluid, fuel, and electrolytes. The joint position of the ACSM, ADA, and DC suggests beverages that provide 6 to 8 percent of carbohydrates or 14 to 18 grams of carbohydrate per cup (250 ml), and 125 to 175 mg of sodium per cup (250 ml), although more sodium may be required by someone who sweats heavily. Potassium status is less affected by

A Word of Caution for Female Athletes

The female athlete triad is a syndrome characterized by the presence of three interrelated conditions: disordered eating, amenorrhea (cessation of menstruation), and osteoporosis. A woman's desire to maintain a very lean appearance can provoke a dangerous cascade of effects, beginning with energy restriction and disordered eating. In response, the body expends its fat stores, triggering hormonal imbalances, amenorrhea, and bone loss.

The syndrome is more common in athletes involved in endurance sports, such as distance running, and aesthetic sports, such as dancing, gymnastics, swimming, and figure skating. While its prevalence is unknown, estimates of eating disorders range from 25 to 62 percent among elite female athletes. Reports of amenorrhea are as high as 69 percent in dancers and 65 percent in long-distance runners. Finally, a literature review on the bone health of female athletes found a prevalence of osteopenia (low bone density), ranging from 22 to 50 percent, and osteoporosis, ranging from 0 to 13 percent.[43]

According to the ACSM, athletes at greatest risk are those who consume energy-restricted diets, who limit the types of foods they eat, who exercise for prolonged periods, or who are vegetarian.[43] Menstrual irregularities have been disproportionately associated with vegetarian athletes,[44, 45] and very high-fiber, low-fat diets have been shown to increase fecal excretion of estrogens and reduce estrogen levels.[46] However, risk doesn't appear to be elevated in weight-stable vegetarians with normal BMIs.[47] Vegetarian diets per se may not be to blame, but rather the restrictive eating behaviors that make vegetarian diets attractive to such athletes (for more information, see pages 390 to 400).

Female vegan athletes need to ensure sufficient intakes of calories, protein, and fat. Energy intakes that fall below 30 calories per kilogram of fat-free body mass per day are associated with the most pronounced adverse effects.[43] For example, a 120-pound (55 kg) athlete with a body fat of 12 percent would have a fat-free body mass of 105.6 pounds (48.4 kg). An energy intake of less than 1,452 calories (30 calories x 48.4 kg) would significantly increase health risk. Athletes with high caloric requirements may find it helpful to incorporate lower-fiber foods, such as tofu, refined grains, and juices, into their diets.[35]

sweating, so a potassium-rich diet may be sufficient to maintain body levels during events. However, some authorities suggest using sports beverages enhanced with potassium, particularly during endurance events.[12]

POST-EVENT FOOD AND FLUID

After an event or training session, the body must rehydrate, reestablish muscle and liver glycogen stores, and ensure maintenance of lean muscle tissue. Food and fluid needs depend on the intensity and duration of the completed event or training session and the timing of the next event. For athletes participating in more than one event in a day, the interval between events is critical; for a single event, the post-event protocol is less significant.

Ideally, athletes should begin to replenish glycogen stores within thirty minutes of an event. Eating carbohydrates at a rate of 1 to 1.5 grams per kilogram of body weight at two-hour intervals for up to six hours is generally recommended, especially if glycogen stores need to be replenished for another event. For example, a 160-pound (73 kg) athlete would eat 70 to 110 grams of carbohydrate immediately after an event, and again at 2.5 hours and 4.5 hours; for a 120-pound (55 kg) athlete, carbohydrate intake would be 55 to 80 grams each time.

Although refueling isn't as important if there are rest days between events or training days, including a post-event meal helps athletes meet energy intake goals. Eating food with a high glycemic index (GI) results in higher glycogen stores following glycogen depletion than consuming food with a low GI. Some authorities suggest a carbohydrate to protein ratio of 3:1 to ensure sufficient protein for muscle-tissue synthesis and repair. Table 3.5 (page 97) shows the relative amounts of calories from carbohydrate and protein in various foods (these reflect relative weights of carbohydrate and protein; grams of protein also are given). Other experts suggest consuming 15 to 25 grams of protein after workouts or events.[12, 35, 37]

After an event or training session, athletes need to replace the fluids and sodium lost in perspiration. Generally 6 cups (1.5 L) of fluid are recommended for every kilogram lost (2.2 lb). This is especially important when athletes participate in multiple events with limited time between events.

Ergogenic Aids 101

T he market for ergogenic aids has been gaining momentum for decades. It's estimated that 76 to 100 percent of athletes in certain sports use these types of supplements.[48] Although the claims associated with nutritional ergogenic aids are substantial, the evidence for associated benefits is disappointing.[12] Regardless, in the United States, the dietary supplement industry is poorly regulated, and claims about effects on body structure or performance are permitted on labels, even if the claims have no validity. Producers aren't responsible for demonstrating safety or effectiveness, although the Food and Drug Administration polices safety. The rules are simple—ingredients (including active ingredients) must be listed, and therapeutic claims about disease prevention or treatment are not permitted. In Canada, supplements are regulated as medicine or natural health products. Producers are free to make performance and disease claims if the scientific evidence to support those claims is deemed sufficient.[12, 49]

National and international sports authorities have rules concerning the permissible use of ergogenic aids and require random testing of athletes to prevent the use and abuse of banned substances. Athletes cannot assume that a product is safe or effective simply because it is marketed over the counter. All products must be scrutinized for safety, purity, and effectiveness. Generally, sports authorities advocate whole foods over dietary supplements.[49]

ARE ERGOGENIC AIDS USEFUL TO VEGAN ATHLETES?

Among the hundreds of ergogenic aids, just a handful hold special interest for vegan athletes. For example, nutrients that may be suboptimal in vegan diets are viewed as possible performance enhancers. (See pages 423 to 425 for information on vitamins and minerals that may be helpful for vegan athletes.) Compounds with ergogenic potential found exclusively or predominantly in meat or dairy products are thought to provide greater benefits for vegans than meat-eating athletes. Athletes are advised to consult with a health care provider before taking any ergogenic aid. These ergogenic aids top the vegan short list.

Carnosine and Beta-alanine

Carnosine is a dipeptide containing beta-alanine (a nonprotein amino acid) and histidine. Naturally produced by the body, it's most concentrated in muscle and brain tissue. Internal carnosine production depends on the supply of beta-alanine, which is less abundant in muscle tissue than histidine. Carnosine is touted for its ability to boost performance in high-intensity exercise by increasing the buffering capacity of muscles during lactic acid buildup, improving muscle contractile performance and defending against reactive oxygen species (unstable oxygen atoms that can quickly oxidize and harm the body on a cellular level).[50, 51] Carnosine is also promoted as an antiaging aid due to its impressive antioxidant and anti-inflammatory properties.[52]

Because carnosine is present only in animal products, carnosine levels tend to be reduced in vegetarians compared to meat eaters. One study found levels in vegetarians to be about half that of omnivores,[53] while a second study reported a 17 to 26 percent reduction in carnosine levels in the leg muscle tissue of vegetarians compared with omnivores.[54]

Although no studies exist that assess the effects of beta-alanine or carnosine supplements in vegan athletes whose muscle levels of carnosine are low, it's reasonable to expect that vegans would enjoy greater benefits of supplementation than meat-eating athletes. Beta-alanine supplements effectively boost muscle carnosine concentrations. However, in doses exceeding 10 mg/kg/day, beta-alanine may cause temporary paraesthesia (a prickling or burning sensation like pins and needles, usually occurring in the feet, legs, arms, and/or hands).[55]

Although most carnosine supplements are less well absorbed than beta-alanine, some newer forms are proving effective. In certain individuals, carnosine supplements disrupt sleep, although well-absorbed forms act more rapidly than beta-alanine and don't cause paraesthesia. It's too soon to make a general recommendation for beta-alanine or carnosine supplementation for vegan athletes; however, evidence suggests benefit for some athletes.

Branched-Chain Amino Acids

The branched-chain amino acids (BCAA)—leucine, isoleucine, and valine—have sparked considerable interest among sports-nutrition scientists due to their effects on muscle recovery and immune function. Although most studies have failed to show enhanced performance with BCAA supplementation, there's reasonable evidence to suggest it can reduce muscle damage, promote muscle-protein synthesis (which decreases muscle soreness and fatigue), and regulate immune function.[53, 54]

Well-designed vegan and nonvegan diets provide sufficient BCAA; however, for elite athletes, BCAA supplementation may be of value. There's no evidence that vegans would benefit more than nonvegans by BCAA supplementation.[3, 12, 56–72]

Carnitine

The amino acid carnitine (also called L-carnitine) is important for fatty-acid and protein metabolism. It is commonly touted for weight loss and athletic performance, is sometimes promoted as a fat burner, and is thought to spare glycogen and reduce lactic acid production.

Carnitine is present in many foods but is much more concentrated in animal products than plant foods. One exception is tempeh, which contains almost 20 mg per 3.5-ounce (100 g) serving. This compares to 95 mg in beef steak, 28 mg in pork, 6 mg in cod, and 4 mg for chicken per 3.5-ounce (100 g) serving. A medium avocado contains about 2 mg, while most other plant foods contain less than 0.5 mg per serving.[58]

Humans produce carnitine in the liver, kidneys, and brain. There's some evidence that adults who habitually consume little carnitine compensate by increasing reabsorption from the kidneys and reducing urinary carnitine excretion. Blood levels of carnitine are still lower among vegans and vegetarians than meat eaters, although overt carnitine deficiency is uncommon.[59, 60] Two decades of research have demonstrated ergogenic benefits from carnitine supplementation only when a carnitine deficiency is present.[61, 62]

Creatine

Creatine is among the most popular ergogenic aids for athletes, especially body builders and other strength athletes. It's also one of the few nutritional supplements that clinical trials have clearly demonstrated to be effective. Creatine supplementation reduces fatigue during short bursts of high-intensity activities, such as sprinting, soccer, and weight lifting, and maximizes lean body gains and muscle strength.[3, 12] However, it's not generally advised for endurance activities.

Creatine is found only in meat, so vegans don't naturally ingest it. The rate-limiting enzymes for creatine synthesis are fully activated by creatine-free vegetarian diets and suppressed by meat consumption.[3] The body manufactures about 1 gram of creatine per day from precursor amino acids; dietary intake in meat eaters is also about 1 gram per day. While internal production helps to compensate for differences in dietary intakes, blood and tissue creatine concentrations have been shown to be lower among vegetarians and vegans than omnivores.[63, 64] Research suggests that vegetarians may enjoy greater benefits from taking creatine than nonvegetarians.[65]

Generally, creatine supplements are synthetically produced and are vegan. Muscle creatine content can be increased by 30 percent or more with the use of supplements, particularly when levels are low. Popular supplementation regimens suggest a three- to seven-day loading phase of 20 to 25 grams of creatine per day, followed by a maintenance dose of about 3 grams per day for four weeks.[3] The effects of long-term creatine supplementation aren't known, although supplementation is generally considered safe for healthy adults. The most common adverse effects of creatine supplements are weight gain (usually fluid), cramps, nausea, and diarrhea.[12]

Taurine

Taurine is a nonessential amino sulfonic acid (different than an amino acid). It's present in animal products, especially meat, fish, and shell fish, and is found only in trace amounts in land plants; however, some sea plants (macro- and microalgae) contain higher amounts.[66, 67] Although the body produces taurine, two studies reported reduced plasma levels in vegans compared to nonvegans (although in one study, there were only slight differences) and decreased urinary taurine excretion.[68, 69] There's some evidence that taurine boosts athletic performance, so it's commonly added to energy drinks and other ergogenic aids. Currently, no studies have assessed the ergogenic effects of taurine supplementation for vegans, but one report suggests that 500 mg of taurine twice daily would be appropriate for vegan athletes who want to try it.[70]

Protein Supplements

Current evidence suggests that protein and amino-acid supplements provide no advantage over food for increasing muscle mass when dietary protein intakes are adequate.[12] However, for vegan athletes who have difficulty consuming sufficient protein from food, supplements are a practical and effective way of meeting needs. Vegan supplements based on hemp, pea, pumpkin seed, rice, and/or soy protein are widely available. For athletes who already consume soy foods in generous quantities (soy milk, tofu, soy-based vegan meat substitutes, for example), selecting protein powders based on other plant proteins may be preferable. Some supplements supply a mix of plant proteins, which can increase the overall quality of the protein.

Other Commonly Used Supplements

Other effective nutritional ergogenic aids are caffeine and sodium bicarbonate (baking soda). Caffeine, a known stimulant, should only be used in moderation. Its use is restricted by some sports authorities, and excess intakes can cause anxiety, jitteriness, rapid heartbeat, gastrointestinal distress, and insomnia. Sodium bicarbonate acts as a blood buffer, helping to prevent fatigue; however, excessive intakes can cause diarrhea.[12]

Several additional ergogenic aids appear promising, although evidence for their benefits is inconclusive. These include glutamine, hydroxymethylbutyrate, and ribose. There is no evidence that any of these ergogenic aids would provide greater benefit to vegans than nonvegans.

Other supplements currently marketed as ergogenic aids lack scientific evidence to support their use. Some ergogenic aids are dangerous, banned, or illegal. Examples include anabolic steroids, *Tribulus terrestris*, ephedra, strychnine, and human growth hormone.[12]

In summary, although ergogenic aids are rarely necessary for athletes, they may enhance physical performance in certain circumstances. If used, they should be taken in conjunction with a nutritionally adequate diet.

Achieving Peak Performance

T he keys to optimizing performance, regardless of dietary pattern, are to eat sufficient quantities of a wide variety of nutrient-dense whole foods and stay well hydrated. The Vegan Plate and menus in chapter 14 provide healthful food choices at various levels of caloric intake. The menus are appropriate for active vegans, including competitive athletes. For most athletes, the 2,500- to 2,800- or 4,000-calorie menus will be most appropriate, although for athletes who require fewer calories or who are trying to lose weight, the lower-calorie menus provide sufficient protein and are nutritionally adequate.

Table 13.6 lists suggested numbers of servings from each food group at various levels of caloric intake. The numbers of servings can be varied to suit

TABLE 13.6. Suggested number of servings from food groups at various caloric intakes

FOOD GROUP (AVERAGE CALORIES*)	SERVING SIZE	2,000 CALO-RIES	2,500 CALO-RIES	3,000 CALO-RIES	4,000 CALO-RIES	5,000 CALO-RIES
Vegetables (30 calories)	½ c (125 ml) raw or cooked vegetables or vegetable juice 1 c (250 ml) raw leafy vegetables	6	8	9	10	12
Fruits (60 calories)	½ c (125 ml) fruit or fruit juice ¼ c (60 ml) dried fruit 1 medium fruit	4	5	6	7	8
Legumes (125 calories)	½ c (125 ml) cooked beans, peas, or lentils, tofu, or tempeh 1 c (250 ml) raw peas or sprouted lentils or peas ¼ c (60 ml) peanuts 2 T (30 ml) peanut butter 2 oz (60 g) vegetarian meat substitute	3	4	5	7	9
Grains (90 calories)	½ c (125 ml) cooked cereal, rice, pasta, quinoa, or other grain 1 slice bread ½ c (125 ml) raw corn or sprouted quinoa, buckwheat, or other grain 1 oz (30 g) ready-to-eat cereal	8	10	12	14	16
Nuts and seeds (200 calories)	¼ cup (60 ml) nuts and seeds 2 T (30 ml) nut or seed butter	2	2	3	4	6
Other choices (80 calories)	2 tsp (10 ml) oil 2 T (30 ml) maple syrup ½ oz (15 g) dark chocolate	1	2	3	4	5

*Calorie estimates are based on an average of several choices, and individual items can vary considerably from these estimates.

Note:
- Starchy vegetables provide at least double the calories of other vegetables.
- Energy content of legume choices varies widely. See table 3.5 (page 97) for more precise calorie counts. Peanuts and peanut butter contain about 200 calories per serving (similar to nuts and seeds).
- Whole grains are heavier and slightly higher in calories than bread.

different eating styles; a minimum number of servings from each group is recommended in The Vegan Plate (see pages 434 and 435). Calcium-rich foods should be selected in every category, meeting the recommended 6 to 8 servings a day at all calorie levels (see pages 439 to 432). "Other choices" refers to added fats, added sugars, or items that don't fit into any of the other food groups. Vegans who prefer not to use these "other choices" can select a greater number of servings from the other food groups to roughly equal the number of calories allotted.

PRACTICAL POINTERS

Vegetables

To avoid difficulty achieving the recommended number of servings from this group, include vegetables at lunch as well as dinner and use a mixture of raw and cooked vegetables. (Cooking condenses vegetables so larger amounts can be eaten.) Keep cut-up, ready-to-eat vegetables handy to enjoy as snacks. Juicing vegetables greatly reduces their bulkiness, making it easier to consume generous portions. Avocado can be added to smoothies. Look for dehydrated vegetable chip recipes online (kale, zucchini, and sweet potatoes work especially well).

Fruits

To increase fruit consumption, add fruit to breakfast cereal, bring a few pieces to enjoy as snacks at work or school, add several pieces to a smoothie, and make fruit-based desserts. Fresh fruit juices and dried fruits can also be used, if desired, and are easier to transport.

Legumes

As the protein powerhouses of the plant kingdom, beans and products made from beans are important for athletes. To consume the suggested number of servings, use white beans in dips and pâtés, add cooked red lentils to spaghetti sauce, and add puréed black beans to brownies and sprouted peas to salads. Snack on peas in the pod. Experiment with ethnic cuisines and use a wide variety of products made from beans, such as tofu, tempeh, and vegan meat substitutes.

Grains

As caloric needs increase, the suggested quantity of grain servings may look daunting. However, one serving is only ½ cup (125 ml) of grains or one slice of bread. It's relatively easy to consume six servings of grains in one meal. For example, 2 cups (500 ml) of rice plus a whole-grain roll, or 2 cups (500 ml) of pasta plus two slices of garlic bread, each provide six servings. At breakfast, 2 cups (500 ml) of oatmeal with two slices of toast provides six servings. For those who prefer to limit grain intake, substitute larger servings of starchy vegetables, such as yams, potatoes, and corn, as well as additional servings from other food groups.

Other Choices

This optional category includes fats and oils, concentrated sweeteners (such as maple syrup and organic blackstrap molasses, which is a great source of iron and calcium), dark chocolate, and other sweet treats. Although it isn't necessary to eat these foods, most people use some, so it's important to include them in the overall calorie count. They can add flavor and variety to meals and snacks and boost calorie intakes for athletes with high energy needs.

Facing Challenges Head On

 eing a vegan athlete can present unique challenges. The following information can allay some common concerns.

As a competitive triathlete, I dread trying to get a decent meal when I'm on the road. What can I do to ensure that I get enough good food when travelling?

Always bring a handy selection of favorites when travelling: individual aseptic containers of nondairy milk, fresh fruit, dried fruit, nuts, seeds, nut butter, oatmeal or other cereal, crackers, bread, energy bars, dehydrated soups (in individual serving containers), and canned single-serving beans with easy-open lids. When staying in a hotel room equipped with a refrigerator, add nondairy yogurt, fresh vegetables, hummus, bean salad, vegetarian sushi rolls, juice, and flavored tofu. Bring a plate, a bowl, and some utensils. Buy nonspill containers of various sizes to transport foods, for leftovers, and for takeout foods from restaurants along the road.

Check for vegan or vegan-friendly restaurants (see Resources on page 450). If there are no vegetarian restaurants, go ethnic. Most ethnic restaurants offer legume or tofu dishes. In an American-style restaurant, ask for a vegan meal. The more requests restaurants receive, the more likely it is that vegan options will appear on their menus later on. If the chef needs ideas, ask for a pasta dish with loads of vegetables and possibly beans as well. Request rice and a vegetable stir-fry (with nuts, if available) or a vegetable plate with baked potatoes. Another option is a large salad with a baked potato. Ask for hummus, nuts, seeds, or beans to complete the meal (or bring a small package of cashews or almonds to add to salads or a stir-fry).

Bring plenty of food when flying. In a pinch, many flights offer nuts, hummus and pita bread, or vegan sandwiches for purchase. Mexican, Chinese, and Japanese restaurants and kiosks at airports offer an assortment of vegan travel meals (see Resources on page 450).

I play college football. I became vegan about six months ago and I've lost about 10 pounds. My coach is not impressed. How can I regain this weight or at least stop any further weight loss?

Vegan foods are less energy dense and more bulky; just eat more. Increase portion sizes and eat more often. Don't skip meals; allow for a few snacks throughout the day. Consider having a nutrition-packed smoothie as an evening snack (see

Exercise for Everybody

Human bodies are meant to move—even those whose owners have no intention of ever being a competitive athlete. Regular exercise is not a luxury—it's a basic necessity, like eating and sleeping. Besides controlling weight and body shape, exercise reduces the risk of death and disease, boosts immune function, suppresses inflammation, sharpens the mind, yields better sleep, provides more energy and endurance, elevates mood—and even improves one's sex life.

To enjoy these benefits, set aside thirty to sixty minutes a day for physical activity and do whatever type of exercise that provides movement and motivation. Three main types of exercise are essential for a fit body: aerobic activity, strength training, and flexibility exercises—incorporate all three into a weekly routine.

The following exercise guidelines are adapted from the *Physical Activity Guidelines for Americans:*[68]

- **Children and adolescents.** One hour or more per day of moderate or vigorous aerobic activity. Include vigorous activity at least three days per week; include strength training at least three days per week.

- **Adults (ages 18 to 64).** A minimum of two and a half hours per week of moderate-intensity activity—with five hours or more per week preferred—or a minimum of one and a quarter hours a week of vigorous-intensity exercise, with two and a half hours or more per week preferred. Include strength training for all large muscle groups at least two days per week.

- **Older adults (age 65+).** Follow the adult guidelines above. If that's not possible, be as active as abilities allow; avoid inactivity. Do exercises that maintain or improve balance if at risk of falling. Do resistance training with light weights.

- **Disabled.** Follow the guidelines for the appropriate age group as much as the disability permits.

- **Pregnant and postpartum.** Healthy women who are not already doing vigorous exercise are advised to get at least two and a half hours of moderate aerobic exercise per week. Women who regularly engage in vigorous aerobic activity can continue if approved by their health care provider.

To maintain a high level of fitness, it's best to exercise daily or almost daily. For people who haven't exercised regularly, start with ten minutes of activity and build slowly from there. Gradually increase the duration, frequency, and intensity of workouts to make fitness goals more achievable, reduce risk of injury, and add an immensely enjoyable dimension to life.[71–73]

page 387 for the Protein Power Smoothie recipe). Choose plenty of higher-calorie vegan options, such as nut and seed butters, tofu, and avocados. Bring convenient snacks to eat throughout the day, especially pre- and post-workout. Trail mix, power bars, sandwiches, and tofu jerky are good options. Bring caloric beverages, such as vegetable and fruit juices or soy milk, as well. (See pages 381 to 390 for more tips on weight gain).

I'm a body builder who recently switched to a vegan diet. My trainer is freaking out. My fellow body builders are all trying to entice me to eat meat. They all think it's impossible to achieve the kind of muscle gains body builders are after on a vegan diet. Is it possible to be a vegan body builder? What can I do to convince them?

The best way to convince skeptics is to prove them wrong. Educate yourself, train hard, and eat well. Check out websites dedicated to vegan bodybuilding (see Resources on page 450), which include extraordinary examples of buff vegans. Share these sites with the trainer. To learn the actual protein content of your diet, consider hiring a dietitian to do a nutritional analysis; this can give you and your trainer confidence. Talk to your health care provider about ergogenic aids, such as protein powder and creatine, especially if protein intake falls below about 1.5 grams per kilogram of body weight per day. Eat more to compensate for the lower energy density of plant foods. Keeping energy intakes up is necessary to allow for muscle gains.

The Vegan Plate and Menus

When you embrace a vegan lifestyle, you become aware of the fact that you have more food choices than ever before . . . When you shift your gaze from one direction to another, an entire world opens up—of new cuisines, new flavors, new textures, new aromas, new experiences.

COLLEEN PATRICK-GOUDREAU, AUTHOR, COMPASSIONATE-LIVING EXPERT

F or those striving toward a truly ethical world, being vegan makes sense. It's a choice that merges compassion for animals with environmental rationality, healthful living and—last, but not least—incredibly delicious, beautiful food. (People who enjoy making sacrifices will have to look elsewhere.)

Yet, transforming the data and recommendations from previous chapters into daily food choices may seem a rather daunting task. One may ask if it's possible to take into account each vitamin, mineral, and essential fat, plus the necessary protein, amino acids, and fiber, and then to develop a plan that meets the nutrient needs of every adult vegan—a plan that fits on a page or two for daily use.

That's what The Vegan Plate is intended to do. By using it as a food guide, vegans will be well nourished and on their way to achieving life-long good health. The following guidelines, tips, and sample menus are designed to make this journey both enjoyable and fruitful.

Food Guides in Perspective

Governments have vested interests in keeping their populations healthy *and* in promoting the products of national agriculture. As nutrition knowledge has advanced over the last century, these dual interests have led to the periodic release of recommendations for healthful eating. The US Department of Agriculture (USDA) has developed and distributed science-based food guides and food buying guides since 1916. These have been presented in a myriad of forms; all were suitable for vegetarians because legumes have always been suggested as meat alternatives.[1]

For example, a 1933 USDA food buying plan—with twelve food groups—was developed to help individuals eat nutritious meals despite the financial hardships imposed by the Depression. During the two previous decades, most of the vitamins had been identified. The guide's various food groupings were centered on specific nutrients, with distinct groups for protein-, iron-, and zinc-rich dry beans, peas, and nuts; for carbohydrate-rich potatoes and sweet potatoes; for vitamin C–rich tomatoes and citrus fruits; for carotenoid (vitamin A)-rich leafy green and yellow vegetables; for other vegetables and fruits; and for B vitamin-rich flours and cereals. Butter, other fats, and sugars formed three groups, and the remaining three groups were milk, meats and fish, and eggs.[1]

In 1943, the USDA issued its *National Wartime Nutrition Guide*, which condensed the number of groups to the "Basic Seven." By 1956, these had been further reduced to the "Basic Four": milk, meat, vegetables and fruit, and cereals and breads. Since 1980, when the USDA and the Department of Health and Human Services issued the first *Dietary Guidelines for Americans*, the food guide has been revised several more times.[1]

In 2011, the first USDA food guide that included an entirely vegan option was presented in MyPlate, a visual representation of the 2010 *Dietary Guidelines for Americans*. The dairy group lists calcium-fortified soy milk (along with twenty-three commonly eaten cow's milk products) as a way to get calcium. Since 2007, *Canada's Food Guide* has also listed fortified soy beverages in its milk and alternatives group.[2]

A footnote to MyPlate states, "Calcium-fortified foods and beverages, such as cereals, orange juice, or rice or almond beverages, may provide calcium, but may not provide the other nutrients found in dairy products."[3] Unfortunately, apart from fortified soy milk, the highly nutritious plant foods that are powerful calcium providers (see page 184) aren't included among these dairy alternatives. However, a foot has been firmly lodged in the door; with a concerted effort and perseverance, the door will be pushed wide open, and a variety of plant foods will take their rightful places in national food guides as calcium sources.

A look at food guides beyond those of the United States and Canada is revealing. Several food guides from other parts of the world are easily adapted to vegan eating. For example, the national food pyramid of the Republic of the Philippines has no milk group because Filipinos don't typically drink milk. This food guide places good sources of plant protein in a group that comprises animal foods, dried beans, and nuts. The model that guides Mexican eating is a circular *El Plato del Bien Comer* (Dish of Good Eating), divided into three equal sections: *cereales* (cereals); *verduras y frutas* (vegetables and fruits); and *leguminosas y alimentos de origen animal* (legumes/pulses and foods of animal origin). As a result, it easily allows for an entirely vegan selection. Meanwhile, China's guide suggests 50 grams of beans as an alternative for 100 milliliters of milk.[4, 5]

Regarding serving sizes, the national guides of the Philippines, Mexico, Portugal, Germany, and Sweden avoid taking a specific quantitative approach. Instead, they suggest which food groups should be eaten in relatively larger amounts. For example, the Swedish *Tallriksmodellen* (Plate Model) suggests larger portions of carbohydrates (potatoes, pasta, rice, and bread) for people who require more energy or calories; it notes that those who are overweight should fill half their plate with vegetables and fruit. In addition, lentils, chickpeas, beans, and tofu are shown as clear alternatives to animal products.[4, 5]

The correct use of any food guide calls for slight or sedentary people to appreciate that they have relatively low needs for calories and certain nutrients, and larger, very active, or growing people to be aware that they'll have greater requirements. People who intend to lose weight face the challenge of taking in fewer calories while getting the full spectrum of essential nutrients.

Plant-Based Food Guides

The peer-reviewed medical literature provides several vegetarian food guides that feature vegan options. For example, experts who attended the Third International Congress on Vegetarian Nutrition in 1997 collaborated on a food guide pyramid with an entirely vegan foundation composed of five food groups (grains, legumes, vegetables, fruits, and nuts and seeds). The pyramid's tip presents optional foods (oils, eggs, dairy products, and sweets). A note recommends the use of vitamin B_{12} supplements for people who don't consume eggs or dairy products.[6–8]

A clean, simple, and straightforward vegan food guide is The Power Plate from the Physicians Committee for Responsible Medicine. This guide includes four food groups of equal size (grains, vegetables, legumes, fruits) and emphasizes in a note below, "Be sure to include a reliable source of vitamin B_{12}, such as any common multiple vitamin or fortified foods."[9]

A joint paper by the Academy of Nutrition and Dietetics (AND, formerly the American Dietetic Association) and Dietitians of Canada (DC) includes a food guide that groups legumes, nuts, and seeds together in a food group called legumes, nuts, and other protein-rich foods; other food groups are grains, vegetables, and fruits. This plan then highlights the foods within each group that provide 100 to 150 mg of calcium per serving. The calcium-rich foods within the legumes, nuts, and other protein-rich foods group are fortified soy milk, tempeh, calcium-set tofu, almonds, almond butter, sesame tahini, soybeans, soy nuts, cow's milk, yogurt, and cheese.[8, 10, 11] Vesanto Melina, coauthor of this book, was a cocreator of that dietary guide and the related scientific article, along with Virginia Messina and Reed Mangels.[11]

The Vegan Plate featured in this chapter has been adapted from the AND/DC dietary guide; it includes five food groups, shown on page 434 in graphic form and on page 435 as a table. A color version is also presented on the back cover and at the becomingvegan.ca/food-guide website.

A column in the table lists the calcium-rich foods within each food group that provide about 100 to 150 mg of calcium per serving. Most plant foods provide some calcium, but the foods listed in the calcium column are especially high in this mineral. (In the graphic, calcium-rich foods are shown in the central circle.) The "other essentials" included in the illustration indicate the need for reliable sources of omega-3 fatty acids, vitamins B_{12} and D, and iodine, which may not be supplied in adequate amounts from the food groups.[12, 13]

As with any diet, it's not essential to meet the minimum intake from every food group every day, though this could be a goal for average intakes over time. In fact, eating patterns can vary greatly and still meet nutrient recommendations. As a result, The Vegan Plate is a versatile tool that can work equally well for individuals whose goal is weight loss, those whose caloric requirements have decreased with age, for athletes with high energy needs, and those in between. It can help in menu planning for couples and families, and even for people on raw vegan diets.

For those new to plant-based diets, the guide appears to recommend a lot of servings, which raises the question: Is it possible to consume that much in one day? The short answer is yes.

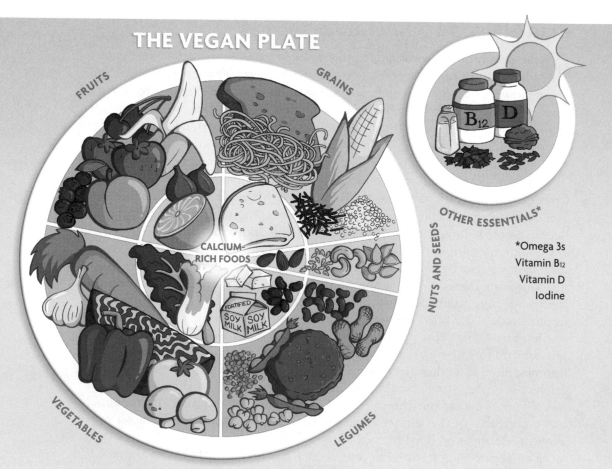

THE VEGAN PLATE

Daily plan for healthful eating.

FOOD GROUP (SERVINGS PER DAY)	FOODS IN THIS GROUP (SERVING SIZE)	CALCIUM-RICH FOODS: CHOOSE 6 TO 8 SERVINGS PER DAY (SERVING SIZE)	NOTES
Vegetables (5 or more servings)	½ c (125 ml) raw or cooked vegetables 1 c (250 ml) raw leafy vegetables ½ c (125 ml) vegetable juice	1 c (250 ml) cooked bok choy, collard greens, napa cabbage, kale, mustard greens, or okra 2 c (500 ml) raw bok choy, collard greens, kale, or napa cabbage ½ c (125 ml) calcium-fortified tomato or vegetable juice	Choose from the full rainbow of colorful vegetables: blue, green, orange, purple, red, yellow, and white. Include at least 2 daily servings of the calcium-rich greens.
Fruits (4 or more servings)	1 medium fruit ½ c (125 ml) fruit or fruit juice ¼ c (60 ml) dried fruit	½ c (125 ml) calcium-fortified fruit juice ½ c (125 ml) dried figs 2 oranges	Fruits are excellent sources of potassium. Select from the full spectrum of colorful fruits; feature them for dessert or treats.
Legumes (3 or more servings)	½ c (125 ml) cooked beans, peas, lentils, tofu, or tempeh 1 c (250 ml) raw peas or sprouted lentils or peas ¼ c (60 ml) peanuts 2 T (30 ml) peanut butter 1 oz (30 g) vegetarian meat substitute	1 c (250 ml) black or white beans ½ c (125 ml) fortified soy milk or soy yogurt ½ c (125 ml) calcium-set tofu (calcium should be included on the ingredient list), cooked soybeans, or soy nuts	Legumes provide generous amounts of iron, magnesium, potassium, zinc, fiber, and protein, with an average of 7 to 9 grams of protein per serving. Include a selection from this group at most meals.
Grains (3 or more servings)	½ c (125 ml) cooked cereal, rice, pasta, quinoa, or other grain or grain product 1 oz (30 g) bread ½ c (125 ml) raw corn or sprouted quinoa, buckwheat, or other grain 1 oz (30 g) ready-to-eat cereal	1 oz (30 g) calcium-fortified cereal 1 calcium-fortified tortilla	Select whole grains as often as possible. Adjust the number of grain servings to suit energy needs. Some fortified cereals and tortillas are particularly high in calcium (check labels).
Nuts and seeds (1 or more servings)	¼ c (60 ml) nuts and seeds 2 T (30 ml) nut or seed butter	¼ c (60 ml) almonds 2 T (30 ml) almond butter or sesame tahini	Seeds and nuts contribute copper, selenium, other minerals, vitamin E, and fat; choose some that are rich in omega-3 fatty acids (see page 436).

As in many other guides, The Vegan Plate clearly states the serving sizes of various foods within each food group. Bear in mind that what's consumed as a "normal" serving varies greatly from one individual to the next, so it's important to become familiar with the interpretation of a "serving" according to the guide. In practice, people often eat more than one serving from a particular food group at a meal. For example, someone who has 1 cup (250 ml) of fortified soy milk, sliced fruit, green peas, cooked oatmeal, pasta, or rice will have consumed two servings of these items. A large salad may count as two or more servings, depending on the quantity of greens and vegetables. In The Vegan Plate, a portion of one of the calcium-rich foods also counts as one or two servings of one of the five food groups listed in the column at the left.

Extras that are high in sugar or fat (but lack other nutrients) can still be enjoyed as occasional treats, though there's limited room for such items in a healthy diet that meets recommended intakes, vegan or not. Following The Vegan Plate means that most of the day's calories will be provided by wholesome, nutritious foods.

OTHER ESSENTIALS

For omega-3 fatty acids, include at least one of the following daily:

- 2 tablespoons (30 ml) of ground flaxseeds or chia seeds
- ¼ cup (60 ml) of hempseeds
- ⅓ cup (85 ml) of walnuts
- 1½ teaspoons (7 ml) of flaxseed oil
- 1½ tablespoons (22 ml) of hempseed oil
- 2½ tablespoons (37 ml) of canola oil

These amounts provide enough alpha-linolenic acid (ALA) for the average man (3.2 grams of ALA) and will provide more than enough for the average woman (who needs only about 2.2 grams of ALA). A vegan docosahexaenoic acid (DHA) supplement of 200 to 300 mg of DHA two to three times a week is optional and may be beneficial for some individuals (such as pregnant women or people with diabetes). A supplement that combines DHA with eicosapentaenoic acid (EPA) also can be used. (For more information on omega-3 fatty acids, see pages 117 to 134.)

For vitamin B_{12}, include at least one of the following; larger amounts may be advisable:

- a daily supplement that provides at least 25 mcg of vitamin B_{12}
- twice a week, a supplement that provides at least 1,000 mcg of vitamin B_{12}
- three servings over the course of a day of vitamin B_{12}-fortified foods, such as nondairy milks, vegan meat substitutes, or breakfast cereals, each fortified with a total of 2 mcg of vitamin B_{12} or 33 percent of the DV (check the label). Two teaspoons (10 ml or 5 g) of Red Star Vegetarian Support Formula

nutritional yeast can qualify as one of these servings. (For more information on vitamin B_{12}, see pages 214 to 222.)[14–16]

For vitamin D, get daily exposure to sunlight, eat fortified foods, take a supplement, or use a combination of these sources:

- **Sunlight.** Expose the face and forearms to warm sunlight (10 a.m. to 3 p.m.) without sunscreen for fifteen minutes for light-skinned people, at least twenty minutes for dark-skinned people, or thirty minutes for the elderly.
- **Fortified foods or supplements.** The recommended daily vitamin D intake from supplements or fortified foods is 15 mcg (600 IU) for people up to age 70 and 20 mcg (800 IU) for people older than 70. Up to 100 mcg (4,000 IU) of vitamin D daily is considered suitable and safe for adults. (For more information on vitamin D, see pages 222 to 230.)

For iodine, take a multivitamin-mineral supplement that contains iodine or consume about $\frac{1}{3}$ teaspoon (2 ml) of iodized salt for the daily recommended intake of 150 mcg of iodine. (Sea salt generally isn't iodized.) Sea vegetables, such as kelp, also contain iodine, though the amount of iodine in these vegetables can vary greatly. (For more information on iodine, see pages 191 to 194.)

For recommended intakes of vitamins and minerals at various ages and during pregnancy and lactation, see the tables in the appendix (pages 446 and 447).

Practical Pointers

To ensure consumption of sufficient nutrients and protective phytochemicals—and to make meals appealing—include a wide variety of plant foods on a daily basis. To plan an optimal diet using The Vegan Plate, follow these guidelines:

- Eat lots of legumes; at least three servings per day should be included.
- Fill at least half the plate with an assortment of vegetables and fruits at each meal.
- Limit intakes of fats, oils, and sugars, if used. Whole foods, such as seeds, nuts, avocados, and fruits, are preferred as sources of fat and sugar.
- Monitor sodium consumption. Regular use of ready-to-eat processed foods can result in high sodium intakes; check labels and balance intakes with fresh, unprocessed items.
- Aim for an hour of physical activity each day for energy balance and overall health. Daily exercise helps to maintain muscle strength, bone density, physical balance, and mental well-being.
- Stay hydrated. Drink water, herbal teas, and vegetable juices to maintain good health and avoid kidney stones and urinary tract infections; take particular care in hot weather.[17]

Menus

Four sample menus for people with different caloric needs follow. Additional guidance on weight management is provided in chapter 12, and nutrition for athletes is addressed in chapter 13. Plus, sample menus are suggested for:

- Pregnant or breastfeeding women (page 297), with 2,135 calories and 97 grams of protein
- Infants at the age of 7 and 11 months (tables 10.2 and 10.3 on pages 317 and 318)
- Children of different weights (table 10.6 on page 335).

Also see:

- Table 9.3 showing foods that provide 15 grams of protein per serving (page 289).
- Table 10.1 showing iron, zinc, and protein contents of foods for infants (page 312).
- Vegan food guide for 1- to 3-year-old children (table 10.1 on page 312).
- Table 10.6 showing fillings for vegan sandwiches (page 334).
- List of easy-to-prepare meals, complete with prep tips (page 356).
- Table 12.2 showing suggested daily food servings for weight gain (page 382).
- Mechanical-eating menu example for eating disorders (page 398).
- Table 12.4 showing protein-rich foods to increase the protein content of meals (page 386).
- Table 13.3 showing vegan foods that provide 10 grams of protein per serving (page 411).
- Table 13.4 showing protein-rich foods to increase the protein content of meals (page 411).
- Table 13.6 showing suggested servings from food groups at various caloric levels (page 426).

The four menus that follow are suitable for people who need 1,600; 2,000; 2,500 to 2,800; or 4,000 calories daily. A nutritional analysis follows each menu. (For recommended intakes of vitamins and minerals for various age groups, see pages 446 and 447.)

After each menu item, a letter indicates the food group it represents: grains (G); vegetables (V); fruit (F); legumes (L); nuts and seeds (N); calcium-rich foods (C); and omega-3 fatty acids (n-3). Due to the nutritional bounty of these whole plant foods, many items represent more than one food group; a summary of the total servings from each food group is shown below each menu. The nutritional analysis below each menu is based on metric measures and, where there is a choice, on the first option listed. Certain nutrients may depend on the product chosen; for example, calcium content differs markedly between brands of tofu. Any of the menus can be modified by substituting another item from that food group.

1,600-CALORIE SAMPLE MENU

This high-protein, low-calorie menu is suitable for small or elderly people or people who want to lose weight. It provides 19 percent of calories from protein, 23 percent of calories from fat, and 58 percent of calories from carbohydrates. Replacing soy milk with other fortified nondairy beverages will reduce the protein in this menu by about 10 to 12 grams.

BREAKFAST

½ cup (125 ml) cooked cereal or 1 ounce (30 g) dry cereal	1 G
½ cup (125 ml) raspberries or other fruit	1 F
½ cup (125 ml) fortified soy milk	1 L, 1 C

LUNCH

Soup of 1 cup (250 ml) cooked lentils plus 1 cup (250 ml) cooked vegetables (onion, carrot, celery)	2 L, 2 V
4 rye wafers or rice crackers	1 G
2 cups (500 ml) raw vegetables (peppers, cherry tomatoes, cucumber, carrots)	2 V
1½ cups (375 ml) watermelon or other fruit	3 F

SUPPER

Stir-fry of 2 cups (500 ml) green vegetables (broccoli, napa cabbage)	2 V, 1 C
with ½ cup (125 ml) cubed calcium-set tofu	1 L, 1 C
and 1 teaspoon (5 ml) sesame oil, 1 teaspoon (5 ml) tamari	—
½ cup (125 ml) cooked whole grain, such as brown rice, millet, or quinoa	1 G
½ cup (125 ml) fortified soy milk	1 L, 1 C

SNACK

Chocolate shake: 1 banana, ½ cup (125 ml) blueberries,	2 F
with 1 cup (250 ml) fortified chocolate soy milk,	2 L, 2 C
¼ cup (60 ml) hempseeds	1 N, 1 n-3

Total servings of food groups: grains: 3; vegetables: 6; fruits: 6; legumes: 7; nuts and seeds: 1; calcium-rich foods: 6; omega-3 fatty acids: 1

Vitamin B_{12} is supplied by three servings of fortified soy milk.

Vitamin D is supplied by fortified soy milk; add sunshine or a supplement.

Nutritional analysis: calories: 1,597; protein: 80 g; fat: 43 g; carbohydrate: 241 g; dietary fiber: 52 g; calcium: 1,964 mg; iron: 22 mg; magnesium: 680 mg; phosphorus: 1,583 mg; potassium: 4,700 mg; sodium: 826 mg; zinc: 14 mg; thiamin: 1.7 mg; riboflavin: 10.9 mg; niacin: 23 mg; vitamin B_6: 2.2 mg; folate: 904 mcg; pantothenic acid: 5.3 mg; vitamin B_{12}: 5.4 mcg; vitamin A: 1,438 mcg RAE (4,746 IU); vitamin C: 283 mg; vitamin D: 10 mcg (400 IU); vitamin E: 13 mg (19.5 IU); omega-6 fatty acids: 13.8 g; omega-3 fatty acids: 9.7 g

2,000-CALORIE SAMPLE MENU

This menu provides 15 percent of calories from protein, 33 percent of calories from fat, and 52 percent of calories from carbohydrate. It has enough protein for adults (including recreational athletes) who weigh up to 168 pounds (76 kg) at a suitable level of 1 gram of protein per kilogram (2.2 lb) of body weight. Almond milk is a source of vitamin E. Blackstrap molasses and sesame tahini are good sources of calcium. Dark chocolate provides iron and magnesium.

BREAKFAST	
2 slices toast (2 ounces/60 g total)	2 G
with 2 tablespoons (30 ml) sesame tahini and 1 tablespoon (15 ml) blackstrap molasses	1 N, 2 C
1 cup (250 ml) calcium-fortified orange juice	2 F, 2 C

LUNCH	
Taco: 1 tortilla and 1 cup (250 ml) black beans, pinto beans, or refried beans	1 G, 2 L, 1 C
with 1 tomato, 1 cup (250 ml) lettuce, ¼ avocado, and salsa	3 V
½ cup (125 ml) fortified almond milk	1 C

SUPPER	
½ cup (125 ml) cooked whole grain, such as brown rice or quinoa, or 1 whole-grain roll (1 ounce/30 g)	1 G
4 cups (1 L) salad of kale, romaine lettuce, and napa cabbage	4 V
with 2 tablespoons (30 ml) Liquid Gold Dressing (page 219)	1 n-3
½ cup (125 ml) cubed tempeh with lemon and ginger or BBQ sauce	1 L

SNACKS	
¼ cup (60 ml) dried figs and 1 orange	2 F, 1 C
¼ cup (60 ml) pumpkin seeds	1 N
½ cup (125 ml) fortified almond milk	1 C
1 ounce (30 g) dark chocolate	—

Total servings of food groups: grains: 4; vegetables: 7; fruits: 4; legumes: 3; nuts and seeds: 2; calcium-rich foods: 8; omega-3 fatty acids: 1

Vitamin B_{12} is supplied by nutritional yeast in Liquid Gold Dressing and fortified nondairy milk.

Vitamin D is supplied by fortified juice and almond milk; add sunshine or a supplement.

Nutritional analysis: calories: 1,958; protein: 76 g; fat: 76 g; carbohydrate: 268 g; dietary fiber: 48 g; calcium: 1,294 mg; iron: 22 mg; magnesium: 808 mg; phosphorus: 1,867 mg; potassium: 4,847 mg; sodium: 1,100 mg; zinc: 12 mg; thiamin: 3.2 mg; riboflavin: 2.2 mg; niacin: 23 mg; vitamin B_6: 2.9 mg; folate: 826 mcg; pantothenic acid: 5 mg; vitamin B_{12}: 5.6 mcg; vitamin A: 1,313 mcg RAE (4,333 IU); vitamin C: 294 mg; vitamin D: 5 mcg (200 IU); vitamin E: 15 mg (22.5 IU); omega-6 fatty acids: 20.9 g; omega-3 fatty acids: 5.8 g

2,500- TO 2,800-CALORIE SAMPLE MENU

This 2,500-calorie menu provides 15 percent of calories from protein, 26 percent of calories from fat, and 59 percent of calories from carbohydrate. To increase the calories to 2,800, add more food, such as a piece of fruit and two cookies. Using the Vega One nutritional shake rather than seeds boosts the levels of most nutrients well above the recommended intake. Convenience foods, such as vegan meat substitutes and canned baked beans or chili, can be high in sodium; users should check the labels—or prepare homemade versions, which are typically lower in sodium.

BREAKFAST	
1 bagel with 2 tablespoons (30 ml) peanut butter or 1 cup (250 ml) whole-grain cereal with nuts	2 G, 1 L
Fruit smoothie: 1 scoop (35.9 g) Vega One nutritional shake or ¼ cup (60 ml) sunflower seeds or hempseeds	1 L, 4 C
with 1 cup (250 ml) calcium-fortified juice (or nondairy milk)	2 F, 2 C
and ½ banana and ½ cup (125 ml) strawberries	2 F

LUNCH	
1½ sandwiches: 3 slices whole-grain bread (3 ounces/90 g total)	3 G
with 3 slices vegan turkey	1.5 L
and 1 tomato and 1 cup (250 ml) lettuce	2 V
and 1 tablespoon (15 ml) vegan mayonnaise	—

SUPPER	
1 cup (250 ml) baked beans or vegetarian chili	2 L
1 cup (250 ml) baked squash or yam	2 V
1 cup (250 ml) steamed broccoli	2 V, 1 C
1 baked potato with 2 tablespoons (30 ml) vegan spread	1 V

SNACKS	
1 cup (250 ml) trail mix: ⅓ cup (85 ml) walnuts, ⅓ cup (85 ml) raisins, ⅓ cup (85 ml) dried apricots	1 N, 2 F, 1 n-3
1 cup (250 ml) calcium-fortified nondairy milk	2 C

Total servings of food groups: grains: 5, vegetables: 7, fruits: 6, legumes: 5.5, nuts and seeds: 1, calcium-rich foods: 9, omega-3 fatty acids: 1

Vitamin B_{12} is supplied by the Vega One nutritional shake and fortified vegan meat substitute, or add a supplement.

Vitamin D is supplied by fortified juice, nondairy milk, and the Vega One nutritional shake; add sunshine or a supplement.

Nutritional analysis: calories: 2,501; protein: 97 g; fat: 75 g; carbohydrate: 395 g; dietary fiber: 59 g; calcium: 1,858 mg; iron: 30 mg; magnesium: 772 mg; phosphorus: 1,793 mg; potassium: 6,841 mg; sodium: 2,200 mg; zinc: 24 mg; thiamin: 2.9 mg; riboflavin: 2.2 mg; niacin: 34 mg; vitamin B_6: 4 mg; folate: 898 mcg; pantothenic acid: 11 mg; vitamin B_{12}: 4.2 mcg; vitamin A: 988 mcg RAE (3,260 IU); vitamin C: 409 mg; vitamin D: 55 mcg (2,200 IU); vitamin E: 27 mg (40.5 IU); omega-6 fatty acids: 20 g; omega-3 fatty acids: 5.6 g

4,000-CALORIE SAMPLE MENU

This menu provides 12 percent of calories from protein, 32 percent of calories from fat, and 56 percent of calories from carbohydrate. Despite the moderate percentage of calories from protein, total protein content is high, without substantial reliance on soy. Other protein-rich alternatives that might be chosen are scrambled tofu for breakfast or soy-based veggie burgers.

BREAKFAST	
2 cups (500 ml) granola or 4 pancakes or waffles with maple syrup	4 G
2 oranges or other fruit	2 F, 1 C
2 cups (500 ml) fortified almond milk or other nondairy milk	4 C

LUNCH	
Burgers: 2 whole wheat hamburger buns	4 G
with 2 fortified black bean burgers	1 G, 1 L
and sliced tomato, red onion, chopped lettuce, and spreads	2 V
1½ cups (375 ml) potato salad	3 V
½ cup (125 ml) mango, or 1 apple or other fruit	1 F

SUPPER	
Stir-fry: 1 cup (250 ml) chickpeas and ⅓ cup (85 ml) cashews	2 L, 1.5 N
with 2 cups (500 ml) greens (such as broccoli, okra, napa cabbage)	4 V, 2 C
and 1 cup (250 ml) carrots or peppers	2 V
and 1 teaspoon (5 ml) sesame oil and 1 teaspoon (5 ml) tamari	—
2 cups (500 ml) noodles or rice	4 G
1 tablespoon (15 ml) olive oil	—

SNACKS	
½ cup (125 ml) hummus	1 L
8 crackers	1 G
1 peach or other fruit	1 F
1 cup (250 ml) fortified almond milk or other nondairy milk (or juice)	2 C
½ cup (125 ml) walnuts	1 N, 1 n-3
1 power bar (68 g) or dessert	

Total servings of food groups: (total does not include choice of power bar or dessert) grains: 14; vegetables: 11, fruits: 4, legumes: 4; nuts and seeds: 2.5, calcium-rich foods: 9, omega-3 fatty acids: 1

Vitamin B_{12} is supplied by the fortified nondairy milk and veggie burger, or add a supplement.

Vitamin D is supplied by fortified nondairy milk; add sunshine or a supplement.

Nutritional analysis: calories: 4,002; protein: 128 g; fat: 152 g; carbohydrate: 584 g; dietary fiber: 88 g; calcium: 1,826 mg; iron: 37 mg; magnesium: 910 mg; phosphorus: 2,589 mg; potassium: 6,258 mg; sodium: 2,300 mg; zinc: 23 mg; thiamin: 7.4 mg; riboflavin: 2.5 mg; niacin: 38 mg; vitamin B_6: 3.9 mg; folate: 1,646 mcg; pantothenic acid: 16 mg; vitamin B_{12}: 3.8 mcg; vitamin A: 1,844 mcg RAE (6,085 IU); vitamin C: 425 mg; vitamin D: 8 mcg (317 IU); vitamin E: 52 mg (78 IU); omega-6 fatty acids: 33 g; omega-3 fatty acids: 6 g

For more menus, see the companion volume, *Cooking Vegan,* by Vesanto Melina and Joseph Forest (Book Publishing Company, 2012). It includes more than 150 delicious recipes and a dozen menus. Each menu is presented at three calorie levels—1,600, 2,000, and 2,500 calories—and every menu and recipe includes a nutritional analysis. Eight of the menus offer recipes based on cuisines from around the world: North American, Asian fusion, East Indian, French, Italian, Japanese, Mexican, and Middle Eastern. The remaining menus focus on raw foods, simple dishes, family meals with children's favorites, and foods for holidays and celebrations.

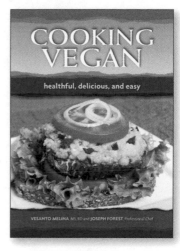

Cooking Vegan includes a chapter on becoming acquainted with new ingredients, which include healthful oils, sweeteners, thickeners, nondairy milks, soy foods, and herbs and spices, along with specific directions for cooking grains and legumes. The book provides instructions on how to substitute vegan for nonvegan items in other recipes, as well as a helpful shopping list, kitchen equipment list, and chef tips.

Recommended Intakes of Vitamins and Minerals

T he Dietary Reference Intakes (DRIs) are a comprehensive set of reference values that indicate recommended daily intakes for vitamins, minerals, and other nutrients for healthy populations. The DRIs have been established by American and Canadian scientists through a review process overseen by the US National Academies, which is an independent, nongovernmental body, and they reflect the current state of scientific knowledge with respect to nutrient requirements. They can be used for assessing and planning diets.

The Recommended Dietary Allowance (RDA) is the average daily dietary intake of a nutrient that is sufficient to meet the requirement of most (97 to 98 percent) healthy persons. This number can be used as a goal for individuals and is likely to exceed the recommended intake for most people within that age or gender group. In the following tables, RDAs are shown in bold type.

Adequate Intake (AI) is the intake level suggested when an RDA cannot be determined due to insufficient data. The AI is more of a good guess or estimate of the amount needed to promote health. In the tables, these are shown in regular rather than bold type.

These and Tolerable Upper Intake Level (UL) are available through the Institute of Medicine of the National Academies online at iom.edu/Activities/Nutrition/SummaryDRIs/~/media/Files/Activity%20Files/Nutrition/DRIs/New%20Material/5DRI%20Values%20SummaryTables%2014.pdf or by scanning the QR code below. Alternate measures sometimes used (such as international units, or IU) can also be found at this website. For additional details and reports, see the website iom.edu. The UL is the highest daily intake of a nutrient, consumed on a continuing basis, that is considered safe; in other words, likely to pose no risks of adverse health effects for most individuals.

For further details on vitamins and essential minerals, see chapters 6 and 7 and the websites:

lpi.oregonstate.edu/infocenter/vitamins.html

lpi.oregonstate.edu/infocenter/minerals.html.

US National Academies DRIs

TABLE A.1. Dietary Reference Intakes for Vitamins

AGE / LIFE STAGE	VIT A mcg	VIT C mg	VIT D mcg	VIT E mg	VIT K mcg	THIAMIN mg	RIBOFLAVIN mg	NIACIN mg	VIT B$_6$ mg	FOLATE mcg	VIT B$_{12}$ mcg	PANTOTHENIC ACID mg	BIOTIN mcg	CHOLINE mg
INFANTS														
0–6 months	400	40	10	4	2.0	0.2	0.3	2	0.1	65	0.4	1.7	5	125
7–12 months	500	50	10	5	2.5	0.3	0.4	4	0.3	80	0.5	1.8	6	150
CHILDREN														
1–3 years	300	15	15	6	30	0.5	0.5	6	0.5	150	0.9	2	8	200
4–8 years	400	25	15	7	55	0.6	0.6	8	0.6	200	1.2	3	12	250
MALES														
9–13 years	600	45	15	11	60	0.9	0.9	12	1.0	300	1.8	4	20	375
14–18 years	900	75	15	15	75	1.2	1.3	16	1.3	400	2.4	5	25	550
19–30 years	900	90	15	15	120	1.2	1.3	16	1.3	400	2.4	5	30	550
31–50 years	900	90	15	15	120	1.2	1.3	16	1.3	400	2.4	5	30	550
51–70 years	900	90	15	15	120	1.2	1.3	16	1.7	400	2.4	5	30	550
> 70 years	900	90	20	15	120	1.2	1.3	16	1.7	400	2.4	5	30	550
FEMALES														
9–13 years	600	45	15	11	60	0.9	0.9	12	1.0	300	1.8	4	20	375
14–18 years	700	65	15	15	75	1.0	1.0	14	1.2	400	2.4	5	25	400
19–30 years	700	75	15	15	90	1.1	1.1	14	1.3	400	2.4	5	30	425
31–50 years	700	75	15	15	90	1.1	1.1	14	1.3	400	2.4	5	30	425
51–70 years	700	75	15	15	90	1.1	1.1	14	1.5	400	2.4	5	30	425
> 70 years	700	75	20	15	90	1.1	1.1	14	1.5	400	2.4	5	30	425
PREGNANCY														
14–18 years	750	80	15	15	75	1.4	1.4	18	1.9	600	2.6	6	30	450
19–30 years	770	85	15	15	90	1.4	1.4	18	1.9	600	2.6	6	30	450
31–50 years	770	85	15	15	90	1.4	1.4	18	1.9	600	2.6	6	30	450
LACTATION														
14–18 years	1,200	115	15	19	75	1.4	1.6	17	2	500	2.8	7	35	550
19–30 years	1,300	120	15	19	90	1.4	1.6	17	2	500	2.8	7	35	550
31–50 years	1,300	120	15	19	90	1.4	1.6	17	2	500	2.8	7	35	550

Key: g = gram; mcg = microgram; mg = milligram; vit = vitamin

TABLE A.2. Dietary Reference Intakes for Minerals

LIFE STAGE / AGE	CALCIUM mg	CHROMIUM mcg	COPPER mcg	FLUORIDE mg	IODINE mcg	IRON mg	MAGNESIUM mg	MANGANESE mg	MOLYBDE-NUM mcg	PHOSPHO-RUS mg	SELENIUM mcg	ZINC mg	POTASSIUM g	SODIUM g	CHLORIDE g
INFANTS															
0–6 months	200	0.2	200	0.01	110	0.27	30	0.003	2	100	15	2	0.4	0.11	0.18
7–12 months	260	5.5	220	0.5	130	11	75	0.6	3	275	20	3	0.86	0.37	0.57
CHILDREN															
1–3 years	700	11	340	0.7	90	7	80	1.2	17	460	20	3	2.0	0.8	1.5
4–8 years	1,000	15	440	1	90	10	130	1.5	22	500	30	5	2.3	1.0	1.9
MALES															
9–13 years	1,300	25	700	2	120	8	240	1.9	34	1,250	40	8	2.5	1.2	2.3
14–18 years	1,300	35	890	3	150	11	410	2.2	43	1,250	55	11	3.0	1.5	2.3
19–30 years	1,000	35	900	4	150	8	400	2.3	45	700	55	11	3.4	1.5	2.3
31–50 years	1,000	35	900	4	150	8	420	2.3	45	700	55	11	3.4	1.5	2.3
51–70 years	1,000	30	900	4	150	8	420	2.3	45	700	55	11	3.4	1.5	2.0
>70 years	1,200	30	900	4	150	8	420	2.3	45	700	55	11	3.4	1.5	1.8
FEMALES															
9–13 years	1,300	21	700	2	120	8	240	1.6	34	1,250	40	8	2.3	1.2	2.3
14–18 years	1,300	24	890	3	150	15	360	1.6	43	1,250	55	9	2.3	1.5	2.3
19–30 years	1,000	25	900	3	150	18	310	1.8	45	700	55	8	2.6	1.5	2.3
31–50 years	1,000	25	900	3	150	18	320	1.8	45	700	55	8	2.6	1.5	2.3
51–70 years	1,200	20	900	3	150	8	320	1.8	45	700	55	8	2.6	1.5	2.0
>70 years	1,200	20	900	3	150	8	320	1.8	45	700	55	8	2.6	1.5	1.8
PREGNANCY															
14–18 years	1,300	29	1,000	3	220	27	400	2.0	50	1,250	60	13	4.7	1.5	2.3
19–30 years	1,000	30	1,000	3	220	27	350	2.0	50	700	60	11	4.7	1.5	2.3
31–50 years	1,000	30	1,000	3	220	27	360	2.0	50	700	60	11	4.7	1.5	2.3
LACTATION															
14–18 years	1,300	44	1,300	3	290	10	360	2.6	50	1,250	70	14	5.1	1.5	2.3
19–30 years	1,000	45	1,300	3	290	9	310	2.6	50	700	70	12	5.1	1.5	2.3
31–50 years	1,000	45	1,300	3	290	9	320	2.6	50	700	70	12	5.1	1.5	2.3

Key: g = gram; mcg = microgram; mg = milligram; vit = vitamin

RESOURCES

WEBSITES

Authors' Websites

Becoming Vegan
(Comprehensive and Express Editions)
becomingvegan.ca

Brenda Davis
brendadavisrd.com

Vesanto Melina
nutrispeak.com

General Nutrition Information

Dietary Reference Intakes
fnic.nal.usda.gov/dietary-guidance/dietary-
    reference-intakes

Estimated Energy Requirements Calculator
globalrph.com/estimated_energy_requirement.cgi

Linus Pauling Institute's Micronutrient Informa-
    tion Center
lpi.oregonstate.edu/infocenter

National Institute of Health. Office of Dietary
    Supplements
ods.od.nih.gov

Nutrition Facts (Dr. Michael Greger, lab tests)
nutritionfacts.org

USDA National Nutrient Database for Standard
    Reference
ndb.nal.usda.gov

Vitamin D Council for self-test kit
vitamindcouncil.org

Plant-Based Nutrition Information

The Plant-Based Dietitian
plantbaseddietitian.com

The Vegan R.D.
theveganrd.com

Vegan Health (Jack Norris, RD)
veganhealth.org

"Vegetarian Diets." Position of the Academy of
    Nutrition and Dietetics (AND)
eatright.org/About/Content.aspx?id=8357

Vegetarian Nutrition Dietary Practice Group of
    the AND (search for vegan friendly dieticians,
    pregnancy, infants, children, and more)
vegetariannutrition.net

Vitamin B_{12}
veganhealth.org/articles/vitaminb12

Food Information

Infant formula section of "Soy: What's the
    Harm?"
veganhealth.org/articles/soy_harm#formula

Infant Formulas for Vegan Families
becomingvegan.ca/faqs

Iodine in Maine Sea Coast Vegetables
seaveg.com

PCRM (search for school lunch issues)
pcrm.org

"Vegetarian Journal's Guide to Food Ingredients"
vrg.org/ingredients

Vegetarian Resource Group (search for preg-
    nancy, infants, children, teen, seniors, Meals
    on Wheels menus, and other topics)
vrg.org

"Wholesome Baby Foods from Scratch"
vrg.org/recipes/babyfood.htm

Growth Charts for Infants,
Children, and Teens

Centers for Disease Control (US)
cdc.gov/growthcharts/who_charts.htm

Centers for Disease Control (US) BMI charts
apps.nccd.cdc.gov/dnpabmi

World Health Organization charts adapted for
    Canada
dietitians.ca/Secondary-Pages/Public/Who-
    Growth-Charts.aspx

Vegan Athletes

Great Vegan Athletes
greatveganathletes.com

No Meat Athlete
nomeatathlete.com

Organic Athlete
organicathlete.org

Vegan Athlete
veganathlete.com

Vegan Body Building
veganbodybuilding.com

Vegan Fitness
veganfitness.net

Eating Disorders

The Eating Disorder Foundation
eatingdisorderfoundation.org

National Eating Disorders Association (NEDA)
nationaleatingdisorders.org

Vegetarian Organizations and Festivals

American Vegan Society
americanvegan.org

International Vegetarian Union (search by region)
ivu.org

Meetups (search for local vegan groups)
meetup.com

North American Vegetarian Society (NAVS)
navs-online.org

Vegetarian Summerfest (NAVS)
vegetariansummerfest.org

Vegan-Friendly Restaurants and Travel

Happy Cow
happycow.net

PCRM Airport Food Reviews
pcrm.org/health/reports/2012-airport-food-re-
view

Vegetarian Dining Worldwide
vegdining.com

Worldwide Veg-Friendly Guide
vegguide.org

Vegan Cuisine

A Dash of Compassion
adashofcompassion.com

Allyson Kramer
allysonkramer.com

Bitter Sweet
bittersweetblog.com

FatFree Vegan Kitchen
blog.fatfreevegan.com

Happy Herbivore
happyherbivore.com

Healthy. Happy. Life.
kblog.lunchboxbunch.com

JL Goes Vegan
jlgoesvegan.com

Maple Spice
maplespice.com

Oh She Glows
ohsheglows.com

PostPunk Kitchen
theppk.com

This Rawsome Vegan Life
thisrawsomeveganlife.com

The Vegan Chickpea
theveganchickpea.com

Vegan Culinary Crusade
veganculinarycrusade.com

VeganFusion
veganfusion.com

Vegan Richa
veganricha.com

Veggie Girl
veggiegirl.com

Yum Universe
yumuniverse.com

Animal Activism

Action for Animals
afa-online.org

Animal Rights: The Abolitionist Approach
abolitionistapproach.com

The Animals Voice
animalsvoice.com

Compassion Over Killing
cok.net

Farm Animal Rights Movement
farmusa.org

Farm Sanctuary
farmsanctuary.org

Humane Society of the United States
humanesociety.org

Mercy for Animals
mercyforanimals.org

People for the Ethical Treatment of Animals
peta.org

United Poultry Concerns
upc-online.org

Viva USA
vivausa.org

Environment/Ecology

Environmental Working Group
ewg.org

United Nations Environmental Programme
unep.org

Worldwatch Institute
worldwatch.org

BOOKS

Vegan Nutrition

Becoming Raw. Brenda Davis and Vesanto Melina, Book Publishing Company, 2010.

Becoming Vegan: Express Edition. Brenda Davis and Vesanto Melina, Book Publishing Company, 2013.

Cooking Vegan. Vesanto Melina and Joseph Forest, Book Publishing Company, 2012.

The Complete Idiot's Guide to Plant-Based Nutrition. Julieanna Hever, Alpha Books, 2011.

The Dietitian's Guide to Vegetarian Diets. Third Edition. Reed Mangels, Virginia Messina, and Mark Messina, Jones and Bartlett Learning, 2011.

The Everything Vegan Pregnancy Book. Reed Mangels, Adams Media, 2011.

Never Too Late to Go Vegan. Carol Adams, Patti Breitman, and Virginia Messina, The Experiment, 2014.

The Plant-Powered Diet. Sharon Palmer, The Experiment, 2012.

Vegan for Her: The Women's Guide to Being Healthy and Fit on a Plant-Based Diet. Ginny Messina and JL Fields, Da Capo Lifelong Books, 2013.

Vegan for Life. Jack Norris and Virginia Messina, Da Capo Lifelong Books, 2011.

Vegan Health and Lifestyle

Defeating Diabetes. Brenda Davis and Tom Barnard, Book Publishing Company, 2000.

Dr. Neal Barnard's Program for Reversing Diabetes. Neal Barnard, Rodale Books, 2008.

Food Allergies: Health and Healing. Jo Stepaniak, Vesanto Melina, and Dina Aronson, Books Alive, 2010.

Food Allergy Survival Guide. Vesanto Melina, Jo Stepaniak, and Dina Aronson, Healthy Living Publications, 2004.

Food Over Medicine. Pamela Popper and Glen Merzer, BenBella Books, 2013.

Goodbye Diabetes. Wes Younbgberg, Hart Books, 2013.

Meatonomics. David Robinson Simon, Conrai Press, 2013.

Power Foods for the Brain. Neal Barnard, Grand Central Life and Style, 2013.

Real-Life Vegan. Victoria Laine, Friesens Printing, 2013.

The 30-Day Vegan Challenge. Colleen-Patrick Goudreau, Ballantine Books, 2011.

Vegan Main Street. Victoria Moran, Tarcher, 2012.

Vegan Athletes

Eat and Run. Scott Jurek, Mariner Books, 2013.

Finding Ultra: Rejecting Middle Age, Becoming One of the World's Fittest Men, and Discovering Myself. Rich Roll, Three Rivers Press, 2012.

Lifelong Running and *Senior Fitness.* Lantern Books, 2005, Ruth Heidrich. (ruthheidrich.com)

No Meat Athlete. Matt Frazier and Matthew Ruscigno, Fair Winds Press, 2013.

Power Vegan: Plant-Fueled Nutrition for Maximum Health and Fitness. Rea Frey, Agate Surrey, 2013.

Thrive: The Vegan Nutrition Guide to Optimal Performance in Sports and Life. Brendan Brazier, The Penguin Group, 2007.

Vegan Bodybuilding and Fitness. Robert Cheeke, Book Publishing Company, 2010.

Vegetarian Sports Nutrition. Enette Larson-Meyer, Human Kinetics, 2007.

Animal Rights

Animal Liberation. Peter Singer, Harper Perennial, 2009.

The Animal Manifesto. Marc Bekoff, New World Library, 2010.

The Animal Rights Debate: Abolition or Regulation. Gary L. Francione and Robert Garner, Columbia University Press, 2010.

The Bond. Wayne Pacelle, William Morrow, 2011.

Dominion. Matthew Scully, St. Martin's Press, 2002.

Eating Animals. Jonathan Safran Foer, Little, Brown and Company 2009.

Empty Cages. Tom Regan, Rowman & Littlefield Publishers, 2003.

Eternal Treblinka. Charles Patterson, Lantern Books, 2002.

The Ethics of What We Eat: Why Our Food Choices Matter. Peter Singer and Jim Mason, Rodale, 2006.

The Face on Your Plate. Jeffery Moussaieff Masson, W. W. Norton & Company, 2009.

Farm Sanctuary. Gene Bauer, Touchstone, 2008.

The Lucky Ones. My Passionate Fight for Farm Animals. Jenny Brown, Avery, 2012.

Making a Killing: The Political Economy of Animal Rights. Bob Torres, AK Press, 2007.

Meat Market by Eric Marcus, Brio Press, 2005.

Second Nature: The Inner Lives of Animals. Johnathon Balcombe and JM Coetzee, Palgrave Macmillan, 2010.

Why We Love Dogs, Eat Pigs, and Wear Cows. Melanie Joy, Conari Press, 2010.

DVDS AND VIDEO DOWNLOADS
Health

Bethany's Story
sanaview.com/bethanys-story.aspx

Fat, Sick & Nearly Dead
fatsickandnearlydead.com

Food, Inc.
takepart.com/foodinc

Foodmatters
foodmatters.tv

Forks Over Knives
forksoverknives.com

The Future of Food
thefutureoffood.com

Simply Raw: Reversing Diabetes in 30 Days
topdocumentaryfilms.com/simply-raw-reversing-diabetes-in-30-days

Supersize Me
snagfilms.com/films/title/super_size_me

Vegucated
getvegucated.com

Animal Rights/Environment

Compassion Over Killing investigation videos
cok.net/investigations

A Cow at My Table
goodknights.org/abbott

Cowspiracy
cowspiracy.com

The Cove
thecovemovie.com

Earthlings
earthlings.com

HSUS videos
video.humanesociety.org

A Life Connected: Vegan. For the People. For the Planet. For the Animals.
nonviolenceunited.org/projects

Meet Your Meat
meat.org

Peaceable Kingdom: The Journey Home, The Witness
tribeofheart.org

PETA documentaries, DVDs, and videos
peta.org

Sharkwater
sharkwater.com

REFERENCES

REFERENCES FOR CHAPTER 1

1. Spencer C. *The Heretic's Feast: A History of Vegetarianism*. Great Britain: Hartnolls Ltd., Bodmin, 1993.

2. Watson D. *Vegan News*. No. 1, November 1944. (Available online at http://ukveggie.com/vegan_news/vegan_news_1.pdf)

3. Stepaniak J. *The Vegan Sourcebook*. Lincolnwood IL: Lowell House, 1998.

4. Dinshah F. The American Vegan Society. Personal communication.

5. Dinshah J. *Out of the Jungle: The Way Of Dynamic Harmlessness*. 5th Ed. Malaga NJ: The American Vegan Society, 1995.

6. Vegan World Network. Directory. www.vegansworldnetwork.org/world_vegan_directory.php.

7. Donald Watson obituary. *The Times*. London England: Dec. 8, 2005.

8. "Vegetus." AZAD Latin to English Dictionary. www.dictionary.com May 27, 2011.

9. Davis J. "Extracts from some journals 1842-48–the earliest known uses of the word 'vegetarian'". *International Vegetarian Union*. July 15, 2010. www.ivu.org/history/vegetarian.html

10. Dimitri C et al. The 20th Century Transformation of U.S. Agriculture and Farm Policy. United States Department of Agriculture. Economic Research Service. *Economic Information Bulletin*. No. 3. June 2005. www.ers.usda.gov/publications/EIB3/eib3.pdf

11. *An HSUS Report: The Welfare of Animals in the Meat, Egg and Dairy Industries*. www.humanesociety.org/assets/pdfs/farm/welfare_overview.pdf

12. Imhoff D. ed. *CAFO: The Tragedy of Industrial Animal Factories*. Berkley and Los Angeles California: Foundation for Deep Ecology, 2010.

13. Safran-Foer J. *Eating Animals*. New York: Back Bay Books, 2009.

14. Humane Society of the United States. *More About Pigs: the underestimated animal*. Nov. 2, 2009. www.humanesociety.org/animals/pigs/pigs_more.html#edn184

15. Helft M. 1997. Pig video arcades critique life in the pen. Wired, June 6. www.wired.com/science/discoveries/news/1997/06/4302.

16. U.S. Department of Agriculture National Agricultural Statistics Service. *Livestock slaughter: 2010 annual summary*. 2011. http://usda.mannlib.cornell.edu/usda/current/LiveSlauSu/LiveSlauSu-04-25-2011.pdf.

17. Foreign Agricultural Service, USDA, Livestock and Poultry: World Markets and Trade, April 2011. www.fas.usda.gov/dlp/circular/ 2011/livestock_poultry.pdf.

18. Food and Agriculture Organization of the UN, "Pigmeat Slaughtered/Production Animals," FAOSTAT Database, 2004.

19. HSUS. *An HSUS Report: The Welfare of Animals in the Pig Industry*. Oct. 26, 2010. www.humanesociety.org/assets/pdfs/farm/welfare_pig_industry.pdf.

20. The Weekly Journal of Rural America. PETA Unveils Hog Farm Abuse Video. Posted on Sept. 19, 2008. Iowa Public Television. www.iptv.org/mtom/story.cfm/lead/116.

21. *The Merck Veterinary Manual*. Respiratory diseases of pigs: introduction. 2011. www.merckvetmanual.com/mvm/index.jsp?cfile=htm/bc/121400.htm

22. Goihl J. "Transport Losses of Market Hogs Studied" *Feedstuffs*. 28 Jan. 2008.

23. Gay L. "Faulty Practices Result in Inhumane Slaughterhouses," *Scripps Howard News Service*, February, 2001.

24. Pew Commission on Industrial Farm Animal Production. *Putting Meat on the Table: Industrial Farm Production in America*. 2008. www.ncifap.org/.

25. Robbins J. *The Food Revolution*. Berkley CA: Conari Press, 2001.

26. Sanghani R. Chickens Cleverer than Toddlers. June 19, 2013. *The Telegraph*. UK. www.telegraph.co.uk/science/science-news/10129124/Chickens-cleverer-than-toddlers.html.

27. HSUS. *An HSUS Report: The Welfare of Animals in the Egg Industry*. www.humanesociety.org/assets/pdfs/farm/welfare_egg.pdf.

28. Striffer S. *Chicken: The Dangerous Transformation of America's Favorite Food*. New Haven: Yale University Press, 2005.

29. HSUS. *An HSUS Report: The Welfare of Animals in the Chicken Industry*. www.humanesociety.org/assets/pdfs/farm/welfare_broiler.pdf.

30. Compassion Over Killing. *A COK Report: Animal Suffering in the Broiler Industry*. 2004. www.cok.net/lit/broiler/main.php.

31. Compassion Over Killing. *A COK Report: Animal Suffering in the Egg Industry*. 2004. www.eggindustry.com/cfi/report/.

32. United Egg Producers. *Animal Husbandry Guidelines for U.S. Egg Laying Flocks*. 2010 Edition. www.uepcertified.com/media/pdf/UEP-Animal-Welfare-Guidelines.pdf.

33. HSUS. *An HSUS Report: The Welfare of Calves in the Beef Industry*. www.humanesociety.org/assets/pdfs/farm/welfare_calves.pdf.

34. Blezinger S. *Cattle today: Rumen function in beef cattle - part 4*. 2000. www.cattletoday.com/archive/2000/May/Cattle_Today91.shtml.

35. Mellon M. Testimony Before the House Committee on Rules on The Preservation of Antibiotics for Medical Treatment Act. H. R. 1549. July 13, 2009. www.ucsusa.org/assets/documents/food_and_agriculture/july-2009-pamta-testimony.pdf.

36. Waters AE et al. Multidrug-Resistant Staphy-lococcus aureus in US Meat and Poultry. *Clinical Infectious Diseases* 2011;52(10):1–4. Downloaded from cid.oxfordjournals.org April 17, 2011.

37. Johnson R, Hanrahan CE. The U.S.-EU Beef Hormone Dispute. *Congressional Research Service*. Dec. 6, 2010.

38. Raloff J. Hormones: Here's the Beef. Environmental concerns reemerge over steroids given to livestock. *Science News*. 2002;161.

39. Best's Underwriting Guide. Meat Packing Plants. 2003. www.ambest.com/sales/bugentry.pdf

40. Schlosser E. Fast Food Nation. New York: Houghton Mifflin Company, 2001.

41. Coppock CE. Selected Features of the U.S. Dairy Industry from 1900 to 2000. Coppock Nutritional Services, San Antonio TX. 2000. www.coppock.com/carl/writings/History_of_Dairy_Production_From_1900_to_2000.htm.

42. HSUS. *An HSUS Report: The Welfare of Cows in the Dairy Industry*. www.humanesociety.org/assets/pdfs/farm/hsus-the-welfare-of-cows-in-the-dairy-industry.pdf

43. HSUS. *An HSUS Report: The Welfare of Animals in the Veal Industry*. www.humanesociety.org/assets/pdfs/farm/hsus-the-welfare-of-animals-in-the-veal-industry.pdf.

44. Mood A. Fishcount.org.uk *Worse things happen at sea: the welfare of wild caught fish*. 2010: chapter 19. www.fishcount.org.uk/published/standard/fishcountfullrptSR.pdf

45. FAO. FAO *Report: The State of World Fisheries and Aquaculture 2010*. www.fao.org/docrep/013/i1820e/i1820e.pdf

46. Myers RA, Worm B. Rapid worldwide depletion of predatory fish communities. *Nature*. 2003;423:280-283.

47. Worm B et al. Impacts of Biodiversity Loss on Ocean Ecosystem Services. *Science*. 2006; 314(5800):787-90.

48. United Nations. Report of the Secretary-General. *The Impacts of Fishing on Vulnerable Marine Ecosystems*. 2006. www.un.org/Depts/los/general_assembly/documents/impact_of_fishing.pdf.

49. Clucas I. Discards and bycatch in shrimp trawl fisheries. *Fisheries Circular*. 1997: No. 928, FIIU/C928. Food and Agriculture Organization. 1997.

50. Yue S. An HSUS Report: Fish and Pain Perception. www.humanesociety.org/assets/pdfs/farm/hsus-fish-and-pain-perception.pdf.

51. Yue Cottee S. Are fish the victims of 'speciesism'? A discussion about fear, pain and animal consciousness. *Fish Physiol Biochem*. 2012;38(1):5-15.

52. Nordgreen J et al. Thermonociception in fish: Effects of two different doses of morphine on thermal threshold and post-test behavior in goldfish (Carassius auratus). *Applied Animal Behavior Science*. 2009;119(1-2):101-107.

53. Rose JD et al. Can fish really feel pain? *Fish and Fisheries*. 2012; doi:10.1111/faf.12010.

54. FAO. 2007. *The State of World Fisheries and Aquaculture 2006*. FAO, Rome. ftp://ftp.fao.org/docrep/fao/009/a0699e/a0699e.pdf.

55. FAO. *The State of World Fisheries and Aquaculture 2010*. Rome, FAO. 2010. www.fao.org/docrep/W6602E/w6602E09.htm.

56. Jenkins DJ et al. Are dietary recommendations for the use of fish oils sustainable? *CMAJ*. 2009;180(6):633-7.

57. Anderson DM. The Growing Problem of Harmful Algae: Tiny plants pose potent threat to those who live in and eat from the sea. *Oceanus Magazine*. Nov. 12, 2004. Updated April 6, 2011. www.whoi.edu/page.do?pid=11913&tid=282&cid=2483.

58. Yue Cottee S, Petersan P. Animal Welfare and Organic Aquaculture in Open Systems. *J Agric Environ Ethics*. 2009;22:437–461. www.humanesociety.org/assets/pdfs/farm/organic_aquaculture.pdf.

59. HSUS. *An HSUS Report: The Welfare of Animals in the Aquaculture Industry*. www.humanesociety.org/assets/pdfs/farm/hsus-the-welfare-of-animals-in-the-aquaculture-industry-1.pdf.

60. WWF. Eating the Earth – graphic. http://assets.panda.org/img/original/good_diet_infographic.png

61. WWF. *Living Planet Report 2012*. http://awsassets.panda.org/downloads/1_lpr_2012_online_full_size_single_pages_final_120516.pdf

62. Attenborough D. "This heaving planet." *New Statesman*. April 27, 2011. www.newstatesman.com/environment/2011/04/human-population-essay-food

63. Leopold A. *"The Land Ethic"*. In Environmental Ethics: the big questions. Ed. Keller D. Singapore: Blackwell Publishing Ltd, 2010.

64. UNEP. *Assessing the Environmental Impacts of Consumption and Production: Priority Products and Materials*, A Report of the Working Group on the Environmental Impacts of Products and Materials to the International Panel for Sustainable Resource Management. 2010. www.unep.org/resourcepanel/Portals/24102/PDFs/PriorityProductsAndMaterials_Report.pdf

65. Carcus, Felicity. UN urges global move to meat and dairy-free diet. *Guardian.co.uk*. June 2, 2010. http://www.guardian.co.uk/environment/2010/jun/02/un-report-meat-free-diet

66. Foley JA. Can we feed the world? *Scientific American*. November 2011:60-65.

67. Seung-Ki M et al. Human contribution to more intense precipitation extremes. *Nature*. 2011;V470:378–381.

68. Pall P et al. Anthropogenic greenhouse gas contribution to flood risk in England and Wales in autumn 2000. *Nature*. 2011;V470:382–385.

69. HSUS. *An HSUS Report: The Impact of Animal Agriculture on Global Warming and Climate Change*. White Papers. www.humanesociety.org/assets/pdfs/farm/animal-agriculture-and-climate.pdf

70. Steinfeld H et al. *Livestock's Long Shadow: Environmental Issues and Options*. Food and Agriculture Organization of the United Nations. 2006.

71. Food and Agriculture Organization of the United Nations. 2010. FAOSTAT. http://faostat.fao.org

72. Koneswaran G, Nierenberg D. Global Farm Animal Production and Global Warming: Impacting and Mitigating Climate Change.

Environmental Health Perspectives. 2008;116(5):578-582. ftp://ftp.fao.org/docrep/fao/010/a0701e/a0701e00.pdf

73. United Nations. *Kyoto Protocol to the United Nations Framework Convention on Climate Change.* Kyoto. Dec. 11, 1997. www.un.org/millennium/law/xxvii-23.htm

74. Weber CL, Matthews HS. Food miles and the relative climate impacts of food choices in the United States. *Enviro Sci & Techn.* 2008;42(10):3508-3513.

75. Powell R. Eat less meat to help the environment, UN climate expert says. *The Telegraph News.* Sept. 7, 2008. www.telegraph.co.uk/news/uknews/2699173/Eat-less-red-meat-to-help-the-environment-UN-climate-expert-says.html

76. Pachauri RK. Meat Production and Climate Change. Powerpoint presentation. Sept. 8, 2008. www.scribd.com/doc/13095652/Dr-Pachauri-Meat-Production-and-Climate-Change

77. Weise Elizabeth. Eating can be energy efficient too. *USA Today.* April 21, 2009. www.usatoday.com/news/nation/environment/2009-04-21-carbon-diet_N.htm

78. King SS, McLaughlin RA. *Soil Facts: Fiber Check Dams and Ployacrylamide for Water Quality Improvement.* North Carolina Cooperative Extension. www.soil.ncsu.edu/publications/Soilfacts/AG439-71W.pdf

79. Pimental D et al. Water resources: Agricultural and environmental issues. *Biosciences.* 2004; 54:909-918.

80. U.S. Environmental Protection Agency. *National Pollutant Discharge Elimination System permit regulation and effluent limitation guidelines and standards for concentrated animal feeding operations (CAFOs); final rule.* Federal Register. Feb. 12, 2003;68(29).

81. U.S. Environmental Protection Agency. *Risk Management Evaluation for Concentrated Animal Feeding Operations.* U.S. EPA National Risk Management Laboratory. May 2004:7. www.epa.gov/nrmrl/pubs/600r04042/600r04042.pdf

82. Schrum C. Hog Confinements Kill Communities: How Industrial-sized Hog Lots are Destroying Rural Iowa. *The Iowa Source.* September 2005. www.iowasource.com/health/CAFO_people_0905.html

83. HSUS. *An HSUS Report: Factory Farming in America: The True Cost of Animal Agribusiness for Rural Communities, Public Health, Families, Farmers, the Environment, and Animals.* White Papers. www.humanesociety.org/assets/pdfs/farm/hsus-factory-farming-in-america-the-true-cost-of-animal-agribusiness.pdf

84. Nikiforuk A. When Water Kills. Maclean's. 2000;113(24),18-21.

85. Gollehon N et al. Confined animal production and manure nutrients. U.S. Department of Agriculture Economic Research Service. *Agriculture Information Bulletin* No. 771. 2001. www.ers.usda.gov/publications/aib771/aib771.pdf

86. Gilchrist MJ et al. The potential role of concentrated animal feeding operations in infectious disease epidemics and antibiotic resistance. *Environ Health Perspect.* 2007;115(2):313-6.

87. Epstein SS. *A Ban on Hormonal Meat is Three Decades Overdue.* February 2010 www.preventcancer.com/publications/ipublications.php

88. Hogan M, Draggan S. *Overgrazing.* In: Encyclopedia of Earth. Eds. Cutler J. Cleveland (Washington DC.: Environmental Information Coalition, National Council for Science and the Environment). [First published in the Encyclopedia of Earth May 1, 2010; Last revised May 5, 2011.] www.eoearth.org/article/Overgrazing?topic=49480

89. Pimental D, Pimentel M. Sustainability of meat-based and plant-based diets and the environment. *Am J Clin Nutr.* 2003;78(suppl):660S–3S.

90. Marler JB, Wallin JR. Human Health, the Nutritional Quality of Harvested Food and Sustainable Farming Systems. *Nutrition Security Institute.* 2006. www.nutritionsecurity.org/PDF/NSI_White%20Paper_Web.pdf

91. Phillips OL et al. Drought Sensitivity of the Amazon Rainforest. Science. 2009: V323(5919): 1344-1347.

92. Union of Concerned Scientists (USC). *Scientists and NGOs: Deforestation and Degradation Responsible for Approximately 15 Percent of Global Warming Emissions.*

Nov. 6, 2009. www.ucsusa.org/news/press_release/scientists-and-ngos-0302.html

93. NASA Facts. *Tropical Deforestation. The Earth Science Enterprise Series.* November 1998. www.msu.edu/user/urquhart/professional/NASA-Deforestation.pdf

94. WWF. Amazon Alive: A Decade of Discovery 1999-2009. 2010. http://wwf.panda.org/what_we_do/where_we_work/amazon/publications/?200056/ AmazonAliveAdecadeofdiscovery1999-2009

95. Butler, Rhett. *Calculating Deforestation Figures for the Amazon.* 2010. http://rainforests.mongabay.com/amazon/deforestation_calculations.html

96. Margulis S. Causes of Deforestation of the Brazilian Amazon. World Bank Working Paper No. 22. The World Bank, Washington DC. 2004. https://openknowledge.worldbank.org/bitstream/handle/10986/15060/277150PAPER0wbwp0no1022.pdf?sequence=1

97. Nierenberg D. Cattle ranching eating up Latin American forests. *World Watch.* FindArticles.com 03 July 2011. http://findarticles.com/p/articles/mi_hb6376/is_5_18/ai_n29203941/

98. Da Silva JMC et al. "The Fate of the Amazonian Areas of Endemism." *Conservation Biology.* 2005;19.3:689-694.

99. Donham KJ. Community and occupational health concerns in pork production: A review. *Journal of Animal Science.* 2010;88(2):1-31.

100. Agrilife Extension Texas A&M. Health Hints: Safe Practices in and around Confined Spaces Health Hints. December 2009– Vol.13,No.12. http://fcs.tamu.edu/health/healthhints/2009/dec/confined-spaces.pdf

101. Patel Raj. The Value of Nothing: *How to Reshape Market Society and Redefine Democracy.* New York: St. Martin's Press, 2009.

102. Stein J. The Rise of the Power Vegans. *Bloomberg Businessweek.* Nov. 4, 2010, 5:00PM EST. www.businessweek.com/magazine/content/10_46/b4203103862097.htm

103. National Restaurant Association. What's Hot 2013 Chef Survey. www.restaurant.org/Downloads/PDFs/News-Research/WhatsHotFood2013.pdf

104. Foxnews. *Going Vegan Getting Easier.* Jan. 6, 2011. www.foxnews.com/leisure/2011/01/06/going-vegan-getting-easier-popular/www.usatoday.com/money/industries/retail/2011-01-24-trends201124_CV_N.htm

105. The Vegetarian Resource Group (VRG). *How many people are vegetarian?* www.vrg.org/nutshell/faq.htm#poll

REFERENCES FOR CHAPTER 2

Nutritional Adequacy

1. American Dietetic Association. Position of the American Dietetic Association: Vegetarian Diets. JADA. 2009;109(7):1266–1282.

2. International Federation of Red Cross and Red Crescent Societies. World Disasters Report 2011: Focus on Hunger and Malnutrition. Imprimerie Chirat, Lyons, France, 2011.

3. Rizzo NS et al. Nutrient profiles of vegetarian and nonvegetarian dietary patterns. *J Acad Nutr Diet.* 2013 Dec;113(12):1610–9.

4. Tonstad S et al. Type of vegetarian diet, body weight, and prevalence of type 2 diabetes. *Diabetes Care.* 2009; May,32(5):791–6.

5. Spencer EA et al. Diet and body mass index in 38000 EPIC-Oxford meat eaters, fish eaters, vegetarians and vegans. *Int J Obes Relat Metab Disord.* 2003;27(6):728–34.

6. Key T, Davey G. Prevalence of obesity is low in people who do not eat meat. *BMJ.* 1996 Sep 28;313(7060):816–7.

7. Rosell M et al. Weight gain over 5 years in 21,966 meat-eating, fish-eating, vege-

tarian, and vegan men and women in EP-IC-Oxford. *Int J Obes.* (Lond). 2006; 30(9):1389–96.

8. Flegal KM et al. Prevalence and Trends in Obesity Among US Adults, 1999–2008. JAMA. 2010;235–241.

9. National Institute of Diabetes and Digestive and Kidney Diseases (NIDDK) of the National Institutes of Health (NIH). Statistics related to overweight and obesity. 2010. http://win.niddk.nih.gov/statistics/

10. Davey GK et al. EPIC-Oxford: lifestyle characteristics and nutrient intakes in a cohort of 33883 meat eaters and 31546 non meat eaters in the UK. *Public Health Nutrition.* 2003;6:259–268.

11. Larsson CL, Johansson GK. Dietary intake and nutritional status of young vegans and omnivores in Sweden. *Am J Clin Nutr.* 2002;76:100–6.

12. Haddad EH et al. Dietary intake and biochemical, hematologic, and immune sta-

tus of vegans compared with nonvegetarians. *Am J Clin Nutr.* 1999;70(suppl):586–93S.

13. Draper A et al. The energy and nutrient intakes of different types of vegetarian: a case for supplements? [published erratum appears in *Br J Nutr.* 1993 Nov;70(3):812]. *Br J Nutr.* 1993; Jan;69(1):3–19.

14. Lockie AH et al. Comparison of four types of diet using clinical, laboratory and psychological studies. *J R Coll Gen Pract.* 1985;35(276):333–6.

15. Ellis FR. Montegriffo VME. Veganism, clinical findings and investigations. *Am J Clin Nutr.* 1970;23:249–55.

16. Guggenheim K et al. Composition and nutritive value of diets consumed by strict vegetarians. *Br J Nutr.* 1962;16:467–71.

17. Hardinge, MG, Stare FJ. Nutritional studies of vegetarians: 1. Nutritional, physical and laboratory studies. *J Clin Nutr.* 1954;2:73–82.

Chronic Disease

18. WHO. Global status report on noncommunicable diseases 2010. WHO Press, Geneva Switzerland. 2011.

19. World Health Organization. The global burden of chronic disease. www.who.int/nutrition/topics/2_background/en/index.html

20. WHO Study Group on Diet, Nutrition and the Prevention of Non-communicable Diseases. *Diet, Nutrition and the Prevention of Chronic Diseases.* Geneva, Tech. Report 797. World Health Organization, 1991.

21. U.S. Department of Agriculture and U.S. Department of Health and Human Services. *Dietary Guidelines for Americans, 2010.* 7th Edition, Washington DC: U.S. Government Printing Office, December 2010.

22. Mangels R et al. *The Dietitian's Guide to Vegetarian Diets: Issues and Applications.* Third Edition. Sudbury MA: Jones and Bartlett Learning, 2011.

23. Orlich MJ et al. Vegetarian dietary patterns and mortality in Adventist Health Study 2. *JAMA Intern Med.* 2013;173(13):1230-8.

Cardiovascular Disease

24. World Health Organization. Cardiovascular diseases (CVDs). Media Centre. Fact sheet No. 317. January 2011. www.who.int/mediacentre/factsheets/fs317/en/index.html

25. Hu FB. Plant-based foods and prevention of cardiovascular disease: an overview. *Am J Clin Nutr.* 2003;78(3 Suppl):544S–551S. Review.

26. Key TJ et al. Mortality in vegetarians and nonvegetarians: detailed findings from a collaborative analysis of 5 prospective studies. *Am J Clin Nutr.* 1999;70(suppl):516S–24S.

27. Thorogood M et al. Risk of death from cancer and ischaemic heart disease in meat and non-meat eaters. *BMJ.* 1994;25;308(6945):1667–70.

28. Fraser GE. Associations between diet and cancer, ischemic heart disease, and all-cause mortality in non-Hispanic white California Seventh-day Adventists. *Am J Clin Nutr.* 1999;70(suppl):532S–8S.

29. Craig WJ. Health effects of vegan diets. *Am J Clin Nutr.* 2009;89(suppl):1627S–33S.

30. Crowe FL et al. Risk of hospitalization or death from ischemic heart disease among British vegetarians and nonvegetarians: results from the EPIC-Oxford cohort study. *Am J Clin Nutr.* 2013;97(3):597–603.

31. Li D. Chemistry behind Vegetarianism. *J Agric Food Chem.* 2011;59(3):777–84.

32. Kelly BB eds. *Promoting Cardiovascular Health in the Developing World: A Critical Challenge to Achieve Global Health.* Washington DC: National Academies Press (US); 2010.

33. Draper A et al. The energy and nutrient intakes of different types of vegetarian: a case for supplements? *Br J Nutr* 1993;69(1):3–19. [published erratum appears in *Br J Nutr.* 1993;70(3):812].

34. Akesson B et al. Content of trans-octadecenoic acid in vegetarian and normal diets in Sweden, analyzed by the duplicate portion technique. *Am J Clin Nutr.* 1981;34(11):2517–20.

35. Astrup A et al. The role of reducing intakes of saturated fat in the prevention of cardio-vascular disease: where does the evidence stand in 2010? *Am J Clin Nutr.* 2011;93(4):684–8.

36. Castelli WP. Making practical sense of clinical trial data in decreasing cardiovascular risk. Am J Cardiol. 2001;88(4A):16F–20F.

37. Vinagre JC et al. Metabolism of triglyceride-rich lipoproteins and transfer of lipids to high-density lipoproteins (HDL) in vegan and omnivore subjects. *Nutr Metab Cardiovasc Dis.* 2013;23(1):61–7.

38. Levy Y et al. Consumption of eggs with meals increases the susceptibility of human plasma and low-density lipoprotein to lipid peroxidation. *Ann Nutr Metab.* 1996;40:243–51.

39. Schwab US et al. Dietary cholesterol increases the susceptibility of low density lipoprotein to oxidative modification. *Atherosclerosis.* 2000;149:83–90.

40. Trapp D et al. Could a vegetarian diet reduce exercise-induced oxidative stress? A review of the literature. *J Sports Sci.* 2010;28(12):1261–8. Review.

41. Rauma A et al. Antioxidant status in long-term adherents to a strict uncooked vegan diet. *American Society for Clinical Nutrition.* 1995;62,1221–1227.

42. Krajcovicová-Kudlácková M et al. Lipid peroxidation and nutrition. *Physiol Res.* 2004;53(2):219–24.

43. Szeto YT et al. Effects of a long-term vegetarian diet on biomarkers of antioxidant status and cardiovascular disease risk. *Nutrition.* 2004;20(10):863–6.

44. Benzie IF, Wachtel-Galor S. Vegetarian diets and public health: biomarker and redox connections. *Antioxid Redox Signal.* 2010;13(10):1575–91.

45. Ahluwalia N et al. Iron status is associated with carotid atherosclerotic plaques in middle-aged adults. *J Nutr.* 2010; Apr; 140(4):812–6.

46. Aderibigbe OR et al. The relationship between indices of iron status and selected anthropometric cardiovascular disease risk markers in an African population: the THUSA study. *Cardiovasc J Afr.* 2011;22(5):249–56.

47. Sanders TA, Key TJ. Blood pressure, plasma renin activity and aldosterone concentrations in vegans and omnivore controls. *Hum Nutr Appl Nutr.* 1987;41(3):204–11.

48. Toohey ML et al. Cardiovascular disease risk factors are lower in African-American vegans compared to lacto-ovo-vegetarians. *J Am Coll Nutr.* 1998;17(5):425–34.

49. Li D et al. The association of diet and thrombotic risk factors in healthy male vegetarians and meat eaters. *Eur J Clin Nutr.* 1999;53(8):612–9.

50. Sacks FM et al. Stability of blood pressure in vegetarians receiving dietary protein supplements. *Hypertension.* 1984;6(2 Pt1):199–201.

51. Appleby PN et al. Hypertension and blood pressure among meat eaters, fish eaters,

vegetarians and vegans in EPIC-Oxford. *Public Health Nutr.* 2002;5(5):645–54.

52. Fraser GE. Vegetarian diets: what do we know of their effects on common chronic diseases? *Am J Clin Nutr.* 2009;89(5):1607S–1612S. Review. Erratum in: *Am J Clin Nutr.* 2009;90(1):248.

53. Pettersen BJ et al. Vegetarian diets and blood pressure among white subjects: results from the Adventist Health Study-2 (AHS-2). *Public Health Nutr.* 2012 Jan;10:1–8.

54. Sacks FM et al. Blood pressure in vegetarians. *Am. J. Epidemiol.* 1974;100:390–8.

55. Armstrong B et al. Blood pressure in Seventh-Day Adventist vegetarians. *Am. J. Epidemiol.* 1977;105:444–9.

56. Armstrong B et al. Urinary sodium and blood pressure in vegetarians. *Am J Clin Nutr.* 1979;32:2472–6.

57. Rouse IL et al. The relationship of blood pressure to diet and lifestyle in two religious populations. *J. Hypertens.* 1983;1:65–71.

58. Liu JC et al. Long-Chain Omega-3 Fatty Acids and Blood Pressure. *Am J Hypertens.* 2011;24(10):1121–6.

59. Houston MC. Role of mercury toxicity in hypertension, cardiovascular disease, and stroke. *J Clin Hypertens.* (Greenwich). 2011;13(8):621–7.

60. Tonstad S et al. Vegetarian diets and incidence of diabetes in the Adventist Health Study-2. *Nutr Metab Cardiovasc Dis.* 2013;23(4):292–9.

61. Ridker PM. Cardiology Patient Page. C-reactive protein: a simple test to help predict risk of heart attack and stroke. *Circulation.* 2003 Sep 23;108(12):e81–5.

62. Chen CW et al. Total cardiovascular risk profile of Taiwanese vegetarians. *Eur J Clin Nutr.* 2008 Jan;62(1):138–44.

63. Szeto YT et al. Effects of a long-term vegetarian diet on biomarkers of antioxidant status and cardiovascular disease risk. *Nutrition.* 2004 Oct;20(10):863–6.

64. Paalani M, Lee JW, Haddad E et al. Determinants of inflammatory markers in a bi-ethnic population. *Ethn Dis.* 2011 Spring;21(2):142–9.

65. Krajcovicova-Kudlackova M, Blazicek P. C-reactive protein and nutrition. *Bratisl Lek Listy.* 2005;106(11):345–7.

66. Chen CW et al. Taiwanese female vegetarians have lower lipoprotein-associated phospholipase A2 compared with omnivores. *Yonsei Med J.* 2011 Jan;52(1):13–9.

67. Fontana L et al. Long-term low-calorie low-protein vegan diet and endurance exercise are associated with low cardiometabolic risk. *Rejuvenation Res.* 2007;10:225–34.

68. Rauma AL et al. Antioxidant status in long-term adherents to a strict uncooked vegan diet. *Am J Clin Nutr.* 1995;(6):1221–7.

69. Rauma AL, Mykkänen H. Antioxidant status in vegetarians versus omnivores. *Nutrition.* 2000;16(2):111–9. Review.

70. Waldmann A et al. Dietary intakes and blood concentrations of antioxidant vitamins in German vegans. *Int J Vitam Nutr Res.* 2005 Jan;75(1):28–36.

71. Krajcovicova-Kudlackova M et al. Free radical disease prevention and nutrition. *Bratisl Lek Listy.* 2003;104(2):64–8.

72. Krajcovicová-Kudláčková M, Dusinská M. Oxidative DNA damage in relation to nutrition. *Neoplasma.* 2004;51(1):30–3.

73. Verhagen H et al. Effect of a vegan diet on biomarkers of chemoprevention in females. *Hum Exp Toxicol.* 1996;15(10):821–5.

74. Haldar S et al. Influence of habitual diet on antioxidant status: a study in a population of vegetarians and omnivores. *Eur J Clin Nutr.* 2007;61(8):1011–22.

75. Nagyová A et al. LDL oxidizability and anti-oxidative status of plasma in vegetarians. *Ann Nutr Metab.* 1998;42(6):328–32.

76. Kesse-Guyot E et al. Associations between dietary patterns and arterial stiffness, carotid artery intima-media thickness and atherosclerosis. European Journal of Cardiovascular Prevention & Rehabilitation. 2010; 17(6):718–724.

77. Yang SY et al. Relationship of carotid intima-media thickness and duration of vegetarian diet in Chinese male vegetarians. *Nutr Metab.* (Lond). 2011;8(1):63.

78. Kwok T et al. Vitamin B-12 supplementation improves arterial function in vegetarians with subnormal vitamin B-12 status. *J Nutr Health Aging.* 2012;16(6):569–73.

79. Koeth RA et al. Intestinal microbiota metabolism of L-carnitine, a nutrient in red meat, promotes atherosclerosis. *Nat Med.* 2013;19(5):576–85.

80. Antoniades C, Antonopoulos AS, Tousoulis D, Marinou K, Stefanadis C. Homocysteine and coronary atherosclerosis: from folate fortification to the recent clinical trials. *Eur Heart J.* 2009;30(1):6–15.

81. Veeranna V et al. Homocysteine and re-classification of cardiovascular disease risk. J Am Coll Cardiol. 2011;58:1025–1033.

82. Toole JF et al. Lowering homocysteine in patients with ischemic stroke to prevent recurrent stroke, myocardial infarction, and death: the Vitamin Intervention for Stroke Prevention (VISP) randomized controlled trial. *JAMA.* 2004;291(5):565–75.

83. Bazzano LA, Reynolds K, Holder KN, He J. Effect of folic acid supplementation on risk of cardiovascular diseases: a meta-analysis of randomized controlled trials. *JAMA.* 2006;296(22):2720–6.

84. Bønaa KH et al; NORVIT Trial Investigators. Homocysteine lowering and cardiovascular events after acute myocardial infarction. N Engl J Med. 2006;354(15):1578–88.

85. Albert CM et al. Effect of folic acid and B vitamins on risk of cardiovascular events and total mortality among women at high risk for cardiovascular disease: a randomized trial. *JAMA.* 2008;299(17):2027–36.

86. Ebbing M et al. Mortality and cardiovascular events in patients treated with homocysteine-lowering B vitamins after coronary angiography: a randomized controlled trial. *JAMA.* 2008;300(7):795–804.

87. Khandanpour N et al. Homocysteine and peripheral arterial disease: systematic review and meta-analysis. *Eur J Vasc Endovasc Surg.* 2009;38(3):316–22. Review.

88. Song Y et al. Effect of homocysteine-lowering treatment with folic Acid and B vitamins on risk of type 2 diabetes in women: a randomized, controlled trial. *Diabetes.* 2009;58(8):1921–8.

89. Loland KH et al. Effect of homocysteine-lowering B vitamin treatment on angiographic progression of coronary artery disease: a Western Norway B Vitamin Intervention Trial (WENBIT) substudy. *Am J Cardiol.* 2010;105(11):1577–84.

90. VITATOPS Trial Study Group. B vitamins in patients with recent transient ischaemic attack or stroke in the VITAmins TO Prevent Stroke (VITATOPS) trial: a randomised, double-blind, parallel, placebo-controlled trial. *Lancet Neurol.* 2010;9(9):855–65.

91. Armitage JM et al. Study of the Effectiveness of Additional Reductions in Cholesterol and Homocysteine (SEARCH) Collaborative Group. Effects of homocysteine-lowering with folic acid plus vitamin B_{12} vs placebo on mortality and major morbidity in myocardial infarction survivors: a randomized trial. *JAMA.* 2010;303(24):2486–94.

92. Holmes MV et al. Effect modification by population dietary folate on the association between MTHFR genotype, homocysteine, and stroke risk: a meta-analysis of genetic studies and randomised trials. *Lancet.* 2011;378(9791):584–94.

93. Wang X et al. Efficacy of folic acid supplementation in stroke prevention: a meta-analysis. *Lancet.* 2007;369(9576):1876–82.

94. Lonn E *et al*: Homocysteine lowering with folic acid and B vitamins in vascular disease. *NEJM.* 2006;354(15):1567–1577.

95. Saposnik G et al. Heart Outcomes Prevention Evaluation 2 Investigators. Homocysteine-lowering therapy and stroke risk, severity, and disability: additional findings from the HOPE 2 trial. *Stroke.* 2009;40(4):1365–72.

96. Lee M et al. Efficacy of homocysteine-lowering therapy with folic acid in stroke prevention: a meta-analysis. *Stroke.* 2010; 41(6):1205–12.

97. Selhub J et al. The use of blood concentrations of vitamins and their respective functional indicators to define folate and vitamin B_{12} status. *Food Nutr Bull.* 2008;29(2 Suppl):S67–73.

98. Oh RC, Brown DL. Vitamin B12 Deficiency. *Am Fam Physician.* 2003;67(5):979–986.

99. Li D et al. Platelet phospholipid n-3 PUFA negatively associated with plasma homocysteine in middle-aged and geriatric hyperlipaemia patients. *Prostaglandins Leukot Essent Fatty Acids.* 2007;76(5):293–7.

100. Haines AP et al. Hemostatic variables in vegetarians and non-vegetarians. *Thromb Res.*1980;19:139–48.

101. Mezzano D et al. Vegetarians and cardiovascular risk factors: hemostasis, inflammatory markers and plasma homocysteine. *Thromb Haemost.* 1999;81:913–7.

102. Li D et al. The association of diet and thrombotic risk factors in healthy male vegetarians and meat eaters. *Eur J Clin Nutr.* 1999;53:612–619.

103. Famodu AA et al. The influence of a vegetarian diet on haemostatic risk factors for cardiovascular disease in Africans. *Thromb Res.* 1999;95:31–6.

104. Ernst E et al. Blood rheology in vegetarians. *Br J Nutr.* 1986;56(3):555–60.

105. Pan W-H et al. Hemostatic factors and blood lipids in young Buddhist vegetarians and omnivores. *Am J Clin Nutr.* 1993;58:354–9.

106. Leu M, Giovannucci E. Vitamin D: Epidemiology of cardiovascular risks and events. *Best Pract Res Clin Endocrinol Metab.* 2011;25(4):633–46.

107. Pilz S et al. Vitamin D, cardiovascular disease and mortality. *Clin Endocrinol.* (Oxf). 2011;25(4):633–46.

108. Artaza JN et al. Vitamin D and the cardiovascular system. *Clin J Am Soc Nephrol.* 2009;4(9):1515–22.

109. Ferdowsian H et al. A Multicomponent Intervention Reduces Body Weight and Cardiovascular Risk at a GEICO Corporate Site. *American Journal of Health Promotion.* [serial online]. 2010;24(6):384–387.

110. Ornish D et al. Can lifestyle changes reverse coronary heart disease? The Lifestyle Heart Trial. *Lancet.* 1990;336:129–33.

111. Ornish D. Avoiding revascularization with lifestyle changes: the Multicenter Lifestyle Demonstration Project. *Am J Cardiol.* 1998;82:72T–6T.

112. Ornish D et al. Intensive lifestyle changes for reversal of coronary heart disease. *JAMA.* 1998;280:2001–7. (5-year follow-up).

113. Esselstyn CB. Updating a 12-year experience with arrest and reversal therapy for coronary heart disease (an overdue requiem for palliative cardiology). *Am J Cardiol.* 1999;84:339–41,A8.

114. Esselstyn CB Jr., Gendy G, Doyle J et al. A way to reverse CAD? *The Journal of Family Practice.* 2014;63(7):356-364b.

115. Ellis FR, Sanders T. Letter: Angina and vegetarian diet. *Lancet.* 1976;1:1190.

116. Ellis FR, Sanders TA. Angina and vegan diet. *Am Heart J.* 1977;93:803–5.

117. Jenkins DJ et al. Effect of a diet high in vegetables, fruit, and nuts on serum lipids. *Metabolism.* 1997;46:530 –537.

118. Jenkins DJ et al. The effect of combining plant sterols, soy protein, viscous fibers, and almonds in treating hypercholesterolemia. *Metabolism.* 2003;52:1478–1483.

119. Jenkins DJ et al. Effects of a dietary portfolio of cholesterol-lowering foods vs lovastatin on serum lipids and C-reactive protein. *JAMA.* 2003;290:502–510.

120. Jenkins DJ et al. Direct comparison of a dietary portfolio of cholesterol-lowering foods with a statin in hypercholesterolemic participants. *Am J Clin Nutr.* 2005;81:380–387.

121. Jenkins DJ et al. Assessment of the longer-term effects of a dietary portfolio of cholesterol lowering foods in hypercholesterolemia. *Am J Clin Nutr.* 2006;83: 582–591.

122. Koebnick C et al. Long-term consumption of a raw food diet is associated with favorable serum LDL cholesterol and triglycerides but also with elevated plasma homocysteine and low serum HDL cholesterol in humans. *J Nutr.* 2005;135(10): 2372–8.

123. Agren JJ et al. Divergent changes in serum sterols during a strict uncooked vegan diet in patients with rheumatoid arthritis. *Br J Nutr.* 2001;85:137–9.

124. Hanninen O et al. Effects of eating an un-cooked vegetable diet for 1 week. *Appetite.* 1992;19:243–54.

Cancer

126. Vossenaar M et al. Agreement between di-etary and lifestyle guidelines for cancer prevention in population samples of Eu-ropeans and Mesoamericans. *Nutrition.* 2011;27(11–12):1146–55.

127. Jemal A et al. Global cancer statistics. *CA Cancer J Clin.* 2011;61(2):69–90.

128. Lanou AJ, Svenson B. Reduced cancer risk in vegetarians: an analysis of recent reports. *Cancer Manag Res.* 2010;3:1–8.

129. Anand P et al. Cancer is a Preventable Dis-ease that Requires Major Lifestyle Chang-es. *Pharm Res.* 2008;25(9):2097–116.

130. World Cancer Research Fund in Associa-tion with American Institute of Cancer Re-search. *Food, Nutrition and the Prevention of Cancer: a Global Perspective.* Menasha WI: Banta Book Group, 1997.

131. World Cancer Research Fund/American In-stitute for Cancer Research. *Food, Nutri-tion, Physical Activity and the Prevention of Cancer: A Global Perspective.* Washing-ton DC: AICR, 2007.

132. Colditz GA et al. Physical activity and re-duced risk of colon cancer: implications for prevention. *Cancer Causes Control.* 1997;8:649–67.

133. Aune D et al. Dietary fibre, whole grains, and risk of colorectal cancer: systematic review and dose-response meta-analysis of prospective studies. *BMJ.* 2011;343.

134. WCRF CUP Press releases. Most author-itative ever report on bowel cancer and diet: Links with meat and fibre confirmed. 23 May 2011 www.wcrf-uk.org/audience/media/press_release.php?recid=153

135. Willet W. Eat like it matters. How diet can prevent disease. *Nutrition Action.* October 2011, page 3.

136. Tantamango-Bartley Y et al. Vegetarian di-ets and the incidence of cancer in a low-risk population. *Cancer Epidemiol Biomarkers Prev.* 2013;22(2):286–94.

125. Hanninen O et al. Vegan diet in physiolog-ical health promotion. *Acta Physiol Hung.* 1999;86:171–80.

137. Key TJ, Appleby PN, Crowe FL, et al. Cancer in British vegetarians: updated analyses of 4998 incident cancers in a co-hort of 32,491 meat eaters, 8612 fifish eat-ers, 18,298 vegetarians, and 2246 vegans. *Am J Clin Nutr.* 2014;100(Supplement 1):378S-385S.

138. Ornish D et al. Intensive lifestyle changes may affect the progression of prostate can-cer. *Journal of Urology.* 2005;174(3): 1065–70.

139. Fontana L et al. Long-term low-protein, low-calorie diet and endurance exercise modu-late metabolic factors associated with cancer risk. *Am J Clin Nutr.* 2006;84(6): 1456–62.

140. Allen NE et al. The Associations of Diet with Serum Insulin-like Growth Factor I and Its Main Binding Proteins in 292 Women Meat eaters, Vegetarians, and Vegans. *Cancer Epidemiology, Biomarkers & Prevention.* 2002;11,1441–1448.

141. Ling WH, Hanninen O. Shifting from a con-ventional diet to an uncooked vegan diet re-versibly alters fecal hydrolytic activities in humans. *J Nutr.* 1992;122(4):924–30.

142. Gaisbauer M et al. [Raw food and immu-nity] [Article in German]. *Fortschr Med.* 1990;108(17):338–40.

143. Peltonen R et al. An uncooked vegan diet shifts the profile of human fecal microflora: computerized analysis of direct stool sample gas-liquid chromatography profiles of bac-terial cellular fatty acids. *Applied and Envi-ronmental Microbiology.* 1992; 58:3660–6.

144. Peltonen, R et al. Faecal microbial flora and disease activity in rheumatoid arthri-tis during a vegan diet. *British Journal of Rheumatology.* 1997; 36:64–68.

145. Ryhanan EL et al. Modification of faecal flora in rheumatoid arthritis patients by lactobacilli rich vegetarian diet. *Milchwis-senschaft.* 1993;48(5):255–259.

146. Nenonen, MT et al. Uncooked, lactoba-cilli-rich, vegan food and rheumatoid arthritis. *British Journal of Rheumatology.* 1998;37:274–281.

147. Key TJ. Endogenous oestrogens and breast cancer risk in premenopausal and postmenopausal women. *Steroids.* 2011;76(8): 812–5.

148. Karelis AD et al. Comparison of sex hormonal and metabolic profiles between omnivores and vegetarians in pre- and postmenopausal women. *Br J Nutr.* 2010;104(2): 222–6.

149. Goldin BR et al. Estrogen excretion patterns and plasma levels in vegetarian and omnivorous women. *N Engl J Med.* 1982 Dec 16;307(25):1542–7.

150. Adlercreutz H et al. Urinary estrogen profile determination in young Finnish vegetarian and omnivorous women. *J Steroid Biochem.* 1986;24(1):289–96.

151. Thomas HV et al. Oestradiol and sex hormone-binding globulin in premenopausal and post-menopausal meat eaters, vegetarians and vegans. *Br J Cancer.* 1999;80(9):1470–5.

152. van Faassen A et al. Bile acids and pH values in total feces and in fecal water from habitually omnivorous and vegetarian subjects. *Am J Clin Nutr.* 1993;58(6):917–22.

153. Reddy S et al. Faecal pH, bile acid and sterol concentrations in premenopausal Indian and white vegetarians compared with white omnivores. *Br J Nutr.* 1998;79(6):495–500.

154. Korpela JT et al. Fecal free and conjugated bile acids and neutral sterols in vegetarians, omnivores, and patients with colorectal cancer. *Scand J Gastroenterol.* 1988;23(3):277–83.

155. Turjman N et al. Diet, nutrition intake, and metabolism in populations at high and low risk for colon cancer. Metabolism of bile acids. *Am J Clin Nutr.* 1984;40(4 Suppl):937–41.

156. Thornton JR. High colonic pH promotes colo-rectal cancer. *Lancet.* 1981;1(8229): 1081–3.

157. Lewin MH et al. Red meat enhances the colonic formation of the DNA adduct O6-carboxymethyl guanine: implications for colorectal cancer risk. *Cancer Res.* 2006;66(3):1859–65.

158. Birkett AM et al. Dietary intake and faecal excretion of carbohydrate by Australians: importance of achieving stool weights greater than 150 g to improve faecal markers relevant to colon cancer risk. *Eur J Clin Nutr.* 1997;51(9):625–32.

159. Davies GJ et al. Bowel function measurements of individuals with different eating patterns. *Gut.* 1986;27(2):164–9.

160. Reddy BS et al. Fecal factors which modify the formation of fecal co-mutagens in high- and low-risk population for colon cancer. *Cancer Lett.* 1980;10(2):123–32.

161. Kuhnlein U et al. Mutagens in feces from vegetarians and non-vegetarians. *Mutat Res.* 1981;85(1):1–12.

162. Johansson G et al. The effect of a shift from a mixed diet to a lacto-vegetarian diet on human urinary and fecal mutagenic activity. *Carcinogenesis.* 1992;13(2):153–7.

163. Johansson G et al. Long-term effects of a change from a mixed diet to a lacto-vegetarian diet on human urinary and faecal mutagenic activity. *Mutagenesis.* 1998; 13(2):167–71.

164. de Kok TM et al. Fecapentaene excretion and fecal mutagenicity in relation to nutrient intake and fecal parameters in humans on omnivorous and vegetarian diets. *Cancer Lett.* 1992;62(1):11–21.

165. Krajcovicová-Kudlácková M et al. Effects of diet and age on oxidative damage products in healthy subjects. *Physiol Res.* 2008; 57(4): 647–51.

166. Sebeková K et al. Association of metabolic syndrome risk factors with selected markers of oxidative status and microinflammation in healthy omnivores and vegetarians. *Mol Nutr Food Res.* 2006;50(9):858-68.

167. Krajcovicova-Kudlackova M et al. Lipid and antioxidant blood levels in vegetarians. *Nahrung.* 1996;40(1):17–20.

168. Rauma A, Mykkanen H. Antioxidant status in vegetarians versus omnivores. *Nutrition.* 2000;16:111–119.

169. Rauma A et al. Antioxidant status in long-term adherents to a strict uncooked vegan diet. *American Society for Clinical Nutrition.* 1995;62:1221–1227.

170. Link LB, Potter JD. Raw versus cooked vegetables and cancer risk. *Cancer Epidemiol Biomarkers Prev.* 2004;13(9):1422–35.Review.

171. Oseni T et al. Selective Estrogen Receptor Modulators and Phytoestrogens *Planta Med.* 2008;74(13):1656–1665.

172. Chen X, Anderson JJB. Isoflavones and bone: Animal and human evidence of efficacy. *J Musculoskel Neuron Interact* 2002; 2(4):352–359.

173. Hilakivi-Clarke L et al. Is soy consumption good or bad for the breast? *J Nutr.* 2010;140(12):2326S–2334S.

174. Korde LA et al. Childhood soy intake and breast cancer risk in Asian-American women. *Cancer Epidemiol Biomarkers Prev.* 2009;18:1050–9.

175. Shu XO et al. Soyfood intake during adolescence and subsequent risk of breast cancer among Chinese women. *Cancer Epidemiol Biomarkers Prev.* 2001;10:483–8.

176. Wu AH et al. Adolescent and adult soy intake and risk of breast cancer in Asian-Americans. *Carcinogenesis.* 2002;23: 1491–6.

177. Thanos J et al. Adolescent dietary phytoestrogen intake and breast cancer risk (Canada). *Cancer Causes Control.* 2006;17: 1253–61.

178. Lee SA et al. Adolescent and adult soy food intake and breast cancer risk: results from the Shanghai Women's Health Study. *Am J Clin Nutr.* 2009;89:1920–6.

179. Butler LM et al. A vegetable-fruit-soy dietary pattern protects against breast cancer among postmenopausal Singapore Chinese women. *Am J Clin Nutr.* 2010 ;91(4): 1013–9.

180. Wu AH et al. Soy intake and breast cancer risk in Singapore Chinese health study. *Br J Cancer.* 2008;99(1):196–200.

181. Yamamoto S et al; Japan Public Health Center-Based Prospective Study on Cancer Cardiovascular Diseases Group. Soy, isoflavones, and breast cancer risk in Japan. *J Natl Cancer Inst.* 2003;95(12):906–13.

182. Travis RC et al. A prospective study of vegetarianism and isoflavone intake in relation to breast cancer risk in British women. *Int J Cancer.* 2008;122(3):705–10.

183. Trock BJ et al. Meta-analysis of soy intake and breast cancer risk. *J Natl Cancer Inst.* 2006 Apr 5;98(7):459–71.

184. Setchell KD, Cole SJ. Method of defining equol-producer status and its frequency among vegetarians. *J Nutr.* 2006;136(8): 2188–93.

185. Lampe JW. Emerging research on equol and cancer. *J Nutr.* 2010 Jul;140(7):1369S–72S. Review.

186. Caan BJ et al. Soy Food Consumption and Breast Cancer Prognosis. *Cancer Epidemiol Biomarkers Prev.* 2011;20(5):854–8.

187. Kang X et al. Effect of soy isoflavones on breast cancer recurrence and death for patients receiving adjuvant endocrine therapy. *CMAJ.* 2010;182(17):1857–62.

188. Shu XO et al. Soy food intake and breast cancer survival. *JAMA.* 2009;302(22): 2437–43.

189. Guha N et al. Soy isoflavones and risk of cancer recurrence in a cohort of breast cancer survivors: the Life After Cancer Epidemiology study. *Breast Cancer Res Treat.* 2009;118(2):395–405.

190. Fink BN et al. Dietary flavonoid intake and breast cancer survival among women on Long Island. *Cancer Epidemiol Biomarkers Prev.* 2007;16(11):2285–92.

191. Boyapati SM et al. Soyfood intake and breast cancer survival: a followup of the Shanghai Breast Cancer Study. *Breast Cancer Res Treat.* 2005;92(1):11–7.

192. Zhang YF et al. Positive effects of soy isoflavone food on survival of breast cancer patients in China. *Asian Pac J Cancer Prev.* 2012;13(2):479–82.

193. Woo HD et al. Differential Influence of Dietary Soy Intake on the Risk of Breast Cancer Recurrence Related to HER2 Status. *Nutr Cancer.* 2012;64(2):198–205.

194. Nechuta SJ et al. Soy food intake after diagnosis of breast cancer and survival: an in-depth analysis of combined evidence from cohort studies of US and Chinese women. *Am J Clin Nutr.* 2012;96(1):123–32.

195. Chi F et al. Post-diagnosis soy food intake and breast cancer survival: a meta-analysis of cohort studies. *Asian Pac J Cancer Prev.* 2013;14(4):2407–12.

196. Ko KP et al. Dietary intake and breast cancer among carriers and noncarriers of BRCA mutations in the Korean Hereditary Breast Cancer Study. *Am J Clin Nutr.* 2013 Oct. 23. [Epub ahead of print].

197. van Die MD et al. Soy and soy isoflavones in prostate cancer: a systematic review and meta-analysis of randomised controlled trials. *BJU Int.* 2013 Sep 5. [Epub ahead of print].

198. Ahmad IU et al. Soy isoflavones in conjunction with radiation therapy in patients with prostate cancer. *Nutr Cancer.* 2010;62(7):996–1000.

199. Yan L, Spitznagel EL. Soy consumption and prostate cancer risk in men: a revisit of a meta-analysis. *Am J Clin Nutr.* 2009; 89:1155–63.

Diabetes

200. Centers for Disease Control and Prevention. Long-term Trends in Diabetes. Slide Show. October 2010. www.cdc.gov/diabetes/statistics/slides/long_term_trends.pdf

201. Centers for Disease Control and Prevention. *National Diabetes Statistics Report: Estimates of Diabetes and Its Burden in the United States, 2014.* Atlanta, GA: U.S. Department of Health and Human Services; 2014.

202. Salas-Salvadó J et al. The role of diet in the prevention of type 2 diabetes. *Nutr Metab Cardiovasc Dis.* 2011;21Suppl 2:B32 Chen X, Anderson JJ. Isoflavones and bone: animal and human evidence of efficacy. *Interact.* 2002;2(4):352–9.

Link LB, Potter JD. Raw versus cooked vegetables and cancer risk. *Cancer Epidemiol Biomarkers Prev.* 2004;13(9):1422–35. Review.

203. Tonstad S et al. Vegetarian diets and incidence of diabetes in the Adventist Health Study-2. *Nutr Metab Cardiovasc Dis.* 2013; 23(4):292-9.

204. Chiu T, et al. Taiwanese vegetarians and omnivores: dietary composition, prevalence of diabetes and IFG. *PLoS One.* 2014 Feb. 11;9(2):e88547.

205. Goff LM et al. Veganism and its relationship with insulin resistance and intramyocellular lipid. *Eur J Clin Nutr.* 2005;59(2):291–8.

206. Barnard ND et al. The effects of a low-fat, plant-based dietary intervention on body weight, metabolism, and insulin sensitivity. *Am J Med.* 2005;118(9):991–7.

207. Waldmann A et al. Overall glycemic index and glycemic load of vegan diets in relation to plasma lipoproteins and triacylglycerols. *Ann Nutr Metab.* 2007;51(4):335–44.

208. Crane MG, Sample C. Regression of diabetic neuropathy with total vegetarian (vegan) diet. *Journal of Nutritional Medicine.* 1994;4(4):431.

209. Kahleova H et al. Vegetarian diet improves insulin resistance and oxidative stress markers more than conventional diet in subjects with Type 2 diabetes. *Diabet Med.* 2011;28(5):549–59.

210. Nicholson AS et al. Toward improved management of NIDDM: A randomized, controlled, pilot intervention using a lowfat, vegetarian diet. *Prev Med.* 1999;29(2): 87–91.

211. Barnard ND et al. A low-fat vegan diet improves glycemic control and cardiovascular risk factors in a randomized clinical trial in individuals with type 2 diabetes. *Diabetes Care.* 2006;29(8):1777–83.

212. Barnard ND et al. A low-fat vegan diet and a conventional diabetes diet in the treatment of type 2 diabetes: a randomized, controlled, 74-wk clinical trial. *Am J Clin Nutr.* 2009;89(suppl):1S–9S.

213. Barnard ND et al. A low-fat vegan diet elicits greater macronutrient changes, but is comparable in adherence and acceptability, compared with a more conventional diabetes diet among individuals with type 2 diabetes. *J Am Diet Assoc.* 2009;109(2):263–72.

214. Turner-McGrievy GM et al. Decreases in dietary glycemic index are related to weight loss among individuals following therapeutic diets for type 2 diabetes. *J Nutr.* 2011;141(8):1469–74.

215. Jiang R et al. Nut and peanut butter consumption and risk of type 2 diabetes in women. *JAMA.* 2002;288:2554–2560.

216. Li T et al. Regular consumption of nuts is associated with a lower risk of cardiovascular disease in women with type 2 diabetes. *J Nutr.* 2009;139(7):1333-8.

217. Griel AE, Kris-Etherton PM. Tree nuts and the lipid profile: a review of clinical studies. *Br J Nutr.* 2006;96(Suppl 2), S68–S78.

218. Jenkins DJ et al. Dose response of almonds on coronary heart disease risk factors: blood lipids, oxidized low-density lipoproteins, lipoprotein(a), homocysteine, and pulmonary nitric oxide: a randomized, controlled, crossover trial. *Circulation.* 2002;106(11):1327–32.

219. Jenkins DJ et al. Almonds decrease postprandial glycemia, insulinemia, and oxidative damage in healthy individuals. *J Nutr.* 2006;136:2987–2992.

220. Ros E. Nuts and novel biomarkers of cardiovascular disease. *Am J Clin Nutr.* 2009; 89:1649S–1656S.

221. Josse AR et al. Almonds and postprandial glycemia—a dose-response study. *Metabolism.* 2007;56, 400–404.

222. Jenkins DJ et al. Nuts as a replacement for carbohydrates in the diabetic diet. *Diabetes Care.* 2011;34(8):1706-11.

223. Kendall CW et al. The glycemic effect of nut-enriched meals in healthy and diabetic subjects. *Nutr Metab Cardiovasc Dis.* 2011;21.(Suppl 1):S34–9.

224. Kendall CW et al. Nuts, metabolic syndrome and diabetes. *Br J Nutr.* 2010;104(4): 465–73. Review.

225. Penckofer S et al. Vitamin D and diabetes: let the sunshine in. *Diabetes Educ.* 200;34(6): 939–40,942,944 passim.

226. Sahin M et al. Effects of metformin or rosiglitazone on serum concentrations of homo-cysteine, folate, and vitamin B12 in patients with type 2 diabetes mellitus. *J Diabetes Complications.* 2007;21(2):118–23.

227. Sun Y et al. Effectiveness of vitamin B12 on diabetic neuropathy: systematic review of clinical controlled trials. *Acta Neurol Taiwan.* 2005;14(2):48–54.

228. Talaei A et al. Vitamin B12 may be more effective than nortriptyline in improving painful diabetic neuropathy. *Int J Food Sci Nutr.* 2009;60.(Suppl 5):71-6.

229. Pouwer F et al. Fat food for a bad mood. Could we treat and prevent depression in Type 2 diabetes by means of omega-3 polyunsaturated fatty acids? A review of the evidence. *Diabet Med.* 2005;22(11):1465–75. Review.

230. Flachs P et al. The effect of n-3 fatty acids on glucose homeostasis and insulin sensitivity. *Physiol Res.* 2014;63.(Suppl 1):S93-S118.

Osteoporosis

231. Miller KV, Marchinton L. *Quality whitetails: the why and how of quality deer management.* Mechanicsburg PA: Stackpole Books, 1995.

232. Katz DL. *Nutrition in Clinical Practice a Comprehensive Evidence-based Manual for the Practitioner.* 2nd Edition. Philadelphia PA: Lippincott Williams and Wilkins, 2008.

233. Marsh AG et al. Vegetarian lifestyle and bone mineral density. Am J Clin Nutr. 1988;48(3 Suppl):837–41.

234. Hu JF et al. Dietary calcium and bone density among middle-aged and elderly women in China. *Am J Clin Nutr.* 1993;58(2): 219–27.

235. Parsons TJ et al. Reduced bone mass in Dutch adolescents fed a macrobiotic diet

in early life. *J Bone Miner Res.* 1997;12(9): 1486–94.

236. Johnson PK. Bone mineral status in vegan, lactoovovegetarian, and omnivorous premenopausal women CA. In: II nutritional status and life cycle issues. *Am J Clin Nutr.* 1999;70(3 Suppl):626S–9S.

237. Outila TA, Lamberg-Allardt CJ. Ergocalciferol supplementation may positively affect lumbar spine bone mineral density of vegans. *J Am Diet Assoc.* 2000;100(6):629.

238. Fontana L et al. Low bone mass in subjects on a long-term raw vegetarian diet. *Arch Intern Med.* 2005;165(6):684–9.

239. Ambroszkiewicz J et al. The influence of vegan diet on bone mineral density and biochemical bone turnover markers. *Pediatr Endocrinol Diabetes Metab.* 2010;16(3):201–4.

240. Hunt IF et al. Bone mineral content in postmenopausal women: comparison of omnivores and vegetarians. *Am J Clin Nutr.* 1989;50(3):517–23.

241. Lau E, et al. Bone mineral density in Chinese elderly female vegetarians, vegans, lacto-vegetarians and omnivores. *Eur J Clin Nutr.* 1998;52(1):60–4.

242. Barr SI et al. Spinal bone mineral density in premenopausal vegetarian and nonvegetarian women: cross-sectional and prospective comparisons. *J Am Diet Assoc.* 1998;98(7):760–5.

243. Wang YF et al. Bone mineral density of vegetarian and non-vegetarian adults in Taiwan. *Asia Pac J Clin Nutr.* 2008;17(1):101–6.

244. Ho-Pham LT et al. Effect of vegetarian diets on bone mineral density: a Bayesian meta-analysis. *Am J Clin Nutr.* 2009;90(4): 943–50.

245. Ho-Pham LT et al.Vegetarianism, bone loss, fracture and vitamin D: a longitudinal study in Asian vegans and non-vegans. *Eur J Clin Nutr.* 2012;66(1):75–82.

246. Chiu JF et al. Long-term vegetarian diet and bone mineral density in postmenopausal Taiwanese women. *Calcified Tissue International.* 1997;60:245–249.

247. Appleby P et al. Comparative fracture risk in vegetarians and nonvegetarians in EPIC-

Oxford. *Eur J Clin Nutr.* 2007;61(12): 1400–6.

248. Scerpella TA et al. Sustained skeletal benefit from childhood mechanical loading. *Osteoporos Int.* 2011;22(7):2205–2210.

249. Guadalupe-Grau A et al. Exercise and bone mass in adults. *Sports Med.* 2009;39(6): 439–68.

250. New SA. Intake of fruit and vegetables: Implications for bone health. *Proc Nutr Soc.* 2003;62:889–899.

251. Arjmandi BH, Smith BJ. Soy isoflavones' osteoprotective role in postmenopausal women: Mechanism of action. *J Nutr Biochem.* 2002;13:130–137.

252. Ma DF et al. Soy isoflavone intake increases bone mineral density in the spine of menopausal women: Meta-analysis of randomized controlled trials. *Clin Nutr.* 2008;27:57–64.

253. Fitzpatrick L, Heaney RP. Got soda? *J Bone Miner Res.* 2003;18:1570–1572.

254. Kerstetter JE et al. Dietary protein, calcium metabolism, and skeletal homeostasis revisited. *Am J Clin Nutr.* 2003;78(3 Suppl): 584S–592S.

255. NIH Osteoporosis and Related Bone Diseases: National Resource Center. Other Nutrients and Bone Health At A Glance. 2004. www.niams.nih.gov/Health_Info/ Bone/Bone_Health/Nutrition/other_nutrients.asp

256. Ströhle A et al. Diet-dependent net endogenous acid load of vegan diets in relation to food groups and bone health-related nutrients: results from the German Vegan Study. *Ann Nutr Metab.* 2011;59(2-4):117–26.

257. Turner RT, Sibonga JD. Effects of alcohol use and estrogen on bone. *Alcohol Res Health.* 2001;25(4):276-81.

258. Chakkalakal DA. Alcohol-induced bone loss and deficient bone repair. *Alcohol Clin Exp Res.* 2005;29:2077–2090.

259. Institute of Medicine. Dietary reference intakes for vitamin A, vitamin K, arsenic, boron, chromium, copper, iodine, iron, manganese, molybdenum, nickel, silicon, vanadium, and zinc. Washington DC: National Academies Press; 2001.

260. Grune T et al. Beta-carotene is an important vitamin A source for humans. *J Nutr.* 2010;140(12):2268S–2285S.

261. NIH Osteoporosis and Related Bone Diseases: National Resource Center. Osteoporosis Handout on Health 2011. www.niams.nih.gov/Health_Info/Bone/Osteoporosis/osteoporosis_hoh.asp

262. Welten DC et al. A meta-analysis of the effect of calcium intake on bone mass in young and middle aged females and males. *J Nutr.* 1995;125:2802–13.

263. Shea B et al. Meta-analyses of therapies for postmenopausal osteoporosis. VII. Meta-analysis of calcium supplementation for the prevention of postmenopausal osteoporosis *Endocr Rev.* 2002;23(4):552–9.

264. Shea B et al. Calcium supplementation on bone loss in postmenopausal women. *Cochrane Database Syst Rev.* 2004;1(1): CD004526

265. Cumming RG et al. Calcium intake and fracture risk: results from the study of osteoporotic fractures. *Am J Epidemiol.* 1997;145(10): 926–34.

266. Bischoff-Ferrari HA et al. Calcium intake and hip fracture risk in men and women: a meta-analysis of prospective cohort studies and randomized controlled trials. *Am J Clin Nutr.* 2007;86:1780–90.

267. Committee to Review Dietary Reference Intakes for Vitamin D and Calcium, Food and Nutrition Board, Institute of Medicine. *Dietary Reference Intakes for Calcium and Vitamin D.* Washington DC: National Academy Press, 2010.

268. Hegsted M et al. Urinary calcium and calcium balance in young men as affected by level of protein and phosphorus intake. *J Nutr.* 1981;111:553–562.

269. Metz JA et al. Intakes of calcium, phosphorus, and protein, and physical-activity level are related to radial bone mass in young adult women. *Am J Clin Nutr.* 1993;58:537–542.

270. Feskanich D et al. Protein consumption and bone fractures in women. *Am J Epidemiol.* 1996;143: 472–479.

271. Cooper C et al. Dietary protein intake and bone mass in women. *Calcif Tissue Int.* 1996;58:320–325.

272. Hannan MT et al. Effect of dietary protein on bone loss in elderly men and women: the Framingham Osteoporosis Study. *J Bone Miner Res.* 2000;15:2504–2512.

273. Wengreen HJ et al. Dietary protein intake and risk of osteoporotic hip fracture in elderly residents of Utah. *J Bone Miner Res.* 2004;19:537–545.

274. Darling AL, Millward DJ, Torgerson DJ et al. Dietary protein and bone health: a systematic review and meta-analysis. *Am J Clin Nutr.* 2009;90:1674–1692.

275. Fenton TR et al. Meta-analysis of the effect of the acid-ash hypothesis of osteoporosis on calcium balance. *J Bone Miner Res.* 2009;24(11):1835–40.

276. Maalouf NM et al. Hypercalciuria associated with high dietary protein intake is not due to Acid load. *J Clin Endocrinol Metab.* 2011;96(12):3733–40.

277. Thorpe MP, Evans EM. Dietary protein and bone health: harmonizing conflicting theories. *Nutrition Reviews.* 2011:69(4): 215–230.

278. Thorpe DL et al. Effects of meat consumption and vegetarian diet on risk of wrist fracture over 25 years in a cohort of peri- and postmenopausal women. *Public Health Nutr.* 2008;11(6):564-72.

Cataracts

279. Appleby PN et al. Diet, vegetarianism, and cataract risk. *Am J Clin Nutr.* 2011;93(5): 1128-35.

Dementia

280. Giem P et al. The incidence of dementia and intake of animal products: Preliminary findings from the Adventist Health Study. *Neuroepidemiology.* 1993;12:28–36.

281. Appleby PN et al. Mortality in British vegetarians. *Public Health Nutr.* 2002;5(1): 29–36.

282. Ho RC et al. Is high homocysteine level a risk factor for cognitive decline in elderly? A systematic review, meta-analysis, and meta-regression. *Am J Geriatr Psychiatry.* 2011;19(7):607–17.

283. Nourhashemi F et al. Alzheimer disease: protective factors. *Am J Clin Nutr.* 2000; 71(2): 643S–649S.

284. Selhub J et al. B vitamins, homocysteine, and neurocognitive function in the elderly. *Am J Clin Nutr.* 2000;71(2):614S–620S.

285. Van Dam F, Van Gool WA. Hyperhomocysteinemia and Alzheimer's disease: A systematic review. *Arch Gerontol Geriatr.* 2009 May-Jun;48(3):425–30.

286. Malouf R, Grimley Evans J. Folic acid with or without vitamin B_{12} for the prevention and treatment of healthy elderly and demented people. *Cochrane Database Syst Rev.* 2008;(4):CD004514.

287. White LR et al. Brain aging and midlife tofu consumption. *J Am Coll Nutr.* 2000; 19:242–55.

288. Rice MM et al. Tofu consumption and cognition in older Japanese American men and women. *J Nutr.* 2000(Suppl):676S. (abstract only.)

289. Hogervorst E et al. High tofu intake is associated with worse memory in elderly Indonesian men and women. *Dement Geriatr Cogn Disord.* 2008;26(1):50–7.

290. Hogervorst E et al. Borobudur revisited: Soy consumption may be associated with better recall in younger, but not in older, rural Indonesian elderly. *Brain Res.* 2011;1379:206–12.

291. File SE et al. Cognitive improvement after 6 weeks of soy supplements in postmenopausal women is limited to frontal lobe function. *Menopause.* 2005 ;12(2):193–201.

292. File SE et al. Eating soya improves human memory. *Psychopharmacology.* (Berl). 2001; 157:430–6.

293. Duffy R et al. Improved cognitive function in postmenopausal women after 12 weeks of consumption of a soya extract containing isoflavones. *Pharmacol Biochem Behav.* 2003;75(3):721–9.

294. Fournier LR et al. The effects of soy milk and isoflavone supplements on cognitive performance in healthy, postmenopausal women. *J Nutr Health Aging.* 2007;11(2): 155–64.

295. Thorp AA et al. Soya isoflavone supplementation enhances spatial working memory in men. *Br J Nutr.* 2009;102(9):1348–54.

296. Kritz-Silverstein D et al. Isoflavones and cognitive function in older women: the Soy and Postmenopausal Health In Aging (SOPHIA) Study. *Menopause.* 2003;10(3): 196–202.

297. Islam F et al. Short-term changes in endogenous estrogen levels and consumption of soy isoflavones affect working and verbal memory in young adult females. *Nutr Neurosci.* 2008;11(6):251–62.

298. Celec P et al. Endocrine and cognitive effects of short-time soybean consumption in women. *Gynecol Obstet Invest.* 2005; 59(2):62–6.

299. Celec P et al. Increased one week soybean consumption affects spatial abilities but not sex hormone status in men. *Int J Food Sci Nutr.* 2007;58(6):424–8.

300. Ostatníková D et al. Short-term soybean intake and its effect on steroid sex hormones and cognitive abilities. *Fertil Steril.* 2007; 88(6):1632–6.

301. Kreijkamp-Kaspers S et al. Effect of soy protein containing isoflavones on cognitive function, bone mineral density, and plasma lipids in postmenopausal women: A randomized controlled trial. *JAMA.* 2004;292:65–74.

302. Ho SC et al. Effects of soy isoflavone supplementation on cognitive function in Chinese postmenopausal women: a double-blind, randomized, controlled trial. *Menopause.* 2007;14(3 Pt 1):489–99.

303. Pilsáková L et al. Missing evidence for the effect one-week phytoestrogen-rich diet on mental rotation in two dimensions. *Neuro Endocrinol Lett.* 2009;30(1):125–30.

Diverticular Disease

304. Sheth AA et al. Diverticular Disease and Diverticulitis. *Am J Gastroenterol*. 2008; 103:1550–1556.

305. Painter NS, Burkitt DP. Diverticular disease of the colon: a deficiency disease of Western civilization. *BMJ*. 1969;2(5759): 450–454.

306. Manousos O et al. Diet and other factors in the aetiology of diverticulosis: an epidemiological study in Greece. *Gut*. 1985; 26:544–9.

307. Aldoori WH et al. A prospective study of diet and the risk of symptomatic diverticular disease in men. *Am J Clin Nutr*. 1994; 60:757–764.

308. Matrana MR, Margolin DA. Epidemiology and pathophysiology of diverticular disease. *Clin Colon Rectal Surg*. 2009; 22(3):141–6.

309. Gear JS, Ware A, Fursdon P et al. Symptomless diverticular disease and intake of dietary fibre. *Lancet*. 1979;1:511–514.

310. Crowe FL, Appleby PN, Allen NE, Key TJ. Diet and risk of diverticular disease in Oxford cohort of European Prospective Investigation into Cancer and Nutrition (EPIC): prospective study of British vegetarians and non-vegetarians. *BMJ*. 2011;343:d4131.

311. Lin OS, Soon M, Wu S, Chen Y, Hwang K, Triadafilopoulos G. Dietary habits and right-sided colonic diverticulosis. *Dis Colon Rectum*. 2000;43:1412–8.

Gallstones

312. Pixley F et al. Effect of vegetarianism on development of gall stones in women. *Br Med J. (Clin Res Ed)*. 1985:291:11–12.

313. Kratzer W et al. Gallstone prevalence in Germany: the Ulm Gallbladder Stone Study. *Dig Dis Sci*. 1998; 43:1285–1291.

314. Kratzer W et al. Prevalence of cholecystolithiasis in South Germany–an ultrasound study of 2498 persons of a rural population. *Z Gastroenterol*. 1999; 37:1157–1162.

315. Kratzer W et al. Gallstone prevalence in relation to smoking, alcohol, coffee consumption, and nutrition. The Ulm Gallstone Study. *Scand J Gastroenterol*. 1997; 32(9):953–8.

316. Walcher T et al; EMIL Study Group. The effect of alcohol, tobacco and caffeine consumption and vegetarian diet on gallstone prevalence. *Eur J Gastroenterol Hepatol*. 2010 Nov;22(11):1345–51.

317. Tsai CJ et al. Dietary protein and the risk of cholecystectomy in a cohort of US women: the Nurses' Health Study. *Am J Epidemiol*. 2004;160:11-18.

318. Tsai CJ et al. Fruit and vegetable consumption and risk of cholecystectomy in women. *Am J Med*. 2006;119:760–767.

319. Tsai CJ et al. Frequent nut consumption and decreased risk of cholecystectomy in women. *Am J Clin Nutr*. 2004;80:76–81.

320. Tsai CJ et al. A prospective cohort study of nut consumption and the risk of gallstone disease in men. *Am J Epidemiol*. 2004 Nov. 15;160(10):961–8.

321. Must A et al. The disease burden associated with overweight and obesity. *JAMA*. 1999;282:1523–1529.

322. Misciagna G et al. Diet, physical activity, and gallstones–a population-based, case-control study in southern Italy. *Am J Clin Nutr*. 1999;69:120–126.

323. Tsai CJ et al. Long-term intake of trans-fatty acids and risk of gallstone disease in men. *Arch Intern Med*. 2005;165: 1011–1015.

324. Tsai CJ et al. Long-chain saturated fatty acids consumption and risk of gallstone disease among men. *Ann Surg*. 2008; 247:95–103.

325. Tsai CJ et al. Dietary carbohydrates and glycaemic load and the incidence of symptomatic gall stone disease in men. *Gut*. 2005;54:823–828.

326. Scaggion G et al. Influence of dietary fibres in the genesis of cholesterol gallstone disease. *Ital J Med.* 1988;4:158-161.

327. Marcus SN, Heaton KW. Effects of a new, concentrated wheat fibre preparation on intestinal transit, deoxycholic acid metab-olism and the composition of bile. *Gut.* 1986;27:893–900.

328. Tsai CJ et al. The effect of long-term intake of cis unsaturated fats on the risk for gallstone disease in men: a prospective cohort study. *Ann Intern Med.* 2004;141:514–522.

Kidney Disease

329. Bernstein AM et al. Are high protein, vegetable-based diets safe for kidney function? A review of the literature. *J Am Diet Assoc.* 2007;107:644–650.

330. Kontessis P et al. Renal, metabolic, and hormonal responses to ingestion of animal and vegetable proteins. *Kidney Int.* 1990; 38:136–144.

331. Kontessis PA et al. Renal, metabolic, and hormonal responses to proteins of different origin in normotensive, nonproteinuric type I diabetic patients. *Diabetes Care.* 1995;18:1233–1239.

332. Barsotti G et al. A low-nitrogen low-phosphorus vegan diet for patients with chronic renal failure. *Nephron.* 1996;74(2): 390–4.

333. Piccoli GB et al. Association of Low-Protein Supplemented Diets with Fetal Growth in Pregnant Women with CKD. *Clin J Am Soc Nephrol.* 2014;Feb27. [Epub ahead of print]

334. Moe SM et al. Vegetarian compared with meat dietary protein source and phosphorus homeostasis in chronic kidney disease. *Clin J Am Soc Nephrol.* 2011; 6(2):257–64.

335. Noori N et al. Organic and inorganic dietary phosphorus and its management in chronic kidney disease. *Iran J Kidney Dis.* 2010;4(2):89–100.

Hypothyroidism

336. Tonstad S et al. Vegan diets and hypothyroidism. *Nutrients.* 2013;5,4642–4652.

Rheumatoid Arthritis (RA)

337. Agren JJ et al. Divergent changes in serum sterols during a strict uncooked vegan diet in patients with rheumatoid arthritis. *British Journal of Nutrition.* 2001;85:137–139.

338. Hanninen O et al. Antioxidants in vegan diet and rheumatic disorders. *Toxicology.* 2000;155(1-3):45–53.

339. Hanninen O et al. Vegan diet in physiological health promotion. *Acta Physiol Hung.* 1999;86(3-4):171–80.

340. Nenonen MT et al. Uncooked, lactobacilli-rich, vegan food and rheumatoid arthritis. *British Journal of Rheumatology.* 1998;37:274–281.

341. Peltonen R et al. Faecal microbial flora and disease activity in rheumatoid arthritis during a vegan diet. British *Journal of Rheumatology.* 1997;36,64–68.

342. Rauma AL et al. Effect of a strict vegan diet on energy and nutrient intakes by Finnish rheumatoid patients. *European Journal of Clinical Nutrition.* 1993;47: 747–749.

343. Ryhanan EL, Mantere-Alhonen S, Nenonen M, Hanninen O. Modification of faecal flora in rheumatoid arthritis patients by lactobacilli rich vegetarian diet. *Milchwissenschaft.* 1993;48 (5): 255–259.

344. Hafstrom I et al. A vegan diet free of gluten improves the signs and symptoms of rheumatoid arthritis: the effects on arthritis correlate with a reduction in antibodies to food antigens. *Rheumatology.* (Oxford). 2001;40(10):1175–9.

345. Elkan AC et al. Gluten-free vegan diet induces decreased LDL and oxidized LDL levels and raised atheroprotective natural antibodies against phosphorylcholine in patients with rheumatoid arthritis: a randomized study. *Arthritis Res Ther.* 2008; 10(2):R34.

346. McDougall J et al. Effects of a very low-fat, vegan diet in subjects with rheumatoid arthritis. *J Altern Complement Med.* 2002;8(1):71–5.

347. Hanninen O et al. Effects of eating an uncooked vegetable diet for 1 week. *Appetite.* 1992;19(3):243–54.

348. Fujita A et al. Effects of a low calorie vegan diet on disease activity and general conditions in patients with rheumatoid arthritis. [Article in Japanese] *Rinsho Byori.* (Japanese journal of clinical pathology). 1999; 47(6): 554–60.

349. Kjeldsen-Kragh J. Rheumatoid arthritis treated with vegetarian diets. *Am J Clin Nutr.* 1999;70:594S–600S.

350. Kjeldsen-Kragh J et al. Antibodies against dietary antigens in rheumatoid arthritis patients treated with fasting and a one-year vegetarian diet. *Clin Exp Rheumatol.* 1995;13:167–72.

351. Kjeldsen-Kragh J et al. Vegetarian diet for patients with rheumatoid arthritis--status: two years after introduction of the diet. *Clin Rheumatol.* 1994;13(3):475–82. Erratum in: *Clin Rheumatol.* 1994.

352. Kjeldsen-Kragh J et al. Controlled trial of fasting and one-year vegetarian diet in rheumatoid arthritis. *Lancet.* 1991: 338:899–902.

353. Peltonen R et al. Changes of faecal flora in rheumatoid arthritis during fasting and one-year vegetarian diet. *Br J Rheumatol.* 1994; 33:638–43.

354. Haugen MA et al. Changes in plasma phospholipid fatty acids and their relationship to disease activity in rheumatoid arthritis patients treated with a vegetarian diet. *Br J Nutr.* 1994;72:555–66.

355. Beri D et al. Effect of dietary restrictions on disease activity in rheumatoid arthritis *Annals of the Rheumatic Diseases.* 1988; 47:69–72.

356. Sköldstam L. Fasting and vegan diet in rheumatoid arthritis. *Scand J Rheum* 1986; 15: 219–221.

357. Sköldstam L et al. Effects of fasting and lactovegetarian diet on rheumatoid arthritis. *Scand J Rheumatol.* 1979;8:249–255.

358. Ebringer A, Rashid T. Rheumatoid arthritis is an autoimmune disease triggered by Proteus urinary tract infection. *Clin Dev Immunol.* 2006;13(1):41–8. Review.

359. Kontogiorgis CA et al. Natural Products from Mediterranean Diet: From Anti-Inflammatory Agents to Dietary Epigenetic Modulators. *Anti-Inflammatory & Anti-Allergy Agents in Medicinal Chemistry.* June 2010; 9(2):101–124.

360. Lopez-Garcia E et al. Consumption of trans fatty acids is related to plasma biomarkers of inflammation and endothelial dysfunction. *J Nutr.* 2005 Mar;135(3): 562–6.

361. Lopez-Garcia E et al. Major dietary patterns are related to plasma concentrations of markers of inflammation and endothelial dysfunction. *Am J Clin Nutr.* 2004; 80(4):1029–35.

362. Pattison DJ et al. Dietary risk factors for the development of inflammatory polyarthritis: evidence for a role of high level of red meat consumption. *Arthritis Rheum.* 2004;50:3804–3812.

363. Grant WB. The role of meat in the expression of rheumatoid arthritis. *Br J Nutr.* 2000, 84:589–595.

364. Benito-Garcia E et al. Protein, iron, and meat consumption and risk for rheumatoid arthritis: a prospective cohort study. *Arthritis Res Ther.* 2007;9:R16.

365. Eerola E et al. Intestinal flora in early rheumatoid arthritis. *Br J Rheumatol.* 1994;33: 1030–8.

366. Sköldstam L et al. Weight reduction is not a major reason for improvement in rheumatoid arthritis from lacto-vegetarian, vegan or Mediterranean diets. *Nutr J*. 2005;4:15.

367. Muller H et al. Fasting followed by vegetarian diet in patients with rheumatoid arthritis: A systematic review. *Scand J Rheumatol*. 2001;30:1-10.

REFERENCES FOR CHAPTER 3

1. Millward DJ. The nutritional value of plant-based diets in relation to human amino acid and protein requirements. *Proc Nutr Soc*. 1999;58:249-60.

2. Young VR et al. Plant proteins in relation to human protein and amino acid nutrition. *Am J Clin Nutr*. 1994;59(5 Suppl):1203S-1212S.

3. Millward DJ. Amino acid scoring patterns for protein quality assessment. *British J. Nutr*. 2012 Aug;108 Suppl 2:S31-43.

4. Millward DJ et al. Protein/energy ratios of current diets in developed and developing countries compared with a safe protein/energy ratio: implications for recommended protein and amino acid intakes. *Public Health Nutr*. 2004;7:387-405.

5. Millward DJ, Director, Centre for Nutrition and Food Safety, School of Biomedical and Life Sciences, University of Surrey, Guildford, England (Vice-Chair). Personal communication. August 2011.

6. Millward DJ. Identifying recommended dietary allowances for protein and amino acids: a critique of the 2007 WHO/FAO/UNU report. *British J. Nutr*. 2012 Aug;108(Suppl 2):S3-21.

7. Tomé D et al. Lysine requirement through the human life cycle. *J Nutr*. 2007;137(6 Suppl 2):1642S-1645S.

8. Bezner Kerr R et al. Effects of a participatory agriculture and nutrition education project on child growth in northern Malawi. *Public Health Nutr*. 2011 Aug;14(8):1466-72.

9. Torres y Torres N et al. The importance of soy in Mexico, its nutritional value and effect on health. *Salud Publica Mex*. 2009 May-Jun;51(3):246-54.

10. Snapp SS et al. Biodiversity can support a greener revolution in Africa. *Proc Natl Acad Sci USA*. 2010 Nov 30;107(48):20840-5.

11. Mangels AR, Messina V, Messina M. *The Dietitians Guide to Vegetarian Diets*. Jones and Bartlett Learning Ltd., 2011.

12. Tomé D. Criteria and markers for protein quality assessment–a review. *Br J Nutr*. 2012; 108(Suppl 2):S222-9.

13. Millward DJ. Macronutrient intakes as determinants of dietary protein and amino acid adequacy. *J. Nut*. 2004 Jun;134(6 Suppl):1588S-1596S.

14. Elango R et al. Evidence that protein requirements have been significantly underestimated. *Curr Opin Clin Nutr Metab Care*. 2010;13(1):52-7.

15. Institute of Medicine. National Research Council. Dietary Carbohydrates, Starches and Sugars. *Dietary Reference Intakes for Energy, Carbohydrate, Fiber, Fat, Fatty Acids, Cholesterol, Protein, and Amino Acids (Macronutrients)*. Washington DC: National Academies Press, 2005. Pages 289, 261.

16. Rand WM et al. Meta-analysis of nitrogen balance studies for estimating protein requirements in healthy adults. *Am J Clin Nutr*. 2003;77(1):109-27.

17. World Health Organization/Food and Agriculture Organization/United Nations University. Expert Consultation. Protein and amino acid requirements in human nutrition. *WHO Technical Report Series – 935*. (World Health Organization/Food and Agriculture Organization). 2007.

18. Doyle MD et al. Observations on nitrogen and energy balance in young men consuming vegetarian diets. *Am J Clin Nutr*. 1965;17(6):367-76.

19. Haddad EH et al. Dietary intake and biochemical, hematologic, and immune status of vegans compared with nonvegetarians. *Am J Clin Nutr*. 1999;70(3 Suppl):586S-593S.

20. Greger M. www.nutritionfacts.org

21. Norris J. www.veganhealth.org/articles/protein

22. Gaffney-Stomberg E et al. Increasing dietary protein requirements in elderly people for optimal muscle and bone health. *J Am Geriatr Soc.* 2009 Jun;57(6):1073-9.

23. Millward DJ. Sufficient protein for our elders? *Am J Clin Nutr.* 2008;88:1187-8.

24. Morais JA et al. Protein turnover and requirements in the healthy and frail elderly. *J Nutr Health Aging.* 2006 Jul-Aug;10(4): 272-83.

25. Paddon-Jones D. Dietary protein and muscle in older persons. *Curr Opin Clin Nutr Metab Care.* 2014 Jan;17(1):5-11.

26. Yáñez E et al. Long-term validation of 1 g of protein per kilogram body weight from a predominantly vegetable mixed diet to meet the requirements of young adult males. *J Nutr.* 1986;116(5):865-72.

27. American Dietetic Association, Dietitians of Canada, and the American College of Sports Medicine: Nutrition and Athletic Performance. *J Am Diet Assoc.* 2009;109 (3)509-527.

28. Fuhrman J et al. Fueling the Vegetarian (Vegan) Athlete. *Curr Sports Med Rep.* 2010; 9(4):233-241.

29. Schaafsma G. The protein digestibility-corrected amino acid score. *J Nutr.* 2000; 130(7):1865S-7S and Schaafsma G. The Protein Digestibility-Corrected Amino Acid Score (PDCAAS)—a concept for describing protein quality in foods and food ingredients: a critical review. *J AOAC Int.* 2005; 88(3):988-94.

30. Synder HE et al. *Soybean Utilization.* New York: Van Nostrand Reinhold Company, 1987.

31. Bishnoi S et al. Protein digestibility of vegetables and field peas (Pisum sativum). Varietal differences and effect of domestic processing and cooking methods. *Plant Foods Hum Nutr.* 1994;46:71–6.

32. Hernot DC et al. In vitro digestion characteristics of unprocessed and processed whole grains and their components. *J Agric Food Chem.* 2008;56:10721–6.

33. Oste RE. Digestibility of processed food protein. *Adv Exp Med Biol.* 1991;289: 371–88.

34. Zia-ur-Rehman et al. The effects of hydrothermal processing on antinutrients, protein and starch digestibility of food legumes. *Int J Food Science Technol.* 2005; 40:695–700.

35. Frias J et al. Evolution of trypsin inhibitor activity during germination of lentils. *J Agric Food Chem.* 1995.43:2231–2234.

36. Ibrahim SS et al. Effect of soaking, germination, cooking and fermentation on antinutritional factors in cowpeas. *Nahrung.* 2002;46:92–5.

37. Sathe SK et al. Effects of germination on proteins, raffinose, oligosaccharides, and antinutritional factors in the Great Northern beans (Phaseolus vulgaris L.). *J Food Sci.* 1983;48:1796–1800.

38. Chang KC et al. Effect of germination on oligosaccharides and nonstarch polysaccharidesin navy and pinto beans. *J Food Science.* 1989; 54(6):1615.

39. Oboh HA et al. Effect of soaking, cooking and germination on the oligosaccharide content of selected Nigerian legume seeds. *Plant Foods Hum Nutr.* 2000;55(2):97–110.

40. Chavan JK et al. Nutritional improvement of cereals by sprouting. *Crit Rev Food Sci Nutr.* 1989;28:401–37.

41. Chavan JK et al. Nutritional improvement of cereals by fermentation. *Crit Rev Food Sci Nutr.* 1989;28:349–400.

42. Millward DJ et al. Protein quality assessment: impact of expanding understanding of protein and amino acid needs for optimal health. *Am J Clin Nutr.* 2008;87(5):1576S–1581S.

43. Furst P et al. What Are the Essential Elements Needed for the Determination of Amino Acid Requirements in Humans? *J Nutr.* 2004 Jun;134(6 Suppl):1558S–1565S.

44. Reeds PJ. Dispensable and indispensable amino acids for humans. *J Nutr.* 2000 Jul;130(7): 1835S–40S.

45. Millward DJ et al. Efficiency of utilization of wheat and milk protein in healthy adults and apparent lysine requirements determined by a single-meal [1-13C] leucine balance protocol. *Am J Clin Nutr.* 2002;76(6): 1326–34.

46. Prolla IR et al. Lysine from cooked white rice consumed by healthy young men is highly metabolically available when assessed using the indicator amino acid oxidation technique. *J Nutr.* 2013 Mar;143(3): 302–6.

47. Khalil MM. Effect of soaking, germination, autoclaving and cooking on chemical and biological value of guar compared with faba bean. *Nahrung.* 2001;45(4): 246–50.

48. Mubarak AE. Chemical, nutritional and sensory properties of bread supplemented with lupin seed (Lupinus albus) products. *Nahrung.* 2001 Aug;45(4):241–5.

49. Davis B et al. *Becoming Raw.* Summertown TN: The Book Publishing Company, 2010.

50. El-Adawy TA. Nutritional composition and antinutritional factors of chickpeas (*Cicer arietinum* L.) undergoing different cooking methods and germination. *Plant Foods for Human Nutrition.* 2002;57: 83–97.

51. Savelkoul FHMG et al. The presence and inactivation of trypsin inhibitors, tannins, lectins and amylase inhibitors in legume seeds during germination. *Plant Foods for Human Nutrition.* 1992;42:71–85.

52. Wilson KA. The proteolysis of trypsin inhibitors in legume seeds. *Crit Rev Biotechnol.* 1988;8:197–216.

53. Richard DM et al. L-Tryptophan: Basic Metabolic Functions, Behavioral Research and Therapeutic Indications. *Int J Tryptophan Res.* 2009 Mar 23;2:45–60.

54. USDA United States Department of Agriculture, Agricultural Research Service. *USDA National Nutrient Database for Standard Reference.*

55. ESHA The Food Processor. Nutrition and Fitness Software. 2014. www.esha.com

56. Naturade protein powder. www.naturade. com

57. Vega protein powder. www. http://myvega. com

58. Krajcovicová-Kudláčková M et al. Correlation of carnitine levels to methionine and lysine intake. *Physiol Res.* 2000;49(3): 399–402.

59. Demarquoy J et al. Radioisotopic determination of l-carnitine content in foods commonly eaten in Western countries. *Food Chemistry.* 2004;86(1):137–142.

60. National Institute of Health, Office of Dietary Supplements. *Dietary Supplement Fact Sheet: Carnitine.*

61. Rebouche CJ et al. Renal adaptation to dietary carnitine in humans. *Am J Clin Nutr.*1993; 58(5):660–5.

62. Rebouche CJ. Kinetics, pharmacokinetics, and regulation of L-carnitine and acetyl-L-carnitine metabolism. *Ann N Y Acad Sci.* 2004;1033:30–41.

63. Rebouche C. Personal communication. June 22, 2011.

64. Chen W et al. Urinary, plasma, and erythrocyte carnitine concentrations during transition to a lactoovovegetarian diet with vitamin B-6 depletion and repletion in young adult women. *Am J Clin Nutr.* 1998 Feb;67(2):221–30.

65. Lombard KA et al. Carnitine status of lacto-ovovegetarians and strict vegetarian adults and children. *Am J Clin Nutr.* 1989;50(2): 301–6.

66. Stanley CA. Carnitine deficiency disorders in children. *Ann NY Acad Sci.* 2004;1033: 42–51.

67. Stephens FB et al. Vegetarians have a reduced skeletal muscle carnitine transport capacity. *Am J Clin Nutr.* 2011 Sep;94(3): 938–44.

68. Baumel S. Personal communication. June 2011

69. Malaguarnera M et al. L-Carnitine supplementation reduces oxidized LDL cholesterol in patients with diabetes. *Am J Clin Nutr.* 2009 Jan;89(1):71–6.

70. Villani RG et al. L-Carnitine supplementation combined with aerobic training does not promote weight loss in moderately obese women. *Int J Sport Nutr Exerc Metab.* 2000 Jun;10(2):199–207.

71. Koeth RA et al. Intestinal microbiota metabolism of l-carnitine, a nutrient in red meat, promotes atherosclerosis. *Nat Med.* 2013;19(5):576–85.

72. Rozan P et al. Amino acids in seeds and seedlings of the genus Lens. *Phytochemistry.* 2001;58(2):281–9.

73. Irving CS et al. *Life Sci.* 1986;38(6):491–5.

74. Sanders TA. Vegetarian diets and children. *Pediatr Clin North Am.* 1995 Aug;42(4): 955–65.

75. Rana SK et al. Taurine concentrations in the diet, plasma, urine and breast milk of vegans compared with omnivores. *Br J Nutr.* 1986 Jul;56(1):17–27.

76. Heird WC. Taurine in neonatal nutrition–revisited. *Arch Dis Child Fetal Neonatal Ed.* 2004 Nov;89(6):F473–4.

77. WHO Consultation FAO. Diet, nutrition, and the prevention of chronic diseases. *WHO Technical Report Series 916.* 2003.

78. Esselstyn CB Jr. Resolving the Coronary Artery Disease Epidemic Through Plant-Based Nutrition. *Prev Cardiol.* 2001;4(4): 171–177.

79. Esselstyn CB Jr. Updating a 12-year experience with arrest and reversal therapy for coronary heart disease (an overdue requiem for palliative cardiology). *Am J Cardiol.* 1999;84(3):339–41, A8.

80. Ornish D et al. Intensive lifestyle changes for reversal of coronary heart disease. *JAMA.* 1998;280(23):2001–7.

81. Craig WJ et al. American Dietetic Association. Position of the American Dietetic Association: Vegetarian Diets. *J Am Diet Assoc.* 2009;109 (7)1266–82.

82. Rizzo NS et al. Nutrient profiles of vegetarian and nonvegetarian dietary patterns. *J Acad Nutr Diet.* 2013 Dec;113(12): 1610–9.

83. Koebnick C et al. Long-term consumption of a raw food diet is associated with favorable serum LDL cholesterol and triglycerides but also with elevated plasma homocysteine and low serum HDL cholesterol in humans. *J Nutr.* 2005;135:2372–8.

84. Center for Disease Control. Dietary Intake of Ten Key Nutrients for Public Health, United States: 1999-2000 *Advance Data Report No. 334.* 2003

85. Statistics Canada. *Overview of Canadians' Eating Habits.* 2004. www.statcan.gc.ca/pub/82-620-m/2006002/4053669-eng.htm and www.statcan.gc.ca/pub/82-620-m/2006002/c-g/4144191-eng.htm

86. Cao JJ. A diet high in meat protein and potential renal acid load increases fractional calcium absorption and urinary calcium excretion without affecting markers of bone resorption or formation in postmenopausal women. *J Nutr.* 2011;141(3):391–397.

87. Darling A et al. Dietary protein and bone health: a systematic review and meta-analysis. *Am J Clin Nutr.* 2009 Dec;90(6): 1674–92.

88. Dawson-Hughes B et al. Alkaline diets favor lean tissue mass in older adults. *Am J Clin Nutr.* 2008;87(3):662–665.

89. Ginty F. Dietary protein and bone health. *Proc Nutr Soc.* 2003;62(4):867–76.

90. Lousuebsakul-Matthews V et al. Legumes and meat analogues consumption are associated with hip fracture risk independently of meat intake among Caucasian men and women: the Adventist Health Study-2. *Public Health Nutr.* 2013 Oct;8:1–11.

91. New SA. Intake of fruit and vegetables: implications for bone health. *Proc Nutr Soc.* 2003 Nov; 62(4):889–99.

92. New SA. Intake of fruit and vegetables: implications for bone health. *Proc Nutr Soc.* 2004 Feb;63(1):187.

93. New SA. Calcium, protein, and fruit and vegetables as dietary determinants of bone health. *Am J Clin Nutr.* 2003 May;77(5): 1340–1.

94. Reddy ST et al. Effect of Low-Carbohydrate High-Protein Diets on Acid-Base Balance, Stone-Forming Propensity, and Calcium Metabolism. *American Journal of Kidney Diseases.* 2002;40:265–274.

95. Sebastian A et al. Dietary ratio of animal to vegetable protein and rate of bone loss and risk of fracture in postmenopausal women. *Am J Clin Nutr.* 2001;74(3): 411–2.

96. Messina M. Insights Gained from 20 Years of Soy Research. *J Nutr.* 2010 Dec;140(12): 2289S–2295S.

97. Marini H et al. Update on genistein and thyroid: an overall message of safety. *Front Endocrinol (Lausanne).* 2012 Jul;31;3:94.

98. Messina M et al. Report on the 8th International Symposium on the Role of Soy in Health Promotion and Chronic Disease Prevention and Treatment. *J Nutr.* 2009; 139(4):796S–802S.

99. Messina V et al. *Vegan for Her.* Da Capo Lifelong. 2013.

100. Adams J et al. *Never Too Late to Go Vegan.* The Experiment. 2014.

101. Hilakivi-Clarke L et al. Is soy consumption good or bad for the breast? *J Nutr.* 2010; 140(12):2326S–2334S.

102. Messina M. Soybean isoflavone exposure does not have feminizing effects on men: a critical examination of the clinical evidence. *Fertil Steril.* 2010;93:2095–104.

103. Hamilton-Reeves JM et al. Clinical studies show no effects of soy protein or isoflavones on reproductive hormones in men: results of a meta-analysis. *Fertil Steril.* 2010;94(3):997–1007.

104. Yan L et al. Soy consumption and prostate cancer risk in men: a revisit of a meta-analysis. *Am J Clin Nutr.* 2009;89:1155–63.

105. Martinez J et al. An unusual case of gynecomastia associated with soy product consumption. *Endocr Pract.* 2008;14(4):415–8.

106. Siepmann T et al. Hypogonadism and erectile dysfunction associated with soy product consumption. *Nutrition.* 2011; 27(7-8):859–862.

107. Young VR. Soy protein in relation to human protein and amino acid nutrition. *J Am Diet Assoc.* 91:828.

107. Melina V et al. *Cooking Vegan.* Summertown TN: The Book Publishing Company, 2011.

REFERENCES FOR CHAPTER 4

1. National Research Council. Dietary Reference Intakes for Energy, Carbohydrate, Fiber, Fat, Fatty Acids, Cholesterol, Protein, and Amino Acids (Macronutrients). Washington DC: The National Academies Press, 2005.

2. American Heart Association Nutrition Committee; Lichtenstein AH, Appel LJ, Brands M, Carnethon M, Daniels S et al. Diet and lifestyle recommendations revision 2006: a scientific statement from the American Heart Association Nutrition Committee. *Circulation.* 2006;114:82–96.

3. Mosca L et al. Evidence-based guidelines for cardiovascular disease prevention in women: 2007 update. *Circulation.* 2007;115:1481–1501.

4. Astrup A et al. The role of reducing intakes of saturated fat in the prevention of cardio-vascular disease: where does the evidence stand in 2010? *Am J Clin Nutr.* 2011;93(4):684–8.

5. Hu FB et al. Types of Dietary Fat and Risk of Coronary Heart Disease: A Critical Review. *JACN.* 2001; 20(1): 5–19.

6. Kris-Etherton PM. AHA Science Advisory. Monounsaturated fatty acids and risk of cardiovascular disease. American Heart Association. Nutrition Committee. *Circulation.* 1999;100(11):1253–8.

7. Sacks FM, Katan M. Randomized clinical trials on the effects of dietary fat and carbohydrate on plasma lipoproteins and cardiovascular disease. *Am J Med.* 2002; 113(Suppl 9B):13S–24S.

8. Ghafoorunissa G. Role of trans fatty acids in health and challenges to their reduction in Indian foods. *Asia Pac J Clin Nutr.* 2008;17 Suppl 1:212–5.

9. Micha R, Mozaffarian D. Trans fatty acids: effects on cardiometabolic health and implications for policy. *Prostaglandins Leukot Essent Fatty Acids.* 2008;79(3–5):147–52.

10. Trans Fat Task Force. *Transforming the food supply*. Ottawa Ontario: Ministry of Health Canada, 2006. www.hc-sc.gc.ca/fn-an/alt_formats/hpfb-dgpsa/pdf/nutrition/tf-gt_rep-rap-eng.pdf

11. Mozaffarian D et al. Trans Fatty Acids and Cardiovascular Disease. New England Journal of Medicine. 2006;354(15):1601–1613.

12. Ascherio A, Willett WC. Health effects of trans fatty acids. *Am J Clin Nutr*. 1997; 66(4 Suppl):1006S–1010S. Review.

13. Risérus U. Trans fatty acids and insulin resistance. *Atheroscler Suppl*. 2006;7(2):37–9.

14. Risérus U et al. Metabolic effects of conjugated linoleic acid in humans: the Swedish experience. *Am J Clin Nutr*. 2004;79(6 Suppl):1146S–1148S.

15. ChartsBin statistics collector team 2011, Contribution of Fats in Total Dietary Consumption. http://chartsbin.com/view/1158

16. Willcox DC et al. The Okinawan diet: health implications of a low-calorie, nutrient-dense, antioxidant-rich dietary pattern low in glycemic load. *J Am Coll Nutr*. 2009; 28(Suppl):500S–516S. Review.

17. Appel LJ. Dietary Patterns and Longevity Expanding the Blue Zones. *Circulation*. 2008;118:214–215.

18. Buettner D. The Blue Zones: Lessons for Living Longer from the People Who've Lived the Longest. *National Geographic*. 2008.

19. Report of a Joint FAO/WHO Expert Consultation. Diet, Nutrition and the Prevention of Chronic Diseases. Geneva, Switzerland: Technical Report Series No. 916, 2003.

20. American Diabetes Association. Nutrition Recommendations and Interventions for Diabetes. A position statement of the American Diabetes Association. *Diabetes Care*. 2008;31:S61–S78.

21. Fontana L et al. Long-term low-protein, low-calorie diet and endurance exercise modulate metabolic factors associated with cancer risk. *Am J Clin Nutr*. 2006;84(6): 1456–62.

22. Ågren JJ et al. Divergent changes in serum sterols during a strict uncooked vegan diet in patients with rheumatoid arthritis. *British Journal of Nutrition*. 2001;85:137–139.

23. Rauma AL et al. Antioxidant status in long-term adherents to a strict uncooked vegan diet. *Am J Clin Nutr*. 1995;62 (6):1221–7.

24. Mangels R et al. *The Dietitian's Guide to Vegetarian Diets: Issues and Applications. Appendix A*. Third Edition. Sudbury MA: Jones and Bartlett Learning, 2011.

25. U.S. Department of Agriculture, Agricultural Research Service. 2008. Nutrient Intakes from Food: Mean Amounts and Percentages of Calories from Protein, Carbohydrate, Fat, and Alcohol, One Day, 2005–2006. www.ars.usda.gov/SP2UserFiles/Place/12355000/pdf/0506/Table_6_NIF_05.pdf

26. Draper A et al. The energy and nutrient intakes of different types of vegetarian: a case for supplements? *Br. J. Nutr*. 1993;69:3–19. (Published erratum appears in *Br J Nutr*. 1993;70:812.)

27. Ornish D et al. Can lifestyle changes reverse coronary heart disease? The Lifestyle Heart Trial. *Lancet*. 1990;336(8708):129–33.

28. McDougall J et al. Rapid reduction of serum cholesterol and blood pressure by a twelve-day, very low fat, strictly vegetarian diet. *J Am Coll Nutr*. 1995;5:491–6.

29. Esselstyn, CB Jr. Updating a 12 year experience with arrest and reversal therapy of coronary heart disease. *Am J Cardiol*. 1999;84(3)339–41.

30. Barnard ND et al. A low fat vegan diet improves glycemic control and cardiovascular risk factors in a randomized clinical trial in individuals with type 2 diabetes. *Diabetes Care*. 2006;29(8):1777–83.

31. Ornish D et al. Intensive lifestyle changes for reversal of coronary heart disease. *J.A.M.A.* 1998;280(23):2001–7.

32. National Research Council. Dietary Reference Intakes for Vitamin C, Vitamin E, Selenium, and Carotenoids. Washington DC: The National Academies Press, 2000.

33. National Research Council. Dietary Reference Intakes for Calcium and Vitamin D. Washington DC: The National Academies Press, 2011.

34. National Research Council. Dietary Reference Intakes for Vitamin A, Vitamin K, Arsenic, Boron, Chromium, Copper, Iodine, Iron, Manganese, Molybdenum, Nickel, Silicon, Vanadium, and Zinc. Washington DC: The National Academies Press, 2001.

35. Gartner C et al. Lycopene is more bioavailable from tomato paste than from fresh tomatoes. *Am J Clin Nutr.* 1997;66:116–122.

36. Siri-Tarino PW et al. Saturated fat, carbohydrate, and cardiovascular disease. *Am J Clin Nutr.* 2010;91(3):502–9.

37. Dagnalie P, Van Staveren W. Macrobiotic nutrition and child health: results of a population-based, mixed-longtitudinal cohort study in the Netherlands. *Am J Clin Nutr.* 1994;59(suppl):1187S–1196S.

38. Shinwell ED, Gorodischer R. Totally vegetarian diets and infant nutrition. *Pediatrics.* 1982;4:582–6.

39. Willet WC. *Eat, Drink, and Be Healthy.* The Harvard Medical School Guide to Healthy Eating. New York: Simon and Schuster Source, 2001.

40. Davis B, Melina V. *Becoming Raw.* Summertown TN: The Book Publishing Company, 2010.

41. Keys A. Wine, garlic, and CHD in seven countries. *Lancet.* 1980;1(8160):145–6.

42. Keys A et al. The diet and 15-year death rate in the Seven Countries Study. *Am. J. Epidemiol.* 1986;124(6):903–15.

43. Sarri K, Kafatos A. The Seven Countries Study in Crete: olive oil, Mediterranean diet or fasting? *Public Health Nutrition.* 2005;8(6),666.

44. Bladbjerg EM et al. Non-fasting factor VII coagulant activity (FVII:C) increased by high fat diet. Thromb Haemost. 1994;71: 755–758.

45. Larsen LF et al. Effects of dietary fat quality and quantity on postprandial activation of blood coagulation factor VII. Arterioscler Thromb Vasc Biol. 1997;17:2904–2909.

46. World Cancer Research Fund/American Institute for Cancer Research. *Food, Nutrition, Physical Activity and the Prevention of Cancer: A Global Perspective.* Washington DC: AICR, 2007.

47. Raatz SK et al. Total fat intake modifies plasma fatty acid composition in humans. *J Nutr.* 2001 Feb;131(2):231–4.

48. Chow CK. *Fatty acids in foods and their health implications.* Third Edition. CRC Press, 2007.

49. Bolton GE, Sanders TH. Effect of Roasting Oil Composition on the Stability of Roasted High-Oleic Peanuts. *JAOCS.* 2002;79(2).

50. MacDonald-Wicks LK, Garg ML. Incorporation of n-3 fatty acids into plasma and liver lipids of rats: importance of background dietary fat. *Lipids.* 2004; 39(6):545–51.

51. Gibson RA et al. Conversion of linoleic acid and alpha-linolenic acid to long-chain polyunsaturated fatty acids (LCPUFAs), with a focus on pregnancy, lactation and the first 2 years of life. *Matern Child Nutr.* 2011;7Suppl 2:17–26.

52. Mann N et al. Fatty acid composition of habitual omnivore and vegetarian diets. *Lipids.* 2006;41(7):637–46.

53. Brenna JT et al. alpha-Linolenic acid supplementation and conversion to n23 long-chain polyunsaturated fatty acids in humans. *Prostaglandins Leukot Essent Fatty Acids.* 2009;80:85–91.

54. Kohli P, Levy BD. Resolvins and protectins: mediating solutions to Inflammation. Review. *British Journal of Pharmacology.* 2009;158, 960–971.

55. Calder PC. Mechanisms of action of (n-3) fatty acids. *J Nutr.* 2012;142(3):592S–599S.

56. Davis B, Kris-Etherton P. Achieving Optimal Essential Fatty Acid Status in Vegetarians: Current Knowledge and Practical Implications. *Am J Clin Nutr.* 2003: 78(suppl); 640S–6S.

57. Kris-Etherton PM et al. Dietary reference intakes for DHA and EPA. *Prostaglandins Leukot Essent Fatty Acids.* 2009;81(2-3): 99–104.

58. Connor WE. Importance of n-3 fatty acids in health and disease. *Am J Clin Nutr.* 2000;71(1 Suppl):171S–5S.

59. Das UN. Essential fatty acids and their meta-bolites could function as endogenous

HMG-CoA reductase and ACE enzyme inhibitors, anti-arrhythmic, anti-hypertensive, anti-atherosclerotic, anti-inflammatory, cytoprotective, and cardioprotective molecules. *Lipids Health Dis.* 2008;7:37.

60. Simopoulos AP. The importance of the omega-6/ omega-3 fatty acid ratio in cardiovascular disease and other chronic diseases. *Experimental Biology and Medicine.* 2008; 233:674–688.

61. Welch AA et al. Dietary intake and status of n-3 polyunsaturated fatty acids in a population of fish-eating and non-fish-eating meat eaters, vegetarians, and vegans and the precursor-product ratio of alpha-linolenic acid to long-chain n-3 polyunsaturated fatty acids: results from the EPIC-Norfolk cohort. *Am J Clin Nutr.* 2010;92(5):1040–51.

62. Rosell MS et al. Long-chain n-3 polyunsaturated fatty acids in plasma in British meat-eating, vegetarian, and vegan men. *Am J Clin Nutr.* 2005;82(2):327–34.

63. Arterburn LM et al. Distribution, interconversion, and dose response of n-3 fatty acids in humans. *Am J Clin Nutr.* 2006;83(6 Suppl):1467S–1476S.

64. Uauy R. Professor of Public Health Nutrition. London School of Hygiene & Tropical Medicine and INTA. University of Chile. Personal communication. March 18, 2012.

65. Harris WS et al. Towards establishing dietary reference intakes for eicosapentaenoic and docosahexaenoic acids. *J Nutr.* 2009;139(4):804S–19S.

66. Burdge GC et al. Eicosapentaenoic and docosapentaenoic acids are the principal products of alpha-linolenic acid metabolism in young men. *Br J Nutr.* 2002;88: 355–64.

67. Burdge GC, Wootton SA. Conversion of alpha-linolenic acid to eicosapentaenoic, docosapentaenoic and docosahexaenoic acids in young women. *Br J Nutr.* 2002;88(4):411–20.

68. Emken EA et al. Effect of dietary docosahexaenoic acid on desaturation and uptake in vivo of isotopelabeled oleic, linoleic and linolenic acids by male subjects. *Lipids.* 1999;34:785–798.

69. Conquer JA, Holub BJ. Supplementation with an algae source of docosahexaenoic acid increases (n-3) fatty acid status and alters selected risk factors for heart disease in vegetarian subjects. *J Nutr.* 1996; 126(12):3032–9.

70. Conquer JA, Holub BJ. Dietary docosahexaenoic acid as a source of eicosapentaenoic acid in vegetarians and omnivores. *Lipids.* 1997;32(3):341–5.

71. Burdge GC, Calder PC. Conversion of alpha-linolenic acid to longerchain polyunsaturated fatty acids in human adults. *Reprod Nutr Dev.* 2005;45:581–97.

72. Simopoulos AP. Genetic variants in the metabolism of omega-6 and omega-3 fatty acids: their role in the determination of nutritional requirements and chronic disease risk. *Exp Biol Med* (Maywood). 2010;235(7):785–795.

73. Truong H et al. Does genetic variation in the Delta6-desaturase promoter modify the association between alpha-linolenic acid and the prevalence of metabolic syndrome? *Am J Clin Nutr.* 2009;89(3):920–5.

74. Marangoni F et al. Cigarette smoke negatively and dose-dependently affects the biosynthetic pathway of the n-3 polyunsaturated fatty acid series in human mammary epithelial cells. *Lipids.* 2004;39:633–637.

75. Das UN. Essential fatty acids: Biochemistry, physiology, and pathology. Biotechnology J. 2006;1:420–439.

76. Simopoulos AP et al. Workshop on the essentiality of and recommended dietary intakes for omega-6 and omega-3 fatty acids, *J Am Coll Nutr.* 1999;18(5):487–9

77. Emken EA et al. Dietary linoleic acid influences desaturation and acylation of deuterium-labeled linoleic and ALAs in young adult males. *Biochim Biophys Acta.* 1994; 1213:277–88.

78. Gerster H. Can adults adequately convert α-linolenic acid (18:3 n-3) to eicosapentaenoic acid (20:5n-3) and docosahexaenoic acid (22:6 n-3)? *Internat J Vit Nutr Res.* 1998;68:159–173.

79. Chan JK et al. Effect of dietary alpha-linolenic acid and its ratio to linoleic acid on

platelet and plasma fatty acids and thrombogenesis. *Lipids* 1993;28:811–817.

80. Bailey N. Current choices in omega 3 supplementation. *Nutrition Bulletin*. 2009;34: 85–91.

81. Siguel EN, Lerman RH. Altered fatty acid metabolism in patients with angiographically documented coronary artery disease. *Metabolism*. 1994;43:982–993.

82. Horrobin DF. Nutritional and medical importance of gamma-linolenic acid. *Prog. Lipid Res*. 1992;31,2:163–194.

83. Harris WS, Lemke SL, Hansen SN et al. Stearidonic acid-enriched soybean oil increased the omega-3 index, an emerging cardiovascular risk marker, *Lipids*. 2008; 43(9):805–11.

84. Callaway JC. Hempseed as a nutritional resource: an overview. *Euphytica*. 2004; 140:65-72.

85. Berti M et al. *Echium: A Source of Stearidonic Acid Adapted to the Northern Great Plains in the US. Issues in new crops and new uses*. J. Janick and A. Whipkey eds. Alexandria VA:ASHA Press, 2007.

86. Traifler H et al. Fractionation of blackcurrant seed oil. *Journal of the American Oil Chemists' Society*. 1988:65(5);755–760.

87. Harnack K, Andersen G, Somoza V. Quantitation of alpha-linolenic acid elongation to eicosapentaenoic and docosahexaenoic acid as affected by the ratio of n6/n3 fatty acids. *Nutr Metab*. (Lond). 2009;6:8.

88. Sanders TA. DHA status of vegetarians. *Prostaglandins Leukot Essent Fatty Acids*. 2009;81(2-3):137–41.

89. Calder PC, Deckelbaumb RJ. Editorial Comment: Harmful, harmless or helpful? The n-6 fatty acid debate goes on. *Current Opinion in Clinical Nutrition and Metabolic Care*. 2011;14:113–114.

90. Liou YA et al. Decreasing linoleic acid with constant α-linolenic acid in dietary fats increases (n-3) eicosapentaenoic acid in plasma phospholipids in healthy men. *J Nutr*. 2007; 137:945–952.

91. Indu M, Ghafoorunissa SA. N-3 Fatty acids in Indian diets: comparison of the effects of precursor (alpha-linolenic acid) vs. product (long chain n-3 polyunsaturated fatty acids). *Nutr Res*. 1992;12:569–82.

92. Masters C. n-3 Fatty acids and the peroxisome. *Mol Cell Biochem*. 1996;165:83–93.

93. Zhao G et al. Dietary a-linolenic acid inhibits proinflammatory cytokine production by peripheral blood mononuclear cells in hypercholesterolemic subjects. *Am J Clin Nutr*. 85:385–391, 2007.

94. Ezaki O et al. Long-term effects of dietary alpha-linolenic acid from perilla oil on serum fatty acids composition and on the risk factors of coronary heart disease in Japanese elderly subjects. *J Nutr Sci Vitaminol*. (Tokyo). 1999;45(6):759–72.

95. Kornsteiner M et al. Very low n-3 long-chain polyunsaturated fatty acid status in Austrian vegetarians and vegans. *Ann Nutr Metab*. 2008;52(1):37–47

96. Sanders TAB, Ellis FR, Dickerson JWT. Studies of vegans: the fatty acid composition of plasma choline phosphoglycerides and some indicators of susceptibility to ischemic heart disease in vegan and omnivore control. *Am J Clin Nutr*. 1978;31: 805–13.

97. Sanders TAB, Roshanai F. Platelet phospholipid fatty acid composition and function in vegans compared with age- and sex-matched omnivore controls. *Eur J Clin Nutr*. 1992;46(11):823–31.

98. Reddy S, Sanders TA, Obeid O. The influence of maternal vegetarian diet on essential fatty acid status of the newborn. *Eur J Clin Nutr*. 1994;48(5):358–68.

99. Krajcovicova-Kudlackova M, Simoncic R, Bederova A, Klvanova J. Plasma fatty acid profile and alternative nutrition. *Ann Nutr Metab*. 1997;41(6):365–70.

100. Ågren J et al. Fatty acid composition of erythrocyte, platelet, and serum lipids in strict vegans. *Lipids*. 1995;30:365–369.

101. Li D et al. Relationship between platelet phospholipid FA and mean platelet volume in healthy men. *Lipids*. 2002;37(9):901–6.

102. Sanders TA, Reddy S. The influence of a vegetarian diet on the fatty acid composition of human milk and the essential

fatty acid status of the infant. *J Pediatr.* 1992;120:S71–7.

103. Mangat I. Do vegetarians have to eat fish for optimal cardiovascular protection? *Am J Clin Nutr.* 2009;89(5):1597S–1601S.

104. Key TJ et al. Mortality in vegetarians and nonvegetarians: detailed findings from a collaborative analysis of 5 prospective studies. *Am J Clin Nutr.* 1999;70(3 Suppl): 516S–524S.

105. Crowe FL et al. Risk of hospitalization or death from ischemic heart disease among British vegetarians and nonvegetarians: results from the EPIC-Oxford cohort study. *Am J Clin Nutr.* 2013;97(3):597–603.

106. Nishida C et al. The joint WHO/FAO expert consultation on diet, nutrition and the prevention of chronic diseases: process, product and policy implications. *Public Health Nutr.* 2004;7(1A): 245–50.

107. Harris WS et al. Towards establishing dietary reference intakes for eicosapentaenoic and docosahexaenoic acids. *J Nutr.* 2009;139(4):804S–19S.

108. Kris-Etherton PM et al. Dietary reference intakes for DHA and EPA. *Prostaglandins Leukot Essent Fatty Acids.* 2009 Aug-Sep;81(2-3):99–104.

109. Calder PC et al. Essential fats for future health. Proceedings of the 9th Unilever Nutrition Symposium, 26-27 May 2010. *Eur J Clin Nutr.* 2010;Suppl 4: S1–13.

110. European Food Safety Authority. Scientific Opinion: Labelling reference intake values for n-3 and n-6 polyunsaturated fatty acids. *The EFSA Journal.* 2009;1176,1–11.

111. Anderson BM, Ma DW. Are all n-3 polyunsaturated fatty acids created equal? *Lipids Health Dis.* 2009;8:33.

112. Chong EW et al. Dietary omega-3 fatty acid and fish intake in the primary prevention of age-related macular degeneration: a systematic review and meta-analysis. *Arch Ophthalmol.* 2008;126(6):826–33. Review.

113. SanGiovanni JP et al. The relationship of dietary omega-3 long-chain polyunsaturated fatty acid intake with incident age-related macular degeneration:

AREDS report no. 23. *Arch Ophthalmol.* 2008;126(9):1274–9.

114. Christen WG et al. Dietary Ω-3 fatty acid and fish intake and incident age-related macular degeneration in women. *Arch Ophthalmol.* 2011;129(7):921–9.

115. Sublette ME et al. Meta-analysis of the effects of eicosapentaenoic acid (EPA) in clinical trials in depression. *J Clin Psychiatry.* 2011;72(12):1577–84.

116. Huffman SL et al. Essential fats: how do they affect growth and development of infants and young children in developing countries? A literature review. *Maternal and Child Nutrition.* 2011;7(Suppl. 3): 44–65.

117. Hoffman DR et al. Toward optimizing vision and cognition in term infants by dietary docosahexaenoic and arachidonic acid supplementation: a review of randomized controlled trials. *Prostaglandins, Leukotrienes, and Essential Fatty Acids.* 2009;81:151–158.

118. Innis SM. Fatty acids and early human development. *Early Human Development.* 2007; 83:761–766.

119. Baylin A et al. a-Linolenic acid, D6-desaturase gene polymorphism, and the risk of nonfatal myocardial infarction. *Am J Clin Nutr.* 2007;85:554–60.

120. Geppert J et al. Microalgal docosahexaenoic acid decreases plasma triacylglycerol in normolipidaemic vegetarians: a randomised trial. *Br J Nutr.* 2006;95(4):779–86.

121. Geppert J et al. Docosahexaenoic acid supplementation in vegetarians effectively increases omega-3 index: a randomized trial. *Lipids.* 2005;40(8):807–14.

122. Lloyd-Wright Z et al. Randomized placebo controlled trial of a daily intake of 200 mg docosahexaenoic acid in vegans. Abstracts of Original Communications. *Proceedings of the Nutrition Society.* 2003;42a.

123. Wu et al. Effects of docosahexaenoic acid supplementation on blood lipids, estrogen metabolism, and in vivo oxidative stress in postmenopausal vegetarian women. *Eur J Clin Nutr.* 2006;60(3):386–92.

124. Geleijnse JM et al. Alpha-linolenic acid: is it essential to cardiovascular health? *Curr Atheroscler Rep.* 2010;12(6):359–67.

125. Gebauer SK et al. n-3 fatty acid dietary recommendations and food sources to achieve essentiality and cardiovascular benefits. *Am J Clin Nutr.* 2006;83(Suppl 6):1526S–1535S.

126. Koletzko B et al. The roles of long-chain polyunsaturated fatty acids in pregnancy, lactation and infancy: review of current knowledge and consensus recommendations. *J Perinat Med.* 2008;36(1):5–14.

127. AOCS. Collected recommendations for long-chain polyunsaturated fatty acid intake, *AOCS Inform.* 2003:762–763.

128. Simopoulos AP. Essential fatty acids in health and chronic disease. *Am J Clin Nutr.* 1999;70(suppl):560s–569s.

129. Pelser C, Mondul AM, Hollenbeck AR, Park Y. Dietary fat, fatty acids, and risk of prostate cancer in the NIH-AARP diet and health study. *Cancer Epidemiol Biomarkers Prev.* 2013;22(4):697–707.

130. Christensen JH et al. Prostate tissue and leukocyte levels of n-3 polyunsaturated fatty acids in men with benign prostate hyperplasia or prostate cancer. *BJU Int.* 2006;97: 270–273.

131. Harvei S, Bjerve KS, Tretli S et al. Prediagnostic level of fatty acids in serum phospholipids: Ω-3 and Ω-6 fatty acids and the risk of prostate cancer. *In. J Cancer.* 1997;71:545–551.

132. Newcomer LM et al. The association of fatty acids with prostate cancer risk. *Prostate.* 2001;47: 262–268.

133. Yang YJ et al. Comparison of fatty acid profiles in the serum of patients with prostate cancer and benign prostatic hyperplasia. *Clin Biochem.* 1999;32:405–409.

134. Gann PH et al. Prospective study of plasma fatty acids and risk of prostate cancer. *J Natl Cancer Inst.* 1994;86:281–286.

135. De Stefani E et al. α-Linolenic acid and risk of prostate cancer: a case-control study in Uruguay. *Cancer Epidemiol. Biomarkers Prev.* 2000;9:335–338.

136. Ramon JM et al. Dietary fat intake and prostate cancer risk: A case-control study in Spain. *Cancer Causes Control.* 2000; 11:679–685.

137. Giovannucci E et al. A prospective study of dietary fat and risk of prostate cancer. *J Natl Cancer Inst.* 1993;85:1571–1579.

138. Giovannucci E et al. Risk factors for prostate cancer incidence and progression in the Health Professionals Follow-up Study. *Int J Cancer.* 2007;121(7):1571–8.

139. Leitzmann MF et al. 2004. Dietary intake of n-3 and n-6 fatty acids and the risk of prostate cancer. *Am J Clin Nutr.* 2004;80:204–216.

140. Azrad M et al. Prostatic alpha-linolenic acid (ALA) is positively associated with aggressive prostate cancer: a relationship which may depend on genetic variation in ALA metabolism. *PLoS One.* 2012;7(12): e53104.

141. Freeman VL et al. Prostatic levels of fatty acids and the histopathology of localized prostate cancer. *J Urol.* 2000;164:2168–2172.

142. Freeman VL et al. 2004. Inverse association between prostatic polyunsaturated fatty acid and risk of locally advanced prostate carcinoma. *Cancer.* 2004;101: 2744–2754.

143. Godley PA et al. Biomarkers of essential fatty acid consumption and risk of prostatic carcinoma. Cancer Epidemiol. *Biomarkers Prev.* 1996;5:889–895.

144. Männistö S et al. Fatty acids and risk of prostate cancer in a nested case-control study in male smokers. *Cancer Epidemiol. Biomarkers Prev.* 2003;12:1422–1428.

145. Chavarro JE et al. A prospective study of polyunsaturated fatty acid levels in blood and prostate cancer risk. *Cancer Epidemiol Biomarkers Prev.* 2007;16:OF1–OF7.

146. Andersson S-O, et al. Energy, nutrient intake and prostate cancer risk: a population-based case-control study in Sweden. *Int J Cancer.* 1996;68:716–722.

147. Bairati I et al. Dietary fat and advanced prostate cancer. *J Urol.* 1998;159:1271–1275.

148. Bidoli E et al. Macronutrients, fatty acids, cholesterol and prostate cancer risk. *Ann Oncol.* 2005;16:152–157.

149. Koralek DO et al. A prospective study of dietary alpha-linolenic acid and the risk of prostate cancer (United States). *Cancer Causes Control.* 2006;17:783–791.

150. Laaksonen DE et al. Serum linoleic and total polyunsaturated fatty acids in relation to prostate and other cancers: a population-based cohort study. *Int J Cancer.* 2004;111: 444–450.

151. Schuurman AG et al. Association of energy and fat intake with prostate carcinoma risk: results from the Netherlands Cohort Study. *Cancer* 1999;86:1019–1027.

152. Carleton AJ et al. Case-control and prospective studies of dietary α-linolenic acid intake and prostate cancer risk: a meta-analysis. *BMJ Open.* 2013;3(5).

153. Sorongon-Legaspi MK et al. Blood level omega-3 Fatty acids as risk determinant molecular biomarker for prostate cancer. *Prostate Cancer.* 2013;2013:875615.

154. Chua ME et al. Relationship of dietary intake of omega-3 and omega-6 Fatty acids with risk of prostate cancer development: a meta-analysis of prospective studies and review of literature. *Prostate Cancer.* 2012; 2012:826254.

155. Carayol M et al. Prospective studies of dietary alpha-linolenic acid intake and prostate cancer risk: a meta-analysis. *Cancer Causes Control.* 2010;21(3):347–55.

156. Shannon J et al. Erythrocyte fatty acids and prostate cancer risk: a comparison of methods. *Prostaglandins Leukot Essent Fatty Acids.* 2010;83(3):161–9.

157. Simon JA et al. The relation of alpha-linolenic acid to the risk of prostate cancer: a systematic review and meta-analysis. *Am J Clin Nutr.* 2009;89(5):1558S–1564S.

158. Lu M et al. Dietary fat intake and early age-related lens opacities. *Am J Clin Nutr.* 2005;81(4):773–9.

159. Lu M et al. Dietary linolenic acid intake is positively associated with five-year change in eye lens nuclear density. *J Am Coll Nutr.* 2007;26(2):133–40.

160. Cho E et al. Prospective study of dietary fat and the risk of age-related macular degeneration. *Am J Clin Nutr.* 2001;73(2): 209–18.

161. Demark Wahnefried W et al. Flaxseed supplementation (not dietary fat restriction) reduces prostate cancer proliferation rates in men presurgery. *Cancer Epidemiol Biomarkers Prev.* 2008;17:3577–3587.

162. Demark Wahnefried W et al. Pilot study to explore effects of low-fat, flaxseed-supplemented diet on proliferation of benign prostatic epithelium and prostate-specific antigen. *Urology.* 2004;63:900–904.

163. Demark-Wahnefried W et al. Pilot study of dietary fat restriction and flaxseed supplementation in men with prostate cancer before surgery: exploring the effects on hormonal levels, prostate specific antigen, and histopathologic features. *Urology.* 2001;58:47–52.

164. He J Bazan HE. Omega-3 fatty acids in dry eye and corneal nerve regeneration after refractive surgery. *Prostaglandins Leukot Essent Fatty Acids.* 2010;82(4-6):319–25.

165. U.S. Department of Agriculture, Agricultural Research Service. 2007. USDA National Nutrient Database for Standard Reference, Release 20. Nutrient Data Laboratory Home Page. www.ars.usda.gov/ba/bhnrc/ndl

166. Sanders T, Lewis F. Review of Nutritional Attributes of GOOD OIL (Cold Pressed Hemp Seed Oil). Nutritional Sciences Division, King's College London. 2008: www.goodwebsite.co.uk/kingsreport.pdf

167. Kushak R et al. Blue-green algae Aphanizomenon flos-aquae as a source of dietary polyunsaturated fatty acids and a hypocholesterolemic agent. *Annual Meeting of the American Chemical Society.* March 1999.

168. Manitoba Harvest Hemp Foods. Nutrition Facts. Hemp Hearts. www.manitobaharvest.com/

169. World Cancer Research Fund/American Institute for Cancer Research. *Food, Nutrition, Physical Activity and the Prevention of Cancer: A Global Perspective.* Washington DC:AICR, 2007.

170. Mente A et al. A systematic review of the evidence supporting a causal link between dietary factors and coronary heart disease. *Arch Intern Med.* 2009;169(7):659–69.

171. Siri-Tarino PW et al. Meta-analysis of prospective cohort studies evaluating the association of saturated fat with cardiovascular disease. *Am J Clin Nutr.* 2010;91:535–46.

172. Micha R, Mozaffarian D. Saturated fat and cardiometabolic risk factors, coronary heart disease, stroke, and diabetes: a fresh look at the evidence. *Lipids.* 2010;45:893–905.

173. Hooper L et al. Reduced or modified dietary fat for preventing cardiovascular disease. *Cochrane Database Syst Rev.* 2012;5:CD002137. Review.

174. Mozaffarian D, Micha R, Wallace S et al, ed. Effects on Coronary Heart Disease of Increasing Polyunsaturated Fat in Place of Saturated Fat: A Systematic Review and Meta-Analysis of Randomized Controlled Trials. *PLoS Medicine.* 2010;7(3):1–10.

175. Danaei G et al. The preventable causes of death in the United States: comparative risk assessment of dietary, lifestyle, and metabolic risk factors. *PLoS Med.* 2009;6(4):e1000058.

176. Skeaff CM, Miller J. Dietary fat and coronary heart disease: summary of evidence from prospective cohort and randomised controlled trials. *Ann Nutr Metab.* 2009;55(1–3):173–201.

177. Jakobsen MU et al. Major types of dietary fat and risk of coronary heart disease: a pooled analysis of 11 cohort studies. *Am J Clin Nutr.* 2009;89 (5):1425–32.

178. Van Horn L et al. The evidence for dietary prevention and treatment of cardiovascular disease. *JADA.* 2008;108(2):287–331.

179. Chanu B. Primary dietetic prevention of ischaemic heart disease. *Archives des Maladies du Coeur et des Vaisseux.* 2003;96(Sp. Iss. 6):21–25.

180. Hu FB, Stamfer MJ. Nut consumption and risk of coronary heart disease: a review of the epidemiologic evidence. Current Atherosclerosis Reports. 1999;1:204–209.

181. Truswell AS. "Review of dietary intervention studies: effect on coronary events and on total mortality". *Australian and New Zealand Journal of Medicine.* 1994;24(1):98–106.

182. Dietary Guidelines Advisory Committee (DGAC). USDA Nutrition Evidence Library, 2010. What is the effect of saturated fat (SFA) intake on increased risk of cardiovascular disease or type 2 diabetes, including effects on intermediate markers such as serum lipid and lipoprotein levels? www.nutritionevidencelibrary.com/conclusion.cfm?conclusion_statement_id=250194

183. Astrup A et al. The role of reducing intakes of saturated fat in the prevention of cardiovascular disease: where does the evidence stand in 2010? *Am J Clin Nutr.* 2011;93:684–8.

184. Barclay AW et al. Glycemic index, glycemic load, and chronic disease risk–a meta-analysis of observational studies. *Am J Clin Nutr.* 2008;87:627–37.

185. Mellen PB et al. Whole grain intake and cardiovascular disease: a meta-analysis. *Nutr Metab Cardiovasc Dis.* 2008;18(4):283–90.

186. Nöthlings U et al. Intake of vegetables, legumes, and fruit, and risk for all-cause, cardiovascular, and cancer mortality in a European diabetic population. *Br J Nutr.* 2009;102(2):285–92.

187. Nagura J et al; JACC Study Group. Fruit, vegetable and bean intake and mortality from cardiovascular disease among Japanese men and women: the JACC Study. *J Nutr.* 2008;138(4):775–81.

188. Tey SL et al. Effects of different forms of hazelnuts on blood lipids and α-tocopherol concentrations in mildly hypercholesterolemic individuals. *Eur J Clin Nutr.* 2011;65(1):117–24.

189. O'Neil CE et al. Nut consumption is associated with decreased health risk factors for cardiovascular disease and metabolic syndrome in U.S. adults: NHANES 1999–2004. Journal of the American College of Nutrition. 2011;30(6):502–510.

190. Sabaté J. Nut consumption, vegetarian diets, ischemic heart disease risk, and all-cause mortality: evidence from epidemiologic studies. *Am J Clin Nutr.* 1999;70(3 Suppl):500S–503S. Review.

191. Fraser GE, Shavik, DJ. Ten years of life: is it a matter of choice? Arch Int Med. 2001;161:1645–1652.

192. Jiang R et al. Nut and peanut butter consumption and risk of type 2 diabetes in women. JAMA. 2002;288:2554–2560.

193. Kendall CW et al. Nuts, metabolic syndrome and diabetes. *Br J Nutr.* 2010; 104(4):465–73. Review.

194. Jenkins DJ et al. Nuts as a replacement for carbohydrates in the diabetic diet. *Diabetes Care.* 2011;34(8):1706–11.

195. Wang X et al. Effects of pistachios on body weight in Chinese subjects with metabolic syndrome. *Nutr J.* 2012;11(1):20.

196. Sabaté J et al. Nut consumption and blood lipid levels: a pooled analysis of 25 intervention trials. *Arch Intern Med.* 2010;170(9): 821–7.

197. Ros E. Health benefits of nut consumption. *Nutrients.* 2010;2(7):652–82. Review

198. Fraser GE et al. A possible protective effect of nut consumption on risk of coronary heart disease. The Adventist Health Study. *Arch Intern Med.* 1992;152:1416–24.

199. Fraser GE. Nut consumption, lipids, and risk of a coronary event. *Clin Cardiol.* 1999;22(7 Suppl):III11–5. Review.

200. Kushi LH et al. Dietary antioxidant vitamins and death from coronary heart disease in postmenopausal women. *N Engl J Med.* 1996;334:1156–62.

201. Ellsworth JL et al. Frequent nut intake and risk of death from coronary heart disease and all causes in postmenopausal women: the Iowa Women's Health Study. *Nutr Metab Cardiovasc Dis.* 2001;11(6):372–7.

202. Hu FB et al. Frequent nut consumption and risk of coronary heart disease in women: prospective cohort study. *BMJ.* 1998; 317:1341–5.

203. Albert CM et al. Nut consumption and decreased risk of sudden cardiac death in the Physicians' Health Study. *Arch Intern Med.* 2002;162:1382–7.

204. Sabaté J, Fraser GE. Nuts: a new protective food against coronary heart disease. *Curr Opin Lipidol.* 1994;5(1):11–6. Review.

205. Mukuddem-Petersen J et al. A systematic review of the effects of nuts on blood lipid profiles in humans. *J Nutr.* 2005; 135(9):2082–9.

206. Griel AE, Kris-Etherton PM. Tree nuts and the lipid profile: a review of clinical studies. *Br J Nutr.* 2006;96 Suppl 2:S68-78. Review.

207. Kris-Etherton PM et al. The role of tree nuts and peanuts in the prevention of coronary heart disease: multiple potential mechanisms. *J Nutr.* 2008;138(9):1746S–1751S.

208. Banel DK, Hu FB. Effects of walnut consumption on blood lipids and other cardiovascular risk factors: a meta-analysis and systematic review. *Am J Clin Nutr.* 2009;90:56–63.

209. Dreher ML. Pistachio nuts: composition and potential health benefits. *Nutr Rev.* 2012;70(4):234–40.

210. Lamarche B et al. Combined effects of a dietary portfolio of plant sterols, vegetable protein, viscous fiber and almonds on LDL particle size. *Br J Nutr.* 2004: 92(4): 654–63.

211. Ros E. Nuts and novel biomarkers of cardiovascular disease. *Am J Clin Nutr.* 2009; 89(5):1649S–56S. Review.

212. Alexiadou K, Katsilambros N. Nuts: antiatherogenic food? *Eur J Intern Med.* 2011; 22(2):141–6.

213. Yochum LA et al. Intake of antioxidant vitamins and risk of death from stroke in post-menopausal women. Am J Clin Nutr. 2000;72:476–483.

214. Bernstein AM et al. Dietary protein sources and the risk of stroke in men and women. *Stroke.* 2012;43(3):637–44.

215. Zhang SM et al. Intakes of vitamins E and C, carotenoids, vitamin supplements, and PD risk. Neurology. 2002;59:1161–9.

216. Gu Y, Scarmeas N. Dietary patterns in Alzheimer's disease and cognitive aging. *Curr Alzheimer Res.* 2011;8(5):510–9.

217. Tsai CJ et al. Frequent nut consumption and decreased risk of cholecystectomy in women. Am J Clin Nutr. 2004;80:76–81.

218. Seddon JM et al. Progression of age-related macular degeneration: association with dietary fat, transunsaturated fat, nuts and fish intake. Archives of Ophthalmology. 2003;121:1728–37.

219. Bes-Rastrollo M et al. Nut consumption and weight gain in a Mediterranean cohort: the SUN study. *Obesity.* 2007;15(1):107–116.

220. Bes-Rastrollo M et al. Prospective study of nut consumption, long-term weight change, and obesity risk in women. *Am J Clin Nutr.* 2009;89(6):1913–1919.

221. Casas-Agustench P et al. Cross-sectional association of nut intake with adiposity in a Mediterranean population. *Nutrition, Metabolism and Cardiovascular Diseases.* 2011; 21(7):518–525.

222. Griel AE et al. Improved diet quality with peanut consumption. *Journal of the American College of Nutrition.* 2004;23(6): 660–668.

223. Phung OJ et al. Almonds have a neutral effect on serum lipid profiles: a meta-analysis of randomized trials. *J Am Diet Assoc.* 2009;109(5):865–73.

224. Casas-Agustench P et al. Effects of one serving of mixed nuts on serum lipids, insulin resistance and inflammatory markers in patients with the metabolic syndrome. *Nutr Metab Cardiovasc Dis.* 2011;21(2): 126–35.

225. Griel AE et al. A macadamia nut-rich diet reduces total and LDL-cholesterol in mildly hypercholesterolemic men and women. *J Nutr.* 2008;138(4):761–7.

226. Mattes RD et al. Impact of peanuts and tree nuts on body weight and healthy weight loss in adults. *J Nutr.* 2008;138(9): 1741S–1745S.

227. Mattes RD, Dreher ML. Nuts and healthy body weight maintenance mechanisms. *Asia Pac J Clin Nutr.* 2010;19(1):137–41.

228. Yaacoub R, Saliba R, Nsouli B, Khalaf G, Birlouez-Aragon I. Formation of lipid oxidation and isomerization products during processing of nuts and sesame seeds. *J Agric Food Chem.* 2008;56(16):7082–90.

229. Lukac H et al. P Influence of roasting conditions on the acrylamide content and the color of roasted almonds. *Journal of Food Science.* 2006;72(1):c033–c038.

230. World Intellectual Property Organization (WO/2005/039322). Edible Testa-on (Skin-on) cashew nuts and methods for preparing same. 2005. www.wipo.int/pctdb/en/wo.jsp?IA=IB2003005287&DISPLAY=DESC

231. Thompson LU, Li T, Chen, J, Goss, PE. Biological effects of dietary flaxseed in patients with breast cancer (abstract). *Breast Cancer Res Treatment.* 2000;64:50.

232. Sung MK et al. Mammalian lignans inhibit the growth of estrogen-independent human colon tumor cells. *Anticancer Res.* 1998;18:1405–1408.

233. Cunnane SC et al. Nutritional attributes of traditional flaxseed in healthy young adults. *Am J Clin Nutr.* 1995;61:62–68.

234. Manda escu S et al. Flaxseed supplementation in hyperlipidemic patients. *Rev Med Chir Soc Med Nat Iasi.* 2005;109(3):502–6.

235. Lucas EA et al. Flaxseed improves lipid profile without altering biomarkers of bone metabolism in postmenopausal women. *J. Clin Endocrinol Metab.* 2002;87: 1527–1532.

236. Jenkins DJA et al. Health aspects of partially defatted flaxseed, including effects on serum lipids, oxidative measures, and ex vivo androgen and progestin activity: A controlled crossover trial. *Am J Clin Nutr.* 1999;69:395–402.

237. Morris D. *Flax: a health and nutrition primer. Fourth Edition.* Flax Council of Canada. 2007.

238. Ayerza R. The seed's protein and oil content, fatty acid composition, and growing cycle length of a single genotype of chia (Salvia hispanica L.) as affected by environmental factors. *J Oleo Sci.* 2009;58(7):347–54.

239. Callaway JC. Hempseed as a nutritional resource: an overview. *Euphytica*. 2004; 140: 65–72.

240. Lu QY et al. California Hass avocado: profiling of carotenoids, tocopherol, fatty acid, and fat content during maturation and from different growing areas. *J Agric Food Chem*. 2009;57(21):10408–13.

241. Duester KC. Avocado fruit is a rich source of beta-sitosterol. *J Am Diet Assoc*. 2001; 101(4):404–5.

242. Colquhoun DM et al. Comparison of the effects on lipoproteins and apolipoproteins of a diet high in monounsaturated fatty acids, enriched with avocado, and a high-carbohydrate diet. *Am J Clin Nutr*. 1992;56(4):671–7.

243. Lu QY, Arteaga JR, Zhang Q et al. Inhibition of prostate cancer cell growth by an avocado extract: role of lipid-soluble bioactive substances. *J Nutr Biochem*. 2005; 16(1):23–30.

244. Ding H et al. Selective induction of apoptosis of human oral cancer cell lines by avocado extracts via a ROS-mediated mechanism. *Nutr Cancer*. 2009;61(3):348–56.

245. D'Ambrosio SM et al. Aliphatic acetogenin constituents of avocado fruits inhibit human oral cancer cell proliferation by targeting the EGFR/RAS/RAF/MEK/ERK1/2 pathway. *Biochem Biophys Res Commun*. 2011;409(3):465–9.

246. Paul R et al. Avocado fruit (Persea americana Mill) exhibits chemo–protective potentiality against cyclophosphamide induced genotoxicity in human lymphocyte culture. *J Exp Ther Oncol*. 2011;9(3):221–30.

247. Castillo-Juarez I et al. Anti- Helicobacter pylori activity of plants used in Mexican traditional medicine for gastrointestinal disorders. *J Ethnopharmacol*. 2009; 122:402–405.

248. Christensen R et al. Symptomatic efficacy of avocado-soybean unsaponifiables (ASU) in osteoarthritis (OA) patients: a meta-analysis of randomized controlled trials. *Osteoarthritis Cartilage*. 2008;16(4):399–408. Review.

249. Ernst E. Avocado-soybean unsaponifiables (ASU) for osteoarthritis - a systematic review. *Clin Rheumatol*. 2003;22:285–288.

250. Visioli F et al. Free radical scavenging properties of olive oil polyphenols. *Biochem Biophys Res Commun*. 1998;247: 60–64.

251. Stupans I et al. Comparison of radical scavenging effect, inhibition of microsomal oxygen free radical generation, and serum lipoprotein oxidation of several natural antioxidants. *J Agric Food Chem*. 2002;50: 2464–2469.

252. Kremastinos DT. Olive and oleuropein. *Hellenic J Cardiol*. 2008;49(4):295–6.

253. Owen RW, Haubner R, Würtele G, Hull E, Spiegelhalder B, Bartsch H. Olives and olive oil in cancer prevention *Eur J Cancer Prev*. 2004 Aug;13(4):319–26.

254. Beauchamp GK et al. Ibuprofen-like activity in extra-virgin olive oil. *Nature*. 2005; 437:45–6.

255. Casado FJ, Montaño A. Influence of processing conditions on acrylamide content in black ripe olives. *J Agric Food Chem*. 2008;56(6):2021–7.

256. Prior IA et al. Cholesterol, coconuts, and diet on Polynesian atolls: a natural experiment: the Pukapuka and Tokelau island studies. *Am J Clin Nutr*. 1981;34(8): 1552–61.

257. Lipoeto NI et al. Contemporary Minangkabau food culture in West Sumatra, Indonesia. *Asia Pac J Clin Nutr*. 2001;10(1): 10–6.

258. Lipoeto NI et al. Dietary intake and the risk of coronary heart disease among the coconut-consuming Minangkabau in West Sumatra, Indonesia. *Asia Pac J Clin Nutr*. 2004;13(4):377–84.

259. Rego Costa AC, Rosado EL, Soares-Mota M. Influence of the dietary intake of medium chain triglycerides on body composition, energy expenditure and satiety: a systematic review. *Nutr Hosp*. 2012 Jan-Feb;27(1):103–8.

260. Hunter JE et al. Cardiovascular disease risk of dietary stearic acid compared with trans, other saturated, and unsaturated fatty acids: a systematic review. *Am J Clin Nutr*. 2010;91(1):46–63.

261. de Roos NM et al. Consumption of a Solid Fat Rich in Lauric Acid Results in a More

Favorable Serum Lipid Profile in Healthy Men and Women than Consumption of a Solid Fat Rich in *trans*-Fatty Acids. Journal of Nutrition. 2001;131:242–245.

262. Mensink RP et al. Effects of dietary fatty acids and carbohydrates on the ratio of serum total to HDL cholesterol and on serum lipids and apolipoproteins: a meta-analysis of 60 controlled trials. *Am J Clin Nutr.* 2003;77:1146–55.

263. DebMandal M, Mandal S. Coconut (Cocos nucifera L.: Arecaceae): in health promotion and disease prevention. *Asian Pac J Trop Med.* 2011;4(3):241–7. Review.

264. Ogbolu DO et al. In vitro antimicrobial properties of coconut oil on Candida species in Ibadan, Nigeria. J Med Food. 2007;10(2):384–7.

265. Erguiza G et al. The effect of virgin coconut oil supplementation for community-acquired pneumonia in children aged 3 months to 60 months admitted at the Phillipine Children's Medical Center: a single blinded randomized controlled trial. *Chest Journal. American College of Chest Physicians.* Oct. 29, 2008.

266. Hierholzer JC, Kabara JJ. In vitro effects of monolaurin compounds on enveloped RNA and DNA viruses. *Journal of Food Safety.* 1982;4:1–12.

267. Carpo BG et al. Novel antibacterial activity of monolaurin compared with conventional antibiotics against organisms from skin infections: an in vitro study. *J Drugs Dermatol.* 2007;6:991–998.

268. Nevin KG, Rajamohan T. Beneficial effects of virgin coconut oil on lipid parameters and in vitro LDL oxidation. *Clin Biochem.* 2004;37(9):830–5.

269. Marina AM, Man YB, Nazimah SA, Amin I. Antioxidant capacity and phenolic acids of virgin coconut oil. *Int J Food Sci Nutr.* 2008; Dec 29:1–10.

270. Troika. Vegetable oil refining plant. www.troikaindia.com/refinery-plant.html

271. Wikipedia. Smoke point. http://en.wikipedia.org/wiki/Smoke_point

272. Quest Network Blue Zones - Longevity Secrets: "Live Longer, Better: Longevity Secrets", Quest Network, 2006. http://en.wikipedia.org/wiki/Blue_Zones

273. Chowdhury R, et al: Association of Dietary, Circulating, and Supplement Fatty Acids With Coronary Risk. A Systematic Review and Meta-analysis. *Annals of Internal Medicine.* 2014;160(6):398–406.

274. Astrup A, et al. The role of reducing intakes of saturated fat in the prevention of cardio-vascular disease: where does the evidence stand in 2010? *Am J Clin Nutr.* 2011; Apr;93(4):684–8. Review.

275. Riccardi G, et al. Dietary fat, insulin sensitivity and the metabolic syndrome. *Clin Nutr.* 2004;23(4):447–56. Review.

REFERENCES FOR CHAPTER 5

1. World Health Organization. *WHO Technical report series 916. Diet, Nutrition and the Prevention of Chronic Diseases.* Report of a joint FAO/WHO Expert Consultation. 2003.

2. Mann J, Cummings JH, Englyst HN. FAO/WHO Scientific Update on carbohydrates in human nutrition: conclusions. *Euro J Clin Nutr.* 2007;61(1):S132–S137.

3. National Research Council. Dietary Carbohydrates, Starches and Sugars. *Dietary Reference Intakes for Energy, Carbohydrate, Fiber, Fat, Fatty Acids, Cholesterol, Protein, and Amino Acids (Macronu-* trients). Washington DC: National Academies Press, 2005:265–338.

4. FAO Food Nutrition Paper. Carbohydrates in human nutrition. *Report of a Joint FAO/WHO Expert Consultation.* 1998; 66:1–140. www.fao.org/docrep/W8079E/W8079E00.htm

5. Wright JD et al. *Dietary Intake of Ten Key Nutrients for Public Health, United States: 1999-2000.* Advance data from vital and health statistics no. 334. Hyattsville MD: National Center for Health Statistics. 2003. www.cdc.gov/nchs/data/ad/ad334.pdf

6. Mangels R et al. *The Dietitian's Guide to Vegetarian Diets: Issues and Applications.* Third Edition. Sudbury MA: Jones and Bartlett Learning, 2011. Data from Appendix A.

7. Davis B et al. *Becoming Raw.* Summertown TN: The Book Publishing Company, 2010.

8. Pedersen AN et al. Health effects of protein intake in healthy adults: a systematic literature review. *Food Nutr Res.* 2013; 57:21245.

9. Fung TT et al. Low-carbohydrate diets and all-cause and cause-specific mortality: two cohort studies. *Ann Intern Med.* 2010;153(5):289–98.

10. Noto H et al. Low-carbohydrate diets and all-cause mortality: a systematic review and meta-analysis of observational studies. *PLoS One.* 2013;8(1):e55030.

11. Gray J. *Dietary Fiber: definition, analysis, physiology and health.* ILSI Europe Concise Monograph Series. Brussels Belgium: ILSI Europe, 2006.

12. Cummings JH, Stephen AM. Carbohydrate terminology and classification. *Eur J Clin Nutr.* 2007;61(Suppl 1):S5–18.

13. U.S. Department of Agriculture, Agricultural Research Service. 2013. USDA National Nutrient Database for Standard Reference, Release 26. Nutrient Data Laboratory Home Page. www.ars.usda.gov/ba/bhnrc/ndl

14. Craig W. Phytochemicals: Guardians of Health. *JADA.* 1997; 97(10):S199–S204.

15. Howlett JF et al. The definition of dietary fiber–discussions at the Ninth Vahouny Fiber Symposium: building scientific agreement. *Food Nutr Res.* 2010;54:10.

16. National Research Council. *Dietary Reference Intakes: Proposed Definition of Dietary Fiber.* Washington DC: The National Academies Press, 2001.

17. Novak M, Vetvicka V. Beta-glucans, history, and the present: immunomodulatory aspects and mechanisms of action. *Journal Of Immunotoxicology.* 2008;5(1):47–57.

18. Englyst KN et al. Nutritional characterization and measurement of dietary carbo-hydrates. *Eur J Clin Nutr.* 2007;61(Suppl 1):S19–39.

19. Pereira MA et al. Dietary fiber and risk of coronary heart disease: a pooled analysis of cohort studies. *Arch Intern Med.* 2004; 164:370–6.

20. Rimm EB et al. Vegetable, fruit, and cereal fiber intake and risk of coronary heart disease among men. *JAMA.* 1996; 275:447–51.

21. Brown L et al. Cholesterol-lowering effects of dietary fiber: a meta–analysis. *Am J Clin Nutr.* 1999; 69:30–42.

22. McKeown NM et al. Carbohydrate nutrition, insulin resistance, and the prevalence of the metabolic syndrome in the Framingham Offspring Cohort. *Diabetes Care.* 2004; 27:538–46.

23. McKeown NM et al. Whole-grain intake is favorably associated with metabolic risk factors for type 2 diabetes and cardiovascular disease in the Framingham Offspring Study. *Am J Clin Nutr.* 2002; 76:390–8.

24. Krishnan S et al. Glycemic index, glycemic load, and cereal fiber intake and risk of type 2 diabetes in US black women. *Arch Intern Med.* 2007;167:2304–9.

25. Schulze MB et al. Glycemic index, glycemic load, and dietary fiber intake and incidence of type 2 diabetes in younger and middle-aged women. *Am J Clin Nutr.* 2004; 80:348–56.

26. Konner M, Eaton SB. Paleolithic nutrition: twenty-fifive years later. *Nutr Clin Pract.* 2010;25(6):594-602.

27. Anderson JW et al. Health benefits of dietary fiber. *Nutr Rev.* 2009;67(4):188–205.

28. Streppel MT et al. Dietary fiber and blood pressure: a meta-analysis of randomized placebo-controlled trials. *Arch Intern Med.* 2005;165(2):150–6.

29. Macfarlane S, Macfarlane GT. Composition and metabolic activities of bacterial biofilms colonizing food residues in the human gut. *Appl Environ Microbiol.* 2006;72(9):6204–11.

30. Winham DM, Hutchins AM. Perceptions of flatulence from bean consumption among adults in 3 feeding studies. *Nutr J.* 2011;10:128.

31. Kavas A, Sedef NEL. Nutritive value of germinated mung beans and lentils. *J Consumer Studies Home Econ.* 1991;15:357–66.

32. Savitri A et al. Effect of spices on in vitro gas production by Clostridium perfringens. *Food Microbiology.* 1986; 3:195–199.

33. USDA Economic Research Service. Briefing Rooms: Dry Beans. www.ers.usda.gov/Briefing/DryBeans/

34. Hardarson et al. (Eds.) *Maximizing the Use of Biological Nitrogen Fixation in Agriculture.* Report of an FAO/IAEA Technical Expert Meeting held in Rome, 13-15 March 2001. Series: Developments in Plant and Soil Sciences. Vol. 99.

35. Theil EC et al. Absorption of iron from ferritin is independent of heme iron and ferrous salts in women and rat intestinal segments. *J Nutr.* 2012;142(3):478–83.

36. Darmadi-Blackberry I et al. Legumes: the most important dietary predictor of survival in older people of different ethnicities. *Asia Pacific J Clin Nutr.* 2004;13(2):217–220.

37. Winham D et al. Beans and good health: Compelling research earns beans expanded roles in dietary guidance. *Nutrition Today.* 2008;43:201–209.

38. Johnson RK et al. Dietary Sugars Intake and Cardiovascular Health : A Scientific Statement From the American Heart Association. *Circulation.* 2009;120:1011–1020.

39. No Author. The Consumption of Sugar. *New York Times.* Sept. 20, 1902. http://query.nytimes.com/mem/archive-free/pdf?res=F20D10FF355414728DDDA90A94D1405B828CF1D3.

40. Wells HF, Buzby JC. The United States Department of Agriculture. Economic Research Service. *Dietary Assessment of Major Trends in U.S. Food Consumption, 1970-2005.* Economic Information Bulletin Number 33. 2008.

41. Tappy L, Le KA. Metabolic Effects of Fructose and the Worldwide Increase in Obesity. *Physiol Rev.* 2010;90:23–46.

42. Lustig RH et al. Public health: The toxic truth about sugar. *Nature.* 2012; 482(7383):27–9.

43. Nseir W et al. Soft drinks consumption and nonalcoholic fatty liver Disease. *World J Gastroenterol.* 2010;16(21):2579-2588.

44. Key TJ, Spencer EA. Carbohydrates and cancer: an overview of the epidemiological evidence. *European Journal of Clinical Nutrition.* 2007;61(Suppl 1):S112–S121.

45. World Cancer Research Fund/American Institute for Cancer Research. *Food, nutrition, physical activity and the prevention of cancer: a global perspective.* Washington DC: AICR; 2007.

46. Kabat GC et al. A longitudinal study of serum insulin and glucose levels in relation to colorectal cancer risk among postmenopausal women. *Br J Cancer.* 2012;106(1):227–32.

47. Gunter MJ et al. Insulin, insulin-like growth factor-I, and risk of breast cancer in postmenopausal women. *J Natl Cancer Inst.* 2009; 101(1):48–60.

48. Krajcik RA et al. Insulin-like Growth Factor I (IGF-I), IGF-binding Proteins, and Breast Cancer. *Cancer Epidemiol Biomarkers Prev.* 2002;11(12):1566–73.

49. Van Dam RM, Seidell JC. Review: Carbohydrate intake and obesity. *European Journal of Clinical Nutrition.* 2007;61(1): S75–S99.

50. Turina M et al. Acute hyperglycemia and the innate immune system: clinical, cellular, and molecular aspects. *Cri Care Med.* 2005;33(7):1624–33.

51. Turina M et al. Short-term hyperglycemia in surgical patients and a study of related cellular mechanisms. *Ann Surg.* 2006; 243(6):845–51; discussion 851–3.

52. Stegenga ME et al. Effect of acute hyperglycaemia and/or hyperinsulinaemia on proinflammatory gene expression, cytokine production and neutrophil function in humans. *Diabet Med.* 2008;25(2):157–64.

53. Luevano-Contreras C, Chpman-Novakofski K. Dietary advanced glycation end products and aging. *Nutrients.* 2010;2(12):1247–65.

54. Sanchez A et al. Role of sugars in human neutrophilic phagocytosis. *The American Journal of Clinical Nutrition.* 1973; 26:1180–1184.

55. Takeuchi M et al. Immunological detection of fructose-derived advanced glycation end-products. *Lab Invest*. 2010 Jul;90(7): 1117–27.

56. U.S. Department of Agriculture and U.S. Department of Health and Human Services. *Dietary Guidelines for Americans, 2010*. 7th Edition, Washington DC: U.S. Government Printing Office, December 2010.

57. Beverage Marketing Corporation. U. S. Liquid Refreshment Beverage Market 2007-2008. Volume by Segment. www.beveragemarketing.com/?section=news&newsID=111

58. Malik VS et al. Intake of sugar-sweetened beverages and weight gain: a systematic review. *Am J Clin Nutr*. 2006;84:274–288.

59. Vartanian LR et al. Effects of soft drink consumption on nutrition and health: a systematic review and meta-analysis. *Am J Pub Health*. 2007;97:667–675.

60. Jacobson MJ. Liquid Candy – How Soft Drinks are Harming Americans' Health. Washington; DC: *Center for Science in the Public Interest*. June 2005. www.cspinet.org/new/pdf/liquid_candy_final_w_new_supplement.pdf

61. Shi Z. et al. Association between soft drink consumption and asthma and chronic obstructive pulmonary disease among adults in Australia. *Respirology*. 2012;17(2): 363–9.

62. White JS. Straight talk about high-fructose corn syrup: what it is and what it ain't. *Am J Clin Nutr*. 2008;88(6):1716S–1721S.

63. Le MT et al. Effects of high-fructose corn syrup and sucrose on the pharmacokinetics of fructose and acute metabolic and hemodynamic responses in healthy subjects. *Metabolism*. 2012;61(5):641–51.

64. American Dietetic Association. Position of the American Dietetic Association: use of nutritive and nonnutritive sweeteners. *J Am Diet Assoc*. 2004;104(2):255–75.

65. Anderson J, Young L. *Sugar and Sweeteners. Fact Sheet No. 9.301*.Food and Nutrition Series/Health. Colorado State University Extension. 9/98. Revised 5/10. www.ext.colostate.edu/pubs/foodnut/09301.PDF

66. Ulbricht C et al. An evidence-based systematic review of stevia by the Natural Standard Research Collaboration. *Cardiovasc Hematol Agents Med Chem*. 2010;8(2): 113–27. Review.

67. Goyal SK et al. Stevia (Stevia rebaudiana) a bio-sweetener: a review. *Int J Food Sci Nutr*. 2010;61(1):1–10. Review.

68. Chatsudthipong V, Muanprasat C. Stevioside and related compounds: therapeutic benefits beyond sweetness. *Pharmacol Ther*. 2009;121(1):41–54.

69. Mattes RD, Popkin BM. Nonnutritive sweetener consumption in humans: effects on appetite and food intake and their putative mechanisms. *Am J Clin Nutr*. 2009; 89:1–14.

70. Yang Q. Gain weight by "going diet?" Artificial sweeteners and the neurobiology of sugar cravings: Neuroscience 2010. *Yale J Biol Med*. 2010;83(2):101–8.

71. Liebman B. Carbo loading: do you overdo refined grains? *Nutrition Action Healthletter*. March 2011.

72. Liu S. Intake of Refined Carbohydrates and Whole Grain Foods in Relation to Risk of Type 2 Diabetes Mellitus and Coronary Heart Disease. *Journal of the American College of Nutrition*. 2002; 21(4): 298–306.

73. Steffen LM, Jacobs Jr. DR, Stevens J et al. Associations of whole-grain, refined-grain, and fruit and vegetable consumption with risks of all-cause mortality and incident coronary artery disease and ischemic stroke: the Atherosclerosis Risk in Communities (ARIC) Study. *Am J Clin Nutr*. 2003;78:383–90.

74. Buyken AE et al. Carbohydrate nutrition and inflammatory disease mortality in older adults. *Am J Clin Nutr*. 2010;92(3): 634–43.

75. Harvard School of Public Health. Carbohydrates: Good carbs guide the way. The Nutrition Source. www.hsph.harvard.edu/nutritionsource/what-should-you-eat/carbohydrates-full-story/

76. Yang F et al. Studies on germination conditions and antioxidant contents of wheat

grain. *International Journal of Food Sciences and Nutrition.* 2001;52: 319–330.

77. Sapone A et al. Divergence of gut permeability and mucosal immune gene expression in two gluten associated conditions: celiac disease and gluten sensitivity. *BMC Medicine.* 2011;9:23. www.biomedcentral.com/1741-7015/9/23

78. Zimmer KP. Nutrition and celiac disease. *Curr Probl Pediatr Adolesc Health Care.* 2011;41(9):244–7.

79. Fric P et al. Celiac disease, gluten-free diet, and oats. *Nutr Rev.* 2011;69(2):107–15.

80. Pulido OM et al. Introduction of oats in the diet of individuals with celiac disease: a systematic review. *Adv Food Nutr Res.* 2009;57:235–85.

81. Alicia Woodward. The latest on gluten sensitivity and celiac disease: Q & A with Alessio Fasano, MD. *Living Without Magazine.* Aug/Sep 2011 Issue. www.livingwithout.com/issues/4_15/qa_aug-sep11-2554-1.html

82. Barclay AW et al. Glycemic index, glycemic load, and chronic disease risk--a meta-analysis of observational studies. *Am J Clin Nutr.* 2008;87(3):627–37.

83. Jenkins, DJA et al. Glycemic Index of Foods: a Physiological Basis for Carbohydrate Exchange. *Am J Clin Nutr.* 1981;34: 362–366.

84. Atkinson FS et al. International tables of glycemic index and glycemic load values: 2008. *Diabetes Care.* 2008;31(12): 2281–3.

85. Gell P. From jelly beans to kidney beans: what diabetes educators should know about the glycemic index. *Diabetes Educ.* 2001;27(4):505–8.

86. Tremblay F et al. Role of Dietary Proteins and Amino Acids in the Pathogenesis of Insulin Resistance. *Annual Review of Nutrition.* 2007;27:293–310.

87. Duke University Medical Center. Too Much Protein, Eaten Along With Fat, May Lead To Insulin Resistance. *ScienceDaily.* April 9, 2009. www.sciencedaily.com/releases/2009/04/090407130905.htm

88. Brand Miller JC. Importance of glycemic index in diabetes. *Am J Clin Nutr.* 1994;59 (supplement: 747S–752S.)

89. Waldmann A et al. Overall glycemic index and glycemic load of vegan diets in relation to plasma lipoproteins and triacylglycerols. *Ann Nutr Metab.* 2007;51(4):335–44.

90. Foster-Powell K, Miller JB. International tables of glycemic index. *Am J Clin Nutr.* 1995;62(4):871S–890S. Review.

91. Foster-Powell K et al. International table of glycemic index and glycemic load values: 2002. *Am J Clin Nutr.* 2002;76(1):5–56.

92. Liljeberg H, Björck I. Delayed gastric emptying rate may explain improved glycaemia in healthy subjects to a starchy meal with added vinegar. *Eur J Clin Nutr.* 1998; 52(5):368–71.

93. Ostman E et al. Vinegar supplementation lowers glucose and insulin responses and increases satiety after a bread meal in healthy subjects. *Eur J Clin Nutr.* 2005; 59(9):983–8.

REFERENCES FOR CHAPTER 6

1. Hambidge KM. Micronutrient bioavailability: Dietary Reference Intakes and a future perspective. *Am J Clin Nutr.* 2010;91(5): 1430S–1432S.

2. Hunt J. Bioavailability of iron, zinc, and other trace minerals from vegetarian diets. *Am J Clin Nutr.* 2003;78(suppl):633S–9S.

3. Institute of Medicine. *Dietary Reference Intakes for Calcium and Vitamin D.* Washington DC: National Academies Press, 2010.

4. Hotz C et al. Traditional Food-Processing and Preparation Practices to Enhance the Bioavailability of Micronutrients in Plant-Based Diets. *J Nutr.* 2007;137(4):1097–100.

5. Kuhnlein HV et al. Composition of traditional Hopi foods. *J Am Diet Assoc.* 1979; 75:37–41.

6. Bohn L et al. Phytate: impact on environment and human nutrition. A challenge for molecular breeding. *J Zhejiang Univ Sci B.* 2008;9(3):165–91.

7. Gibson RS et al. Improving the bioavailability of nutrients in plant foods at the household level. *Proceedings of the Nutrition Society.* 2006;65(2):160–168.

8. Hurrell R et al. Iron bioavailability and dietary reference values. *Am J Clin Nutr.* 2010;91(5):1461S–1467S.

9. Lönnerdal B. Dietary factors influencing zinc absorption. *J Nutr.* 2000;130(5S Suppl):1378S–83S.

10. Viadel B et al. Effect of cooking and legume species upon calcium, iron and zinc uptake by Caco-2 cells. *J Trace Elem Med Biol.* 2006;20(2):115–20.

11. Coulibaly A et al. Phytic acid in cereal grains: structure, healthful or harmful ways to reduce phytic acid in cereal grains, and their effects on nutritional quality. *Am J Plant Nutr and Fertilization Technology.* 2011;1(1):1–22.

12. Urbano G et al. The role of phytic acid in legumes: antinutrient or beneficial function? *J Physiol Biochem.* 2000;56(3):283–94.

13. Markiewicz LH et al. Diet shapes the ability of human intestinal microbiota to degrade phytate - in vitro studies. *J Appl Microbiol.* 2013;115(1):247–59.

14. United States Department of Agriculture. *Oxalic Acid Content of Selected Vegetables.* 2009.

15. Bonsmann MS et al. Oxalic acid does not influence nonhaem iron absorption in humans: a comparison of kale and spinach meals. *Eur J Clin Nutr.* 2008;62(3):336–41.

16. Sotelo A et al. Role of oxate, phytate, tannins and cooking on iron bioavailability from foods commonly consumed in Mexico. *Int J Food Sci Nutr.* 2010;61(1):29–39.

17. Chai W et al. Effect of different cooking methods on vegetable oxalate content. *J Agric Food Chem.* 2005;53:3027–30.

18. Massey LK. Food oxalate: factors affecting measurement, biological variation, and bioavailability. *J Am Diet Assoc.* 2007;107:1191–4.

19. Heilberg IP et al. Optimum nutrition for kidney stone disease. *Adv Chronic Kidney Dis.* 2013;20(2):165–74.

20. Linus Pauling Institute. *Micronutrient Research for Optimum Health.* Online at http://lpi.oregonstate.edu/infocenter/minerals

21. Eaton SB et al. Paleolithic nutrition. A consideration of its nature and current implications. *N Engl J Med.* 1985;312:283–9.

22. Eaton SB et al. Calcium in evolutionary perspective. *Am J Clin Nutr.* 1991;54(1 Suppl):281S–7S.

23. Frassetto L et al. Diet, evolution and aging–the pathophysiologic effects of the post-agricultural inversion of the potassium-to-sodium and base-to-chloride ratios in the human diet. *Eur J Nutr.* 2001;40:200–13.

24. Lomer MC et al. Review article: lactose intolerance in clinical practice–myths and realities. *Aliment Pharmacol Ther.* 2008;27(2):93–103.

25. Lanham-New S.A. Importance of calcium, vitamin D and vitamin K for osteoporosis prevention and treatment. *Proc Nutr Soc.* 2008;67:163–176.

26. Ho-Pham LT et al. Vegetarianism, bone loss, fracture and vitamin D: a longitudinal study in Asian vegans and non-vegans. *Eur J Clin Nutr.* 2012;66(1):75–82.

27. Kohlenberg-Mueller K et al. Calcium balance in young adults on a vegan and lacto-vegetarian diet. *J Bone Miner Metab.* 2003;21(1):28–33.

28. Lanham-New SA. Is "vegetarianism" a serious risk factor for osteoporotic fracture? *Am J Clin Nutr.* 2009;90(4):910–1.

29. Mangels AR et al. *The Dietitians Guide to Vegetarian Diets.* Jones and Bartlett Learning Ltd. 2011.

30. Rizzo NS et al. Nutrient profiles of vegetarian and nonvegetarian dietary patterns. *J Acad Nutr Diet.* Dec. 2013;113(12):1610–9.

31. Appleby P et al. Comparative fracture risk in vegetarians and nonvegetarians in EPIC-Oxford. *Eur J Clin Nutr.* 2007;61(12):1400–6.

32. Mangano KM et al. Calcium intake in the United States from dietary and supplemental sources across adult age groups: new estimates from the National Health and Nutrition Examination Survey 2003-2006. *J Am Diet Assoc*. 2011;111(5):687–95.

33. Tang AL et al. Calcium absorption in Australian osteopenic post-menopausal women: an acute comparative study of fortified soymilk to cows' milk. *Asia Pac J Clin Nutr*. 2010;19(2):243–9.

34. Zhao Y et al. Calcium bioavailability of calcium carbonate fortified soymilk is equivalent to cow's milk in young women. *J Nutr*. 2005 Oct;135(10):2379–82.

35. Guillemant J et al. Mineral water as a source of dietary calcium: acute effects on parathyroid function and bone resorption in young men. *Am J Clin Nutr*. 2000; 71(4):999–1002.

36. Forouhi NG et al. Elevated serum ferritin levels predict new-onset type 2 diabetes: results from the EPIC-Norfolk prospective study. *Diabetologia*. 2007;50(5):949–56.

37. Geissler C et al. Iron, meat and health. *Nutrients*. 2011;3(3):283–316.

38. Institute of Medicine. National Research Council. *Dietary Reference Intakes for Vitamin A, Vitamin K, Arsenic, Boron, Chromium, Copper, Iodine, Iron, Manganese, Molybdenum, Nickel, Silicon, Vanadium, and Zinc*. Washington DC: National Academies Press, 2001.

39. Jiang R et al. Body iron stores in relation to risk of type 2 diabetes in apparently healthy women. *JAMA*. 2004;291(6):711–7.

40. Kim MH et al. Postmenopausal vegetarians' low serum ferritin level may reduce the risk for metabolic syndrome. *Biol Trace Elem Res*. 2012;149(1):34–41.

41. Cooper M et al. Iron sufficiency of Canadians. Component of Statistics Canada Catalogue no. 82-003-X Health Reports, 2012.

42. Norris J et al. *Vegan for Life*. Da Capo Long Life Publ, 2011.

43. Cook JD et al. Assessment of the role of nonheme-iron availability in iron balance. *Am J Clin Nutr*. 1991;54:717–22.

44. Suárez-Ortegón MF et al. Body iron stores as predictors of insulin resistance in apparently healthy urban Colombian men. *Biol Trace Elem Res*. 2012;145(3):283–5.

45. Hua NW et al. Low iron status and enhanced insulin sensitivity in lacto-ovo vegetarians. *Br J Nutr*. 2001;86(4):515–9.

46. Waldmann A et al. Dietary iron intake and iron status of German female vegans: results of the German vegan study. *Ann Nutr Metab*. 2004;48(2):103–8.

47. Collings R et al. The absorption of iron from whole diets: a systematic review. *Am J Clin Nutr*. 2013;98(1):65–81.

48. Theil EC et al. Absorption of Iron from Ferritin Is Independent of Heme Iron and Ferrous Salts in Women and Rat Intestinal Segments. *J Nutr*. 2012;142(3):478–83.

49. Saunders AV. Iron and vegetarian diets. *MJA Open*. 2012;1(Suppl 2):11–16.

50. Gliszczynska-Swigło A et al. Changes in the content of health-promoting compounds and antioxidant activity of broccoli after domestic processing. *Food Addit Contam*. 2006;23(11):1088–98.

51. Davis B et al. *Becoming Raw*. Summertown TN: The Book Publishing Company, 2010.

52. Gautam S et al. Higher bioaccessibility of iron and zinc from food grains in the presence of garlic and onion. *J Agric Food Chem*. 2010;58(14):8426–9.

53. Brown KH et al. International Zinc Nutrition Consultative Group (IZiNCG) technical document #1. Assessment of the risk of zinc deficiency in populations and options for its control. *Food Nutr Bull*. 2004;25(1 Suppl 2):S99–203.

54. Reinhold JG et al. Decreased Absorption of Calcium, Magnesium, Zinc and Phosphorus by Humans due to Increased Fiber and Phosphorus Consumption as Wheat Bread. *J Nutr*. 1976;106(4) 493–503.

55. Prasad AS. Zinc deficiency in women, infants and children. *J Am Coll Nutr*. 1996; 15(2):113–20.

56. Slavin J et al. Plausible mechanisms for the protectiveness of whole grains. *A J Clin Nutr.* 1999;70(3):459S–463S.

57. Baer MT et al. Tissue zinc levels and zinc excretion during experimental zinc depletion in young men. *Am J Clin Nutr.* 1984;39(4):556–70.

58. Lönnerdal B et al. Dietary Factors Influencing Zinc Absorption. *J Nutr.* 2000;130(5S Suppl):1378S–83S.

59. Prasad AS et al. Zinc status and serum testosterone levels of healthy adults. *Nutrition.* 1996;12(5):344–8.

60. Fulgoni VL 3rd et al. Foods, fortificants, and supplements: Where do Americans get their nutrients? *J Nutr.* 2011;141(10):1847–54.

61. Leung AM et al. History of U.S. iodine fortification and supplementation. *Nutrients.* 2012;4(11):1740–6.

62. Fields C et al. Iodine-deficient vegetarians: a hypothetical perchlorate-susceptible population? *Regul Toxicol Pharmacol.* 2005;42:37–46.

63. Geelhoed GW. Health care advocacy in world health. *Nutrition.* 1999;15:940–3.

64. Geelhoed GW. Metabolic maladaptation: individual and social consequences of medical intervention in correcting endemic hypothyroidism. *Nutrition.* 1999;15:908–32; discussion 939.

65. Miller D. Extrathyroidal benefits of iodine. *J Amer Physicians Surgeons.* 2006;119:106–10.

66. Perrine CG. Some Subgroups of Reproductive Age Women in the United States May Be at Risk for Iodine Deficiency. *J Nutr.* 2010;140(8):1489–94.

67. Leung AM et al. Iodine Status and Thyroid Function of Boston-Area Vegetarians and Vegans. *J Clin Endocrinol Metab.* 2011;96(8):E1303–7.

68. Dasgupta PK et al. Iodine nutrition: iodine content of iodized salt in the United States. *Environ Sci Technol.* 2008;42(4):1315–23.

69. Teas J et al. Variability of iodine content in common commercially available edible seaweeds. *Thyroid.* 2004;14(10):836–41.

70. Cunnane SC. Hunter-gatherer diets-a shore-based perspective. *Am J Clin Nutr.* 2000;72:1584–8. Comment on: *Am J Clin Nutr.* 2000;71:665–7. *Am J Clin Nutr.* 2000;71:682–92.

71. Walsh S. *Plant Based Nutrition and Health.* The Vegan Society. St Leonards-on-Sea, U.K., 2003.

72. Eden Foods. www.edenfoods.com

73. ESHA. The Food Processor. Nutrition and Fitness Software. 2014. www.esha.com

74. Crohn DM. Perchlorate controversy calls for improving iodine nutrition. *Vegetarian Nutrition Update.* 2005. XIV (2)1, 6–8. American Dietetic Association, Vegetarian Nutrition Network. Online at http://vegetariannutrition.net

75. Maine Sea Coast Vegetables www.seaveg.com

76. U.S. Department of Agriculture, Agricultural Research Service. *USDA National Nutrient Database for Standard Reference, Release 26.* Nutrient Data Laboratory Home Page. http://ndb.nal.usda.gov/ndb/foods/list

77. Marini H et al. Update on genistein and thyroid: an overall message of safety. *Front Endocrin.* 2012; 3:94.

78. Teas J et al. Seaweed and soy: companion foods in Asian cuisine and their effects on thyroid function in American women. *J Med Food.* 2007;10(1):90–100.

79. Shomburg L et al. On the importance of selenium and iodine metabolism for thyroid hormone biosynthesis and human health. *Mol Nutr Food Res.* 2008;52(11):1235–46.

80. Rauma AI et al. Iodine status in vegans consuming a living food diet. *Nutr Res.* 1994;14:1789–95.

81. National Institute of Health. Office of Dietary Supplements. *Dietary Supplement Fact Sheets.* Chromium. http://ods.od.nih.gov/factsheets/Chromium-HealthProfessional/

82. Bergman C et al. What is next for the Dietary Reference Intakes for bone metabolism related nutrients beyond calcium:

phosphorus, magnesium, vitamin D, and fluoride? *Crit Rev Food Sci Nutr.* 2009; 49:136–44.

83. Fine KD et al. Intestinal absorption of magnesium from food and supplements. *J Clin Invest.* 1991;88:396–402.

84. Institute of Medicine. National Research Council. Dietary Reference Intakes for Sodium and Potassium. Washington DC: National Academies Press, 2019.

85. Ogra Y et al. Selenometabolomics explored by speciation. *Biol Pharm Bull.* 2012;35(11):1863–9.

86. Hoeflich J et al. The choice of biomarkers determines the selenium status in young German vegans and vegetarians. *Br J Nutr.* 2010;104(11):1601–4.

87. Chang JC. Selenium content of brazil nuts from two geographic locations in Brazil. *Chemosphere.* 1995;30:801–802.

88. U.S. Department of Agriculture, Agricultural Research Service. *Selenium Content of Selected Foods.* www.nal.usda.gov/fnic/foodcomp/Data/SR20/nutrlist/sr20w317.pdf

89. Institute of Medicine. *Dietary Reference Intakes for Vitamin C, Vitamin E, Selenium, and Carotenoids.* Washington DC: National Academies Press, 2000.

90. Lanham-New SA et al. Potassium. *Adv Nutr.* 2012;3(6):820–1.

91. Institute of Medicine. National Academies. Sodium Intake in Populations: Assessment

of Evidence. Washington DC: National Academies Press, 2013.

92. Frassetto L et al. Adverse effects of sodium chloride on bone in the aging human population resulting from habitual consumption of typical American diets. *J Nutr.* 2008;138(2): 419S–422S.

93. Saunders AV et al. Zinc and vegetarian diets. *MJA Open.* 2012;1(Suppl 2):17–21.

94. Ma DF et al. Soy isoflavone intake increases bone mineral density in the spine of menopausal women: meta-analysis of randomized controlled trials. *Clin Nutr.* 2008;27(1):57–64.

95. Tonstad S et al. Vegan diets and hypothyroidism. *Nutrients.* 2013;5,4642–4652.

96. Craig WJ et al. Position of the American Dietetic Association: vegetarian diets. *J Am Diet Assoc.* 2009;109(7):1266–82.

97. Hunt JR et al. Apparent copper absorption from a vegetarian diet. *Am J Clin Nutr.* 2001;74(6):803–7.

98. U.S. Food and Drug Administration. Guidance for Industry: A Food Labeling Guide (14. Appendix F: Calculate the Percent Daily Value for the Appropriate Nutrients). 2013.

99. Murphy SP et al. Recommended Dietary Allowances should be used to set Daily Values for nutrition labeling. *Am J Clin Nutr.* 2006;83(suppl):1223S–7S.

100. Weaver CM et al. Dietary calcium: adequacy of a vegetarian diet. *Am J Clin Nutr.* 1994;59(5 Suppl):1238S–1241S.

REFERENCES FOR CHAPTER 7

1. Heymann W. Scurvy in children. *J Am Acad Dermatol.* 2007 Aug;57(2):358–9.

2. Institute of Medicine. National Research Council. *Dietary Reference Intakes for Thiamin, Riboflavin, Niacin, Vitamin B$_6$, Folate, Vitamin B$_{12}$, Pantothenic Acid, Biotin, and Choline.* The National Academies Press,1998

3. Lanska DJ. Chapter 29: historical aspects of the major neurological vitamin defi-

ciency disorders: overview and fat-soluble vitamin A. *Handb Clin Neurol.* 2010;95: 435–44.

4. Linus Pauling Institute. *Micronutrient Information Center. Vitamins.* http://lpi.oregonstate.edu/infocenter/vitamins.html

5. Stabler SP et al. Vitamin B12 deficiency as a worldwide problem. *Annu Rev Nutr.* 2004; 24:299–326.

6. Iqtidar N et al. Misdiagnosed vitamin B_{12} deficiency a challenge to be confronted by use of modern screening markers. *J Pak Med Assoc.* 2012 Nov;62(11):1223–9.

7. Herrmann W et al. Enhanced bone metabolism in vegetarians–the role of vitamin B_{12} deficiency. *Clin Chem Lab Med.* 2009; 47(11):1381–7.

8. Aaron S et al. Clinical and laboratory features and response to treatment in patients presenting with vitamin B_{12} deficiency-related neurological syndromes. *Neurol India.* 2005;53:55–8.

9. Antony AC. Vegetarianism and vitamin B-12 (cobalamin) deficiency. *Am J Clin Nutr.* 2003;78(1):3–6.

10. Oh R et al. Vitamin B12 deficiency. *Am Fam Physician.* 2003 Mar;1;67(5):979–86.

11. Molloy AM et al. Maternal vitamin B_{12} status and risk of neural tube defects in a population with high neural tube defect prevalence and no folic acid fortification. *Pediatrics.* 2009;123:917–23.

12. Pepper MR et al. B12 in fetal development. *Semin Cell Dev Biol.* 2011 Aug;22(6): 619–23.

13. Abu-Kishk I et al. Infantile encephalopathy due to vitamin deficiency in industrial countries. *Childs Nerv Syst.* 2009;25(11): 1477–80.

14. Roschitz B et al. Nutritional infantile vitamin B_{12} deficiency: pathobiochemical considerations in seven patients. *Arch Dis Child Fetal Neonatal Ed.* 2005 May;90(3):F281–2.

15. Carmel R et al. Update on Cobalamin, Folate, and Homocysteine. *Hematology Am Soc Hematol Educ Program.* 2003:62–81.

16. Norris J. *Veganhealth.org.* www.veganhealth.org/b12/values.

17. Mangels R et al. *The Dietitians' Guide to Vegetarian Diets,* Third Edition. Jones and Bartlett, 2011.

18. Pawlak R et al. How prevalent is vitamin B_{12} deficiency among vegetarians? *Nutr Rev.* 2013 Feb;71(2):110–7.

19. Chen X et al. Influence of cobalamin deficiency compared with that of cobalamin absorption on serum holo-transcobalamin II. *Am J Clin Nutr.* 2005 Jan;81(1):110–4.

20. Heil SG et al. Screening for metabolic vitamin B_{12} deficiency by holotranscobalamin in patients suspected of vitamin B_{12} deficiency: a multicentre study. *Ann Clin Biochem.* 2012 Mar;49(Pt 2):184–9.

21. Herbert V. Staging vitamin B-12 (cobalamin) status in vegetarians. *Am J Clin Nutr.* 1994 May;59(5 Suppl):1213S–1222S.

22. Herrmann W et al. Functional vitamin B_{12} deficiency and determination of holotranscobalamin in populations at risk. *Clin Chem Lab Med.* 2003;41:1478–88.

23. National Institutes of Health. Office of Dietary Supplements. *Dietary Supplement Fact Sheet: Vitamin B_{12}.* http://ods.od.nih.gov/factsheets/vitaminb12-HealthProfessional/

24. Dagnelie PC. *J Nutr.* 1997 Feb;127:379; author reply 380. Comment on: Rauma A. Some algae are potentially adequate sources of vitamin B-12 for vegans. *J Nutr.* 1995 Oct;125:2511–5.

25. Mitsuyama Y et al. Serum and cerebrospinal fluid vitamin B_{12} levels in demented patients with CH3- B_{12} treatment–preliminary study. *Jpn J Psychiatry Neurol.* 1988 Mar;42(1): 65–71.

26. Zeuschner C. Vitamin B_{12} and vegetarian diets. *MJA Open.* 2013;1(2)27–32.

27. Wahlin A et al. Reference values for serum levels of vitamin B_{12} and folic acid in a population-based sample of adults between 35 and 80 years of age. *Public Health Nutrition.* 2002;5(3),505–511.

28. Bor MV et al. Daily intake of 4 to 7 lg dietary vitamin B-12 is associated with steady concentrations of vitamin B-12–related biomarkers in a healthy young population. *Am J Clin Nutr.* 2010 Mar;91(3):571–7.

29. Donaldson MS. Hallelujah vegetarians and nutritional science: answering your questions. Personal communication. 2005.

30. LeSaffre Yeast Corporation. (Red Star). Personal communication. 2012. http://lesaffre-yeast.com/red-star/vsf.html

31. Desmukh US et al. Effect of physiological doses of oral vitamin B_{12} on plasma ho-

mocysteine – A randomized, placebo-controlled, double-blind trial in India. *Eur J Clin Nutr.* 2010 May; 64(5):495–502.

32. Scott JM. Bioavailability of vitamin B12. *Eur J Clin Nutr.* 1997 Jan;51(Suppl 1): S49–53.

33. Greger M. *NutritionFacts.org* http://nutritionfacts.org

34. Heyssel RM et al. Vitamin B12 turnover in man. The assimilation of vitamin B_{12} from natural foodstuff by man and estimates of minimal daily dietary requirements. *Am J Clin Nutr.* 1966 Mar;18(3):176–84.

35. Medline Plus. National Institutes of Health. *Vitamin B_{12}. Are There Safety Concerns?* Online at www.nlm.nih.gov/medlineplus/druginfo/natural/926.html#Safety

36. Committee on Toxicity of Chemicals in Food. *Consumer Products and the Environment.* 2006. http://cot.food.gov.uk/pdfs/cotstatementapricot200615.pdf

37. Hill MH et al. A Vitamin B-12 Supplement of 500 µg/d for Eight Weeks Does Not Normalize Urinary Methylmalonic Acid or Other Biomarkers of Vitamin B-12 Status in Elderly People with Moderately Poor Vitamin B-12 Status. *J Nutr.* 2013 Feb;143(2):142–7.

38. Vegan Society (UK). *What Every Vegan Should Know About Vitamin B_{12}.* Online at www.vegansociety.com/lifestyle/nutrition/b12.aspx

39. Graham ID et al. Oral cobalamin remains medicine's best kept secret. *Arch Gerontol Geriatr.* 2007 Jan-Feb;44(1):49–59.

40. Gilsing AM et al. Serum concentrations of vitamin B_{12} and folate in British male omnivores, vegetarians and vegans: results from a cross-sectional analysis of the EPIC-Oxford cohort study. *Eur J Clin Nutr.* 2010 Sep;64(9):933–9.

41. Herrmann W et al. Vitamin B-12 status, particularly holotranscobalamin II and methylmalonic acid concentrations, and hyperhomocysteinemia in vegetarians. *Am J Clin Nutr.* 2003 Jul;78(1):131–6.

42. Rizzo NS et al. Nutrient profiles of vegetarian and nonvegetarian dietary patterns. *J Acad Nutr Diet.* 2013 Dec;113(12): 1610–9.

43. Donaldson MS. Metabolic vitamin B_{12} status on a mostly raw vegan diet with follow-up using tablets, nutritional yeast, or probiotic supplements. *Ann Nutr Metab.* 2000;44:229–34.7.

44. ESHA. *The Food Processor SQL, Nutrition and Fitness Software.* 2014. www.esha.com/foodprosql

45. USDA United States Department of Agriculture. National Nutrient Database for Standard Reference. www.ars.usda.gov/main/site_main.htm?modecode=12-35-45-00

46. Tucker KL et al. Breakfast cereal fortified with folic acid, vitamin B_6, and vitamin B-12 increases vitamin concentrations and reduces homocysteine concentrations: a randomized trial. *Am J Clin Nutr.* 2004; 79(5)805–811.

47. Baroni L et al. Effect of a Klamath algae product ("AFA- B_{12}") on blood levels of vitamin B_{12} and homocysteine in vegan subjects: a pilot study. *Int J Vitam Nutr Res.* 2009 Mar;79(2):117–23.

48. Chen JH et al. Determination of cobalamin in nutritive supplements and chlorella foods by capillary electrophoresis-inductively coupled plasma mass spectrometry. *J Agric Food Chem.* 2008;56:1210–5.

49. Kittaka-Katsura H et al. Purification and characterization of a corrinoid compound from Chlorella tablets as an algal health food. *J Agric Food Chem.* 2002;50:4994–7.

50. Nakano S et al. Chlorella pyrenoidosa supplementation reduces the risk of anemia, proteinuria and edema in pregnant women. *Plant Foods Hum Nutr.* 2010 Mar;65(1):25–30.

51. Watanabe F et al. Characterization and bioavailability of vitamin B_{12}-compounds from edible algae. *J Nutr Sci Vitaminol.* (Tokyo). 2002;48:325–31.

52. Watanabe F et al. Biologically active vitamin B_{12} compounds in foods for preventing deficiency among vegetarians and elderly subjects. *J Agric Food Chem.* 2013 Jul; 17; 61(28):6769–75.

53. Allen LH. How common is vitamin B-12 deficiency? *Am J Clin Nutr.* 2009 Feb; 89(2):693S–6S.

54. Andrès E et al. Oral cobalamin (vitamin B$_{12}$) treatment. An update. *Int J Lab Hematol.* 2009 Feb;31(1):1–8.

55. Su TC et al. Arterial function of carotid and brachial arteries in postmenopausal vegetarians. *Vasc Health Risk Manag.* 2011;7: 517–23.

56. Hughes CF et al. Vitamin B12 and ageing: current issues and interaction with folate. *Ann Clin Biochem.* 2013 Jul;50(Pt4):315–29.

57. Elmadfa I et al. Vitamin B-12 and homocysteine status among vegetarians: a global perspective. *Am J Clin Nutr.* 2009 May; 89(5):1693S–1698S.

58. Moore E et al. Cognitive impairment and vitamin B12: a review. *International Psychogeriatrics.* 2012;24(4)541–556.

59. Almeida OP et al. Homocysteine and depression in later life. *Arch Gen. Psychiatry.* 2008 Nov;65(11):1286–94.

60. Obeid R et al. Holotranscobalamin in laboratory diagnosis of cobalamin deficiency compared to total cobalamin and methylmalonic acid. *Clin Chem Lab Med.* 2007; 45(12):1746–50.

61. Obersby D et al. Plasma total homocysteine status of vegetarians compared with omnivores: a systematic review and meta-analysis. *Br J Nutr.* 2013 Mar;14;109(5): 785–94.

62. Chaplin G et al. Vitamin D and the evolution of human depigmentation. *Am J Phys Anthropol.* 2009 Aug;139(4):451–61.

63. Holick M. Resurrection of vitamin D deficiency and rickets. *J Clin Invest.* 2006; 116(8):2062–2072.

64. Holick M. Shining light on the vitamin D Cancer connection IARC report. *Dermatoendocrinol.* 2009;1(1): 4–6.

65. Holick MF. Vitamin D deficiency. *N Engl J Med.* 2007;357(3):266-81

66. Institute of Medicine, National Research Council. *Dietary Reference Intakes for Calcium and Vitamin D.* 2011.

67. Loomis WF. *Rickets.* Impact of Human Nutrition on Health and Disease. *Scientific American.* W.H. Freeman. 1970.

68. Rajakumar K. Vitamin D, Cod-Liver Oil, Sunlight, and Rickets: A Historical Perspective. *Pediatrics.* 2003;112(2)132–135.

69. Heaney R. Vitamin D and calcium interactions: functional outcomes. *Am J Clin Nutr.* 2008;88(2):541S–544S.

70. Tang BM et al. Use of calcium or calcium in combination with vitamin D supplementation to prevent fractures and bone loss in people aged 50 years and older: a meta-analysis. *Lancet.* 2007;370(9588):657–66.

71. Heaney RP. Health is better at serum 25(OH) D above 30ng/mL. *J Steroid Biochem Mol Biol.* 2013;136:224–8.

72. Heaney RP. Vitamin D–the iceberg nutrient. *J Musculoskelet Neuronal Interact.* 2006 Oct-Dec;6(4):334–5.

73. Prietl B et al. Vitamin D and immune function. *Nutrients.* 2013;5(7):2502–21.

74. Giovannucci E et al. Prospective study of predictors of vitamin D status and cancer incidence and mortality in men. *J Natl Cancer Inst.* 2006;98(7):451–9.

75. Institute of Medicine. *Dietary Supplement Fact Sheet: Vitamin D.* Online at http://ods.od.nih.gov/factsheets/VitaminD-Health Professional/

76. Lee DM et al. Association between 25-hydroxy-vitamin D levels and cognitive performance in middle-aged and older European men. *J Neurol Neurosurg Psychiatry.* 2009;80(7):722–9.

77. Souberbielle JC et al. Vitamin D and musculoskeletal health, cardiovascular disease, autoimmunity and cancer: Recommendations for clinical practice. *Autoimmun Rev.* 2010;9(11):709–15.

78. Suda T et al. Vitamin D and bone. *J Cell Biochem.* 2003;88:259–66.

79. Thacher TD et al. Vitamin D insufficiency. *Mayo Clin Proc.* 2011;86(1):50–60.

80. Webb AR et al. Influence of season and latitude on the cutaneous synthesis of vitamin D$_3$: exposure to winter sunlight in Boston

and Edmonton will not promote vitamin D$_3$ synthesis in human skin. *J Clin Endocrinol Metab.* 1988;67(2):373–8.

81. Chan J et al. Determinants of serum 25 hydroxyvitamin D levels in a nationwide cohort of blacks and non-Hispanic whites. *Cancer Causes Control.* 2010; 21(4): 501–11.

82. Grant WB. In defense of the sun: An estimate of changes in mortality rates in the United States if mean serum 25-hydroxyvitamin D levels were raised to 45 ng/mL by solar ultraviolet-B irradiance. *Dermatoendocrinol.* 2009;1(4):207–14.

83. Grant WB et al. Health benefits of higher serum 25-hydroxyvitamin D levels in The Netherlands. *J Steroid Biochem Mol Biol.* 2010;121(1-2):456–8.

84. Lamberg-Allardt C et al. Low serum 25-hydroxyvitamin D concentrations and secondary hyperparathyroidism in middle-aged white strict vegetarians. *Am J Clin Nutr.* 1993;58(5):684–9.

85. Schwalfenberg G. Not enough vitamin D: health consequences for Canadians. *Can Fam Physician.* 2007;53(5):841–54.

86. Chan J et al. Serum 25-hydroxyvitamin D status of vegetarians, partial vegetarians, and nonvegetarians: the Adventist Health Study-2. *Am J Clin Nutr.* 2009 May;89(5):1686S–1692S.

87. Friedman CF et al. Vitamin D Deficiency in Postmenopausal Breast Cancer Survivors. *Journal of Women's Health.* April 2012; 21(4): 456–462.

88. Holick M. Deficiency of sunlight and vitamin D. *British Medical Journal.* June 2008; 14;336(7657):1318–1319.

89. Binkley N et al. Low Vitamin D Status despite Abundant Sun Exposure. *J Clin Endocrinol Metab.* 2007 Jun;92(6):2130–5.

90. Jacobs ET et al. Vitamin D insufficiency in southern Arizona. *Am J Clin Nutr.* 2008 Mar;87(3):608–13.

91. Kimlin M et al. Does a high UV environment ensure adequate vitamin D status? *J Photochem Photobiol B.* 2007;89:139–47.

92. Nowson CA et al. Vitamin D intake and vitamin D status of Australians. *Med J Aust.* 2002;177:149–52.

93. Schoenmakers I et al. Abundant sunshine and vitamin D deficiency. *Br J Nutr.* 2008; 99:1171–3.

94. Craig WJ et al. Position of the American Dietetic Association: vegetarian diets. *J Am Diet Assoc.* 2009 Jul;109(7):1266–82.

95. Yetley EA. Assessing the vitamin D status of the US population. *Am J Clin Nutr.* 2008; 88:558S–64S.

96. Biancuzzo RM et al. Fortification of orange juice with vitamin D$_2$ or vitamin D$_3$ is as effective as an oral supplement in maintaining vitamin D status in adults. *Am J Clin Nutr.* 2010 Jun;91(6):1621–6.

97. Binkley N at al. Evaluation of Ergocalciferol or Cholecalciferol Dosing, 1,600 IU Daily or 50,000 IU Monthly in Older Adults. *JCEM.* 2011;96:981–988.

98. Phillips KM et al. Vitamin D and sterol composition of 10 types of mushrooms from retail suppliers in the United States. *J Agric Food Chem.* 2011;59(14):7841–7853.

99. Urbain P et al. Bioavailability of vitamin D$_2$ from UV-B-irradiated button mushrooms in healthy adults deficient in serum 25-hydroxy-vitamin D: A randomized controlled trial. *Eur J Clin Nutr.* 2011;65(8):965–971.

100. Davis B et al. *Becoming Raw.* Summertown TN: The Book Publishing Company, 2010.

101. Aloia JF et al. Vitamin D intake to attain a desired serum 25-hydroxyvitamin D concentration. *Am J Clin Nutr.* 2008 Jun;87(6): 1952–8.

102. Engelsen O et al. Daily duration of vitamin D synthesis in human skin with relation to latitude, total ozone, altitude, ground cover, aerosols and cloud thickness. *Photochem Photobiol.* 2005 Nov-Dec;81(6):1287–90.

103. Vitamin D council test kit. www.vitamindcouncil.org/about-vitamin-d/vitamin-d-deficiency/am-i-vitamin-d-deficient/

104. Crowe FL et al. Plasma concentrations of 25-hydroxyvitamin D in meat eaters, fish eaters, vegetarians and vegans: results from the EPIC-Oxford study. *Public Health Nutr.* 2011 Feb;14(2):340–6.

105. Fontana L et al. Low Bone Mass in Subjects on a Long-term Raw Vegetarian Diet. *Arch Intern Med.* 2005;165:684–9.

106. Ho-Pham LT et al. Vegetarianism, bone loss, fracture and vitamin D: a longitudinal study in Asian vegans and non-vegans. *Eur J Clin Nutr.* 2012 Jan;66(1):75–82.

107. Ströhle A et al. Diet-Dependent Net Endogenous Acid Load of Vegan Diets in Relation to Food Groups and Bone Health-Related Nutrients: Results from the German Vegan Study. *Ann Nutr Metab.* 2011; 59:117–126.

108. Outila TA et al. Dietary intake of vitamin D in premenopausal, healthy vegans was insufficient to maintain concentrations of serum 25-hydroxyvitamin D and intact parathyroid hormone within normal ranges during the winter in Finland. *J Am Diet Assoc.* 2000 Apr;100(4):434–41.

109. Yetley EA et al. Dietary reference intakes for vitamin D: justification for a review of the 1997 values. *Am J Clin Nutr.* 2009 Mar;89(3):719–27.

110. Michaëlsson K et al. Plasma vitamin D and mortality in older men: a community-based prospective cohort study. *Am J Clin Nutr.* 2010 Oct;92(4):841–8.

111. Dyett PA et al. Vegan lifestyle behaviors: an exploration of congruence with health-related beliefs and assessed health indices. *Appetite.* 2013 Aug;67:119-24.

112. Dagnelie PC et al. High prevalence of rickets in infants on macrobiotic diets. *Am J Clin Nutr.* 1990 Feb;51(2):202-8.

113. German Nutrition Society. New reference values for vitamin D. *Ann Nutr Metab.* 2012;60(4):241–6.

114. Binkley N et al. Low vitamin D status: definition, prevalence, consequences, and correction. *Endocrinol Metab Clin North Am.* 2010 Jun;39(2):287–301.

115. Umhau JC et al. Low Vitamin D Status and Suicide: A Case-Control Study of Active Duty Military Service Members. *PLoS One.* 2013; 8(1):e51543.

116. Institute of Medicine. National Research Council. *Dietary Reference Intakes for Vitamin C, Vitamin E, Selenium, and Carotenoids.* 2000.

117. Institute of Medicine. National Research Council. *Dietary Reference Intakes for Vitamin A, Vitamin K, Arsenic, Boron, Chromium, Copper, Iodine, Iron, Manganese, Molybdenum, Nickel, Silicon, Vanadium, and Zinc.* 2001.

118. Adzersen KH et al. Raw and cooked vegetables, fruits, selected micronutrients, and breast cancer risk: a case-control study in Germany. *Nutr Cancer.* 2003;46:131–7.

119. Bland JS. Oxidants and antioxidants in clinical medicine: past, present and future potential. *J Nutr Environ Med.* 1995; 5:255–80.

120. Liska DJ. The detoxification enzyme systems. *Altern Med Rev.* 1998;3:187–98.

121. Randhir R et al. Phenolics, their antioxidant and antimicrobial activity in dark germinated fenugreek sprouts in response to peptide and phytochemical elicitors. *Asia Pac J Clin Nutr.* 2004;13:295–307.

122. Szeto YT et al. Total antioxidant and ascorbic acid content of fresh fruits and vegetables: implications for dietary planning and food preservation. *Br J Nutr.* 2002;87:55–9.

123. Maiani G et al. Carotenoids: actual knowledge on food sources, intakes, stability and bioavailability and their protective role in humans. *Mol Nutr Food Res.* 2009;53: 000–000.

124. Milner JA. Incorporating basic nutrition science into health interventions for cancer prevention. *J Nutr.* 2003;133(11 Suppl 1):3820S–6S.

125. Bland J. Managing biotransformation: introduction and overview. *Altern Ther Health Med.* 2007;13:S85–7.

126. Murray M. Altered CYP expression and function in response to dietary factors: po-

tential roles in disease pathogenesis. *Curr Drug Metab.* 2006;7:67–81.

127. Shapiro TA. Chemoprotective Glucosinolates and Isothiocyanates of Broccoli Sprouts Metabolism and Excretion in Humans. *Cancer Epidemiol Biomarkers Prev.* 2001 May;10(5):501–8.

128. Stipanuk MH. Detoxification and Protective Functions of Nutrients. In Stipanuk MH ed. *Biochemical and Physiological Aspects of Human Nutrition.* Philadelphia: WB Saunders Company, 2000:909–12.

129. Zmrzljak UP et al. Circadian regulation of the hepatic endobiotic and xenobitoic detoxification pathways: the time matters. *Chem Res Toxicol.* 2012 Apr16;25(4): 811–24.

130. Rauma AL et al. Antioxidant status in long-term adherents to a strict uncooked vegan diet. *Am J Clin Nutr.* 1995;62:1221–7.

131. Beecher CW. Cancer preventive properties of varieties of Brassica oleracea: a review. *Am J Clin Nutr.* 1994;59(5 Suppl): 1166S–70S.

132. Gill CI et al. Watercress supplementation in diet reduces lymphocyte DNA damage and alters blood antioxidant status in healthy adults. *Am J Clin Nutr.* 2007; 85:504–10.

133. Pool-Zobel B et al. Modulation of xenobiotic metabolising enzymes by anticarcinogens–focus on glutathione S-transferases and their role as targets of dietary chemoprevention in colorectal carcinogenesis. *Mutat Res.* 2005;591:74–92.

134. Link LB et al. Raw versus cooked vegetables and cancer risk. *Cancer Epidemiol Biomarkers Prev.* 2004;13:1422–35.

135. Nestle M. Broccoli sprouts as inducers of carcinogen-detoxifying enzyme systems: clinical, dietary, and policy implications. *Proc Natl Acad Sci USA.* 1997;94: 11149–51.

136. van Het Hof KH et al. Dietary factors that affect the bioavailability of carotenoids. *J Nutr.* 2000;130:503–6.

137. Benzie IF et al. Antioxidants in food: content, measurement, significance, action, cautions, caveats, and research needs. *Adv Food Nutr Res.* 2014;71:1–53.

138. Calzuola I et al. Synthesis of antioxidants in wheat sprouts. *J Agric Food Chem.* 2004; 52:5201–6.

139. Sheweita SA et al. Cancer and phase II drug-metabolizing enzymes. *Curr Drug Metab.* 2003;4:45–58.

140. Wargovich MJ et al. Diet, individual responsiveness and cancer prevention. *J Nutr.* 2003;133(7 Suppl):2400S–3S.

141. Institute of Medicine. National Research Council. *Dietary Supplement Fact Sheet: Vitamin A and Carotenoids.* http://ods. od.nih.gov/factsheets/VitaminA-Health-Professional

142. Grune T et al. b-Carotene Is an Important Vitamin A Source for Humans. *J Nutr.* 2010 Dec;140(12):2268S–2285S.

143. Davis B et al. *Becoming Raw.* Summertown TN: The Book Publishing Company, 2010.

144. Meinke MC et al. Bioavailability of natural carotenoids in human skin compared to blood. *Eur J Pharm Biopharm.* 2010 Oct;76(2):269–74.

145. Byers T. Anticancer vitamins du Jour–The ABCED's so far. *Am J Epidemiol.* 2010 Jul 1;172(1):1–3.

146. Maserejian N et al. Intakes of vitamins and minerals in relation to urinary incontinence, voiding, and storage symptoms in women: a cross-sectional analysis from the Boston Area Community Health survey. *Eur Urol.* 2011 Jun;59(6):1039–47.

147. Maserejian N et al. Dietary, but not supplemental, intakes of carotenoids and vitamin C are associated with decreased odds of lower urinary tract symptoms in men. *J Nutr.* 2011 Feb;141(2):267–73.

148. Feskanich D et al. Vitamin A intake and hip fractures among postmenopausal women. *JAMA.* 2002 Jan 2;287(1):47–54.

149. Garcia AL et al. Long-term strict raw food diet is associated with favourable plasma beta-carotene and low plasma lycopene concentrations in Germans. *Br J Nutr.* 2008 Jun;99(6):1293–300.

150. Wang Y et al. Dietary total antioxidant capacity is associated with diet and plasma antioxidant status in healthy young adults.

J Acad Nutr Diet. 2012 Oct;112(10): 1626–35.

151. Heymann W. Scurvy in children. *J Am Acad Dermatol.* 2007 Aug;57(2):358–9.

152. Mandl J et al. Vitamin C: update on physiology and pharmacology. *Br J Pharmacol.* 2009 Aug;157(7):1097–110.

153. Donaldson, MS. Food and nutrient intake of Hallelujah vegetarians. *Nutrition & Food Science.* 2001;31:293-303. www.hacres.com/diet/research/nutrient_intake.pdf

154. Hoffmann I. Long-term strict raw food diet is associated with favourable plasma beta-carotene and low plasma lycopene concentrations in Germans. *Br J Nutr.* 2008; 99:1293–300.

155. Koebnick C et al. Long-term consumption of a raw food diet is associated with favorable serum LDL cholesterol and triglycerides but also with elevated plasma homocysteine and low serum HDL cholesterol in humans. *J Nutr.* 2005;135:2372–8.

156. Crinnion WJ. Organic foods contain higher levels of certain nutrients, lower levels of pesticides, and may provide health benefits for the consumer. *Altern Med Rev.* 2010 Apr;15(1):4–12.

157. Hallberg L et al. The role of vitamin C in iron absorption. *Int J Vitam Nutr Res Suppl.* 1989;30:103–8.

158. Hurrell R. Iron bioavailability and dietary reference values. *Am J Clin Nutr.* 2010; 91(suppl):1461S–7S.

159. Kovacs CS. Vitamin D in pregnancy and lactation: maternal, fetal, and neonatal outcomes from human and animal studies. *Am J Clin Nutr.* 2008 Aug;88(2):520S–528S.

160. Institute of Medicine. National Research Council. *Dietary Supplement Fact Sheet: Vitamin E.* http://ods.od.nih.gov/factsheets/Vitamine-HealthProfessional

161. Fulgoni V et al. Avocado consumption is associated with better diet quality and nutrient intake, and lower metabolic syndrome risk in US adults: results from the National Health and Nutrition Examination Survey (NHANES) 2001-2008. *Nutr J.* 2013 Jan 2;12:1.

162. Fulgoni V et al. Foods, fortificants, and supplements: Where do Americans get their nutrients? *J Nutr.* 2011 Oct;141(10): 1847–54.

163. Lanham-New SA. Importance of calcium, vitamin D and vitamin K for osteoporosis prevention and treatment. *Proc Nutr Soc.* 2008 May;67(2):163–76.

164. Neogi T, Felson DT, Sarno R. Vitamin K in hand osteoarthritis: results from a randomised clinical trial. *Ann Rheum Dis.* 2008 Nov;67(11):1570–3.

165. Yaegashi Y et al. Association of hip fracture incidence and intake of calcium, magnesium, vitamin D, and vitamin K. *Eur J Epidemiol.* 2008;23(3):219–25.

166. Sanders TA, Roshanai F. Platelet phospholipid fatty acid composition and function in vegans compared with age- and sex-matched omnivore controls. *Eur J Clin Nutr.* 1992 Nov;46(11):823–31.

167. Kamao M et al. Vitamin K content of foods and dietary vitamin K intake in Japanese young women. *J Nutr Sci Vitaminol.* (Tokyo). 2007 Dec;53(6):464–70.

168. Suttie JW. *Vitamin K in Health and Disease.* Boca Raton FL: CRC Press, 2009.

169. Weber P. Vitamin K and bone health. *Nutrition.* 2001;17(10):880–7.

170. Carter KC. The Germ Theory, berieberi, and the deficiency theory of disease. *Medical History.* 1977;21:119–136.

171. Lanska DJ. Chapter 30: historical aspects of the major neurological vitamin deficiency disorders: the water-soluble B vitamins. *Handb Clin Neurol.* 2010;95:445–76.

172. Hamilton MJ et al. Germination and nutrient composition of alfalfa seeds. *J Food Science.* 1979;44:443–5.

173. Kavas A et al. Nutritive value of germinated mung beans and lentils. *J Consumer Studies and Home Economics.* 1991; 15:357–366.

174. Kylen AM et al. Nutrients in seeds and sprouts of alfalfa, lentils, mung beans, and soybeans. *J Food Science.* 1975;40:1008–9.

175. Rauma AL et al. Effect of a strict vegan diet on energy and nutrient intakes by

Finnish rheumatoid patients. *Eur J Clin Nutr.* 1993 Oct;47(10):747–9.

176. Berry RJ et al. Fortification of flour with folic acid. *Food Nutr Bull.* 2010 Mar;31(1 Suppl):S22–35.

177. Ebben M et al. Effects of pyridoxine on dreaming: a preliminary study. *Perceptual & Motor Skills.* 2002;94(1):135–140.

178. Goodyear-Smith F et al. What can family physicians offer patients with carpal tunnel syndrome other than surgery? A systematic review of nonsurgical management. *Ann Fam Med.* 2004 May-Jun;2(3):267–73.

179. Parr J. Autism. *Clin Evid (Online).* 7;2010; 1–19.pii:0322.

180. Lombard KA et al. Biotin nutritional status of vegans, lactoovovegetarians, and nonvegetarians. *Am J Clin Nutr.* 1989 Sep; 50(3):486–90.

181. Bailey SW et al. The extremely slow and variable activity of dihydrofolate reductase in human liver and its implications for high folic acid intake. *Proc Natl Acad Sci USA.* 2009 Sep 8;106(36):15424–9.

182. Furhman J. Is Supplemental Folic Acid Harmful? *Dr. Fuhrman's Vitamin Advisor.* Online at www.sound-diet.com/general-health/supplements/folate-a-folic-acid/671-is-supplemental-folic-acid-harmful-by-dr-joel-fuhrman-md.html

183. Fekete K et al. Effect of folate intake on health outcomes in pregnancy: a systematic review and meta-analysis on birth weight, placental weight and length of gestation. *Nutr J.* 2012 Sep;19;11:75.

184. Zeisel SH et al. Concentrations of choline-containing compounds and betaine in common foods. *J Nutr.* 2003 May;133(5): 1302–7.

185. Food and Nutrition Board, National Research Council. *Dietary Reference Intakes (DRIs): Vitamins.* 2013.

186. Ohrvik VE et al. Human folate bioavailability. *Nutrients.* 2011 Apr;3(4):475–90.

187. Katina K et al. Fermentation-induced changes in the nutritional value of native or germinated rye. *J Cereal Science.* 2007; 46:348–355.

188. McKillop DJ et al. The effect of different cooking methods on folate retention in various foods that are amongst the major contributors to folate intake in the UK diet. *Br J Nutr.* 2002;88:681–688.

189. National Institutes of Health. *Folate: Dietary Supplement Fact Sheet.* http://ods.od.nih.gov/factsheets/Folate-HealthProfessional/

190. Patterson et al. *USDA Database for the Choline Content of Common Foods.* 2008. www.ars.usda.gov/SP2UserFiles/Place/12354500/Data/Choline/Choln02.pdf

191. Yacoubou J. *Vegetarian Journal's Guide To Food Ingredients.* www.vrg.org/ingredients/

192. Engelson O. UV Radiation, Vitamin D and Human Health: An Unfolding Controversy. Daily Duration of Vitamin D Synthesis in Human Skin with Relation to Latitude, Total Ozone, Altitude, Ground Cover, Aerosols and Cloud Thickness. *Photochemistry and Photobiology.* 2005;81:1287–1290.

193. Smith AG et al. Plants need their vitamins too. *Current Opinion in Plant Biology.* 2007;10:266–275.

194. Carmel R. Diagnosis and management of clinical and subclinical cobalamin deficiencies: why controversies persist in the age of sensitive metabolic testing. *Biochimie.* 2013 May;95(5):1047–55.

195. Simpson JL et al. Micronutrients and women of reproductive potential: required dietary intake and consequences of dietary deficiency or excess. Part I–Folate, Vitamin B12, Vitamin B$_6$. *J Matern Fetal Neonatal Med.* 2010 Dec;23(12):1323–43.

REFERENCES FOR CHAPTER 8

1. World Cancer Research Fund/American Institute for Cancer Research. Food, nutrition, physical activity and the prevention of cancer: a global perspective. Washington DC: AICR, 2007.

2. Davis B and Melina V. *Becoming Raw.* Summertown TN; The Book Publishing Company, 2010.

3. Winter C, Davis S. Organic foods: scientific status summary. *J Food Sci.* 2006;71.

4. Zhao X et al. Does organic production enhance phytochemical content of fruit and vegetables? Current knowledge and prospects for research. *HortTechnology.* 2006; 16:449–56.

5. Getahun SM, Chung FL. Conversion of glucosinolates to isothiocyanates in humans after ingestion of cooked watercress. *Cancer Epidemiol Biomarkers Prev.* 1999; 8:447–51.

6. Conaway CC et al. Disposition of glucosinolates and sulforaphane in humans after ingestion of steamed and fresh broccoli. *Nutr Cancer.* 2000;38:168–78. Erratum in: *Nutr Cancer.* 2001;41:196.

7. Shapiro TA et al. Chemoprotecitve clucosinolates and isothiocyanates of broccoli sprouts; metabolism and excretion in humans. *Cancer Epidemiol Biomarkers Prev.* 2001;10:501–8.

8. Vermeulen M et al. Association between consumption of cruciferous vegetables and condiments and excretion in urine of isothiocyanate mercapturic acids. *J Agric Food Chem.* 2006;54:5350–8.

9. Ferracane R et al. Effects of different cooking methods on antioxidant profile, antioxidant capacity, and physical characteristics of artichoke. *J Agric Food Chem.* 2008;56: 8601–8.

10. Miglio C et al. Effects of different cooking methods on nutritional and physicochemical characteristics of selected vegetables. *J Agric Food Chem.* 2008;56: 139–47.

11. Dewanto V et al. Thermal processing enhances the nutritional value of tomatoes by increasing total antioxidant activity. *J Agric Food Chem.* 2000;50:3010–4.

12. Bugianesi R et al. Effect of domestic cooking on human bioavailability of naringenin, chlorogenic acid, lycopene and b-carotene in cherry tomatoes. *Eur J Nutr.* 2004; 43:360e6.

13. Porrini M et al. Absorption of lycopene from single or daily portions of raw and processed tomato. *Br J Nutr.* 1998;80:353e61.

14. Gartner C, Stahl W, Sies H. Lycopene is more bioavailable from tomato paste than from fresh tomatoes. *Am J Clin Nutr.* 1997; 66:116–22.

15. Stahl W et al. Cis-trans isomers of lycopene and beta-carotene in human serum and tissues. Arch Biochem Biophys. 1992; 294:173–7.

16. Dietz JM et al. Reversed phase HPLC analysis of alpha and beta-carotene from selected raw and cooked vegetables. Plant Food Hum Nutr. 1988;38:333–41.

17. Reboul E et al. Bioaccessibility of carotenoids and vitamin E from their main dietary sources. *J Agric Food Chem.* 2006; 54:8749–55.

18. Khachik F et al. Effect of food preparation on qualitative and quantitative distribution of major carotenoid constituents of tomatoes and several green vegetables. *J Agric Food Chem.* 1992;40:390–8.

19. Prince MR, Frisoli JK. Beta-carotene accumulation in serum and skin. *Am J Clin Nutr.* 1993;57:175–81.

20. Jalal F et al. Serum retinol concentrations in children are affected by food sources of beta-carotene, fat intake, and anthelmintic drug treatment. *Am J Clin Nutr.* 1998; 68:623–9.

21. van Het Hof KH et al. Dietary factors that affect the bioavailability of carotenoids. *J Nutr.* 2000;130:503–6.

22. Brown MJ et al. Carotenoid bioavailability is higher from salads ingested with full-fat than with fat-reduced salad dressings as measured with electrochemical detection. *Am J Clin Nutr.* 2004;80:396–403.

23. Unlu NZ et al. Carotenoid absorption from salad and salsa by humans is enhanced by the addition of avocado or avocado oil. *J Nutr.* 2005;135:431–6.

24. Maiani G et al. Carotenoids: actual knowledge on food sources, intakes, stability and bioavailability and their protective role in humans. *Mol Nutr Food Res.* 2008;53(2): S194–218.

25. Rock CL et al. Bioavailability of -carotene is lower in raw than in processed carrots and spinach in women. *J Nutr.* 1998;128:913–6.

26. McEligot AJ et al. Comparison of serum carotenoid responses between women consuming vegetable juice and women consuming raw or cooked vegetables. *Cancer Epidemiol Biomarkers Prev.* 1999;8:227–31.

27. Katina K, Liukkonen K-H, Kaukovirta-Norja A et al. Fermentation-induced changes in the nutritional value of native or germinated rye. *J Cereal Sci.* 2007;46:348–55.

28. Lee SU et al. Flavonoid content in fresh, home-processed, and light-exposed onions and in dehydrated commercial onion products. *J Agric Food Chem.* 2008;56:8541–8.

29. Fahey JW et al. Broccoli sprouts: an exceptionally rich source of inducers of enzymes that protect against chemical carcinogens. *Proc Natl Acad Sci USA.* 1997;94:10367–72.

30. Yang F et al. Studies on germination conditions and antioxidant contents of wheat grain. *Int J Food Sci Nutr.* 2001;52:319–30.

31. Falcioni G et al. Antioxidant activity of wheat sprouts extract "in vitro": inhibition of DNA oxidative damage. *J Food Sci.* 2002;67:2918–2922.

32. Calzuola, I et al. Synthesis of antioxidants in wheat sprouts. *J Agric Food Chem.* 2004;52:5201–6.

33. Marsili V et al. Nutritional relevance of wheat sprouts containing high levels of organic phosphates and antioxidant compounds. *J Clin Gastroenterol.* 2004;38(6 Suppl):S123–6.

34. Liukkonen KH et al. Process-induced changes on bioactive compounds in whole grain rye. *Proc Nutr Soc.* 2003;62:117–22.

35. Randhir R et al. Phenolics, their antioxidant and antimicrobial activity in dark germinated fenugreek sprouts in response to peptide and phytochemical elicitors. *Asia Pac J Clin Nutr.* 2004;13:295–307.

36. Fahey JW et al. Sulforaphane inhibits extracellular, intracellular, and antibiotic-resistant strains of Helicobacter pylori and prevents benzo[a]pyrene-induced stomach tumors. *Proc Natl Acad Sci USA.* 2002;99(11):7610–5.

37. Galan MV et al. Oral broccoli sprouts for the treatment of Helicobacter pylori infection: a preliminary report. *Dig Dis Sci.* 2004;49:1088–90.

38. Bahadoran Z et al. Effect of broccoli sprouts on insulin resistance in type 2 diabetic patients: a randomized double-blind clinical trial. *Int J Food Sci Nutr.* 2012;63(7):767–71.

39. Boddupalli S et al. Induction of phase 2 antioxidant enzymes by broccoli sulforaphane: perspectives in maintaining the antioxidant activity of vitamins a, C, and e. *Front Genet.* 2012;3:7.

40. Fimognari C et al. Chemoprevention of cancer by isothiocyanates and anthocyanins: mechanisms of action and structure-activity relationship. *Curr Med Chem.* 2008;15:440–7.

41. Zhang Y, Callaway EC. High cellular accumulation of sulphoraphane, a dietary anticarcinogen, is followed by rapid transporter-mediated export as a glutathione conjugate. *Biochem J.* 2002;364(Pt 1):301–7.

42. Tapiero H et al. Organosulfur compounds from alliaceae in the prevention of human pathologies. *Biomed Pharmacother.* 2004;58:183–93.

43. Verkerk R, Dekker M. Glucosinolates and myrosinase activity in red cabbage (Brassica oleracea L. var. Capitata f. rubra DC.) after various microwave treatments. *J Agric Food Chem.* 2004;52(24):7318–23.

44. Song K, Milner JA. The influence of heating on the anticancer properties of garlic. *J Nutr.* 2001;131:1054S–7S.

45. Kong F, Singh RP. Disintegration of solid foods in human stomach. *J Food Sci.* 2008;73:R67–80.

46. Collins PJ et al. Proximal, distal and total stomach emptying of a digestible solid meal in normal subjects. *Br J Radiol.* 1988;61:12–8.

47. Hodge C et al. Amylase in the saliva and in the gastric aspirates of premature infants: its potential role in glucose polymer hydrolysis. *Pediatr Res.* 1983;17:998–1001.

48. Fried M et al. Passage of salivary amylase through the stomach in humans. *Dig Dis Sci.* 1987;32:1097–103.

49. Kotz CM et al. Factors affecting the ability of a high beta-galactosidase yogurt to enhance lactose absorption. *J Dairy Sci.* 1994;77:3538–44.

50. Martini MC et al. Lactose digestion by yogurt beta-galactosidase: influence of pH and microbial cell integrity. *Am J Clin Nutr.* 1987;45:432–6.

51. Martini MC et al. Lactose digestion from yogurt: influence of a meal and additional lactose. *Am J Clin Nutr.* 1991;53(5):1253–8.

52. Racette SB et al. Phytosterol-deficient and high-phytosterol diets developed for controlled feeding studies. *J Am Diet Assoc.* 2009;109(12):2043–51.

53. Izar MC et al. Phytosterols and phytosterolemia: gene-diet interactions. *Genes Nutr.* 2011;6(1):17–26.

54. Chen CY, Blumberg JB. Phytochemical composition of nuts. *Asia Pac J Clin Nutr.* 2008; 17(Suppl 1):329–32. Review.

55. Jenkins DJ et al. The Garden of Eden--plant based diets, the genetic drive to conserve cholesterol and its implications for heart disease in the 21st century. *Comp Biochem Physiol A Mol Integr Physiol.* 2003;136(1):141–51.

56. Agren JJ et al. Divergent changes in serum sterols during a strict uncooked vegan diet in patients with rheumatoid arthritis. *Br J Nutr.* 2001;85(2):137–9.

57. Pai R, Kang G. Microbes in the gut: a digestable account of host-symbiont interactions. *Indian J Med Res.* 2008;128(5):587–94.

58. Sears CL. A dynamic partnership: celebrating our gut flora. *Anaerobe.* 2005;11(5): 247–51.

59. Gray J. *Dietary Fiber: definition, analysis, physiology and health.* ILSI Europe Concise Monograph Series. Brussels Belgium: ILSI Europe, 2006.

60. Tang Yet al. G-protein-coupled receptor for short-chain fatty acids suppresses colon cancer. *Int J Cancer.* 2011;128(4):847–56.

61. Harris K et al. Is the gut microbiota a new factor contributing to obesity and its metabolic disorders? *J Obes.* 2012;2012:879151. Erratum in *J Obesity.* 2012;2012:782920.

62. Blaut M, Klaus S. Intestinal microbiota and obesity. *Handb Exp Pharmacol.* 2012;(209):251–73.

63. Marik PE. Colonic flora, Probiotics, Obesity and Diabetes. *Front Endocrinol.* (Lausanne). 2012;3:87.

64. de Vrese M, Schrezenmeir J. Probiotics, prebiotics, and synbiotics. *Adv Biochem Eng Biotechnol.* 2008;111:1–66.

65. Roberfroid M et al. Prebiotic effects: metabolic and health benefits. *Br J Nutr.* 2010; 104 Suppl 2:S1–63.

66. Moshfegh AJ et al. Presence of inulin and oligofructose in the diets of Americans. *J Nutr.* 1999;129(7 Suppl):1407S–11S.

67. Goldin BR, Gorbach SL. Clinical indications for probiotics: an overview. *Clin Infect Dis.* 2008;46(Suppl 2):S96–100; discussion S144–51.

68. Douglas LC, Sanders ME. Probiotics and prebiotics in dietetics practice. *J Am Diet Assoc.* 2008;108(3):510–21.

69. Timmerman HM et al. Monostrain, multistrain and multispecies probiotics–A comparison of functionality and efficacy. *Int J Food Microbiol.* 2004 ;96(3):219–33.

70. Kligler B, Cohrssen A. Probiotics. *Am Fam Physician.* 2008;78(9):1073–1078.

71. Food Allergy and Anaphalaxis Network (FAAN) www.foodallergy.org/section/allergens

72. Vickerstaff Joneja JM. Food Allergies: The Immune Response. *Today's Dietitian.* 2007; 9(7):10.

73. Guandalini S, Newland C. Differentiating food allergies from food intolerances. *Curr Gastroenterol Rep.* 2011;13(5):426–34.

74. Johansson SG et al. Revised nomenclature for allergy for global use: Report of the Nomenclature Review Committee of the World Allergy Organization, October 2003. *J Allergy Clin Immunol.* 2004;113(5):832–6.

75. Melina V, Stepaniak J, Aronson D. *Food Allergy Survival Guide*. Healthy Living Publications, 2004.

76. Tomovich Jacobsen M. *5 Surprising Facts About Kids & Food Allergies*. July 1, 2010 www.raisehealthyeaters.com/2010/07/5-surprising-facts-about-kids-food-allergies/

77. Lomer MC et al. Review article: lactose intolerance in clinical practice—myths and realities. *Aliment Pharmacol Ther*. 2008;15;27(2):93–103.

78. Raiten DJ et al. Executive Summary from the Report: Analysis of Adverse Reactions to Monosodium Glutamate (MSG). *J Nutr*. 1995;125:2892S–2906S.

79. Fasano A. Zonulin and its regulation of intestinal barrier function: the biological door to inflammation, autoimmunity, and cancer. *Physiol Rev*. 2011;91(1):151–75.

80. Fasano A. Leaky gut and autoimmune diseases. *Clin Rev Allergy Immunol*. 2012; 42(1):71–8.

81. Karper WB. Intestinal permeability, moderate exercise, and older adult health. *Holist Nurs Pract*.

82. Rapin JR, Wiernsperger N. Possible links between intestinal permeability and food processing: A potential therapeutic niche for glutamine. *Clinics*. (Sao Paulo). 2010; 65(6):635–43.

83. Maes M et al. Increased IgA and IgM responses against gut commensals in chronic depression: Further evidence for increased bacterial translocation or leaky gut. *J Affect Disord*. 2012;141(1):55–62.

84. Hijazi Z et al. Intestinal permeability is increased in bronchial asthma. *Arch Dis Child*. 2004;89(3):227–9.

85. Kidd PM. Autism, an extreme challenge to integrative medicine. Part: 1: The knowledge base. *Altern Med Rev*. 2002 Aug;7(4): 292-316.

86. Sandek A et al. The emerging role of the gut in chronic heart failure. *Curr Opin Clin Nutr Metab Care*. 2008;11(5):632–9.

87. Visser J et al. Tight junctions, intestinal permeability, and autoimmunity: celiac disease and type 1 diabetes paradigms. *Ann N Y Acad Sci*. 2009;1165:195–205.

88. Maes M, Leunis JC. Normalization of leaky gut in chronic fatigue syndrome (CFS) is accompanied by a clinical improvement: effects of age, duration of illness and the translocation of LPS from gram-negative bacteria. *Neuro Endocrinol Lett*. 2008;29(6):902–10.88.

89. Vaarala O et al. The "perfect storm" for type 1 diabetes: the complex interplay between intestinal microbiota, gut permeability, and mucosal immunity. *Diabetes*. 2008;57(10):2555–62.

90. de Kort S et al. Leaky gut and diabetes mellitus: what is the link? *Obes Rev*. 2011; 12(6):449–58.

91. Gecse K et al. Leaky gut in patients with diarrhea-predominant irritable bowel syndrome and inactive ulcerative colitis. *Digestion*. 2012;85(1):40–6.

92. El-Tawil AM. Zinc supplementation tightens leaky gut in Crohn's disease. *Inflamm Bowel Dis*. 2012 Feb;18(2):E399.

93. Tang Y et al. Nitric oxide-mediated intestinal injury is required for alcohol-induced gut leakiness and liver damage. *Alcohol Clin Exp Res*. 2009;33(7):1220–30.

94. Terjung B, Spengler U. Atypical p-ANCA in PSC and AIH: a hint toward a "leaky gut"? *Clin Rev Allergy Immunol*. 2009; 36(1):40–51.

95. Casanova MF. The minicolumnopathy of autism: A link between migraine and gastrointestinal symptoms. *Med Hypotheses*. 2008;70(1):73–80.

96. Dunn JM, Wilkinson JM. Naturopathic management of rheumatoid arthritis. *Mod Rheumatol*. 2005;15(2):87–90.

97. Picco P et al. Increased gut permeability in juvenile chronic arthritides. A multivariate analysis of the diagnostic parameters. *Clin Exp Rheumatol*. 2000;18(6):773–8.

98. Miraglia del Giudice M Jr. et al. Probiotics and atopic dermatitis. A new strategy in atopic dermatitis. *Dig Liver Dis*. 2002; 34 Suppl 2:S68–71.

99. Hamilton I et al. Small intestinal permeability in dermatological disease. *Q J Med*. 1985; 56(221):559–67.

100. WHO 2012. Chemical risks in food. www.who.int/foodsafety/chem/jmpr/en/index.html

101. Stadler RH, Blank I, Varga N et al. Acrylamide from Maillard reaction products. *Nature.* 200;419:449-50.

102. National Cancer Institute. National Institutes of Health. Acrylamide in Food and Cancer Risk. www.cancer.gov/cancertopics/factsheet/Risk/acrylamide-in-food.

103. Food and Agriculture Organization of the United Nations. World Health Organization. Joint FAO/WHO Expert Committee on Food Additives (JECFA). Seventy-second meeting. Rome, 16-25 Feb. 2010. Summary and Conclusions. www.who.int/foodsafety/chem/summary72_rev.pdf

104. Goldberg T, Cai W, Peppa M et al. Advanced glycoxidation end products in commonly consumed foods. *JADA.* 2004;104: 1287-91.

105. Vlassara H, Uribarri J. Advanced Glycation End Products (AGE) and Diabetes: Cause, Effect, or Both? *Curr Diab Rep.* 2014 Jan;14(1):453.

106. Zhang Q, Ames JM, Smith RD et al. A perspective on the Maillard reaction and the analysis of protein glycation by mass spectrometry: probing the pathogenesis of chronic disease. *J Proteome Res.* 2009; 8:754-69.

107. Cleland B et al. Arsenic exposure within the Korean community (United States) based on dietary behavior and arsenic levels in hair, urine, air, and water. *Environ Health Perspect.* 2009;117(4):632–8.

108. Kapaj S et al. Human health effects from chronic arsenic poisoning–a review. *J Environ Sci Health A Tox Hazard Subst Environ Eng.* 2006;41(10):2399–428.

109. Guha Mazumder D, Dasgupta UB. Chronic arsenic toxicity: studies in West Bengal, India. *Kaohsiung J Med Sci.* 2011;27(9): 360–70.

110. EPA. Rice Consumption May Expose Children to Arsenic. www.epa.gov/ncer/events/news/2012/09_25_12_feature.html

111. Arnold LE et al. Artificial food colors and attention-deficit/hyperactivity symptoms: conclusions to dye for. *Neurotherapeutics.* 2012;9(3):599–609.

112. Stevens LJ et al. Dietary sensitivies and ADHD symptoms: thirty-five years of research. *Clin Pediatr.* (Phila). 2011;50(4): 279–93.

113. McCann D et al. Food additives and hyperactive behaviour in 3-year-old and 8/9-year-old children in the community: a randomised, double-blinded, placebo-controlled trial. *Lancet.* 2007;370(9598): 1560–7.

114. Weiss B. Synthetic food colors and neurobehavioral hazards: the view from environmental health research. *Environ Health Perspect.* 2012 Jan;120(1):1-5.

115. Humphries P et al. Direct and indirect cellular effects of aspartame on the brain. *Eur J Clin Nutr.* 2008;62(4):451–62.

116. Magnuson BA et al. Aspartame: a safety evaluation based on current use levels, regulations, and toxicological and epidemiological studies. *Crit Rev Toxicol.* 2007; 37(8):629–727.

117. Pretorius E. GUT bacteria and aspartame: why are we surprised? *Eur J Clin Nutr.* 2012;66(8):972.

118. FDA. Bisphenol A (BPA): Use in Food Contact Application. January 2010; Updated March 2013. www.fda.gov/NewsEvents/PublicHealthFocus/ucm064437.htm

119. NIH National Toxicology Program. NTP-CERHR Monograph on the Potential Human Reproductive and Developmental Effects of Bisphenol A. September 2008. http://ntp.niehs.nih.gov/ntp/ohat/bisphenol/bisphenol.pdf

120. CDC Factsheet. Dichlorodiphenyltrichloroethane. 2013. www.cdc.gov/biomonitoring/DDT_FactSheet.html

121. EPA 2013 Lead Environmental Protection Agency (EPA). Learn about Lead. 2013. http://www2.epa.gov/lead/learn-about-lead

122. CDC Website. Lead. www.cdc.gov/nceh/lead/

CDC Factsheet. Lead. 2009. www.cdc.gov/biomonitoring/Lead_FactSheet.html

123. FDA 2008 Pesticide Residue Monitoring Program Results and Discussion FY 2006. Food and Drug Administration. June 1, 2008. www.fda.gov/Food/FoodSafety/FoodContaminantsAdulteration/Pesticides/

ResidueMonitoringReports/ucm125187.
htm#reg06 Last updated 11/09/2011.

124. EPA Pesticide Website Environmental Protection Agency (EPA). Pesticide Website. www.epa.gov/pesticides/

125. Phthalates U.S. National Library of Medicine. Tox Town. Phthalates. http://toxtown.nlm.nih.gov/text_version/chemicals.php?id=24

126. CDC Fact Sheet. Phthalates. 2009. www.cdc.gov/biomonitoring/Phthalates_FactSheet.html.

127. European Commission Health and Consumer Protection Directorate. Polycyclic Aromatic Hydrocarbons – Occurrence in foods, dietary exposure and health effects. 4 December 2002. http://ec.europa.eu/food/fs/sc/scf/out154_en.pdf

128. Martí-Cid R et al. Evolution of the dietary exposure to polycyclic aromatic hydrocarbons in Catalonia, Spain. *Food Chem Toxicol*. 2008;46(9):3163–71.

129. Grotheer P et al. Sulfites: Separating Fact from Fiction. U.S. Department of Agriculture, University of Florida. Dean. Publication #FCS8787. 2011. http://edis.ifas.ufl.edu/fy731

130. Health Canada. Sulphites - One of the ten priority food allergens. 2012. www.hc-sc.gc.ca/fn-an/pubs/securit/2012-allergen_sulphites-sulfites/index-eng.php

131. FAO 2009 www.cdc.gov/nceh/ehs/Docs/Understanding_CAFOs_NALBOH.pdfFood and Agriculture Organization of the United Nations. Evaluation of certain veterinary drug residues in food. *World Health Organ Tech Rep Ser*. 2009;(954):1–134.

132. EPA Fact Sheet. Cadmium. CAS Number: 7440-43 9. www.epa.gov/wastes/hazard/wastemin/minimize/factshts/cadmium.pdf

133. EPA Fact Sheet. Dioxins and Furans. www.epa.gov/osw/hazard/wastemin/minimize/factshts/dioxfura.pdf

134. WHO Fact Sheet No. 225. Dioxins and their effects on human health. May 2010. www.who.int/mediacentre/factsheets/fs225/en/

135. National Cancer Institute. National Institutes of Health. Chemicals in Meat Cooked at High Temperatures and Cancer Risk. Fact Sheet. 2010. www.cancer.gov/cancertopics/factsheet/Risk/cooked-meats

136. Hribar C. Understanding Concentrated Animal Feeding Operations and Their Impact on Communities. National Association of Local Boards of Health. 2010.

137. European Commission, the Scientific Committee on Veterinary Measures Relating to Public Health, Assessment of Potential Risks to Human Health from Hormone Residues in Bovine Meat and Meat Products. 1999:16–22. http://ec.europa.eu/fs/sc/scv/out21_en.pdf

138. Food and Agriculture Organization of the United Nations and World Health Organization. JointFAO/WHO Expert Committee on Food Additives. Seventy-eighth meeting (Residues of veterinary drugs). Summary and Conclusions. Geneva, 5–14, November 2013.

139. Bernhoft RA. Mercury toxicity and treatment: a review of the literature. *J Environ Public Health*. 2012;2012:460508.

140. FDA, Mercury Levels in Commercial Fish and Shellfish (1990–2010) www.fda.gov/Food/FoodSafety/Product-SpecificInformation/Seafood/FoodbornePathogensContaminants/Methylmercury/ucm115644.htm FDA (Food and Drug Administration). 2008.

141. Hoffman DJ et al eds. Handbook of Ecotoxicology, Second Edition. "Ecotoxicology of Mercury," Chapter 16 (409–463). Boca Raton FL: CRC Press.

142. Wisconsin Department of Health Services. Polychlorinated Biphenyls (PCBs) and Your Health. 2012. www.dhs.wisconsin.gov/eh/hlthhaz/fs/pcblink.htm

143. EPA. Polychlorinated Biphenyols (PCBs). CAS Number: 1336-36-3. www.epa.gov/osw/hazard/wastemin/minimize/factshts/pcb-fs.pdf

144. de la Monte SM et al. Epidemilogical trends strongly suggest exposures as etiologic agents in the pathogenesis of sporadic Alzheimer's disease, diabetes mellitus, and non-alcoholic steatohepatitis. *J Alzheimers Dis*. 2009;17(3):519–29.

145. Brender JD et al; National Birth Defects Prevention Study. Nitrosatable drug ex-

posure during the first trimester of pregnancy and selected congenital malformations. *Birth Defects Res A Clin Mol Teratol.* 2012;94(9):701–13.

146. Hedlund M et al. Evidence for a human-specific mechanism for diet and antibody-mediated inflammation in carcinoma progression. *Proc Natl Acad Sci USA.* 2008; 105(48):18936–41.

147. Taylor RE, Gregg CJ, Padler-Karavani V et al. Novel mechanism for the generation of human xeno-autoantibodies against the nonhuman sialic acid N-glycolylneuraminic acid. *J Exp Med.* 2010;207(8): 1637–46.

148. Dórea JG. Vegetarian diets and exposure to organochlorine pollutants, lead, and mercury. *Am J Clin Nutr.* 2004;80(1):237–8.

149. Norén K. Levels of organochlorine contaminants in human milk in relation to the dietary habits of the mothers. *Acta Paediatr Scand.* 1983;72:811–6.

150. Hergenrather J, Hlady G, Wallace B, Savage E. Pollutants in breast milk of vegetarians. *N Engl J Med.* 1981;Mar 26;304(13): 792.

151. Somogyi A, Beck H. Nurturing and breastfeeding: exposure to chemicals in breast milk. *Environ Health Perspect.*1993; 101 (Suppl 2):45–52.

152. Mustafa M et al. Maternal and cord blood levels of aldrin and dieldrin in Delhi population. *Environ Monit Assess.* 2010;171(1-4):633–8.

153. Rozati R et al. Role of environmental estrogens in the deterioration of male factor fertility. *Fertil Steril.* 2002;78:1187–94.

154. Dickman MD et al. Hong Kong male subfertility links to mercury in human hair and fish. *Sci Total Environ.* 1998;214:165–74.

155. Srikumar TS et al. Trace element status in healthy subjects switching from a mixed to a lactovegetarian diet for 12 mo. *Am J Clin Nutr.* 1992;55:885–90.

156. Ji K et al. Influence of a five-day vegetarian diet on urinary levels of antibiotics and phthalate metabolites: a pilot study with "Temple Stay" participants. *Food Addit Contam Part A Chem Anal Control Expo Risk Assess.* 2009;26(10):1372–88.

157. Van Audenhaege M et al. Impact of food consumption habits on the pesticide dietary intake: comparison between a French vegetarian and the general population. *Environ Monit Assess.* 2010;171(1-4):633–8.

158. Paleo Plan Website (paleoplan.com/resources/sampler-menu-meal-plan/).

159. Eaton SB et al. Paleolithic Nutrition Revisited: A Twelve-Year Retrospective on Its Nature and Implications. *Euro J Clin Nutr.* 1997; 51(4):207–216 .

160. Konner M, Eaton SB. Paleolithic Nutrition: Twenty-Five Years Later. *Nutr Clin Prac.* 2010; 25:594–602.

161. Revedin A et al. Thirty thousand-year-old evidence of plant food processing. *Proc Natl Acad Sci.* 2010;107(44):18815–18819.

REFERENCES FOR CHAPTER 9

1. Craig WJ et al. American Dietetic Association. Position of the American Dietetic Association: vegetarian diets. *J Am Diet Assoc.* 2009 Jul;109(7):1266-82.

2. Institute of Medicine. National Research Council. *Dietary Reference Intakes for Energy, Carbohydrate, Fiber, Fat, Fatty Acids, Cholesterol, Protein, and Amino Acids (Macronutrients).* Washington DC: National Academy Press, 2002.

3. Han Z et al. Maternal underweight and the risk of preterm birth and low birth weight:

a systematic review and meta-analyses. *Int J Epidemiol.* 2011 Feb;40(1):65–101.

4. Messina V et al. Vegan for Her: The Women's Guide to Being Healthy and Fit on a Plant-Based Diet. Da Capo Press 2013.

5. Ebisch IM et al. The importance of folate, zinc and antioxidants in the pathogenesis and prevention of subfertility. *Hum Reprod Update.* 2007 Mar-Apr;13(2):163–74.

6. Mangels R. *The Everything Vegan Pregnancy Book.* Avon MA: Adams Media, 2011.

7. Institute of Medicine. Weight gain during pregnancy: reexamining the guidelines. National Academies Press, 2009.

8. Majchrzak D. B-vitamin status and concentrations of homocysteine in Austrian omnivores, vegetarians and vegans. *Ann Nutr Metab.* 2006;50(6):485–91.

9. Quinlan JD et al. Nausea and Vomiting of Pregnancy. *American Family Physician.* 2003;68(1): 121–128.

10. Zur E. Nausea and vomiting in pregnancy: a review of the pathology and compounding opportunities. *Int J Pharm Compd.* 2013 Mar-Apr;17(2):113–23.

11. Institute of Medicine. *Dietary Reference Intakes Summaries.* www.iom.edu/Home/Global/News%20Announcements/~/media/Files/Activity%20Files/Nutrition/DRIs/DRI_Summary_Listing.pdf

12. Institute of Medicine. National Research Council. *Dietary reference intakes for calcium and vitamin D.* Washington DC: The National Academies Press. 2011.

13. Institute of Medicine. National Research Council. *Dietary Reference Intakes for Vitamin A, Vitamin K, Arsenic, Boron, Chromium, Copper, Iodine, Iron, Manganese, Molybdenum, Nickel, Silicon, Vanadium, and Zinc.* Washington DC: National Academies Press, 2000.

14. Institute of Medicine. National Research Council. *Dietary Reference Intakes for Thiamin, Riboflavin, Niacin, Vitamin B_6, Folate, Vitamin B_{12}, Pantothenic Acid, Biotin, and Choline.*

15. Linus Pauling Institute. *Micronutrient Information Center.* Online at http://lpi.oregonstate.edu/infocenter/

16. Rasmussen KM et al, eds. Institute of Medicine and National Research Council Committee to Reexamine IOM Pregnancy Weight Guidelines. *Weight Gain During Pregnancy: Reexamining the Guidelines.* Washington DC: National Academies Press (US), 2009.

17. ESHA. *The Food Processor. Nutrition and Fitness Software.* 2014. www.esha.com

18. U.S. Department of Agriculture, Agricultural Research Service. *USDA National Nutrient Database for Standard Reference, Release 26.* Nutrient Data Laboratory Home Page. http://ndb.nal.usda.gov/ndb/foods/list

19. USDA United States Department of Agriculture. *USDA Database for the Choline Content of Common Foods.* 2008 online at www.ars.usda.gov/SP2UserFiles/Place/12354500/Data/Choline/Choln02.pdf

20. Morse NL. Benefits of docosahexaenoic acid, folic acid, vitamin D and iodine on foetal and infant brain development and function following maternal supplementation during pregnancy and lactation. *Nutrients.* 2012 Jul;4(7):799–840.

21. Ohrvik VE et al. Human Folate Bioavailability. *Nutrients.* 2011,3,475–490.

22. Koebnick C et al. Folate Status during Pregnancy in Women Is Improved by Long-term High Vegetable Intake Compared with the Average Western Diet. *J Nutr.* 2001; 131:733–739.

23. Bailey SW et al. The extremely slow and variable activity of dihydrofolate reductase in human liver and its implications for high folic acid intake. *Proc Natl Acad Sci USA.* 2009;106(36):15424–9.

24. Hung J et al. Additional food folate derived exclusively from natural sources improves folate status in young women with the MTHFR 677 CC or TT genotype. *J Nutr Biochem.* 2006;17:728–34.

25. Lucock M et al. Folic acid-vitamin and panacea or genetic time bomb? *Nat Rev Genet.* 2005;6(3):235–40.

26. Haider BA et al. Anaemia, prenatal iron use, and risk of adverse pregnancy outcomes: systematic review and meta-analysis. *BMJ.* 2013 Jun 21;346:f3443.

27. Alwan NA et al. Dietary iron intake during early pregnancy and birth outcomes in a cohort of British women. *Hum Reprod.* 2011 Apr;26(4):911–9.

28. Baker RD et al. Committee on Nutrition American Academy of Pediatrics. Diagnosis and prevention of iron deficiency and iron-deficiency anemia in infants and young children (0-3 years of age). *Pediatrics.* 2010 Nov;126(5):1040–50.

29. Haddad EH et al. Dietary intake and biochemical, hematologic, and immune status of vegans compared with nonvegetarians. *Am J Clin Nutr.* 1999 Sep;70(3 Suppl):586S–593S.

30. Shao J et al. Maternal serum ferritin concentration is positively associated with newborn iron stores in women with low ferritin status in late pregnancy. *J Nutr.* 2012 Nov;142(11):2004–9.

31. Mangels AR et al. *The Dietitians Guide to Vegetarian Diets.* Jones and Bartlett Learning Ltd., 2011.

32. Rizzo NS et al. Nutrient profiles of vegetarian and nonvegetarian dietary patterns. *J Acad Nutr Diet.* 2013 Dec;113(12):1610–9.

33. [No authors listed.] Non anaemic pregnant women should not take iron supplements. *Prescrire Int.* 2009 Dec;18(104):261–2.

34. Amit M. Vegetarian diets in children and adolescents. *Paediatr Child Health.* 2010 May; 15(5):303–14.

35. Maslova E et al. Peanut and tree nut consumption during pregnancy and allergic disease in children-should mothers decrease their intake? Longitudinal evidence from the Danish National Birth Cohort. *J Allergy Clin Immunol.* 2012;130(3):724–32.

36. Fields C et al. Iodine-deficient vegetarians: a hypothetical perchlorate-susceptible population? *Regul Toxicol Pharmacol.* 2005 Jun;42(1):37–46.

37. Perrine CG et al. Some subgroups of reproductive age women in the United States may be at risk for iodine deficiency. *J Nutr.* 2010 Aug;140(8):1489–94.

38. Nishiyama S et al. Transient hypothyroidism or persistent hyperthyrotropinemia in neonates born to mothers with excessive iodine intake. *Thyroid.* 2004 Dec;14(12):1077–83.

39. Leung AM et al. Iodine Status and Thyroid Function of Boston-Area Vegetarians and Vegans. *J Clin Endocrinol Metab.* 2011;May 25.

40. Public Health Committee of the American Thyroid Association et al. Iodine supplementation for pregnancy and lactation-United States and Canada: recommendations of the American Thyroid Association. *Thyroid.* 2006 Oct;16(10):949–51.

41. Dasgupta PK et al. Iodine nutrition: iodine content of iodized salt in the United States. *Environ Sci Technol.* 2008 Feb15; 42(4):1315–23.

42. Crawford BA et al. Iodine toxicity from soy milk and seaweed ingestion is associated with serious thyroid dysfunction. *Med J Aust.* 2010 Oct;4;193(7):413–5.

43. Kovacs CS. Vitamin D in pregnancy and lactation: maternal, fetal, and neonatal outcomes from human and animal studies. *Am J Clin Nutr.* 2008 Aug;88(2):520S–528S.

44. Weaver CM et al. Choices for achieving adequate dietary calcium with a vegetarian diet. *Am J Clin Nutr.* 1999 Sep;70(3 Suppl):543S–548S.

45. Bodnar LM et al. Maternal vitamin D deficiency increases the risk of preeclampsia. *J Clin Endocrinol Metab.* 2007 Sep;92(9): 3517–22.

46. Song SJ et al. The high prevalence of vitamin D deficiency and its related maternal factors in pregnant women in Beijing. *PLoS One.* 2013 Dec 26;8(12):e85081.

47. Pepper MR et al. B_{12} in fetal development. *Semin Cell Dev Biol.* 2011 Aug;22(6): 619–23.

48. Roschitz B et al. Nutritional infantile vitamin B_{12} deficiency: pathobiochemical considerations in seven patients. *Arch Dis Child Fetal Neonatal Ed.* 2005 May;90(3):F281–2.

49. Zeuschner CL et al. Vitamin B_{12} and vegetarian diets. *MJA Open.* 2012; 1 Suppl 2: 27–32.

50. Bor MV et al. Daily intake of 4 to 7 micrograms of dietary vitamin B-12 is associated with steady concentrations of vitamin B-12-related biomarkers in a healthy young population. *Am J Clin Nutr.* 2010 Mar;91(3):571–7.

51. Scott JM. Bioavailability of vitamin B_{12}. *Eur J Clin Nutr.* 1997 Jan;51 Suppl 1:S49–53.

52. Watanabe F. Vitamin B_{12} sources and bioavailability. *Exp Biol Med (Maywood).* 2007;232(10):1266–74.

53. Heysell RM et al. Vitamin B$_{12}$ turnover in Man. *Am J Clin Nutr.* 1966;18:176–184.

54. Takimoto H et al. Relationship between dietary folate intakes, maternal plasma total homocysteine and B-vitamins during pregnancy and fetal growth in Japan. *Eur J Nutr.* 2007 Aug;46(5):300–6.

55. American Academy of Pediatrics, Committee on Nutrition. *Pediatric Nutrition Handbook, 6th ed.* Elk Grove Village: American Academy of Pediatrics, 2009.

56. Burdge GC et al. Conversion of alpha-linolenic acid to longer-chain polyunsaturated fatty acids in human adults. *Reprod Nutr Dev.* 2005 Sep-Oct;45(5):581–97.

57. Carlson SE. Docosahexaenoic acid supplementation in pregnancy and lactation. *Am J Clin Nutr.* 2009;89(2):678S–84S.

58. Haggarty P. Effect of placental function on fatty acid requirements during pregnancy. *Eur J Clin Nutr.* 2004 Dec;58(12):1559–70.

59. Sanders TAB. Essential fatty acid requirements of vegetarians in pregnancy, lactation, and infancy. *Am J Clin Nutr.* 1999; 70(suppl):555S–9S.

60. Zhao JP et al. Circulating Docosahexaenoic Acid Levels Are Associated with Fetal Insulin Sensitivity. *PLoS One.* 2014.

61. AOCS. Collected recommendations for long-chain polyunsaturated fatty acid intake, *AOCS Inform.* 2003;762–763.

62. Koletzko B et al. The roles of long-chain polyunsaturated fatty acids in pregnancy, lactation and infancy: review of current knowledge and consensus recommendations, *J. Perinat. Med.* 36;(2008)5–14.

63. Simopoulos, AP. Essential fatty acids in health and chronic disease. *Am J Clin Nutr.* 1999;70(suppl):560s–569s.

64. Academy of Nutrition and Dietetics. Vegetarian Nutrition. (Search for pregnancy) http://vegetariannutrition.net/

65. Carter JP et al. Preeclampsia and reproductive performance in a community of vegans. *South Med J.* 1987 Jun;80(6):692–7.

66. O'Connell JM et al. Growth of vegetarian children: The Farm study. *Pediatrics.* 1989;84: 475–481.

67. Thomas J et al. The health of vegans during pregnancy. *Proc Nutr Soc.* 1977 May; 36(1):46A.68. van Staveren WA et al. Food consumption, growth, and development of Dutch children fed on alternative diets. *Am J Clin Nutr.* 1988 Sep;48(3 Suppl):819–21.

69. Roed C et al. [Severe vitamin B$_{12}$ deficiency in infants breastfed by vegans]. [Article in Danish] Ugeskr Laeger. 2009 Oct 19;171(43):3099–101.

70. Roschitz B et al. Nutritional infantile vitamin B$_{12}$ deficiency: pathobiochemical considerations in seven patients. *Arch Dis Child Fetal Neonatal Ed.* 2005 May; 90(3):F281–2.

71. Minnes S et al. Prenatal tobacco, marijuana, stimulant, and opiate exposure: outcomes and practice implications. *Addict Sci Clin Pract.* 2011 Jul;6(1):57–70.

72. Arunkumar R et al. Quercetin inhibits invasion, migration and signalling molecules involved in cell survival and proliferation of prostate cancer cell line (PC-3). *Cell Biochem Funct.* 2011;29:87–95.

73. Ko KP et al. Dietary intake and breast cancer among carriers and noncarriers of BRCA mutations in the Korean Hereditary Breast Cancer Study. *Am J Clin Nutr.* 2013; 98(6):1493–501.

74. Canadian Paediatric Society, Dietitians of Canada, and Health Canada. Consultation - *Nutrition for Healthy Term Infants: Recommendations from Birth to Six Months.* Online at www.hc-sc.gc.ca/fn-an/consult/infant-nourrisson/recommendations/index-eng.php

75. Smith JD et al. Pharmacists' guide to infant formulas for term infants. *J Am Pharm Assoc.* (2003). 2011 May-Jun;51(3):e28–35; quiz e36–7.

76. World Health Organization. *Infant and young child feeding: model chapter for textbooks for medical students and allied health professionals.* Geneva: World Health Organization; 2009. www.who.int/nutrition/publications/infantfeeding/9789241597494/en/index.html

77. World Health Organization. *Global strategy for infant and young child feeding.* Geneva, Switzerland: World Health Or-

ganization and UNICEF. 2003. www.who.int/nutrition/publications/infantfeeding/9241562218/en/index.html

78. Gartner LM et al. Breastfeeding and the use of human milk. *Pediatrics*. 2005 Feb; 115(2):496–506.

79. Institute of Medicine. National Research Council. *Nutrition during lactation*. Washington DC: National Academy Press, 1991.

80. Picciano MF et al. Lactation. In: Shils ME et al eds. *Modern nutrition in health and disease*. Philadelphia PA: Lippincott Williams & Wilkins, 2006:784–796.

81. Hergenrather J et al. Pollutants in breast milk of vegetarians. *N Engl J Med*. 1981 Mar 26;304(13):792.

82. Mangels AR et al. Considerations in planning vegan diets: infants. *J Am Diet Assoc*. 2001 Jun;101(6):670–7.

83. Rogan WJ et al. Should the presence of carcinogens in breast milk discourage breast feeding? *Regul Toxicol Pharmacol*. 1991 Jun;13(3):228–40.

84. Setchell KD et al. Exposure of infants to phyto-oestrogens from soy-based infant formula. *Lancet*. 1997 Jul 5;350(9070):23–7.

85. Allen LH. Impact of vitamin B-12 deficiency during lactation on maternal and infant health. *Adv Exp Med Biol*. 2002;503:57–67.

86. Dror DK et al. Effect of vitamin B_{12} deficiency on neurodevelopment in infants: current knowledge and possible mechanisms. *Nutr Rev*. 2008;66(5):250–255.

87. Hartmann H et al. Correspondence (letter to the editor): Risk group includes infants. *Dtsch Arztebl Int*. 2009 Apr;106(17):290–1; author reply 291.

88. Specker BL et al. Vitamin B-12: low milk concentrations are related to low serum concentrations in vegetarian women and to methylmalonic aciduria in their infants. *Am J Clin Nutr*. 1990 Dec;52(6):1073–6.

89. Specker BL et al. Increased urinary methylmalonic acid excretion in breast-fed infants of vegetarian mothers and identification of an acceptable dietary source of vitamin B-12. *Am J Clin Nutr*. 1988;47(1):89–92.

90. Manley BJ et al. High-dose docosahexaenoic acid supplementation of preterm infants: respiratory and allergy outcomes. *Pediatrics*. 2011 Jul;128(1):e71–7.

91. Bhatia J, Greer F for the American Academy of Pediatrics Committee on Nutrition. Use of soy protein-based formulas in infant feeding. *Pediatrics*. 2008;121(5): 1062–1068.

92. Lasekan JB et al. Growth of newborn, term infants fed soy formulas for 1 year. *Clin Pediatr*. (Phila). 1999 Oct;38(10):563–71.

93. Merritt RJ et al. Safety of soy-based infant formulas containing isoflavones: the clinical evidence. *J Nutr*. 2004 May;134(5): 1220S–1224S.

94. National Toxicology Program (U.S.). *NTP Brief on Soy Infant Formula*. 2010. Online at http://ntp.niehs.nih.gov/ntp/ohat/genistein-soy/soyformulaupdt/finalntpbriefsoyformula_9_20_2010.pdf#search=soy formula

95. Tome D. Criteria and markers for protein quality assessment—a review. *Br J Nutr*. 2012 Aug;108 Suppl 2:S222–9.

96. Herring SJ et al. Optimizing weight gain in pregnancy to prevent obesity in women and children. *Diabetes Obes Metab*. 2012;14(3):195–203.

97. Carmel R. Diagnosis and management of clinical and subclinical cobalamin deficiencies: why controversies persist in the age of sensitive metabolic testing. *Biochimie*. 2013;95(5):1047–55.

98. Simpson JL et al Micronutrients and women of reproductive potential: required dietary intake and consequences of dietary deficiency or excess. Part I—Folate, Vitamin B_{12}, Vitamin B_6. *J Matern Fetal Neonatal Med*. 2010;23(12):1323–43.

99. Sanders TAB et al. Platelet phospholipid fatty acid composition and function in vegans compared with age- and sex-matched omnivore controls. *Eur J Clin Nutr*. 1992; 46(11):823–31.

100. Norris J. Infant Formula. www.veganhealth.org/articles/soy_harm#formula

REFERENCES FOR CHAPTER 10

1. Craig WJ et al. American Dietetic Association. Position of the American Dietetic Association: Vegetarian Diets. *J Am Diet Assoc.* 2009;109(7)1266–82.

2. Baker RD et al. Committee on Nutrition American Academy of Pediatrics. Diagnosis and prevention of iron deficiency and iron-deficiency anemia in infants and young children (0-3 years of age). *Pediatrics.* 2010;126(5):1040–50.

3. Bhatia J et al for the American Academy of Pediatrics Committee on Nutrition. Use of soy protein-based formulas in infant feeding. *Pediatrics.* 2008;121(5):1062–1068.

4. Canadian Paediatric Society, Dietitians of Canada, and Health Canada. Consultation - *Nutrition for Healthy Term Infants: Recommendations from Birth to Six Months.* Online at www.hc-sc.gc.ca/fn-an/consult/infant-nourrisson6-24/recommendations/index-eng.php#c

5. Institute of Medicine. National Research Council. *Dietary Reference Intakes for Thiamin, Riboflavin, Niacin, Vitamin B6, Folate, Vitamin B12, Pantothenic Acid, Biotin, and Choline.* Washington DC: National Academy Press, 2000.

6. Koplin JJ et al. Optimal timing for solids introduction–why are the guidelines always changing? *Clin Exp Allergy.* 2013 Aug;43(8):826–34.

7. Lasekan JB et al. Growth of newborn, term infants fed soy formulas for 1 year. *Clin Pediatr.* (Phila). 1999 Oct;38(10):563–71.

8. Norris J. *Vitamin B$_{12}$.* www.veganhealth.org/b12/rec

9. Smith JD et al. Pharmacists' guide to infant formulas for term infants. *J Am Pharm Assoc.* (2003). 2011 May-Jun;51(3):e28-35; quiz e36–7.

10. National Toxicology Program (U.S.). *NTP Brief on Soy Infant Formula.* 2010. http://ntp.niehs.nih.gov/ntp/ohat/genistein-soy/soyformulaupdt/finalntpbriefsoyformula_9_20_2010.pdf#search=soy formula

11. Joneja J. *The Health Professional's Guide to Food Allergies and Intolerances.* Academy of Nutrition and Dietetics. 2013.

12. Mišak Z. Infant nutrition and allergy. *Proc Nutr Soc.* 2011 Nov;70(4):465–71.

13. Huh SY et al. Timing of solid food introduction and risk of obesity in preschool-aged children. *Pediatrics.* 2011;127(3):e544–51.

14. Möller LM et al. Infant nutrition in relation to eating behaviour and fruit and vegetable intake at age 5 years. *Br J Nutr.* 2012 May 4:1–8.

15. Robison RG et al. Chapter 23: Food allergy. *Allergy Asthma Proc.* 2012 May-Jun; 33(Suppl 1):S77–9.

16. Fiocchi A et al. Adverse Reactions to Foods Committee; American College of Allergy, Asthma and Immunology. Food allergy and the introduction of solid foods to infants: a consensus document. Adverse Reactions to Foods Committee, American College of Allergy, Asthma and Immunology. *Ann Allergy Asthma Immunol.* 2006 Jul;97(1):10-20; quiz 21,77.

17. FDA U.S. Food and Drug Administration. *Questions & Answers: Arsenic in Rice and Rice Products.* www.fda.gov/Food/FoodborneIllnessContaminants/Metals/ucm319948.htm

18. Hurrell R. Use of ferrous fumarate to fortify foods for infants and young children. *Nutrition Reviews.* 2012;68(9):522–530.

19. Hurrell R et al. Iron bioavailability and dietary reference values. *Am J Clin Nutr.* 2010; 91(5):1461S–1467S.

20. United States Department of Agriculture, Agricultural Research Service. *USDA National Nutrient Database for Standard Reference, Release 26.* Nutrient Data Laboratory Home Page. http://ndb.nal.usda.gov/ndb/foods/list

22. Agarwal U. Rethinking Red Meat as a Prevention Strategy for Iron Deficiency. *ICAN: Infant, Child, & Adolescent Nutrition.* 2013; 5(4):231–235.

23. Lönnerdal B. Soybean ferritin: implications for iron status of vegetarians. *Am J Clin Nutr.* 2009;89(suppl):1680S–1685S.

24. Theil EC et al. Absorption of iron from ferritin is independent of heme iron and

ferrous salts in women and rat intestinal segments. *J Nutr.* 2012;142(3):478–83.

25. Health Canada. *Iron-rich complementary foods help to prevent iron deficiency.* 2014 www.hc-sc.gc.ca/fn-an/consult/infant-nourrisson6-24/recommendations/index-eng.php#f

26. Palmer DJ et al. Introducing solid foods to preterm infants in developed countries. *Ann Nutr Metab.* 2012;60(Suppl 2):31–8.

27. Hay G et al. Iron status in a group of Norwegian children aged 6-24 months. *Acta Paediatr.* 2004 May;93(5):592–8.

28. Strazzullo P et al. Does salt intake in the first two years of life affect the development of cardiovascular disorders in adulthood? *Nutr Metab Cardiovasc Dis.* 2012 Jun 30.

29. Peterson K. S. *Wholesome Baby Foods from Scratch.* 2003. Online at www.vrg.org/recipes/babyfood.htm

30. Pedersen TP et al. Fruit and vegetable intake is associated with frequency of breakfast, lunch and evening meal: cross-sectional study of 11-, 13-, and 15-year-olds. *Int J Behav Nutr Phys Act.* 2012 Feb;6;9:9.

31. Health Canada, Canadian Paediatric Society, Dietitians of Canada, and Breastfeeding Committee for Canada. DRAFT–Nutrition for Healthy Term Infants: Recommendations from Six to 24 Months. 2014. Online at www.hc-sc.gc.ca/fn-an/consult/infant-nourrisson6-24/recommendations/index-eng.php#f

32. Guandalini S. The influence of gluten: weaning recommendations for healthy children and children at risk for celiac disease. *Nestle Nutr Workshop Ser Pediatr Program.* 2007;60:139–51; discussion 151–5.

33. Szajewska H. Early nutritional strategies for preventing allergic disease. *Isr Med Assoc J.* 2012 Jan;14(1):58-62.

34. von Berg A. Dietary interventions for primary allergy prevention - what is the evidence? *World Rev Nutr Diet.* 2013;108:71-8.

35. Institute of Medicine, National Research Council. Food and Nutrition Board. *Di-*

etary Reference Intakes for Calcium and Vitamin D. 2011.

36. Elmadfa I et al. Vitamins for the first 1000 days: preparing for life. *Int J Vitam Nutr Res.* 2012 Oct;82(5):342–7.

37. AOCS. Collected recommendations for long-chain polyunsaturated fatty acid intake, *AOCS Inform.* 2003;762–763.

38. Koletzko B et al. The roles of long-chain polyunsaturated fatty acids in pregnancy, lactation and infancy: review of current knowledge and consensus recommendations, *J. Perinat Med.* 2008; (36):5–14.

39. Simopoulos A.P. Essential fatty acids in health and chronic disease. *Am J Clin Nutr.* 1999;70(suppl):560s–569s.

40. Gröber U et al. Vitamin D: Update 2013: From rickets prophylaxis to general preventive healthcare. *Dermatoendocrinol.* 2013 Jun 1;5(3):331–347.

41. *Children's Tall Tree Multi-Vitamin and Mineral* by Country Life. http://store.veganessentials.com/childrens-tall-tree-multi-vitamin-and-mineral-by-country-life-p1517.aspx

42. *PixieVites.* www.drfuhrman.com/shop/pdf_product_factsheets/DrFuhrmans_Pixie_Vites.pdf

43. *VegLife Vegan Kids Multiple.* http://store.veganessentials.com/veglife-vegan-kids-multiple-vitamin-and-mineral-p1792.aspx

44. Whittaker P et al. Iron and folate in fortified cereals. *J Am Coll Nutr.* 2001 Jun; 20(3):247–54.

45. Laroche HH et al. Changes in diet behavior when adults become parents. *J Acad Nutr Diet.* 2012 Jun;112(6):832–9.

46. Maynard M et al. What influences diet in early old age? Prospective and cross-sectional analyses of the Boyd Orr cohort. *Eur J Public Health.* 2006 Jun;16(3):316–24.

47. About.com Pediatrics. *Understanding Growth Charts.* Part of the New York Times. http://pediatrics.about.com/cs/growthcharts2/l/aa050802a.htm

48. Centers for Disease Control and Prevention. *Clinical Growth Charts. Children 2*

to 20 years (5th-95th percentile) www.cdc.
gov/growthcharts/clinical_charts.htm#Set1

49. O'Connell JM et al. Growth of vegetarian children: The Farm study. *Pediatrics.* 1989;84:475-481.

50. Messina M et al. Early intake appears to be the key to the proposed protective effects of soy intake against breast cancer. *Nutr Cancer.* 2009;61:792–798.

51. Messina V et al. *Vegan for Her.* Da Capo Lifelong, 2013.

52. *The Vegetarian Resource Group.* www.vrg.org/

53. Centers for Disease Control and Prevention. *Childhood Obesity Facts.* 2012 www.cdc.gov/healthyyouth/obesity/facts.htm

54. U.S. Department of Health and Human Services. *Childhood Obesity.* Online at http://aspe.hhs.gov/health/reports/child_obesity/

55. United States Department of Agriculture. *Choose My Plate.* 2014. www.choosemyplate.gov/

56. Wang N et al. Effects of television viewing on body fatness among Chinese children and adolescents. *Chin Med J (Engl).* 2012 Apr;125(8):1500–3.

57. Gajre NS et al. Breakfast eating habit and its influence on attention-concentration, immediate memory and school achievement. *Indian Pediatr.* 2008 Oct;45(10): 824–8.

58. *Nature's Path Organic Waffles.* www.naturespath.com and www.naturespath.com/products/waffles?tid=9&brand=All&nutri=All

59. ESHA. *The Food Processor. Nutrition and Fitness Software.* 2014. www.esha.com

60. Dasgupta PK et al. Iodine nutrition: iodine content of iodized salt in the United States. *Environ Sci Technol.* 2008 Feb 15;42(4):1315-23.

61. Robinson-O'Brien R et al. Adolescent and young adult vegetarianism: better dietary intake and weight outcomes but increased risk of disordered eating behaviors. *J Am Diet Assoc.* 2009 Apr;109(4):648–55.

62. Cheng G et al. Beyond overweight: nutrition as an important lifestyle factor influencing timing of puberty. *Nutr Rev.* 2012 Mar;70(3):133–52.

63. Grant R et al. The relative impact of a vegetable-rich diet on key markers of health in a cohort of Australian adolescents. *Asia Pac J Clin Nutr.* 2008;17(1):107–15.

64. Sabaté J et al. Vegetarian diets and childhood obesity prevention. *Am J Clin Nutr.* 2010 May;91(5):1525S–1529S.

65. Sonneville KR et al. Vitamin D, Calcium, and Dairy Intakes and Stress Fractures Among Female Adolescents. *Arch Pediatr Adolesc Med.* 2012; 166(7)595–600.

66. Centers for Disease Control and Prevention. Iron deficiency: United States, 1999–2000. *MMWR Morb Mortal Wkly Rep.* 2002;51(40):897–899.

67. Lanham-New SA. Importance of calcium, vitamin D and vitamin K for osteoporosis prevention and treatment. *Proc Nutr Soc.* 2008 May;67(2):163–76.

68. Whitehead RD et al. Appealing to vanity: could potential appearance improvement motivate fruit and vegetable consumption? *Am J Public Health.* 2012 Feb;102(2): 207–11.

69. World Health Organization. *The WHO Growth Charts. Birth to 24 months.* www.cdc.gov/growthcharts/who_charts.htm

70. Barnard ND et al. Diet and sex-hormone binding globulin, dysmenorrhea, and premenstrual symptoms. *Obstet Gynecol.* 2000 Feb;95(2):245–50.

71. Chocano-Bedoya PO et al. Dietary B vitamin intake and incident premenstrual syndrome. *Am J Clin Nutr.* 2011 May;93(5): 1080–6.

72. Deligiannidis KM et al. Complementary and alternative medicine for the treatment of depressive disorders in women. *Psychiatr Clin North Am.* 2010 Jun;33(2): 441–63.

73. Bayles B et al. Evening primrose oil. *Am Fam Physician.* 2009 Dec 15;80(12):1405–8.

74. Bertone-Johnson ER et al. Dietary vitamin D intake, 25-hydroxyvitamin D_3 levels and premenstrual syndrome in a college-aged

population. *J Steroid Biochem Mol Biol.* 2010 Jul;121(1-2):434–7.

75. Bryant M et al. Modest changes in dietary intake across the menstrual cycle: implications for food intake research. *Br J Nutr.* 2006 Nov;96(5):888–94.

76. Cheng SH et al. Factors associated with premenstrual syndrome–a survey of new female university students. *Kaohsiung J Med Sci.* 2013 Feb;29(2):100–5.

77. Kiesner J. Affective response to the menstrual cycle as a predictor of self-reported affective response to alcohol and alco-

hol use. *Arch Womens Ment Health.* 2012 Dec;15(6):423–32.

78. Pinar G et al. Premenstrual Syndrome in Turkish college students and its effects on life quality. *Sex Reprod Health.* 2011 Jan;2(1):21–7.

79. Daiya Foods. www.daiyafoods.com/

80. Amit M. Vegetarian diets in children and adolescents. *Paediatr Child Health.* 2010 May;15(5):303–14.

81. Craig WJ. Health effects of vegan diets. *Am J Clin Nutr.* 2009 May;89(5):1627S–1633S.

REFERENCES FOR CHAPTER 11

1. Vincent GK et al. The Next Four Decades: The Older Population in the United States: 2010 to 2050. United States Census Bureau. 2010. www.census.gov/prod/ 2010pubs/ p25-1138.pdf

2. Bernstein M et al. Position of the academy of nutrition and dietetics: food and nutrition for older adults: promoting health and wellness. *J Acad Nutr Diet.* 2012;112(8): 1255–77.

3. Key TJ et al. Health effects of vegetarian and vegan diets. *Proc Nutr Soc.* 2006;65(1): 35–41.

4. Mukherjee M. Association of shorter telomeres with coronary artery disease in Indian subjects. *Heart.* 2009 Apr;95(8):669–73.

5. Stahler C. How Often Do Americans Eat Vegetarian Meals? and How Many Adults in the U.S. Are Vegetarian? 2012. National Harris Poll. *Vegetarian Resource Group.* Online at www.vrg.org/blog/2012/05/18/ how-often-do-americans-eat-vegetarian-meals-and-how-many-adults-in-the-u-s-are-vegetarian/

6. Craig WJ. Health effects of vegan diets. *Am J Clin Nutr.* 2009 May;89(5):1627S–1633S.

7. Craig WJ et al. American Dietetic Association. Position of the American Dietetic Association: vegetarian diets. *J Am Diet Assoc.* 2009 Jul;109(7):1266–82.

8. Mangels R et al. *The Dietitians' Guide to Vegetarian Diets,* Third Edition. Jones and Bartlett, 2011.

9. Institute of Medicine. National Research Council. *Dietary Reference Intakes for Energy, Carbohydrate, Fiber, Fat, Fatty Acids, Cholesterol, Protein, and Amino Acids (Macronutrients).* Washington DC: The National Academies Press, 2005.

10. Gallagher D et al. Appendicular skeletal muscle mass: effects of age, gender, and ethnicity. *J Appl Physiol.* 1997 Jul;83(1):229–39.

11. Manini TM. Energy Expenditure and Aging. *Ageing Res Rev.* 2010 January ; 9(1):1.12. Farmer B et al. A vegetarian dietary pattern as a nutrient-dense approach to weight management: an analysis of the national health and nutrition examination survey 1999-2004. *J Am Diet Assoc.* 2011 Jun;111(6):819–27.

13. Heidrich R. *Senior Fitness.* NY: Lantern Books, 2012.

14. Heidrich R. *Lifelong Running.* NY: Lantern Books, 2005. Agarwal R. Vitamin B_{12} deficiency & cognitive impairment in elderly population. *Indian J Med Res.* 2011 Oct;134:410–2.

15. Timmerman KL et al. A moderate acute increase in physical activity enhances nutritive flow and the muscle protein anabolic response to mixed nutrient intake in older adults. *Am J Clin Nutr.* 2012 Jun;95(6):1403–12.

16. U.S. Department of Health and Human Services. 2008 physical activity guidelines

for Americans. www.health.gov/paguidelines/guidelines

17. Elsawy B et al. Physical activity guidelines for older adults. *Am Fam Physician.* 2010 Jan 1;81(1):55–9. www.aafp.org/afp/2010/0101/p55.html

18. Tomioka M et al. Replicating the Enhance Fitness physical activity program in Hawaii's multicultural population, 2007-2010. *Prev Chronic Dis.* 2012;9:E74.

19. Centers for Disease Control and Prevention. *Physical activity for everyone. How much physical activity do older adults need?* www.cdc.gov/physicalactivity/everyone/guidelines/olderadults.html

20. Groessl EJ et al. cost analysis of a physical activity intervention for older adults. *J Phys Act Health.* 2009 Nov;6(6):767–74.

21. Haub MD et al. Beef and soy-based food supplements differentially affect serum lipoprotein-lipid profiles because of changes in carbohydrate intake and novel nutrient intake ratios in older men who resistive-train. *Metabolism.* 2005 Jun;54(6):769–74.

22. Haub MD et al. Effect of protein source on resistive-training-induced changes in body composition and muscle size in older men. *Am J Clin Nutr.* 2002 Sep;76(3):511–7.

23. Andrich DE et al. Relationship between essential amino acids and muscle mass, independent of habitual diets, in pre- and postmenopausal US women. *Int J Food Sci Nutr.* 2011 Nov;62(7):719–24.

24. Gaffney-Stomberg E et al. Increasing dietary protein requirements in elderly people for optimal muscle and bone health. *J Am Geriatr Soc.* 2009 Jun;57(6):1073–9.

25. Morais JA et al. Protein turnover and requirements in the healthy and frail elderly. *J Nutr Health Aging.* 2006 Jul-Aug;10(4):272–83.

26. Paddon-Jones D et al. Role of dietary protein in the sarcopenia of aging. *Am J Clin Nutr.* 2008 May;87(5):1562S–1566S.

27. Rizzo NS et al. Nutrient profiles of vegetarian and nonvegetarian dietary patterns. *J Acad Nutr Diet.* 2013 Dec;113(12):1610–9.

28. Institute of Medicine. National Research Council. *Dietary Reference Intakes for Vitamin A, Vitamin K, Arsenic, Boron, Chromium, Copper, Iodine, Iron, Manganese, Molybdenum, Nickel, Silicon, Vanadium, and Zinc.* Washington DC: National Academies Press, 2001.

29. Norris J et al. *Vegan for Life.* Da Capo Press, 2011.

30. Saunders AV. Iron and vegetarian diets. *MJA Open.* 2012;1(Suppl 2):11–16.

31. Cook JD et al. Assessment of the role of nonheme-iron availability in iron balance. *Am J Clin Nutr.* 1991;54:717–22.

32. Chernoff R. Micronutrient requirements in older women. *Am J Clin Nutr.* 2005. May;81(5):1240S–1245S.

33. Eisenstaedt R et al. Anemia in the elderly: current understanding and emerging concepts. *Blood Rev.* 2006 Jul;20(4):213–26.

34. Penninx BW et al. Anemia in old age is associated with increased mortality and hospitalization. *J Gerontol A Biol Sci Med Sci.* 2006 May;61(5):474–9.

35. Tussing-Humphreys L et al. Anemia in postmenopausal women: dietary inadequacy or nondietary factors? *J Am Diet Assoc.* 2011 Apr;111(4):528–31.

36. Lanham-New SA. Importance of calcium, vitamin D and vitamin K for osteoporosis prevention and treatment. *Proc Nutr Soc.* 2008 May;67(2):163–76.

37. Linus Pauling Institute. Micronutrient Information Center. http://lpi.oregonstate.edu/infocenter/minerals/calcium/

38. Ströhle A, Waldmann A, Koschizke J et al. Diet-dependent net endogenous acid load of vegan diets in relation to food groups and bone health-related nutrients: results from the German Vegan Study. *Ann Nutr Metab.* 2011;59(2-4):117–26.

39. Holick MF. Vitamin D Deficiency. *N Engl J Med.* 2007;357:266–81.

40. Verbrugge FH et al. Who should receive calcium and vitamin D supplementation? *Age Ageing.* 2012 Sep;41(5):576–80.

41. Dawson-Hughes B. Racial/ethnic considerations in making recommendations for

vitamin D for adult and elderly men and women. *Am J Clin Nutr.* 2004 Dec;80(6 Suppl):1763S–6S.

42. Garcia MN et al. One-year effects of vitamin D and calcium supplementation on chronic periodontitis. *J Periodontol.* 2011 Jan;82(1):25–32.

43. Pilz S et al. Low 25-hydroxyvitamin D is associated with increased mortality in female nursing home residents. *J Clin Endocrinol Metab.* 2012 Apr;97(4):E653–7.

44. Leblanc ES et al. Associations Between 25-Hydroxyvitamin D and Weight Gain in Elderly Women. *J Womens Health.* (Larchmt). 2012 Jun 25. 2012 Oct;21(10): 1066–73.

45. Holick MF. Vitamin D: a d-lightful solution for health. *J Investig Med.* 2011;59(6): 872–80.

46. Heaney RP et al. Amount and type of protein influences bone health. *Am J Clin Nutr.* 2008 May;87(5):1567S–1570S.

47. Bolton-Smith C et al. A two-year randomized controlled trial of vitamin K_1 (phylloquinone) and vitamin D_3 plus calcium on the bone health of older women. *J Bone Miner Res.* 2007; 22: 509–519.

48. U.S. Department of Agriculture. *Nutrient Data Laboratory.* www.ars.usda.gov/main/site_main.htm?modecode=12-35-45-00

49. Institute of Medicine.National Research Council. *Dietary Reference Intakes for Thiamin, Riboflavin, Niacin, Vitamin B_6, Folate, Vitamin B_{12}, Pantothenic Acid, Biotin, and Choline.* Washington DC: The National Academies Press, 1998.

50. Hill MH et al. A vitamin B-12 supplement of 500 µg/d for eight weeks does not normalize urinary methylmalonic acid or otherbiomarkers of vitamin B-12 status in elderly people with moderately poor vitamin B-12 status. *J Nutr.* 2013 Feb;143(2): 142–7.

51. Norris J. *Elderly Vegetarians.* www.veganhealth.org/b12/elder

52. Linus Pauling Institute. Micronutrient Information Center. Vitamins. Online at http://lpi.oregonstate.edu/infocenter/vitamins.html

53. Agarwal R. Vitamin B deficiency & cognitive impairment in elderly population. *Indian J Med Res.* 2011 Oct;134:410–412.

54. Hin H et al. Clinical relevance of low serum vitamin B_{12} concentrations in older people: the Banbury B_{12} Study. *Age and Ageing.* 2006; 35: 416–422.

55. Hughes CF, Ward M, Hoey L et al. Vitamin B_{12} and ageing: current issues and interaction with folate. *Ann Clin Biochem.* 2013 Jul;50(Pt 4):315–29.

56. Kwok T et al. Vitamin B-12 supplementation improves arterial function in vegetarians with subnormal vitamin B-12 status. *J Nutr Health Aging.* 2012;16(6):569–73. www.ncbi.nlm.nih.gov/pubmed/22659999

57. Heok KE et al. The many faces of geriatric depression. *Curr Opin Psychiatry.* 2008 Nov;21(6):540–5.

58. Ho RC et al. Is high homocysteine level a risk factor for cognitive decline in elderly? A systematic review, meta-analysis, and meta-regression. *Am J Geriatr Psychiatry.* 2011 Jul; 19(7):607–17.

59. Andrès E et al. Vitamin B_{12} (cobalamin) deficiency in elderly patients. *CMAJ.* 2004 Aug 3;171(3):251–9.

60. Graham ID et al. Oral cobalamin remains medicine's best kept secret. *Arch Gerontol Geriatr.* 2007 Jan-Feb;44(1):49–59.

61. Adams CJ et al. *Never Too Late to Go Vegan.* The Experiment, 2014.

62. Appleby P et al. Diet, vegetarianism, and cataract risk. *Am J Clin Nutr.* 2011;93: 1128–35.

63. Crowe FL et al. Diet and risk of diverticular disease in Oxford cohort of European Prospective Investigation into Cancer and Nutrition (EPIC): prospective study of British vegetarians and non-vegetarians. *BMJ.* 2011 Jul 19;343:d4131.

64. Kim MS at al. Strict vegetarian diet improves the risk factors associated with metabolic diseases by modulating gut microbiota and reducing intestinal inflammation. *Environ Microbiol Rep.* 2013 Oct;5(5):765–75.

65. Toivanen P et al. A vegan diet changes the intestinal flora. *Rheumatology (Oxford).* 2002 Aug;41(8):950–1.

66. Zimmer J et al. A vegan or vegetarian diet substantially alters the human colonic faecal microbiota. *Eur J Clin Nutr.* 2012 Jan; 66(1):53–60.

67. Zeeb H et al. The role of vitamin D in cancer prevention: does UV protection conflict with the need to raise low levels of vitamin D? *Dtsch Arztebl Int.* 2010 Sep; 107(37):638–43.

68. Tang AL et al. Calcium absorption in Australian osteopenic post-menopausal women: an acute comparative study of fortified soymilk to cows' milk. *Asia Pac J Clin Nutr.* 2010;19(2):243–9.

69. Darmadi-Blackberry I et al. Legumes: the most important dietary predictor of survival in older people of different ethnicities. *Asia Pac J Clin Nutr.* 2004;13(2):217–20.

70. Izumi T et al. Oral intake of soy isoflavone aglycone improves the aged skin of adult women. *J Nutr Sci Vitaminol.* (Tokyo). 2007 Feb;53(1):57–62.

71. Ali T et al. WM. Long-term safety concerns with proton pump inhibitors. *Am J Med.* 2009 Oct;122(10):896–903.

72. Happycow Mobile To-Go version. www.happycow.net/mobile.html

73. Senior Farmers' Market Nutrition Program. www.fns.usda.gov/wic/seniorfmnp/SFMNPcontacts.htm

74. Vegetarian Resource Group. *4-Week Vegetarian Menu Set for Meals On Wheels Sites.* Online at www.vrg.org/fsupdate/fsu974/fsu974menu.htm#WEEK1

75. U.S. Department of Health and Human Services Administration on Aging. Online at www.aoa.gov/AoARoot/AoA_Programs/index.aspx

76. U.S. Department of Agriculture. *SNAP (Supplemental Nutrition Assistance Program).* Note: other funding programs are Food Distribution Programs on Indian Reservations, Commodity Supplemental Food Programs, Seniors' Farmers Market Nutrition Programs, and Child and Adult Food Programs. Online at www.fns.usda.gov/snap/ and www.fns.usda.gov

77. Durrett C. *Senior Cohousing: A Community Approach to Independent Living.* New Society Publishers, 2009.

78. Seventh-day Adventist Church. www.adventist.org/

79. Living Well Bistro, Pavilion of Adventist Health, 10000 SE Main St., Portland, OR 97216.

80. Berkoff N. Vegetarian Resource Group. *Vegan in Volume.* The Vegetarian Resource Group, Baltimore MD 2000. www.vrg.org/press/2000marvolume.htm

81. Dietetic associations. (Search national websites using the word vegetarian or vegan). Vegetarian Dietary Practice Group, US: http://vegetariannutrition.net/rd/; Dietitians of Canada: www.dietitians.ca/Find-a-Dietitian.aspx; Australia: http://daa.asn.au/; U.K. http://www.freelancedietitians.org; International Confederation of Dietetic Associations: www.internationaldietetics.org/

82. Pribis P et al. Beliefs and attitudes toward vegetarian lifestyle across generations. *Nutrients.* 2010 May;2(5):523–31.

83. Carmel R. Diagnosis and management of clinical and subclinical cobalamin deficiencies: why controversies persist in the age of sensitive metabolic testing. *Biochimie.* 2013;95(5):1047–55.

84. World Cancer Research Fund/American Institute for Cancer Research. Food, Nutrition, Physical Activity and the Prevention of Cancer: A Global Perspective. Washington DC: AICR, 2007.

85. WCRF CUP Press releases. Most authoritative ever report on bowel cancer and diet: Links with meat and fibre confirmed. 2011. www.wcrf-uk.org/audience/media/press_release.php?recid=153

REFERENCES FOR CHAPTER 12

Weight Matters Introductory Section

1. United States Department of Health and Human Services; Center for Disease Control and Prevention, and National Center for Health Statistics. Health, United States,

2012: With Special Feature on Emergency Care. Hyattsville MD 2013.

2. Ogden CL et al. Prevalence of obesity in the United States, 2009–2010. NCHS data brief, no 82. Hyattsville MD: National Center for Health Statistics, 2012. www.cdc.gov/nchs/data/databriefs/db82.pdf

3. Fryar CD, Ogden CL. Prevalence of Underweight Among Adults Aged 20 Years and Over: United States, 2007–2008. Division of Health and Nutrition Examination Surveys. June 2010. www.cdc.gov/nchs/data/hestat/underweight_adult_07_08/underweight_adult_07_08.htm

4. National Eating Disorders Association. Anorexia Nervosa. 2005. www.nationaleatingdisorders.org/

5. Stöppler MC. Bulimia. MedicineNet.com. 2008. www.medicinenet.com/bulimia/article.htm

6. Jackson AS et al. Body mass index bias in defining obesity of diverse young adults: the Training Intervention and Genetics of Exercise Response (TIGER) study. Br J Nutr. 2009;102(7):1084–90.

7. Campbell MC, Tishkoff SA. African genetic diversity: implications for human demographic history, modern human origins, and complex disease mapping. *Annu Rev Genomics Hum Genet.* 2008;9:403–33.

8. Shiwaku K et al. Overweight Japanese with body mass indexes of 23.0-24.9 have higher risks for obesity-associated disorders: a comparison of Japanese and Mongolians. *Int J Obes Relat Metab Disord.* 2004; 28(1):152–8.

9. Revision of Body Mass Index (BMI) Cut-Offs in Singapore. 16 March 2005 www.hpb.gov.sg/hpb/default.asp?TEMPORARY_DOCUMENT=1769&TEMPORARY_TEMPLATE=2

Overweight

10. Newby PK et al. Risk of overweight and obesity among semivegetarian, lactovegetarian, and vegan women. *Am J Clin Nutr.* 2005;81(6): 1267–74.

11. Mangels R et al. *The Dietitian's Guide to Vegetarian Diets: Issues and Applications.* Third Edition. Sudbury MA: Jones and Bartlett Learning, 2010.

12. Spencer EA et al. Diet and body mass index in 38000 EPIC-Oxford meat-eaters, fish-eaters, vegetarians and vegans. *Int J Obes Relat Metab Disord.* 2003;27(6):728–34.

13. Tonstad S et al. Type of Vegetarian Diet, Body Weight and Prevalence of Type 2 Diabetes. *Diabetes Care.* 2009;32(5):791–6.

14. Gibbs BB et al. Short- and long-term eating habit modification predicts weight change in overweight, postmenopausal women: results from the WOMAN Study. J Acad Nutr Diet. 2012;112:1347–1355.

15. Vergnaud AC et al. Meat consumption and prospective weight change in participants of the EPIC-PANACEA study. *Am J Clin Nutr.* 2010;92(2):398–407.

16. Ebbeling CB et al. Effects of dietary composition on energy expenditure during weight loss maintenance. *JAMA.* 2012;307(24): 2627–34.

17. Corsica JA, Pelchat ML. Food addiction: true or false? *Curr Opin Gastroenterol.* 2010; 26(2):165–9.

18. Ifland JR et al. Refined food addiction: a classic substance use disorder. *Med. Hypotheses.* 2009;72(5):518–26.

19. Liu Y et al. Food addiction and obesity: evidence from bench to bedside. *J Psychoactive Drugs.* 2010;42(2):133–45.

20. Center for Disease Control (CDC). The New (Ab)Normal Infographic. http://makinghealtheasier.org/newabnormal

21. Morselli L et al. Role of sleep duration in the regulation of glucose metabolism and appetite. *Best Pract Res Clin Endocrinol Metab.* 2010;24(5):687–702.

22. Finkelstein EA et al. Annual medical spending attributable to obesity: payer-and service-specific estimates. Health Aff (Millwood). 2009;28(5):w822–31.

23. Kramer CK, Zinman B, Retnakaran R. Are Metabolically Healthy Overweight and Obesity Benign Conditions?: A Systematic Re-

view and Meta-analysis. *Ann Intern Med.* 2013;159(11):758–69.

24. National Heart, Lung, and Blood Institute (NHLBI). National Institutes of Health (NIH). Clinical Guidelines on the Identification, Evaluation, and Treatment of Overweight and Obesity in Adults–The Evidence Report. *Obes Res.* 1998;6 Suppl 2:51S–209S.

25. Guh DP et al. The incidence of co-morbities related to obesity and overweight: a systematic review and meta-analysis. *BMC Public Health.* 2009;9:88.

26. Choi HK et al. Obesity, weight change, hypertension, diuretic use, and risk of gout in men: the health professionals follow-up study. *Arch Intern Med.* 2005;165(7):742–8.

27. Matheson EM et al. Healthy lifestyle habits and mortality in overweight and obese individuals. *J Am Board Fam Med.* 2012; 25(1):9–15.

28. Ouchi N et al. Sfrp5 is an anti-inflammatory adipokine that modulates metabolic dysfunction in obesity. *Science.* 2010; 329(5990):454–7.

29. Rapin JR, Wiernsperger N. Possible links between intestinal permeability and food processing: A potential therapeutic niche for glutamine. *Clinics* (Sao Paulo). 2010; 65(6):635–43.

30. Catalioto RM et al. Intestinal epithelial barrier dysfunction in disease and possible therapeutical interventions. *Curr Med Chem.* 2011;18(3):398–426.

31. Macdonald TT, Monteleone G. Immunity, inflammation, and allergy in the gut. *Science.* 2005;307(5717):1920–5. Review.

32. Fasano A. Leaky gut and autoimmune diseases. *Clin Rev Allergy Immunol.* 2012; 42(1):71–8.

33. de Kort S et al. Leaky gut and diabetes mellitus: what is the link? *Obes. Rev.* 2011; 12(6):449-58.

34. Lambert GP et al. Effect of aspirin dose on gastrointestinal permeability. *Int J Sports Med.* 2012;33(6):421–5.

35. Harris K et al. Is the gut microbiota a new factor contributing to obesity and its metabolic disorders? *J Obes.* 2012;2012: 879151.

36. Blaut M, Klaus S. Intestinal microbiota and obesity. *Handb Exp Pharmacol.* 2012;(209):251–37. Marik PE. Colonic flora, Probiotics, Obesity and Diabetes. *Front Endocrinol.* (Lausanne). 2012;3:87.

38. Walker AW, Parkhill J. Fighting Obesity with Bacteria. *Science.* 2013; 341(6150): 1069–1070.

39. Ji K, Lim Kho Y, Park Y, Choi K. Influence of a five-day vegetarian diet on urinary levels of antibiotics and phthalate metabolites: a pilot study with "Temple Stay" participants. *Environ Res.* 2010;110(4):375–82.

40. Hergenrather J et al. Pollutants in breast milk of vegetarians. *N Engl J Med.* 1981; 304(13):792.

41. Tamer G et al. Relative vitamin D insufficiency in Hashimoto's thyroiditis. *Thyroid.* 2011;21(8):891–6.

42. Saranac L et al. Why is the thyroid so prone to autoimmune disease? *Horm Res Paediatr.* 2011;75(3):157–65.

43. Andrews RC et al. Abnormal cortisol metabolism and tissue sensitivity to cortisol in patients with glucose intolerance. *The Journal of Clinical Endocrinology* 2002; 87(12): 5587–5593.

44. Epel E et al. Stress may add bite to appetite in women: a laboratory study of stress-induced cortisol and eating behavior. *Psychoneuroendocrinology.* 2001;26:37–49.

45. Jones A et al. Adiposity is associated with blunted cardiovascular, neuroendocrine and cognitive responses to acute mental stress. *PLoS One.* 2012;7(6):e39143.

46. Diamanti-Kandarakis E et al. Pancreatic beta-cells dysfunction in polycystic ovary syndrome. *Panminerva Med.* 2008;50(4): 315–25.

47. Pasquali R et al. Obesity and infertility. *Curr Opin Endocrinol Diabetes Obes.* 2007; 14(6):482–7.

48. Martínez-González MA, Bes-Rastrollo M. Nut consumption, weight gain and obesity: Epidemiological evidence. *Nutr Metab Cardiovasc Dis.* 2011;21(Suppl 1):S40–5.

49. Rudelle S et al. Effect of a thermogenic beverage on 24-hour energy metabolism in humans. *Obesity*. (Silver Spring). 2007:15(2):349–55.

Underweight

50. Rosell M et al. Weight gain over 5 years in 21,966 meat-eating, fish-eating, vegetarian, and vegan men and women in EPIC-Oxford. *Int J Obes*. (Lond). 2006;30(9): 1389–96.

51. Thomas EL et al. An in vivo 13C magnetic resonance spectroscopic study of the relationship between diet and adipose tissue composition. *Lipids*. 1996;31:145–51.

52. Ross JK et al. Dietary and hormonal evaluation of men at different risks for prostate cancer: fiber intake, excretion, and composition, with in vitro evidence for an association between steroid hormones and specific fiber components. *Am J Clin Nutr*. 1990;51(3):365–70.

53. Janelle KC, Barr SI. Nutrient intakes and eating behavior scores of vegetarian and nonvegetarian women. *J Am Diet Assoc*. 1995;95(2):180-6,189,quiz 187–8.

54. Koebnick C et al. Consequences of a long-term raw food diet on body weight and menstruation: results of a questionnaire survey. *Ann Nutr*. 43:69–79.

55. Donaldson, MS. Food ad nutrient intake of Halelujah vegetarians. *Nutrition and Food Science*. 2001;31(6):293-303.

56. Bradbury KE, et al. Serum concentrations of cholesterol, apolipoprotein A-I and apolipoprotein B in a total of 1694 meat-eaters, fish-eaters, vegetarians and vegans. *Eur J Clin Nutr*. 2014;68(2):178-83.

57. Wändell PE et al. The association between BMI value and long-term mortality. *Int J Obes*. (Lond). 2009;33(5):577–82.

58. Thorogood M, et al. Relation between body mass index and mortality in an unusually slim cohort. *J Epidemiol Community Health*. 2003;57(2):130-3.

59. Jee SH et al. Body-mass index and mortality in Korean men and women. *N Engl J Med*. 2006;355(8):779–787.

60. Flegal KM et al. Cause-specific excess deaths associated with underweight, overweight, and obesity. *JAMA*. 2007;298(17): 2028–37.

61. Chandra RK. Nutrition and the immune system: an introduction. *Am J Clin Nutr*. 1997;66(2):460S–463S.

62. Hewison M. Vitamin D and immune function: Autocrine, paracrine or endocrine? *Scand J Clin Lab Invest Suppl*. 2012;243: 92–102.

63. Meydani SN, Erickson KL. Nutrients as regulators of immune function: Introduction. *FASEB J*. 2001;15(14):2555.

64. Marcos A et al. Changes in the immune system are conditioned by nutrition. *Eur J Clin Nutr*. 2003;57(Suppl 1):S66–9.

65. Tsai IH et al. Associations of the pre-pregnancy body mass index and gestational weight gain with pregnancy outcomes in Taiwanese women. *Asia Pac J Clin Nutr*. 2012;21(1):82–7.

66. Loucks AB et al. Low energy availability, not stress of exercise, alters LH pulsatility in exercising women. *J Appl Physiol*. 1998;84(1):37–46.

67. Qin DD et al. Do reproductive hormones explain the association between body mass index and semen quality? *Asian J Androl*. 2007;9(6):827–34.

68. Misra M, Klibanski A. Bone metabolism in adolescents with anorexia nervosa. *J Endocrinol Invest*. 2011;34(4):324–32.

69. Rauh MJ et al. Relationships among injury and disordered eating, menstrual dysfunction, and low bone mineral density in high school athletes: a prospective study. *J Athl Train*. 2010;45(3):243–52.

70. Anderson RM, Weindruch R. The caloric restriction paradigm: implications for healthy human aging. *Am J Hum Biol*. 2012;24(2):101–6. Review.

71. Fontana L, Meyer TE, Klein S, Holloszy JO. Long-term calorie restriction is highly effective in reducing the risk for atherosclerosis in humans. *Proc Natl Acad Sci. USA*. 2004;101:6659–6663.

72. Meyer TE, Kovacs SJ, Ehsani AA et al. Long-term caloric restriction ameliorates the decline in diastolic function in humans. *J Am Coll Cardiol*. 2006;47:398–402.

Eating Disorders

73. U.S. Department of Agriculture, Agricultural Research Service. 2007. USDA National Nutrient Database for Standard Reference, Release 20. Nutrient Data Laboratory www.ars.usda.gov/ba/bhnrc/ndl

74. Sullivan PF. Mortality in anorexia nervosa. *Am J Psychiatry*. 1995;152(7):1073–4.

75. American Psychiatric Association..Diagnostic and statistical manual of mental disorders (5th ed.). Arlington VA: American Psychiatric. Publishing, 2013.

76. Hoek HW, van Hoeken D. Review of the prevalence and incidence of eating disorders. *International Journal of Eating Disorders*. 2003;34(4):383–96.

77. Crow SJ et al. Increased mortality in bulimia nervosa and other eating disorders. *Am J Psychiatry*. 2009;166(12):1342–6.

78. National Eating Disorders Association. Bulimia Nervosa. 2005. www.nationaleatingdisorders.org/

79. NIH. Understanding Eating Disorders: Anorexia, Bulimia, and Binge-Eating. *NIH Medline Plus*. 2008;3(2):17–19. www.nlm.nih.gov/medlineplus/magazine/issues/spring08/articles/spring08pg18.html

80. Uher R, Rutter M. Classification of feeding and eating disorders: review of evidence and proposals for ICD-11. *World Psychiatry*. 2012;11(2):80–92.

81. Mazzeo SE, Bulik CM. Environmental and genetic risk factors for eating disorders: what the clinician needs to know. *Child Adolesc Psychiatr Clin N Am*. 2009;18(1):67–82.

82. Birch LL et al. Learning to overeat: maternal use of restrictive feeding practices promotes girls' eating in the absence of hunger. *Am J Clin Nutr*. 2003;78(2):215–20.

83. Fitzgerald N. TV's Big Lie: They're some of your favorite television stars, but these actresses' bodies are sending teens the wrong message about how young women are supposed to look. *Scholastic Choices*. 2002. FindArticles.com. 19 June, 2012. http://findarticles.com/p/articles/mi_hb3415/is_7_17/ai_n28909309/?tag=content;col1

84. Lindeman M et al. Vegetarianism and eating-disordered thinking. Eating Disorders. 2000; 8(2):157–165.

85. Bas M et al. Vegetarianism and eating disorders: Association between eating attitudes and other psychological factors among Turkish adolescents. Appetite. 2005; 44(3):309–315.

86. Klopp SA et al. Self-reported vegetarianism may be a marker for college women at risk for disordered eating. Journal of the American Dietetic Association. 2003; 103(6):745–747.

87. Neumark-Sztainer D et al. Adolescent vegetarians. A behavioral profile of a school-based population in Minnesota. Archives of Pediatrics and Adolescent Medicine. 1997; 151(8):833–838.

88. Robinson-O'Brien R et al. Adolescent and young adult vegetarianism: better dietary intake and weight outcomes but increased risk of disordered eating behaviors. *J Am Diet Assoc*. 2009;109(4):648–55.

89. Bardone-Cone AM et al. The inter-relationships between vegetarianism and eating disorders among females. *J Acad Nutr Diet*. 2012;112(8):1247–52.

90. Amit M. Canadian Paediatric Society, Community Paediatrics Committee. Vegetarian diets in children and adolescents. *Paediatr Child Health*. 2010;15(5):303–314.

91. O'Connor MA et al. Vegetarianism in anorexia nervosa? A review of 116 consecutive cases. The Medical Journal of Australia. 1987;147(11-12):540–542.

92. Forestell CA et al. To eat or not to eat red meat. A closer look at the relationship between restrained eating and vegetarianism in college females. *Appetite*. 2012;58(1): 319–25.

93. Timko CA et al. Will the real vegetarian please stand up? An investigation of di-

etary restraint and eating disorder symptoms in vegetarians versus non-vegetarians. *Appetite.* 2012;58(3):982–90.

94. Levine JA. Nonexercise activity thermogenesis–liberating the life-force. *J Intern Med.* 2007; 262(3):273–87.

95. Høstmark AT et al. Postprandial light physical activity blunts the blood glucose increase. *Prev Med.* 2006;42(5):369–71.

96. Aadland E, Høstmark AT. Very Light Physical Activity after a Meal Blunts the Rise in Blood Glucose and Insulin *The Open Nutrition Journal.* 2008;2:94–99.

97. Thayer KA et al. Role of environmental chemicals in diabetes and obesity: a national toxicology program workshop review. *Environ Health Perspect.* 2012;120(6): 779–89.

REFERENCES FOR CHAPTER 13

1. Nieman DC. Physical fitness and vegetarian diets: is there a relation? *Am J Clin Nutr.* 1999;70(3 Suppl):570S–575S.

2. Barr SI, Rideout CA. Nutritional considerations for vegetarian athletes. *Nutrition.* 2004;20(7–8):696–703. Review.

3. Venderley AM, Campbell WW. Vegetarian diets: nutritional considerations for athletes. *Sports Med.* 2006;36(4):293–305. Review.

4. Hood DA, Terjung RL. Amino acid metabolism during exercise and following endurance training. *Sports Med.* 1990;9(1):23–35.

5. Larson-Meyer DE, Niemeyer MH. Optimal Nutrition for Active Vegetarians and Vegetarian Athletes. In: *The Complete Vegetarian.* University of Illinois Press, 2009: 288–316.

6. ExRx.net. Substrate Utilization. www.exrx.net/Nutrition/Substrates.html.

7. van Loon LJ et al. Intramyocellular lipids form an important substrate source during moderate intensity exercise in endurance-trained males in a fasted state. *J Physiol.* 2003;553(Pt 2):611–25.

8. Hultman E. Fuel selection, muscle fibre. *Proc Nutr Soc.* 1995;54(1):107–21.

9. Watt MJ et al. Intramuscular triacylglycerol, glycogen and acetyl group metabolism during 4 h of moderate exercise in man. *J Physiol.* 2002;541(Pt 3):969–978.

10. Hargreaves M. Skeletal muscle metabolism during exercise in humans. *Clin Exp Pharmacol Physiol.* 2000;27(3):225–8.

11. Coyle EF. Substrate utilization during exercise in active people. *Am J Clin Nutr.* 1995; 61(4 Suppl):968S–979S.

12. American Dietetic Association; Dietitians of Canada; American College of Sports Medicine, Rodriguez NR, Di Marco NM, Langley S. American College of Sports Medicine position stand. Nutrition and athletic performance. *Med Sci Sports Exerc.* 2009; 41(3):709–31.

13. Dunford M, Doyle JA. *Nutrition for Sport and Exercise.* Edition 2. Belmont CA: Cengage Learning, 2011.

14. Bittman M. Diet and exercise to the extremes. *New York Times.* Sports. 2010; May 13: B14.

15. Toth MJ, Poehlman ET. Sympathetic nervous system activity and resting metabolic rate in vegetarians. *Metabolism.* 1994; 43(5):621–5.

16. Poehlman ET et al. Resting metabolic rate and postprandial thermogenesis in vegetarians and nonvegetarians. *Am J Clin Nutr.* 1988;48(2):209–13.

17. Bissoli L et al. Resting metabolic rate and thermogenic effect of food in vegetarian diets compared with Mediterranean diets. Ann *Nutr Metab.* 1999;43(3):140–4.

18. Mangels AR et al. *The Dietitians Guide to Vegetarian Diets.* Jones and Bartlett Learning Ltd., 2011.

19. Food and Nutrition Board. Institute of Medicine. Dietary Reference Intakes for Energy, Carbohydrate, Fiber, Fat, Fatty Acids, Cholesterol, Protein, and Amino Acids (Macronutrients). Washington DC: The National Academies Press, 2005.

20. Nutrition Working Group of the Medical Commission of the International Olympic Committee. *Nutrition for athletes.* June

2003. www.olympic.org/Documents/Reports/EN/en_report_1251.pdf

21. U.S. Department of Agriculture, Agricultural Research Service. 2007. USDA National Nutrient Database for Standard Reference, Release 20. Nutrient Data Laboratory www.ars.usda.gov/ba/bhnrc/ndl

22. Manitoba Harvest Hemp Foods. Nutrition Facts. Hemp Hearts. www.manitoba harvest.com/

23. Fisher-Wellman K, Bloomer RJ. Acute exercise and oxidative stress: a 30 year history. *Dyn Med.* 2009;13(8):1.

24. Rauma AL et al. Antioxidant status in long-term adherents to a strict uncooked vegan diet. *Am J Clin Nutr.* 1995;62(6):1221–7.

25. Rauma AL, Mykkänen H. Antioxidant status in vegetarians versus omnivores. *Nutrition.* 2000;16(2):111–9.

26. Brownlie T 4th, Utermohlen V, Hinton PS et al. Tissue iron deficiency without anemia impairs adaptation in endurance capacity after aerobic training in previously untrained women. *Am J Clin Nutr.* 2004;79(3):437–43.

27. Wells AM et al. Comparisons of vegetarian and beef-containing diets on hematological indexes and iron stores during a period of resistive training in older men. *J Am Diet Assoc.* 2003;103(5):594–601.

28. Snyder AC et al. Influence of dietary iron source on measures of iron status among female runners. *Med Sci Sports Exerc.* 1989;21:7–10.

29. Telford RD et al. Footstrike is the major cause of hemolysis during running. *J Appl Physiol.* 2003;94(1):38–42.

30. Waller MF, Haymes EM. The effects of heat and exercise on sweat iron loss. *Med Sci Sports Exerc.* 1996;28:197–203.

31. Robertson J et al. Faecal blood loss in response to exercise. *BMJ.* 1987;295:303–305.

32. Micheletti A et al. Zinc status in athletes: relation to diet and exercise. *Sports Med.* 2001;31(8):577–82.

33. National Research Council. Dietary Reference Intakes for Calcium, Phosphorus, Magnesium, Vitamin D, and Fluoride. Washington DC: The National Academies Press, 1997.

34. Nielsen FH, Lukaski HC. Update on the relationship between magnesium and exercise. *Magnes Res.* 2006;19(3):180–9.

35. Larson DE. Vegetarian Diet for Exercise and Athletic Training and Performing: An Update. A Continuing Education Article. *VNDPG.* http://vndpg.org/articles/Vegetarian-Nutrition-For-Athletes.php

36. IAFF Medical Manual. Chapter 6: Nutrition and Athlete Health. 2012. www.iaaf.org/about-iaaf/documents/medical#nutrition-in-athletics

37. International Olympic Committee Consensus Statement on Sports Nutrition. Oct. 27, 2010. Available at: www.olympic.org/Documents/Reports/EN/CONSENSUS-FINAL-v8-en.pdf

38. Cohen D. The truth about sports drinks. *BMJ.* 2012;345:e4737.

39. Bailey SJ et al. Dietary nitrate supplementation reduces the O2 cost of low-intensity exercise and enhances tolerance to high-intensity exercise in humans. J Appl Physiol. 2009;107:1144–1155.

40. Vanhatalo A et al. Acute and chronic effects of dietary nitrate supplementation on blood pressure and the physiological responses to moderate-intensity and incremental exercise. Am J Physiol Regul Integr Comp Physiol. 2010;299(4):R1121–R1131.

41. Lansley KE et al. Acute dietary nitrate supplementation improves cycling time trial performance. Med Sci Sports Exerc. 2011;43(6): 1125–1131.

42. ESHA Research. The Food Processor nutrition analysis system.

43. The American College of Sports Medicine. Position Stand. The Female Athlete Triad. *Medicine & Science in Sports & Exercise.* 2007;39(10):1867–1882.

44. Slavin J, Lutter J, Cushman S. Amenorrhoea in vegetarian athletes. *Lancet.* 1984;1:1474–5.

45. Brooks SM et al. Diet in athletic amenorrhoea. *Lancet.* 1984;1:559–60.

46. Goldin BR et al. Estrogen excretion patterns and plasma levels in vegetarian and omnivorous women. *N Engl J Med*. 1982: 16; 307(25):1542–7.

47. Barr SI. Vegetarianism and menstrual cycle disturbances: is there an association? *Am J Clin Nutr*. 1999;70(3 Suppl):549S–54S.

48. Ahrendt DM. Ergogenic Aids: Counseling the Athlete. *Am Fam Physician*. 2001; 63(5):913–923.

49. Buell JL et al. National Athletic Trainers' Association. National Athletic Trainers' Association position statement: evaluation of dietary supplements for performance nutrition. *J Athl Train*. 2013;48(1):124–36.

50. Caruso J et al. Ergogenic Effects of ß-Alanine and Carnosine: Proposed Future Research to Quantify Their Efficacy. *Nutrients*. 2012;4(7):585–601.

51. Derave W et al. Muscle carnosine metabolism and beta-alanine supplementation in relation to exercise and training. *Sports Med*. 2010;40(3):247–63.

52. Hipkiss AR. Carnosine and its possible roles in nutrition and health. *Adv Food Nutr Res*. 2009;57:87–154.

53. Harris RC, Jones G, Hill CA et al. The carnosine content of V Lateralis in vegetarians and omnivores. The FASEB Journal. 2007; 21:769.20.

54. Everaert I et al. Vegetarianism, female gender and increasing age, but not CNDP1 genotype, are associated with reduced muscle carnosine levels in humans. *Amino Acids*. 2011;40(4):1221–9.

55. Harris RCet al. Determinants of muscle carnosine content. *Amino Acids*. 2012; 43(1):5–12.

56. Matsumoto K et al. Branched-chain amino acid supplementation attenuates muscle soreness, muscle damage and inflammation during an intensive training program. *J Sports Med Phys Fitness*. 2009;49(4):424–31.

57. Negro M et al. Branched-chain amino acid supplementation does not enhance athletic performance but affects muscle recovery and the immune system. *J Sports Med Phys Fitness*. 2008;48(3):347–51.

58. Wikipedia. Carnitine. http://en.wikipedia.org/wiki/Carnitine.

59. Chen W et al. Urinary, plasma, and erythrocyte carnitine concentrations during transition to a lactoovovegetarian diet with vitamin B-6 depletion and repletion in young adult women. *Am J Clin Nutr*. 1998;67(2): 221–30.

60. Lombard KA et al. Carnitine status of lacto-ovovegetarians and strict vegetarian adults and children. *Am J Clin Nutr*. 1989; 50(2):301–6.

61. President's Council on Physical Fitness and Sports (PCPFS) Research Digests. *Nutritional Erogogenics & Sports Performance*. Washington DC, 2012. www.fitness.gov/digest_jun1998.htm

62. National Institutes of Health. Office of Dietary Supplements. *Dietary Supplement Fact Sheet: Carnitine*. June 15, 2006. http://ods.od.nih.gov/factsheets/Carnitine-HealthProfessional/#en39.

63. Shomrat A et al. Effect of creatine feeding on maximal exercise performance in vegetarians. *Eur J Appl Physiol*. 2000;82(4): 321–5.

64. Delanghe J et al. Normal reference values for creatine, creatinine, and carnitine are lower in vegetarians. *Clin Chem*. 1989;35(8): 1802–3.

65. Burke DG et al. Effect of creatine and weight training on muscle creatine and performance in vegetarians. *Med Sci Sports Exerc*. 2003; 35(11):1946–55.

66. Wang JT, Douglas AE. Nutrients, Signals, and Photosynthate Release by Symbiotic Algae (The Impact of Taurine on the Dinoflagellate Alga Symbiodinium from the Sea Anemone Aiptasia pulchella). *Plant Physiol*. 1997;114(2):631–636.

67. Czerpak R et al. The influence of acetylcholine and taurine on the content of some metabolites in the alga Chlorella vulgaris. *International Journal of Ecohydrology and Hydrobiology*. 2003:3(2), 223–229.

68. Rana SK, Sanders TA. Taurine concentrations in the diet, plasma, urine and breast milk of vegans compared with omnivores. *Br J Nutr*. 1986 Jul;56(1):17–27.

69. Laidlaw SA et al. Plasma and urine taurine levels in vegans. *Am J Clin Nutr.* 1988;47(4):660–3.

70. Fuhrman J, Ferreri DM. Fueling the vegetarian (vegan) athlete. *Curr Sports Med Rep.* 2010;9(4):233–41.

71. U.S. Department of Health and Human Services. Physical Activity Guidelines for Americans. 2008. www.health.gov/paguidelines/guidelines/default.aspx#toc

72. National Institutes of Health (NIH). National Heart, Lung, and Blood Institute (NHLBI). *Your Guide to Physical Activity and Your Heart.* NIH Publication No. 06-5714. June 2006. www.nhlbi.nih.gov/health/public/heart/obesity/phy_active.pdf

73. Garber CE et al; American College of Sports Medicine. American College of Sports Medicine position stand. Quantity and quality of exercise for developing and maintaining cardiorespiratory, musculo-skeletal, and neuromotor fitness in apparently healthy adults: guidance for prescribing exercise. *Med Sci Sports Exerc.* 2011;43(7):1334–59.

74. Nadimi H et al. Association of vegan diet with RMR, body composition and oxidative stress. *Acta Sci Pol Technol Aliment.* 2013;12(3):311–8.

REFERENCES FOR CHAPTER 14

1. United States Department of Agriculture. Human Nutrition Information Service. *Miscellaneous Publication 1514.USDA's Food Guide Background and Development.* 1993. www.cnpp.usda.gov/Publications/MyPyramid/OriginalFoodGuidePyramids/FGP/FGPBackgroundAndDevelopment.pdf

2. Britten P et al. Updated US Department of Agriculture Food Patterns meet goals of the 2010 dietary guidelines. *J Acad Nutr Diet.* 2012 Oct;112(10):1648–55.

3. USDA. *ChooseMyPlate.* 2012. www.choosemyplate.gov/food-groups/dairy.html

4. Painter J et al. Comparison of international food guide pictorial representations. *J Am Diet Assoc.* 2002 Apr;102(4):483–9.

5. Wikipedia. *List of nutrition guides.* 2012. http://en.wikipedia.org/wiki/List_of_nutrition_guides

6. Loma Linda University, School of Public Health, Department of Nutrition. *The Vegetarian Food Guide Pyramid.* www.vegetariannutrition.org/food-pyramid.pdf

7. Venti CA et al. Modified food guide pyramid for lactovegetarians and vegans. *J Nutr.* 2002 May;132(5):1050–4.

8. Wikipedia. *Vegetarian Diet Pyramids.* http://en.wikipedia.org/wiki/Vegetarian_Diet_Pyramid

9. Physician's Committee for Responsible Medicine. The Power Plate. http://pcrm.org/health/diets/pplate/power-plate

10. Mangels R et al. *The Dietitians' Guide to Vegetarian Diets*, Third Edition. Jones and Bartlett, 2011.

11. Messina V et al, A new food guide for North American vegetarians. *J Am Diet Assoc.* 2003 Jun;103(6):771–5.

12. Davis et al. *Becoming Vegan: Express Edition.* Summertown TN: The Book Publishing Company, 2013.

13. Davis et al. The Vegan Plate. http://becomingvegan.ca/food-guide/

14. LeSaffre Yeast Corporation. (Red Star). Personal communication. 2012. http://lesaffre-yeast.com/red-star/vsf.html

15. Norris J. *Vitamin B_{12} Recommendations.* www.veganhealth.org/b12/rec

16. Scott JM. Bioavailability of vitamin B_{12}. *Eur J Clin Nutr.* 1997 Jan;51(Suppl 1): S49–53.

17. Popkin BM et al. Water, hydration, and health. *Nutr Rev.* 2010 Aug;68(8):439–58. www.ncbi.nlm.nih.gov/pmc/articles/PMC2908954/?tool=pubmed

INDEX

gluten sensitivity and, 171
magnesium and, 197, 416
premenstrual cramps, 339
sodium (salt) and, 201
solid foods and, 417
cravings for foods, 368, 369,
370–71
C-reactive protein, rheumatoid
arthritis (RA) and, 79
creatine, 346, 424
Crete (Greece), coronary
artery disease and, 115
cretinism, iodine and, 192, 293
Crohn's disease, 223, 267
Crowe, Francesca, 137
CR Society (Calorie
Restriction Society), 379
cruciferous vegetables, 78,
232, 261–62, 372
crystallinity of foods, glycemic
index (GI) and, 175
culture, eating disorders and,
393
cultured food, 263, 264, 265
CUP (Continuous Update
Project), 45, 48
cured meat, sodium nitrate/
nitrite in, 272
curry paste, as seasoning, 357
Curtis, Stanley, 8
CVD (cardiovascular disease).
See cardiovascular disease
(CVD)/heart disease
cyanide, 218
cyanocobalamin, 214, 217,
217–18, 219
cyanogenic glycosides, 140
cysteine, 95, 232, 245
cytochrome-c oxidase, copper
and, 195
cytochrome P-450,
detoxification and, 232
cytokines, 300, 380
Czech Republic diabetes'
study, 62

D
daidzein, 54
daily value (DV)
calcium, 185
folate (vitamin B9, folic
acid), 248

recommended intakes, 182
vitamin B12, 217, 221, 295,
304, 322, 436
vitamin D, 227
dairy products. *See also*
specific types of
antibiotics in, 271
arachidonic acid (AA) and,
117
breast-feeding and, 301
calcium and, 179, 183
carbohydrates and, 147
cholesterol and, 135
DDT in, 270
diabetes and, 58, 59
dioxins in, 271
eating disorders and, 398
ethics and, 2, 13–14
food guide and, 432
global warming and, 21
hormones in, 271
insulin resistance and, 135
iodine and, 192
lactose in, 266
leaky-gut syndrome and, 371
methane/nitrous-oxide
related emissions and, 21
nutrition and, 29
osteoporosis and, 65
Paleolithic ("paleo") diets
and, 279
phthlates in, 270
polychlorinated biphenyls
(PCBs) in, 272
production of, 5
rheumatoid arthritis (RA)
and, 80
saturated fat and, 108, 135
vegan replacements for, 384
Dakotas, selenium in soil and,
200
d-alpha-tocopherol, 238
dandelion greens, 184, 239,
278
Danzig, Mac, 404
dark chocolate
caffeine and, 299
as healthy choice, 428, 440
iron and, 188, 348, 440
magnesium and, 440
weight and, 383, 383, 384
dates, 92, 157, 166, 278

Davey study, 31
Davis, Brenda
animal compassion and,
5–6
Barnard, Tom, and
(Defeating Diabetes), 355
Marshall Islands, diabetes'
treatment program and,
57
and Vesanto Melina
(Becoming Raw: The
Essential Guide to Raw
Vegan Diets)
antioxidants and, 353
cancer and, 53
children and, 330
fiber and, 157
fibromyalgia/rheumatoid
arthritis and, 355
food enzymes and, 262
Green Giant Juice and,
103, 212
menus/recipes and, 212
nutrition and, 277
treats and, 385
Vesanto Melina,and Cherie
Soria (The Raw Food
Revolution Diet), 277, 353
Davis, Steph, 404
DC (Dietitians of Canada).
See Dietitians of Canada
(DC)
DDT, 124, 269, 270, 301
death (mortality)
anemia and, 347
anorexia nervosa and, 391
cancer and, 35, 44–45, 45,
380
carbohydrates and, 148–49
cardiovascular disease
(CVD)/heart disease and,
35, 380
diabetes and, 35, 56, 380
diet and, 36, 45
eating disorders and, 390,
397
fiber and, 155
fruits/vegetables and, lack
of, 380
inactivity and, 380
kidney diseases and, 380
legumes (beans) and, 159

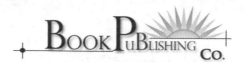

Book Publishing Co.

books that educate, inspire, and empower

To find your favorite books on plant-based cooking and nutrition,
living foods lifestyle, and healthy living, visit:
BookPubCo.com

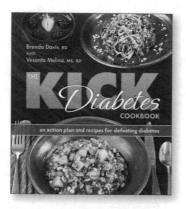

The Kick Diabetes Cookbook
An Action Plan and Recipes
for Defeating Diabetes
Brenda Davis, RD
Vesanto Melina, MS, RD
978-1-57067-359-7
$22.95

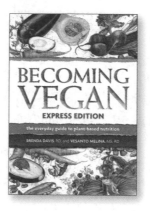

Becoming Vegan:
Express Edition
Brenda Davis, RD,
Vesanto Melina, MS, RD
978-1-57067-295-8
$19.95

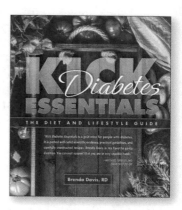

Kick Diabetes Essentials
The Diet and Lifestyle Guide
Brenda Davis, RD
978-1-57067-376-4
$24.95

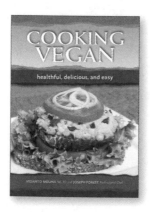

Cooking Vegan
Vesanto Melina, MS, RD,
and Joseph Forest
978-1-57067-267-5
$19.95

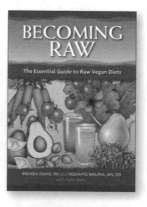

Becoming Raw
Brenda Davis, RD,
Vesanto Melina, MS, RD,
with Rynn Berry
978-1-57067-238-5
$24.95

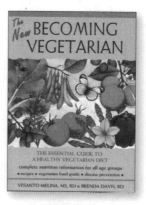

The New
Becoming Vegetarian
Vesanto Melina, MS, RD,
and Brenda Davis, RD
978-1-57067-144-9
$21.95

Purchase these health titles and cookbooks from your local bookstore or natural food store,
or you can buy them directly from:

Book Publishing Company • P.O. Box 99 • Summertown, TN 38483 • 1-888-260-8458

Free shipping and handling on all orders.